Handbook of
Feline Medicine

Edited by

JOSEPHINE WILLS
Waltham Centre for Pet Nutrition, Leicestershire

and

ALICE WOLF
Texas Veterinary Medical Center, Texas A&M University

PERGAMON PRESS

OXFORD · NEW YORK · SEOUL · TOKYO

U.K.   Pergamon Press, Headington Hill Hall,
        Oxford OX3 0BW, England

U.S.A. Pergamon Press, Inc., 660 White Plains Road,
        Tarrytown, New York 10591–5153, U.S.A.

KOREA   Pergamon Press Korea, KPO Box 315, Seoul 110–603,
        Korea

JAPAN   Pergamon Press Japan, Tsunashima Building Annex,
        3–20–12 Yushima, Bunkyo-ku, Tokyo 113, Japan

First edition 1993

Library of Congress Cataloging-in-Publication Data
Handbook of feline medicine / edited by Josephine Wills and Alice Wolf.
1st ed.
p.   cm. — (Pergamon veterinary handbook series)
1. Cats—Diseases—Handbooks, manuals, etc.
I. Wills, Jo. II. Wolf, Alice. III. Series.
SF985.H36 1993
636.8'089—dc20   92–31279

ISBN 0–08–040829 X Hardcover
ISBN 0–08–040830 3 Flexicover

DISCLAIMER

Whilst every effort is made by the Publishers to see that no inaccurate or misleading data, opinion or statement appear in this book, they wish to make it clear that the data and opinions appearing in the articles herein are the sole responsibility of the contributor concerned. Accordingly, the Publishers and their employees, officers and agents accept no responsibility or liability whatsoever for the consequences of any such inaccurate or misleading data, opinion or statement.

Drug and Dosage Selection: The Authors have made every effort to ensure the accuracy of the information herein, particularly with regard to drug selection and dose. However, appropriate information sources should be consulted, especially for new or unfamiliar drugs or procedures. It is the responsibility of every veterinarian to evaluate the appropriateness of a particular opinion in the context of actual clinical situations, and with due consideration to new developments.

Printed in Great Britain by BPCC Wheaton & Co. Ltd., Exeter

Handbook of
Feline Medicine

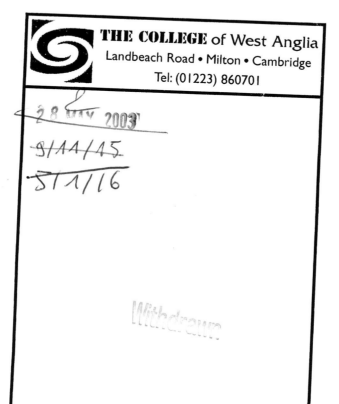

THE COLLEGE of West Anglia
Landbeach Road • Milton • Cambridge
Tel: (01223) 860701

28 MAY 2003

9/11/15

5/1/16

Withdrawn

LEARNING Centre

The card holder is responsible for the return of this book

Fines will be charged on ALL late items

Pergamon Veterinary Handbook Series

Series Editor: A. T. B. Edney

This series of practical and authoritative handbooks covers topics of interest to the practising veterinary surgeon, to veterinary students and to veterinary nurses. The text is authoritative, yet written in a clear and accessible form, and there are numerous photographs and specially commissioned line drawings to enhance understanding. The volumes in this Series will be valuable additions to any practice bookshelf.

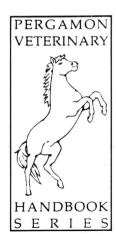

ANDERSON & EDNEY
Practical Animal Handling

BROWN
Aquaculture for Veterinarians: Fish Husbandry and Medicine

EMILY & PENMAN
Handbook of Small Animal Dentistry

GORREL, PENMAN & EMILY
Handbook of Small Animal Oral Emergencies

SHERIDAN & McCAFFERTY
The Business of Veterinary Practice

Other books

BURGER
The Waltham Book of Companion Animal Nutrition

GOLDSCHMIDT & SHOFER
Skin Tumors of the Dog and Cat

ROBINSON
Genetics for Cat Breeders, 3rd Edition
Genetics for Dog Breeders, 2nd Edition

THORNE
The Waltham Book of Dog and Cat Behaviour

WOLDEHIWET & RISTIC
Rickettsial and Chlamydial Diseases of Domestic Animals

Journal

Veterinary Dermatology
The official journal of the European Society of Veterinary Dermatology and the American College of Veterinary Dermatology

Contents

List of Contributors

J. August Department of Small Animal Medicine and Surgery, College of Veterinary Medicine, Texas A&M University, College Station, Texas 77843-4474, USA

D. Bennett Small Animal Clinic, University of Liverpool, Crown Street, Liverpool L7 7EX, UK

S. Center New York State College of Veterinary Medicine, Cornell University, Ithaca, NY-14853, USA

S. Donoghue Box 189, Pembroke, VA 24136, USA

K. Earle Waltham Centre for Pet Nutrition, Waltham-on-the-Wolds, Leics, LE14 4RT, UK

G. Guilford Department of Veterinary Clinical Sciences, Massey University, Palmerston North 5301, New Zealand

T. Graves 753 E Livingston Avenue R, Columbus, OH 43205, USA

T. Gruffydd-Jones Department of Veterinary Medicine, Bristol University, Langford House, Langford, Avon BS18 7DU, UK

J. Hoskins Department of Veterinary Clinical Sciences, School of Veterinary Medicine, Louisiana State University, Baton Rouge, Louisiana 70803, USA

G. Kunkle Department of Small Animal Clinical Sciences, University of Florida, College of Veterinary Medicine, Box J-126, Health Science Center, Gainesville, Florida 32610-0126, USA

D. Kronfeld Box 189, Pembroke, VA 24136, USA

C. Little Department of Veterinary Pathology, University of Glasgow, Bearsden, Glasgow G61 1QH, UK

S. Mayer Director of Science, Greenpeace, Canonbury Villas, London N1 2PN, UK

C. Mooney Department of Veterinary Science, University of Glasgow, Bearsden, Glasgow G61 1QH, UK

J. Mould Department of Veterinary Surgery, University of Glasgow, Bearsden, Glasgow G61 1QH, UK

P. Neville c/o Bristol University, Department of Veterinary Medicine, Langford House, Langford, Avon BS18 7DU, UK

M. Peterson Animal Medical Center, 510 East 62nd Street, New York 10021, USA

S. Petersen-Jones University of Edinburgh, Royal (Dick) School of Veterinary Science, Summerhall, Edinburgh EH9 1QH, UK

A. Rebar Research Programmes Development and Veterinary Medicine, Purdue University Lynn 113, 47907 Lafayette, Indiana, USA

D. Senior School of Veterinary Medicine, Louisiana State University, Baton Rouge, Louisiana 70803-8410, USA

A. Sparkes Department of Veterinary Medicine, Bristol University, Langford House, Langford, Avon BS18 7DU, UK

W. Ware Veterinary Clinical Sciences, Veterinary Teaching Hospital, Iowa State University, Ames, IA 50011, USA

S.J. Wheeler Department of Small Animal Medicine and Surgery, Royal Veterinary College, North Mymms, Herts AL9 7TA, UK

J. Wills Waltham Centre for Pet Nutrition, Waltham-on-the-Wolds, Leics LE14 4RT, UK

A. Wolf College of Veterinary Medicine, Texas A&M University, College Station, Texas 77843-4474, USA

1

Handling

JOSEPHINE WILLS

Many cats can be difficult to handle. They are agile and quick and their independent nature inevitably means that they may tolerate handling for only short periods. In addition to sharp teeth, cats also have four sets of claws that the handler needs to consider. The degree of restraint exercised is very dependent on the individual cat. Most cats respond best to a loose and gentle approach rather than forceful restraint. Much can be achieved by an unhurried but firm technique.

HANDLING

A cat should be approached in a calm but confident manner, speaking to it quietly. When a stranger tries to remove a frightened cat from a cage or basket, the cat may well adopt an instinctive defensive posture. However, unless the cat warns the handler either by hissing or growling, it is usually safe to put a hand on top of the cat's head. Stroking the top of a cat's head and running the hand confidently along its back will normally reassure it. The cat can then be lifted up.

Cats can be lifted in a number of ways, depending on their age and body weight, whether the cat is passive or fractious, whether it is in a cage, basket or on the floor, and the individual preference of the handler. The cat may be lifted up by passing one hand over the chest wall and supporting the sternum, whilst the other hand supports the abdomen from the other side (Fig. 1.1). Once picked up, the cat should be held firmly towards the handler's body (Fig. 1.2). This method is suitable for a relaxed cat. If it is not possible to pick a cat up directly from above, for example when it is in a cage or basket, it can be lifted by grasping both forelegs from the elbows and gently pulling it free from the cage. It can then be tucked under one arm, with the hand of that arm holding the forelegs and with the second hand stroking the cat's head (Fig. 1.3) or gently 'scruffing' it (Fig.

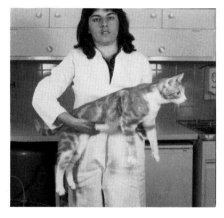

FIG. 1.1 Lifting a cat, with one hand supporting the sternum and the other supporting the abdomen.

1.4). Kittens can be handled similarly, but those lifted or carried gently by their scruff will often adopt a very relaxed, submissive posture. Cats of dubious temperament can be lifted up by the scruff, with the legs pointing away from the handler and the second hand supporting the cat at the sternum (Fig. 1.5) or taking the weight on the hind quarters.

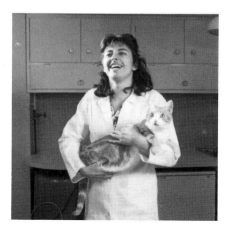

FIG. 1.2 Holding a cat firmly.

1

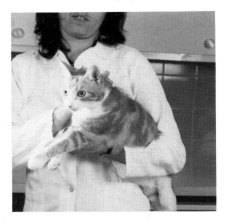

FIG. 1.3   A cat tucked under one arm, with the other hand stroking its head.

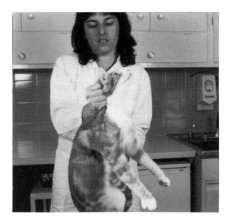

FIG. 1.5   Lifting a cat by the scruff.

Holding for general examination

As before, techniques that can be used for holding a cat for general examination depend on whether the cat is amenable to handling, whether the examiner is single handed, the area to be examined, the nature and extent of the treatment or sampling required, and individual preference. In general, cats respond best to light restraint. However, if the handler is single-handed, firmer restraint may be necessary by, for example, scruffing the cat with one hand whilst leaving the other free to examine the body. If assistance is available, the cat can be presented to the examiner in different ways depending on the site to be examined. For examination of the head, an assistant holds the cat's forelegs to protect the examiner from the front claws, facing the cat towards the examiner (Fig. 1.6). The body of the cat can be restrained in the assistant's arms. This leaves the examiner able to hold the cat's head or scruff with one hand, and have the other hand free for examination, sampling or dosing. For examination of the rest of the body, passive cats can be restrained by gently holding the cat's shoulders and forelegs with both hands with the cat facing the assistant (Fig. 1.7).

If the cat becomes restless or less amenable, the grip can be changed to be more firm by either holding the head under the jaw or scruffing it with one hand, whilst the other hand holds the cat's forelegs and restrains it against the assistant's body

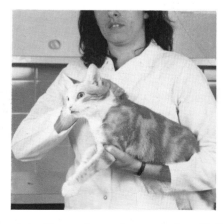

FIG. 1.4   The neck may be gently 'scruffed'.

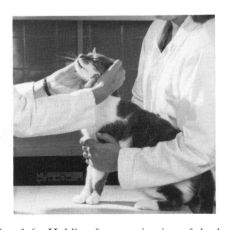

FIG. 1.6   Holding for examination of the head.

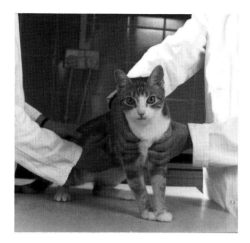

FIG. 1.7   Holding for examination of the body.

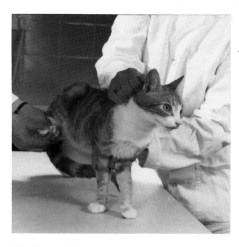

FIG. 1.9   Restraining a restless cat by using the scruff.

(Figs 1.8 and 1.9). If the cat is particularly difficult, it can be held in lateral recumbency with one hand gripping the scruff, whilst the other hand grasps the hind legs (Fig. 1.10). It is best to use only as much restraint as necessary, provided that firmer control can be applied rapidly.

Temporary immobilization of some cats has been achieved by some workers by placing an elastic band around the base of both the cat's ears.[2] The cat then usually assumes a semi-crouched position and remains relatively motionless for a period. In the author's experience, this method is unreliable and should never be used for more than a few minutes.

Restraint of a fractious cat

It may not be possible to restrain a fractious cat safely just by scruffing it and grasping the hind legs. Some cats are capable of letting their neck sink into their shoulders so that the 'scruff' disappears. Also, adult tom cats often have very thickened scruffs which can be difficult to grasp firmly for any length of time. In these cases, it is often advisable to wrap the cat in a large, thick towel. For examination of the head, the whole body can be firmly wrapped in the towel, making sure the forelegs and hind legs are secure (Fig. 1.11). The assistant can then hold the enveloped

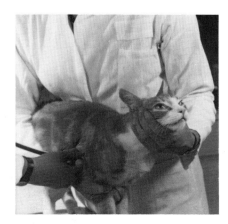

FIG. 1.8   Restraining a restless cat by holding the jaw.

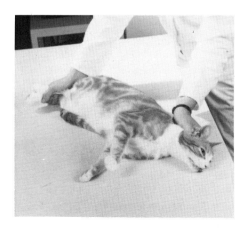

FIG. 1.10   Holding a difficult cat in lateral recumbency.

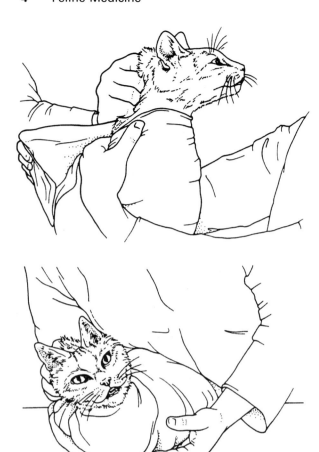

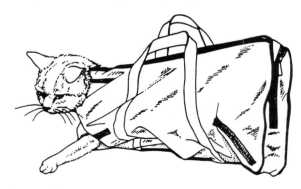

FIG. 1.11   Securely wrapping a cat in a towel.

cat firmly, leaving the examiner free to control the head. It is best not to let the cat have sight of the towel or blanket beforehand. This is a very useful method of restraint which owners can learn to use. It can protect them from being scratched; it can also be used when any medication has to be given at home, such as the administration of ear or eye medication, liquid medicines or tablets.

The wrapping-up-in-a-towel method has been used in the design of restraining bags. These bags are usually made from strong nylon material and are waterproof. The cat is placed in the bag which is then zipped up, leaving only the head showing. There are four leg holes which can be unzipped to allow exposure of a leg for treatment (Fig. 1.12). These bags are also used for cephalic venepuncture. Towels can be utilized to pack the area around the

cat's head so that any biting can be directed on to the towel and not the assistant or examiner.

Restraint of a vicious cat can be a considerable problem. Even if the cat has been grasped by the scruff successfully, or it may contort itself and succeed in striking the handler with its hind legs. A cat which behaves in this way can often be restrained by crowding it into a corner with a thick towel or blanket, then grasping it through the protective layer. Alternatively, a thick pair of gardening or animal gauntlets can be used to protect the handler's hands, but the arms must be well protected as well. The cat's claws must also be kept away from people's faces.

Catching and handling feral cats

Occasionally, it may be necessary to catch a feral cat that is injured or as part of a control scheme for neutering, identification and treatment. Feral cats are usually extremely difficult to handle, despite the recommendations set out above. They are very frightened, not used to man or to any quick or unexpected movements. The most satisfactory method of capturing a feral cat is to use a cat trap with a squeeze-back facility.[3] The captured cat is then pressed against the mesh on the side of the cage, so that an injection of an immobilising agent can be given, and then the cat may be handled safely.

If the cat is presented in a conventional cat basket, a thick blanket can be pushed into the cage, through a narrowly opened lid, to press the cat against the mesh for the injection to be given. If injection techniques are not possible due to the

FIG. 1.12   A cat in a restraining bag, with foreleg extended.

design of the cat basket or carrier, then it will be necessary to use gaseous anaesthesia to immoblize the cat by placing the carrier in a suitable polythene bag, and introducing the gaseous anaesthetic into the bag. The cat can be removed as soon as anaesthesia has reached a level sufficient to immobilize it.

Occasionally it may be necessary to catch a feral cat without the aid of a cat trap, e.g. a feral cat which has escaped from its container and is loose in the veterinary hospital. The cat will often seek refuge under a cupboard. Once the cat is cornered, a set of cat-catchers or cat tongs can be used to catch and restrain it. When used correctly they do not cause injury to the cat.

Specific restraint techniques

Most of the procedures that involve giving medication or taking a sample are best carried out with two people. One person restrains the cat in a way in which the medication can be given accurately and quickly, providing full protection for themselves and the second person who is giving the medication. In certain circumstances, procedures may have to be carried out single-handedly, in which case the restraint procedure has to be adapted so that one person can restrain the cat and carry out the procedure quickly and effectively, whilst protecting themselves from the teeth and claws of an unco-operative cat.

Taking the rectal temperature

Clinical examination of a cat often involves taking the rectal temperature with a thermometer. If assistance is available, then the cat can be presented to the clinician who can then grip the base of the cat's tail with one hand, to control movement of the cat's hind quarters, and use the other hand to insert the rectal thermometer. If single-handed, the handler can restrain the cat by holding it towards the body with the elbow, using the hand of the same arm to grip the base of the tail. This leaves a free hand to take the temperature (Fig. 1.13).

Liquid feeding or medication

Liquid medication, such as an anthelmintic, anti-diarrhoeal agent or antibiotic, is best administered

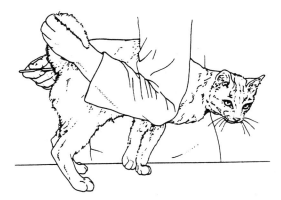

FIG. 1.13   Taking a cat's rectal temperature.

using a plastic syringe. If assistance is available, then a cat can be presented to the clinician as in Fig. 1.6. The assistant presents the cat to the clinician whilst holding the cat's forelegs to prevent it from scratching. The clinician can then restrain the cat's head with one hand, and introduce the end of the syringe through the side of the cat's mouth. If single-handed, the most comfortable way of administering medication or liquid food is to sit down with the cat in sternal recumbency on a towel on the lap, facing away from the handler. One hand can be used to grip the cat's upper jaw and bend the head backwards slightly, whilst the other hand is used to introduce the food into the side of the cat's mouth gradually, via the syringe (Fig. 1.14). If the cat becomes fractious, further control can be obtained by pressing in on the cat with the elbows and chest. The towel can be used to wrap around the cat's forelegs if it tries to claw the syringe. Should the cat become too difficult to handle with these minimal restraint procedures, then it can be wrapped fully in the towel, as in Fig. 1.11, before the medication is given.

Giving a tablet

If an assistant is available, then the cat can be restrained by the forelegs, as described previously. The cat's head is then gripped with one hand, with the thumb and forefinger at the angle of the cat's jaw. The head is tilted well back and pressure at the angle of the jaw will ease the mouth open. With the other hand, the tablet is held with the

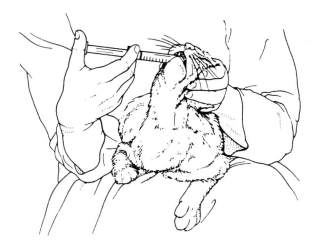

FIG. 1.14   Giving a liquid diet via a syringe, single-handed.

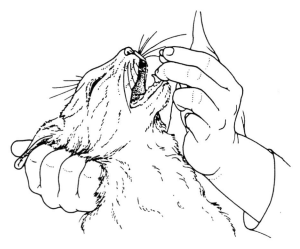

FIG. 1.16   Giving a tablet single-handed.

thumb and forefinger and the second and third fingers are used to press down on the lower jaw (Fig. 1.15). The tablet can then be placed or dropped as far back on the tongue as possible. Usually, a tablet placed far enough on the back of the tongue will induce a swallowing reflex but, if this does not occur, the cat's mouth is closed and held closed. Keeping the cat's head tilted upwards, the cat's throat is gently stroked until it swallows.

A tablet can be given successfully even if the handler is single-handed. The cat is sat on a table

facing the handler. The head is held with one hand with the thumb and fingers gripping the cat's ear and scruff (Fig. 1.16). The cat's head is then rotated until the nose points upwards. The mouth can then be opened as before and the tablet given. If there is a serious danger of being bitten, a tablet doser can be used. This can be made out of a plastic syringe, with the end cut off to allow the tablet to fit into the barrel. The plunger is retained to 'fire' the tablet at the back of the throat.

Giving ear medication

If assistance is available, then the cat can be restrained by the forelegs facing the handler as described previously. With the forefinger and thumb of one hand, the pinna of the affected ear can be held so that the head can be gently rotated so that it faces upwards (Fig 1.17). For more control, the scruff can be incorporated in the holding hand. The medication can then be applied with the free hand.

Ear medication can be administered by one person, by lying the cat on its sternum, facing away from the handler. Grasping the cat's scruff with one hand, the head is tilted so that the affected ear is uppermost. The forearm and elbow can be used to give additional restraint, pressing the cat towards the body (Fig. 1.18). The medication is given with the other hand.

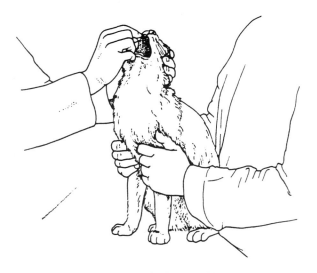

FIG. 1.15   Giving a tablet.

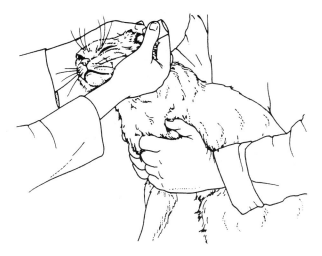

FIG. 1.17 Applying ear medication.

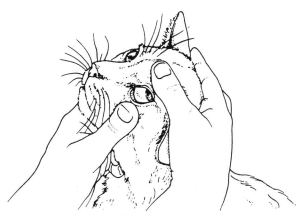

FIG. 1.19 Examination of the conjunctivae.

Giving eye medication

Examination of the eye and conjunctiva is best achieved with an assistant facing the cat towards the handler and restraining the cat by its forelegs and elbows. The conjunctival epithelium can be examined by cupping the cat's head in both hands, and using the thumb of one hand gently to pull down the lower lid so that it is everted. Meanwhile the thumb of the other hand applies gentle pressure to the upper lid (Fig. 1.19). This procedure results in the third eyelid coming across the eye.

Eye medication can be given when there is no assistance available. The cat is sat on the table facing away from the handler. Its body is tucked against the handler's and restrained by the forearms and elbows (Fig. 1.20). The cat's head is restrained in one hand, with the thumb pressing on the top eyelid to keep it open. With the free hand, the third finger is used to open the lower lid, whilst the medication is given with the thumb and forefinger.

Subcutaneous injection

This procedure is best carried out with no assistance. The cat is placed in sternal recumbency on the table, facing away. With one hand grasping the cat by its scruff, the injection is given with the

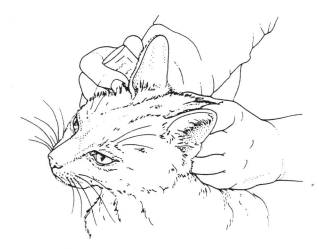

FIG. 1.18 Applying ear medication single-handed.

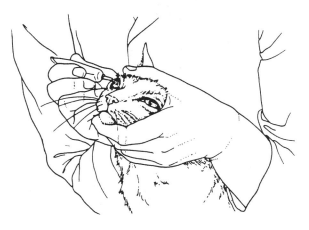

FIG. 1.20 Application of eye medication single-handed.

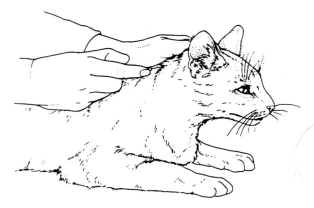

FIG. 1.21   Subcutaneous injection into the scruff of the neck.

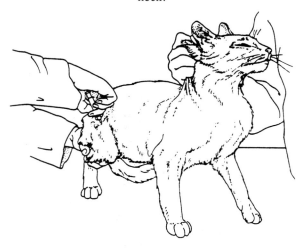

FIG. 1.22   Intramuscular injection.

other hand into the raised skin of the scruff (Fig. 1.21). Most cats tolerate this procedure well, but additional restraint can be achieved with the forearms and elbows and pressing down onto the cat with the chest.

Intramuscular injection

The safest way to give an intramuscular injection is first to have the cat adequately restrained. The most satisfactory muscle mass for an intramuscular injection is the quadriceps group anterior to the femur. The assistant faces the cat's hind quarters towards the clinician, and grasps the cat's scruff with the one hand. The clinician restrains the hind leg with one hand, and gives the injection with the other (Fig. 1.22). Intramuscular injections

can be given to feral or fractious cats, through the mesh of a cage with a squeeze-back facility (see section on catching and handling feral cats).

Intravenous injection

In cats, the cephalic vein is the most convenient way to give an intravenous injection. The cat is sat on a table, facing the clinician. The assistant holds the cat's head under its chin with one hand and uses both forearms and chest to hold the cat. The cat's foreleg is pushed forward at the elbow with the other hand. The thumb and forefinger are used at the crook of the cat's elbow to apply a tourniquet effect, to raise the cephalic vein (Fig. 1.23). The cat can be restrained further by changing the grip from around the chin to one scruffing and twisting the cat's head away from the clinician's face (Fig. 1.24).

After the needle has entered the vein, the assistant releases the thumb pressure on the vein, so that the intravenous injection can be given, whilst still pushing the cat's foreleg forward at the elbow (Fig. 1.25).

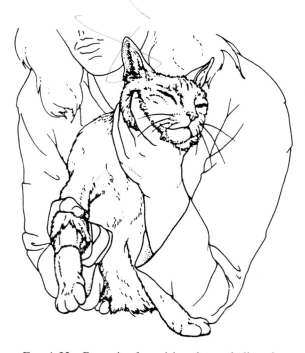

FIG. 1.23   Restraint for raising the cephalic vein.

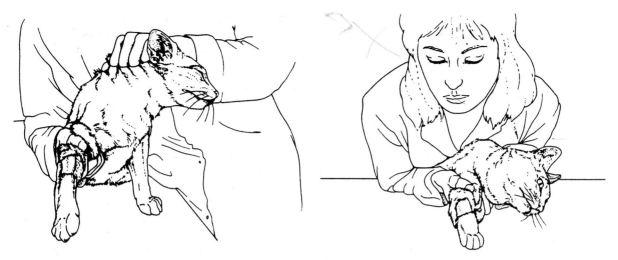

FIG. 1.24   Firmer restraint for raising the cephalic vein.

Blood sampling

Blood samples can be taken safely from conscious cats, either from the cephalic or the jugular vein. The cephalic vein is commonly used (Fig. 1.26). The jugular vein can be used if comparatively large volumes of blood are required quickly, e.g. from a cat used as a blood donor, and is better than the cephalic vein in kittens under six weeks old.

The method of restraint for taking a blood

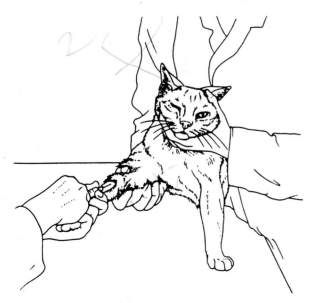

FIG. 1.25   Releasing thumb pressure, for intravenous injection.

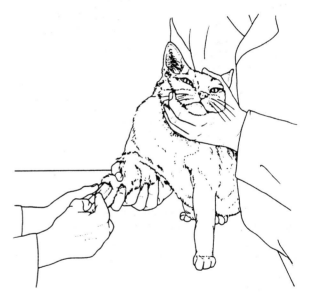

FIG. 1.26   Obtaining a blood sample from the cephalic vein.

sample from the cephalic vein is the same as that described for intravenous injection as illustrated in Figs 1.24 and 1.25. However, the thumb and forefinger remain as a tourniquet throughout the procedure (Fig. 1.26). Wrapping in a towel can be useful for more difficult cats, leaving a foreleg free for sampling (Fig. 1.27).

Jugular venepuncture is tolerated well by most cats. The cat is restrained in dorsal recumbency and placed on the lap of the assistant who sits on

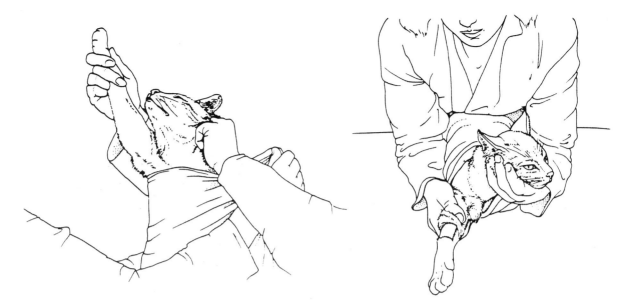

FIG. 1.27   Wrapping a cat in a towel, for intravenous injection or blood sample from the cephalic vein.

a chair (Fig. 1.28). If the right jugular vein is used, the assistant holds all four legs in his right hand. The thumb of the assistant's left hand is placed in the jugular furrow and pressure is applied to raise the jugular vein. The clinician restrains the cat's head by its chin with one hand, and uses the other hand to take the blood sample. The positions are reversed for left-handed operators.

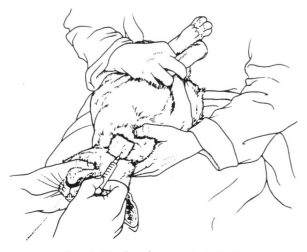

FIG. 1.28   Jugular venepuncture.

Carrying and transporting cats

Domestic cats are usually transported from the home to a cattery or hospital in either a cat-carrying basket, cage or box. A wide range of suitable cat-carrying baskets is readily available from the pet trade and veterinarians. Materials used include wickerwork, fibreglass, wood, plastic and plastic-coated wire mesh. Veterinarians often stock cardboard carrying boxes which are reasonably priced, although they have a limited life span.

Before a cat is removed from a basket to a cage and *vice versa*, it is essential to ensure that all doors and windows are closed as well as securing all cat flaps, fireplaces, chimneys and other possible exits, to prevent the cat from escaping if the grip on the cat is relaxed. Cats can be carried within a room as shown in Figs 1.2, 1.3 and 1.4. However, a cat should only be moved from one room to another, or from the veterinary hospital to the owner's car, in a proper basket and not be carried loose. When a cat is to be removed from a basket, the lid should be raised gently: if the cat does not appear to be vicious, a hand is slipped into the basket to restrain the cat before the lid is folded back fully. When a cat is placed in a basket, it is put in rear-end first, and one hand is kept

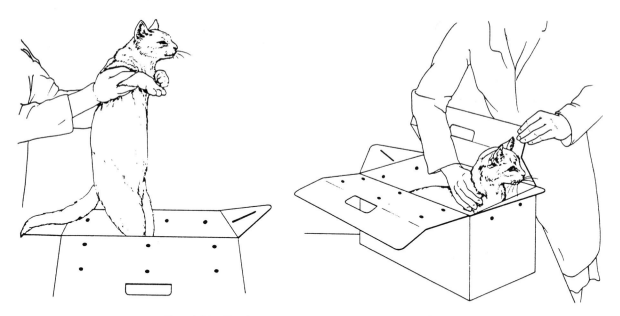

FIG. 1.29   Putting a cat into a cardboard carrying box.

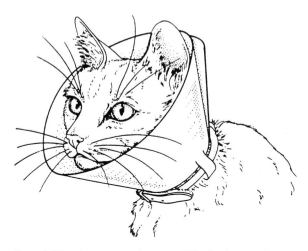

FIG. 1.30   A cat wearing an 'Elizabethan collar' to prevent it from scratching its face and licking areas of the body.

firmly on its back while the lid is shut with the other hand.

Recommendations for the transportation of large numbers of cats over medium-range journeys (e.g. within continental Europe) can be found in the UFAW Handbook.[1] Transportation by road is preferable to rail or air. Fibreglass containers (e.g. length 61–68 cm, breadth 36–44 cm, height 40 cm) can be used to accommodate one or two cats. All four sides should have adequate ventilation with holes which cover 10–15 per cent of the surface area. Absorbent bedding should be provided, together with water and food for long journeys.

REFERENCES

1. Hurni, H. and Rossback, W. (1987) The laboratory cat, in *The UFAW Handbook on the Care and Management of Laboratory Animals*, Editor Poole T. 6th Edition, pp. 476–492.
2. Leedy, M.G. Fishelson, B.A. and Cooper, L.L. (1983) A simple method of restraint for use with cats. *Feline Practice* **13**, 32–33.
3. Universities Federation for Animal Welfare (UFAW) (1981) Feral cats: notes for veterinary surgeons. *Vet Rec.* **108**, 301–303.

2

Husbandry Practices for Multiple-cat Households

JOHN R. AUGUST

As the cat gains popularity as a pet, veterinarians are providing health care for more multiple-cat households than ever before. Some owners enjoy the distinct variations in character that occur among their cats, and are entertained by the constant interaction of their pets. Health problems in these households with modest numbers of cats are usually no more severe than in homes with a single cat.

The increase in the cat population has resulted in more stray or feral animals, and some multiple-cat households arise out of good intentions to care for this abandoned group. Unfortunately, serious health problems are often prevalent in these environments, and the preventive health care measures established for the individual cat are often ineffective in reducing morbidity and mortality in these large groups. The number of cats is often inappropriately high and new cats are introduced frequently into the group. The owner usually has inadequate funds to provide the proper level of nutrition and preventive health care, and the recommendations of the attending veterinarian to dispose of sick and infectious animals are often ignored on humane grounds.

Annual physical examinations and vaccinations, neutering, proper grooming, regular attention to dental hygiene, control of intestinal and external parasites, testing for feline leukaemia virus (FeLV) and feline immunodeficiency virus (FIV) infections, and simple nutritional counselling, are usually effective in maintaining the health of an individual pet cat. To reduce the prevalence of disease in households with many random-source cats, other husbandry practices must be instituted, based more on the concepts of herd health than on the care of the individual animal.[1]

HEALTH PROBLEMS OF MULTIPLE-CAT HOUSEHOLDS

Multiple-cat households have been defined as those homes with three or more cats.[11] Major health problems that may be observed in households with large populations of cats include viral diseases, parasitic diseases, nutritional deficiencies, and behavioural disorders.

By nature, cats are solitary creatures, comingling only at times of mating and territorial disputes. Most of the health problems seen in multiple-cat households result from the artificial environment in which the cats must exist, with overcrowding facilitating the spread of infectious agents, exacerbating the level of stress, and forcing competition for food.[9]

HUSBANDRY PRACTICES FOR MULTIPLE-CAT HOUSEHOLDS

Population management

Efforts to reduce morbidity and mortality in multiple-cat households start with determining if the number of cats is appropriate for the living space and for the financial resources of the owner. Overcrowding may result in an increased concentration of pathogens, with a greater risk of exposure to these organisms through close contact and environmental contamination. Weaker members of the group, or those with special nutritional needs, may have marginal nutrition. Abnormal levels of stress may give rise to behaviour such as urine spraying, obsessive self-grooming, or defecation outside the litter tray. The presence of one or more of these abnormalities may be an important indication that the population density is too high, and the owner should be advised that other husbandry measures may be ineffective as long as overcrowding persists.

Disease problems in multiple-cat households will be reduced by maintaining a closed environment, spaying or neutering all of the cats, adding no new cats to the group, and preventing contact with other cats. Unfortunately, this advice is not likely to be heeded by the 'good Samaritan' whose well-intentioned but misdirected goal is to provide shelter and sustenance for every feral and stray cat in the neighbourhood. Nevertheless, the introduction of new cats of random background into the household is fraught with great risk.[6]

In addition to the likelihood that it may be suffering from an infectious disease, the new cat may introduce strains of micro-organisms against which the group has no inherent resistance, leading to an epizootic of acute disease.[9] Similarly, the new cat is suddenly exposed to the resident microbial strains of the household and may develop acute illness soon after arrival.

The stress associated with introduction into a new social group may cause recrudescence of shedding from latent infections such as FeLV and feline rhinotracheitis virus, exposing the residents of the household to these pathogens. In addition, the new cat will probably disrupt the fragile social order that is present in the group, exacerbating the existing level of stress-associated problems.[10]

The introduction of stray or feral kittens poses the greatest risk to the group.[9] Random-source kittens are very likely to be suffering from infectious diseases and shed large quantities of the organisms with which they are infected. For this reason, limiting the number of kittens in the household will help to reduce the prevalence of infectious diseases.[10] In addition, kittens exposed to pathogenic micro-organisms are more likely to suffer severe clinical signs, or remain chronic carriers, or die.[8] When the owner feels compelled to add cats of unknown background to the group, the introduction of adult animals poses the lesser risk to the other cats.[9]

Under ideal circumstances, random-source cats should be isolated for six weeks before being introduced to the group. The cats in quarantine should be housed in a different facility, because it may be difficult to keep them separated in the rooms of the house.[11] During quarantine, they should be observed for signs of any recrudescent respiratory disease that may have been induced by the stress of re-housing; they should be vaccinated; and faecal examinations should be performed every three weeks. Treatment should be given against any intestinal parasites, and a weekly shampooing with a parasiticidal product to remove external parasites. To prevent the introduction of dermatophyte infections by a sub-clinical carrier, brushings of the haircoat should be taken for fungal culture. Cats should only be introduced to the group if tests for FeLV antigen and FIV antibody are negative at the beginning and end of quarantine, and if no coronavirus antibody is detected at each of these times.

The expense and logistics of these recommendations make it very unlikely that they will be followed by the 'good Samaritan' on a limited budget. However, they may be persuasive enough to deter a rational owner with several healthy cats from adopting a stray or feral cat unless these strict criteria have been fulfilled.

Reduction of stress

Stress is greatly underestimated as a predisposing factor to disease in cats. The veterinarian should make every effort to identify and reduce the unique stresses that may be affecting the household under investigation. In the author's experience, it is very difficult to assess the level of stress by observing the cats, which may appear outwardly to be content and placid. Specific physiological, haematological, biochemical and endocrine abnormalities associated with stress may be identified when diagnostic laboratory tests are performed on individual sick cats from the group.[5]

Detection of the secondary complications of stress is the most reliable indication that the problem is present. Inappropriate levels of stress decrease resistance to disease, especially local immunity affecting the mucous membranes, and therefore a high prevalence of chronic forms of respiratory, conjunctival and enteric infections may be an important indicator of this problem.[8] Other complications of stress include a predisposition to chronic infections with the dermatophyte

Microsporum canis,[7] changes in eating habits, chronic vomition or diarrhoea of non-organic origin, self-mutilation, and urine spraying.[3]

Control of infectious diseases

Factors of practical importance that may increase the prevalence and severity of infectious diseases in multiple-cat households include the mixing of cats of different age groups. the presence of undetected carriers, the accumulation of pathogens due to poor sanitation, the uncontrolled introduction of new cats into the group, stress and overcrowding, and inadequate nutrition.[1]

Cats that are potentially infectious include: those with overt acute illness, asymptomatic animals that are incubating infection, cats that are undergoing re-infection, those that are chronically infected and have low-grade clinical signs, and asymptomatic carriers. Susceptible cats are exposed to pathogens in the excretions, secretions, and exfoliations of these infected animals.[10] Most infectious diseases are transmitted by one or more of the following methods: direct nose-to-nose contact, contact with contaminated fomites, aerosol transmission via sneezed moisture droplets, biting, or congenital transmission from queen to kittens.[11]

Aggressive efforts should be made to identify every cat that may be capable of transmitting infectious diseases and to determine if it may be removed from the home, depending on its emotional value to the owner. As noted previously, kittens with infectious diseases create the greatest hazard to the group, due to the severity of their clinical signs and the large quantities of pathogens that they shed.

Using this knowledge of the causes and spread of infectious diseases in multiple-cat households with poor husbandry, the following basic principles of disease control may be implemented.[1,11] The vaccination programmes should be evaluated to determine if they meet the special needs of the group. Traditional parenteral vaccination may be ineffective in preventing clinical disease in young cats in overcrowded households. Early parenteral vaccination with killed products or early intranasal vaccination may be necessary to reduce the incidence of severe upper respiratory disease in young cats.[2] The concentration of viruses in the environment should be reduced by isolating acutely ill animals until completely recovered, with the permanent removal of carriers, and attention to sanitation. Most well-intentioned owners underestimate the epizootiological importance of the chronically infected cat with low-grade clinical signs, and remain unconvinced that these reasonably healthy animals should be removed from the group. Attempts should be made to isolate susceptible young cats from potentially infectious animals until at least two weeks after their initial vaccination series is completed. Quarantine measures, as described previously, should be recommended. Lastly, and most importantly, overcrowding should be corrected by reducing the number of cats to that which is appropriate for the space available and for the budget of the owner.[11]

Control of parasites

The high concentrations of intestinal parasites and ectoparasites in overcrowded multiple-cat households may produce overt clinical disease in younger animals. Faeces should be removed from the litter trays daily so that infective eggs and oocysts do not accumulate. In the United States, the most prevalent small intestinal parasite of cats is *Toxocara cati*. Patent infections with *T. cati* occur most commonly in young kittens as a result of transmammary transmission.[12] Infections with the roundworm *Toxascaris leonina* are less common. Because the feline hookworm *Ancylostoma tubaeformae* may also infect young cats in households with a high population density, routine anthelmintic treatments for kittens should be effective against roundworms and hookworms.[12]

Oocysts from the coccidia *Isospora felis* and *Isospora rivolta* are often found in the faeces of kittens, with or without diarrhoea. When clinical signs attributable to coccidiosis fail to disappear after appropriate therapy, the veterinarian should determine if other intestinal diseases are present that allow continued production of oocysts. In overcrowded situations, the veterinarian should look carefully for intestinal parasitic diseases (such as giardiasis) that are not detected routinely on faecal flotation.

Flea infections may cause pruritic skin disease in cats of all ages, and anaemia in young kittens. Fleas are the intermediate hosts for the tapeworm *Dipylidium caninum*, and they may facilitate the transmission of *M. canis* between cats by allowing the penetration of arthrospores into abraded skin.[7] If fleas are enzootic in the household, the attending veterinarian should implement a comprehensive regimen of topical and environmental insecticide application, choosing a parasiticide that is non-toxic to humans and cats of all ages.

Infections with the ear mite *Otodectes cynotis* are common in young cats, often causing otic and cutaneous discomfort. The ears of all cats in the household should be examined regularly to determine if *O. cynotis* infections are present, and infected cats should be treated with parasiticidal ear drops and shampoos for no less than four weeks.

A healthy environment

An inspection of the physical environment in the home may reveal problems that predispose the group to infectious diseases. Adult cats thrive comfortably at temperatures of 65–70°F and a relative humidity of 35% or less.[1] The prevalence and severity of infectious diseases are increased markedly by cold damp conditions[10] or wide fluctuations in temperature and relative humidity.[9] The viability of many microbial pathogens is maintained longer in a damp environment.

The environment of the overcrowded multiple-cat household will be heavily contaminated with the secretions, excretions, and exfoliations of the animals.[10] The most severe contamination will occur in areas where cats congregate – such as litter trays, food and water dishes and the floors around them, and window sills. The cats may be exposed to a heavy challenge of pathogens when they frequent these areas; the outcome of this exposure will be most severe for young cats that are immunologically immature.

A routine sanitation programme should be instituted to reduce the prevalence of infectious diseases caused by fomite contamination. Carpets and upholstered furniture should be vacuumed regularly to prevent the build-up of hair and dander, and to remove fleas and fungal spores.

The spores of *M. canis* can remain viable in the environment for up to 18 months.[7]

Impermeable surfaces should be cleaned at least once weekly with a hot solution of soap and water to remove organic debris that may contain microbial pathogens and parasites, and then rinsed with warm water. Heavily used areas should then be disinfected with a 1:32 dilution of household bleach (5.25% sodium hypochlorite) which should be allowed to dry thoroughly before the cats are allowed access to the area. The litter tray should be cleaned and disinfected regularly in the same manner; however, disposable liners provide a more convenient solution to the problem of litter tray contamination.

Feed and water bowls should be washed daily in a solution of hot soap and water and then rinsed. At least once weekly after cleaning, the bowls should be disinfected in a 1:32 bleach solution for 5–10 minutes and rinsed thoroughly with water.[11]

Nutrition

The overcrowded conditions in many multiple-cat households create special nutritional needs for many of the animals. Marginal or subclinical nutritional deficiencies are common, especially in cats with specific nutritional needs, and are often complicated by gastrointestinal disturbances due to frequent and abrupt changes in diet.

The dietary energy requirements of growing kittens and lactating queens are up to three times higher than the maintenance requirement of the mature cat (see Chapter 4). Malnutrition slows the growth rate of the young animal, and impairs cell-mediated immune function, predisposing the kitten to infectious diseases. Debilitation from infection worsens the malnutrition by decreasing the intake of nutrients. For example, malnutrition may be an important factor in predisposing cats to *M. canis* infection.[7]

To minimise these complications, the cats should be fed a consistent premium-quality diet that is palatable, highly digestible, nutritionally complete, and formulated for their life stage. The potent effects of malnutrition and the special nutritional needs of the stressed cat provide strong arguments for the use of such diets in the multiple-cat household. The costs of treating the disease complications of malnourished animals will be substantially reduced by feeding a good quality, nutritionally balanced diet, offsetting the increased cost of the premium food.

SUMMARY

Health maintenance in multiple-cat households requires the implementation of husbandry practices not normally considered for the individual animal. Because of the artificial environment in which they live, these cats are at high risk for developing microbial, parasitic, nutritional, or behavioural diseases. The health of the group may be improved substantially by maintaining the population at a number appropriate for the living space in the house and for the budget of the owner; controlling infectious diseases through population management, vaccination, and environmental sanitation; and meeting the special nutritional needs of the cats.

REFERENCES

1. August J.R. (1988) Maintaining a healthy cattery. In *Proceedings*, 12th Kal Kan Forum, 49–52.
2. August J.R. (1989) Feline viral diseases. In: Ettinger S.J. (ed.) *Textbook of Veterinary Internal Medicine*, 3rd edn, pp 312–340. W.B. Saunders Co., Philadelphia.
3. Beaver B.V. (1991) Psychogenic manifestations of environmental disturbances. In: August J.R. (ed.) *Consultations in Feline Internal Medicine*, pp 19–24. W.B. Saunders Co., Philadelphia.
4. Buffington C.A. (1991) Nutrition and nutritional disorders. In: Pedersen N.C. (ed.) *Feline Husbandry. Diseases and Management in the Multiple-Cat Environment*, pp 325–356. American Veterinary Publications Inc., Goleta, California.
5. Greco D.C. (1991) The effect of stress on the evaluation of feline patients. In: August J.R. (ed.) *Consultations in Feline Internal Medicine*, pp 13–17. W.B. Saunders Co., Philadelphia.
6. Hart B.L., Pedersen, N.C. (1991) Behavior. In: Pedersen N.C. (ed.) *Feline Husbandry. Diseases and Management in the Multiple-Cat Environment*, pp 289–323. American Veterinary Publications Inc., Goleta, California.
7. Moriello K.A. (1991) Management of dermatophytosis in catteries. In: August J.R. (ed.) *Consultations in Feline Internal Medicine*, pp 89–94. W.B. Saunders Co., Philadelphia.
8. Pedersen N.C. (1987) Basic and clinical immunology. In: Holzworth J. (ed.) *Diseases of the Cat. Medicine and Surgery*, pp 146–181. W.B. Saunders Co., Philadelphia.
9. Pedersen N.C. (1991) Common infectious diseases of multiple-cat environments. In: Pedersen N.C. (ed.) *Feline Husbandry. Diseases and Management in the Multiple-Cat Environment*, pp 163–288. American Veterinary Publications Inc., Goleta, California.
10. Pedersen N.C., Wastlhuber J. (1991) Cattery design and management. In: Pedersen N.C. (ed.) *Feline Husbandry. Diseases and Management in the Multiple-Cat Environment*, pp 393–437. American Veterinary Publications Inc., Goleta, California.
11. Scott F.W., Saidla J.E. (1990) Control of feline infectious diseases within catteries, shelters, and multicat households. *Sheba Forum* **1**(2): 3–9.
12. Zajac A. (1991) Treatment of gastrointestinal parasitic infections. In: August J.R. (ed.) *Consultations in Feline Internal Medicine*, pp 425–433. W.B. Saunders Co., Philadelphia.

3

Nutrition and Nutritional Disorders

JOSEPHINE M. WILLS and KAY E. EARLE

Over the last twenty years there has been an increase in the level of awareness of certain key nutrients which are known to be essential in the diet of the domestic cat and can only be supplied adequately from materials of animal origin. It is these interesting nutritional peculiarities which make the cat distinct from the other companion animals and clearly classify it as an obligate carnivore. The science of nutrition encompasses a whole variety of interlinked factors which include not only the levels of essential nutrients, but also the energy content, digestibility and palatability of the food.

NUTRITIONAL PECULIARITIES OF THE CAT

The minimum recommended daily nutrient allowances have been documented for cats and are listed in Fig. 3.1. Any diet that is considered nutritionally complete for cats must satisfy all these minima and allowance must be made for products which are of low digestibility and where the availability of certain nutrients is reduced. Dietary requirements for an individual cat will vary according to its stage of life, level of activity and physiological status.

Protein

Of the major nutrients, protein is required in greater amounts by the cat than most other mammals. The metabolic explanation for this higher protein requirement is the increased activity of the nitrogen catabolising enzymes in the liver of the cat. The level of activity of the hepatic enzymes which metabolise the non-essential amino-acids (alanine amino transferase and glutamate dehydrogenase) is greater than that of either the dog or the rat. In contrast, the level of enzyme activity for the breakdown of the essential amino-acids is lower in the cat. This differential pattern of enzyme activity results in a poor level of nitrogen conservation within the body pool which therefore requires a constant and high dietary input. Even when ingesting a low protein diet, the cat's enzyme activity is unaltered and the result is a negative nitrogen balance as no hepatic adaptation takes place.[13]

During their phase of rapid growth, kittens require more protein per se than adult cats (240 g/kg diet as compared to 140 g/kg diet); this requirement may decline with advancing years but there is little evidence for this effect.

In addition to a high total protein requirement, a number of the individual amino-acids are of particular interest. The cat is unusual in its metabolism of arginine, a deficiency of which rapidly results in a failure of the urea cycle. A total lack of arginine, in an otherwise high protein semi-purified diet, will lead to the development of hyperammonaemia from amino-acid breakdown and can result in death within hours.

Taurine, an amino-sulphonic acid, is synthesised in the liver from the essential amino-acids methionine and cystine. The decarboxylation steps in the taurine anabolic pathway are severely reduced in the cat and consequently taurine synthesis is limited. Without sufficient pre-formed taurine in the diet, blood levels will fall and bile formation will be compromised; the cat is totally dependent on the conjugation of taurine with cholic acid to form its bile salts. Circulating plasma taurine concentrations below 40 µmol/l are considered indicative of taurine deficiency and any diet giving rise to these low levels should be changed or adequately supplemented.

Finally, protein can substitute for carbohydrate in the diet if the concentration is sufficiently high to provide the gluconeogenic amino-acids in the required amounts. Under conditions of high dietary protein, the cat has no known requirement for carbohydrate. However, there may be advantages

MINIMUM RECOMMENDED DAILY NUTRIENT ALLOWANCE			
Nutrient	**Unit**	**Growing kittens**[a]	**All life stages**[b]
Fat[c]	g	–	90
linoleic acid	g	5	10
arachidonic acid	mg	200	–
Protein[d] (Nx6.25)	g	240	280
arginine	g	10	–
histidine	g	3	–
isoleucine	g	5	–
leucine	g	12	–
lysine	g	8	–
methionine + cystine	g	7.5	–
methionine	g	4	–
phenylalanine + tyrosine	g	8.5	–
phenylalanine	g	4	–
taurine	mg	400	–
threonine	g	7	–
tryptophan	g	1.5	–
valine	g	6	–
Minerals			
calcium	g	8	10
phosphorus	g	6	8
magnesium	mg	400	500
potassium[e]	g	4	3
sodium	mg	500	500
chloride	g	1.9	0.8
iron	mg	80	100
copper	mg	5	5
iodine	µg	350	1000
zinc	mg	50	30
manganese	mg	5	10
selenium	µg	100	100
Vitamins			
A	mg	1(3,333IU)	3(10,000IU)
D	µg	12.5(500IU)	25(1000IU)
E[f]	mg	30(30IU)	80(80IU)
K[g]	µg	100	–
thiamin	mg	5	5
riboflavin	mg	4	5
vitamin B6	mg	4	–
niacin	mg	40	45
pantothenic acid	mg	5	10
folic acid[g]	µg	800	1000
biotin[g]	µg	70	50
vitamin B12	µg	20	20
choline[h]	g	2.4	2.0

Notes
[a] Based on a diet with ME concentration of 5.0 kcal/g dry matter, NRC 1986.
[b] Based on a diet with ME concentration of 4.0 kcal/g dry matter, NRC 1978.
[c] No requirement for fat is known apart from the need for essential fatty acids and as a carrier of fat-soluble vitamins.
[d] Assuming that all minimum essential amino acid requirements are met.
[e] The minimum potassium requirement increases with protein intake.
[f] This minimum would increase three-to-four-fold with a high PUFA diet.
[g] These vitamins may not be required unless antimicrobial or antivitamin components are present in the diet.
[h] Choline is not essential in the diet but if this quantity of choline is not present the methionine requirement should be increased to provide the same quantity of methyl groups.

FIG. 3.1   Minimum recommended daily nutrient allowance (per kg diet, dry basis).

in supplying carbohydrate at times of metabolic stress – for example, during lactation.

Fat

Fat is the other major nutrient known to be required in the diet of the cat, although a precise requirement is difficult to assess. The only demonstrable need for fat is as a provider of the essential fatty acids – in particular, the 18 carbon linoleic and linolenic acids. The metabolism of these nutrients is unusual in the cat because of the lack of the $\triangle 6$-desaturase which is the rate-limiting enzyme for most mammals.[8,12] Longer chain polyunsaturated fatty acids (>C18) are produced by an alternative pathway involving the $\triangle 5$ and $\triangle 8$-desaturases but the rate of production is lower in the cat than many other mammals.[10]

Cats cannot sustain normal reproductive performance when maintained on a diet that contains linoleic acid as the sole source of fatty acids: they exhibit a dietary requirement for arachidonic acid in addition to linoleic acid. The exact role of alpha linolenic acid in the metabolism of polyunsaturated fatty acids in the cat is unknown.

Vitamins

The requirement for pre-formed vitamin A in the diet of the cat results from a lack of the dioxygenase enzyme needed to convert beta-carotene to vitamin A. However, excessive quantities must be avoided in the diet (no more than 57,000 IU/kg body-weight) as this fat soluble vitamin is stored in the liver and will lead to hepatic damage and the typical skeletal changes of hypervitaminosis A (see later, and Chapter 17).[14]

Conversely, high dietary concentrations of the water-soluble vitamins will have no deleterious effect on the cat; of these, niacin, pyridoxine and thiamin are particularly important because of their role in protein metabolism. Niacin, for example, is usually synthesised from the amino-acid tryptophan, making a dietary source unnecessary. However, high levels of the enzyme picolinic carboxylase in the liver of the cat result in a diversion of the pathway intermediary, 3 hydroxy-anthranilic acid, to produce an excess of glutamate and may result in a deficiency of niacin. A dietary source of niacin is therefore required to avoid a deficiency of the metabolically active form of this vitamin, nicotinamide. Nicotinamide adenine dinucleotide (NAD) is involved in oxidation/reduction reactions in the utilisation of all major nutrients.

High levels of dietary pyridoxine are necessary for the production of the co-enzyme pyridoxal phosphate. Pyridoxal phosphate is the prosthetic group of the enzymes which decarboxylate the essential amino-acids tyrosine, arginine and glutamic acid. Other functions include the deamination of serine and threonine and the regulation of kynureninase which aids the transfer of amino acids into cells.[1]

The other important water-soluble vitamin is thiamin, which acts as a coenzyme in the oxidation pathway of glucose and in the metabolism of branched-chain amino-acids.[3] Insufficient dietary supplies of thiamin result in an initial accumulation of pentose sugars in the erythrocytes to three times their normal levels before clinical signs of thiamin deficiency are evident.

Dietary supplementation is usually necessary if the diet consists of raw fish containing naturally occurring thiaminases or if the cat's food is over-processed, as thiamin is a heat labile vitamin. The higher turnover of dietary protein in the cat necessitates an increased requirement for all these water-soluble vitamins. For senior cats, there may be an advantage in increasing the concentration of the antioxidant vitamins, as there is some evidence that these nutrients inhibit certain degenerative processes.

Minerals

There is a paucity of data available on the mineral requirements of the cat. Nevertheless calcium, phosphorus, sodium, potassium, magnesium, iron, copper, zinc and iodine are all indispensable in this species; their presence is essential for the maintenance of acid-base balance and tissue structure and as enzyme cofactors. The overall balance of the diet is affected not only by the finite levels of these minerals but also by the interactions between them. For example, the ratio of calcium: phosphorus is important in the maintenance of bone and cellular integrity; in cats, this should be

FIG. 3.2 Nutrient content of home-cooked foods commonly given to domestic cats.

per 100 kcal	Beef[a]	Chicken[b]	Cod[c]	Liver[d]	NRC[e]
NUTRIENT CONTENT OF HOME-COOKED FOODS					
Protein (g)	10	16	22	11	5
Fat (g)	7	4	1	6	2
Linoleic acid (g)	122	508	–	2	100
Arachidonic acid (g)	61	27	31	2	4
Vitamin A (IU)	–	–	–	26,900	61
Thiamin (mg)	22	33	73	1	100
Calcium (mg)	7	6	23	4	160
Magnesium (mg)	9	14	27	11	80
Taurine (mg)	3	5	17	12	10

[a] 100 kcal beef approximately 80g
[b] 100 kcal chicken approximately 50g
[c] 100 kcal cod approximately 150g
[d] 100 kcal liver approximately 60g
[e] Minimum requirement from NRC 1986

within the acceptable range of 0.5:1 to 2:1. A mineral excess may therefore be as harmful as a deficiency. Home prepared, meat-rich diets may well require mineral supplementation as meat is a poor source of calcium but a relatively rich source of phosphorus (see later, and Chapter 17).

Magnesium is also a key mineral in cat nutrition because of its role in the formation of struvite uroliths (magnesium ammonium phosphate). There may be advantages in restricting the level of magnesium to reduce the formation of these uroliths, without compromising its normal physiological role in the neuromuscular system.

DIET FORMULATION

Achieving the correct balance of nutrients in the diet of a cat is difficult without an extensive knowledge of their individual nutrient requirements. Figure 3.2 shows a selection of meats typically fed to cats and compares their nutrient content with the National Research Council (NRC) minimum recommendations. Supplementation of the diet would be necessary if these foods were used regularly as the sole source of nutrients. Prepared pet foods are formulated to a high specification which allows for the inclusion of all the key nutrients at optimum levels, taking into account their biochemical interactions, and

dispenses with the need for additional dietary supplementation.

Energy

Dietary energy content is determined by the protein, fat and carbohydrate content of the raw materials in the food. If the exact concentration of these nutrients in a particular diet is known, the energy content may be calculated by the following formulae.

Dry type diet:

calculated metabolisable energy content (kcal/100g) = [protein (kcal/100g) × 5.65 + fat (kcal/100g) × 9.4 + nitrogen-free extract (kcal/100g) × 4.15] 0.99 − 126

Canned type diet:

calculated metabolisable energy content (kcal/100g) = [protein (kcal/100g) × 3.9 + fat (kcal/100g) × 7.7 + nitrogen-free extract (kcal/100g) × 3] − 5

The energy requirement of the cat can be calculated from its body-weight (BW) and an adult is known to require 70–90 kcal/kg BW/day,

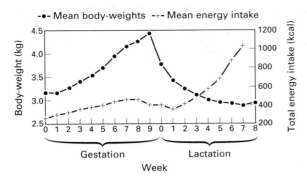

FIG. 3.3   Body-weights and energy intakes of queens during gestation and lactation.

ANALYSIS OF MILK SAMPLES		
% content as fed	Cat	Cow[a]
Moisture	81.5	87.6
Protein	8.1	3.3
Fat	5.1	3.8
Lactose	6.9	4.7
Calcium	0.04	0.12
Phosphorus	0.07	0.10
Energy (kcal/100ml)	142	66

[a] Baines (1981)

FIG. 3.4   Analysis of milk samples from the cat and the cow.

HOME-PREPARED MILK REPLACER
225ml unhomogenised whole milk
10g dried, skimmed milk powder
15g egg yolk

FIG. 3.5   Recipe for a home-prepared milk replacer.

depending on its level of activity. Inactive and obese cats require less energy (50–60 kcal/kg BW) to maintain a steady body-weight.[4] Cats have the ability to regulate their energy intake from day to day and will adjust the amount of food they eat to achieve this. However, if the opportunity for exercise is limited and the diet very palatable, the balance of energy may be affected and obesity will result. The nutrient profile of the diet must be balanced in relation to its overall energy content to ensure the correct intake of each nutrient.

The energy demands of growing and pregnant animals are greater than those of the adult. Figure 3.3 shows the steady increases in energy intake and body-weight following mating that have been observed in queens within the Waltham Centre colony. After parturition, their energy intake continues to rise to provide the extra energy needed for lactation. In order to produce milk of the necessary quantity and quality, the energy requirement of the queen may be as much as three to four times her normal maintenance requirement.

Figure 3.4 shows a comparison between the analysis of milk from the cat and the cow. Queen's milk is more calorie dense than that of the cow and therefore unsupplemented cow's milk would be a nutrient-poor diet for an orphan kitten. Commercial milk-replacers are available, and their use is described in Chapter 5. A suitable home-prepared milk-replacement recipe is shown in Fig. 3.5. At 10 weeks of age, kittens require 250 kcal/kg BW per day but this declines slowly over a period of 10–12 months until they reach

their adult maintenance requirement (Fig. 3.6). The feeding regimen for these young animals must include several small meals a day of a nutritionally balanced food in order to ensure an adequate energy and nutrient intake for growth. The energy requirement of older cats is thought to vary depending on the clinical status of the animal. There may be advantages in providing a diet of higher energy density because of reduced appetite in older pets. Conversely, it may be advantageous to limit energy intake in some inactive, older cats to reduce the risk of obesity. Each individual case must be considered in context of the health status and lifestyle of the senior cat.

Digestibility

Once the nutrient profile of a feline diet has been correctly balanced relative to its energy content, the next factor to consider is the digestibility of the food. This cannot be assessed without recourse to feeding trials with faecal collection. The gross nutrient content of the diet is subjected to the usual mechanical and physiochemical properties of the digestive tract which enable the uptake of the individual components. The digestive tract of

ENERGY REQUIREMENTS OF YOUNG GROWING CATS				
Age (weeks)	**Expected Body-weight (kg)**		**Mean Caloric Intake (kcal/day)**	
	Female	**Male**	**Female**	**Male**
4	0.2	0.3	10	15
6	0.3	0.5	25	30
8	0.6	0.9	80	100
10	0.8	1.2	175	280
12	1.0	1.4	222	275
14	1.2	1.6	235	300
16	1.4	1.9	246	325
18	1.6	2.2	274	355
20	1.8	2.5	280	375
24	2.1	2.8	269	363
28	2.3	3.1	288	395
32	2.5	3.4	301	403
36	2.7	3.7	313	426
40	2.9	4.0	316	436
44	3.0	4.1	300	401
48	3.0	4.2	257	364
52	3.0	4.3	240	344

the cat is relatively short and is usually calculated to be only three times its relative body length, as opposed to a factor of five for man and the dog. This shorter tract has an effect on overall digestive efficiency: the cat is significantly less efficient than the dog at digesting all the major nutrients.[9]

An important factor affecting the digestibility of a particular nutrient in the diet is the form in which it is present – for example, the quality of the protein. Protein material is available in many forms (from hoof or feather to muscle meat) and the quality of each is determined by its amino-acid profile. Cats have a higher requirement for the essential amino-acids than many other mammals, which must be satisfied by their dietary protein intake, and therefore only high grade protein sources should be used.

Bioavailability

There may be interactions between dietary components which reduce their bioavailability from the digestive tract – for example, the effect of high fibre diets on mineral availability. High fibre diets that contain phytate (primarily inositol hexaphosphate) have an adverse effect on the availability of zinc and calcium from the diet of the dog, but very little information is available for the cat.

The range of recommended daily allowance for an individual nutrient may well change, depending on the overall dietary composition. Dietary fibre may be a beneficial component to aid the passage of digesta through the gastrointestinal tract but it will increase the volume of faecal output. Typically cats produce 60–80 g faeces per day when fed commercial cat foods but the inclusion of 9% dietary fibre in the form of cellulose may result in a faecal output of up to 200–250 g per day. The overall effect is a reduction in the availability of all key nutrients, most importantly energy. Caution is therefore advised when advocating the use of dietary fibre in the diet of healthy cats.

Palatability

The palatability of a diet must be considered: there is nothing less nutritious than a food a cat will not eat. Very little information is available on the sensory aspects of a cat's food intake but this is likely to be a major contributing factor in their food choice. They can distinguish between sweet and bitter tastes but show neither a positive nor negative response to the addition of glucose in their food.[2,15] In general, meat is very palatable to cats and its acceptance can often be further enhanced by the addition of fat. Animal fats are preferable to vegetable fats as they are usually more palatable and they contain arachidonic acid, an essential nutrient for the cat.

Cereals in their raw state are not very palatable to cats, but acceptance and digestibility will be enhanced by cooking, which improves the digestion of starch. The acceptance of foodstuffs is also affected by factors such as the size and shape of individual components and the degree of stickiness of the food but, as in many other respects, all cats are individuals, with their own dietary likes and dislikes.

Feeding behaviour

Environmental factors are known to affect the volume of food a particular animal will eat. Most cats do not like food straight from the refrigerator and prefer to eat food that is close to their own body temperature and that of freshly killed prey. This response may reflect a behavioural strategy in the wild which ensures that only the freshest prey is eaten.

The timing of food consumption is influenced by the cat's behaviour, especially when there is ad libitum access to food. Cats will eat many small meals a day (between 12 and 20) and show no preference for day or night in initiating a feeding response.[11] They will, however, adapt to alternative feeding routines implemented by their owners and are most commonly given two meals per day. Nevertheless, if feeding time is restricted then sufficient food must be provided to satisfy their daily nutrient and energy requirements.

NUTRITION AND DISEASE

As in all species, nutrition and disease have a complex inter-relationship in the cat. Broadly speaking, nutrition-related disorders may be classified in one of two ways: those which are

related to dietary errors, and those which respond to dietary management. Nutritional errors may result from either an excess or a deficiency of one or more elements of the diet, whereas diet-responsive conditions are not caused by the diet per se and are due to the specific limitations of the affected animal. However, some overlap between these two classifications does occur, particularly where there are individual variations in susceptibility to a condition.

Numerous diet-related syndromes have been produced experimentally but in this section, discussion will be limited to those of practical importance to the small animal clinician. Many of the conditions described here are covered in more detail elsewhere in this book.

CONDITIONS INDUCED BY DIETARY ERROR

Nutritional errors are frequently induced by well-meaning owners who may have ill-conceived ideas about a cat's requirements. Oversupplementation of the diet with fish oils or indulgence of an apparent 'addiction' may lead to dietary imbalances. Inadequate diets are likely to be erroneous in a number of respects and deficiencies of certain nutrients rarely occur in isolation, making diagnosis on clinical grounds difficult. Notable exceptions do occur and are discussed below. The consequences of many errors in nutrition are most apparent in cats during the critical life stages, such as growth, pregnancy and lactation or at other times of stress or debilitation.

Vitamin A

Although the cat has a requirement for a dietary source of pre-formed vitamin A, specific deficiencies of this vitamin are rare in practice as cats are unlikely to eat diets which are low in fat and vitamin A content.[7] However, experimentally induced deficiencies have resulted in anorexia; weakness; ataxia; weight loss; abnormalities of the squamous epithelium with the possibility of epithelial infections; and ocular lesions (although these may have been complicated by a concurrent taurine deficiency). Bony effects of hypovitaminosis A are described in Chapter 17.

Hypervitaminosis A is far more likely to be

a problem (see Chapter 17). This condition is typically seen in cats whose diets have been oversupplemented with, for example, cod-liver oil, and those which have been fed excessive amounts of liver which is highly palatable to cats and may result in an apparent 'addiction'. Signs of toxicity, which usually develops from feeding the diet over a period of months or years, do not develop until the prolonged daily intake exceeds 17mg (57,000 IU)/kg BW.

Excesses of this fat-soluble vitamin are stored in the liver and a toxicity can lead to hepatic damage due to lipid infiltration. Clinically, the most recognisable signs of hypervitaminosis A are those related to the skeletal changes that occur, particularly in the cervical vertebrae and the long bones of the forelimb. The periosteum appears to be particularly sensitive to high levels of vitamin A and subperiosteal hyperplasia occurs around the bony insertions of tendons and ligaments in response to physical forces exerted in these areas. Bony exostoses result and may invade joints, causing enlargement and ankylosis.

Initial signs may be of stiffness and pain, particularly of the neck and forelegs, and the owner may first observe the cat's reluctance to groom itself. This may be accompanied by anorexia, lethargy, weight loss and an unkempt appearance. The painful lesions may induce an affected cat to adopt a sitting 'kangaroo' posture in order to avoid weight bearing by the anterior regions.

Treatment consists primarily of dietary correction and the provision of a normal diet; supplementation with fish oils is strictly contraindicated. Non-steroidal anti-inflammatory drugs are useful in the initial stages for the control of pain, and food dishes may be elevated to facilitate eating and drinking. Early treatment may bring about a resolution of clinical signs and halt the progression of the disease, but established ankyloses are irreversible.

Vitamin E

A deficiency of vitamin E (α-tocopherol) in cats results in pansteatitis (yellow fat disease) which is a painful inflammatory condition of the subcutaneous fat. Vitamin E has an anti-oxidant function in the body and is vital for maintaining the stability of cell membranes. In the diet, it limits the peroxidation of dietary lipids and the development of rancidity; greater amounts of this vitamin are thus required when the diet contains high levels of polyunsaturated fatty acids, which are easily oxidised. The condition is usually associated with diets of oily fish (especially red tuna) which are rich in polyunsaturated fatty acids or with feeding rancid, oxidised fat. There is individual variation between cats in their dietary requirements for vitamin E, which can also be affected by dietary levels of selenium, sulphur amino-acids, other anti-oxidants and pro-oxidants in prepared foods, and by individual susceptibility to peroxidation.

The clinical signs of vitamin E deficiency are related to the deposition of ceroid, the end product of lipid peroxidation, in adipose tissue. This provokes a foreign body reaction and results in inflammation, with massive neutrophilic infiltration, and fat cell necrosis. Fat thus affected is firm, painful and nodular on palpation; in the latter stages of the disease it assumes a dirty orange or mustard yellow colour attributable to the ceroid pigment. Subcutaneous fat is most notably affected, but fat within the body cavities may have a similar appearance.

Initially, the affected cat will be inappetent and show pain and hypersensitivity to touch. A fever develops, which is related to the inflammatory and necrotic lesions, and is unresponsive to antimicrobial therapy. Abdominal pain is apparent and vomiting may occur. Subsequently, the nodular character of the subcutaneous fat may be detected on palpation but this procedure may be vigorously resented by the cat.

Dietary correction is required and additional supplementation with 75–100 mg α-tocopherol acetate per day PO may be given initially to replace body stores. Short-term therapy with prednisolone at 1 mg/kg/day is valuable in controlling the inflammatory reaction. Parenteral nutritional support may be necessary, but this should be administered intravenously as subcutaneous fluid therapy is likely to be painful and absorption reduced. Recovery is slow and may demand several weeks or even months of continued therapy. Occasionally, severely affected cases do not respond to treatment and they continue to deteriorate until they either die or are euthanased. Rarely, sudden death occurs.

Thiamin

Thiamin (vitamin B_1) is a water-soluble vitamin, with limited storage in the body, which plays an essential part in energy metabolism and neural impulse transmission. It can be destroyed during prolonged storage; interaction with high levels of glutamate, such as those present in vegetable protein, can lead to a thiamin deficiency; and it is progressively, but not immediately, destroyed by high temperatures and under certain conditions of processing. Most cat food manufacturers supplement their products to compensate for possible losses, but some home prepared diets may require additional thiamin. A deficiency of thiamin can also occur when cats are fed large amounts of certain types of raw fish which contain the enzyme thiaminase, although this is destroyed by cooking.

Initial signs of thiamin deficiency appear within 1–2 weeks of the introduction of a deficient diet and include salivation and a failure to eat despite being interested in food.[6] Weight loss, vomiting and mild ataxia may also be apparent. This progresses to a critical stage in which there are severe neurological disturbances with impaired righting reflexes and short tonic convulsions with ventroflexion of the neck. Mydriasis, circling, dysmetria and spinal hypersensitivity may also be observed. Eventually, there is a spasticity of all the limbs such that the cat appears to be 'walking on its toes' and there may be cardiac irregularities. The terminal stage of the disease is characterised by semi-coma, continuous crying, opisthotonos and, ultimately, death.

Provided the cat is not in extremis, response to therapy can be quite dramatic. Treatment with 5 mg thiamin PO or 1 mg IM can result in the disappearance of all signs within 24 hours although therapy may be continued for several days. A deficient diet should be corrected in order to maintain an adequate thiamin intake.

Vitamin D

Although it is possible to induce rickets in kittens experimentally, natural occurrence of this condition is rare. Cats appear to have an extremely low dietary requirement for vitamin D provided that they have exposure to some sunlight and are otherwise well nourished. However, vitamin D toxicity can be produced relatively easily and is usually the result of overzealous dietary supplementation with, for example, cod-liver oil. As with all fat-soluble vitamins, excesses are stored in the body and their effects are cumulative. The resulting hypercalcaemia and hyperphosphataemia lead to soft tissue calcification, which may be demonstrated radiologically, and to multiple organ dysfunction. There may be neuromuscular abnormalities, typified by general weakness and poor motor reflexes, and resorption of bone resulting in pathological fractures. Cases are normally presented because of the most obvious signs of renal failure, and the prognosis is always guarded. Treatment is symptomatic and the cat should be encouraged to eat a balanced diet without additional supplementation.

Taurine deficiency

Although once thought of as a minor metabolite whose only role was in the conjugation of bile acids, the significance of this amino-sulphonic acid is becoming increasingly apparent. Cats have a unique dietary requirement for pre-formed taurine as they have an exceptionally high physiological demand for this nutrient and they are unable to synthesise sufficient quantities for their needs. Their high demand stems from their inability to conjugate bile acids with the alternative, glycine, to any great extent. There may also be competition between taurine and felinine (which is found in cat urine) for the precursor, cysteine, in their respective biosynthetic pathways. Taurine is found almost exclusively in animal-derived material, hence the obligatory carnivorous nature of the cat.

Taurine deficiency in cats is associated with the characteristic lesions (Fig. 3.7) of Feline Central Retinal Degeneration, FCRD (see Chapter 20); reproductive failure in breeding queens due to foetal resorption, abortion, stillbirth and low birthweight of live kittens; developmental abnormalities in kittens such as retarded growth rates, thoracic kyphosis (flat-chested kittens),

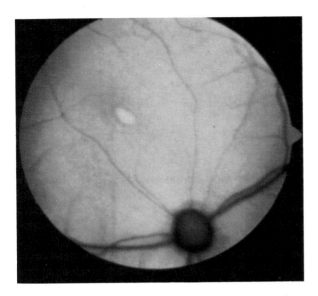

FIG. 3.7   Lesions of feline central retinal degeneration.

paresis with excessive abduction of the hind limbs ('swimmers'), hearing abnormalities and delayed maturation of the nervous system; and compromised immune function. Dilated cardiomyopathy in cats (see Chapter 11) has now been linked with low plasma levels of taurine which have been shown to result in low myocardial taurine concentrations. However, other contributory factors may be involved and recent studies have suggested that one of these may be concurrent potassium depletion. Dietary correction, in combination with taurine supplementation, can halt the progression of FCRD but cannot reverse the existing retinopathy. Cases of dilated cardiomyopathy which are due to taurine deficiency will respond within 10 days of initiating taurine supplementation and, provided they survive the first critical week, an almost complete recovery can be achieved within 4 months.

Previously, clinical cases of taurine deficiency were reported in cats which were fed on cereal-based commercial dog foods with an inadequate taurine content. However, dilated cardiomyopathy associated with low plasma taurine was diagnosed in cats that had been fed commercial cat foods containing levels at the minimum recommended by the NRC. This led to the recognition that processing somehow affected the bioavailability of taurine and this was more marked in canned than in dry diets. The current recommendations are that commercial dry diets for cats should contain at least 1000 mg taurine per kg diet and that canned diets should contain at least 2500 mg per kg diet on a dry matter basis.[5]

Nutritional secondary hyperparathyroidism

Nutritional secondary hyperparathyroidism is the result of feeding a diet which is deficient in calcium. This gives rise to a subtle hypocalcaemia and stimulates the production of parathyroid hormone which acts with vitamin D to restore circulating levels of calcium. This is achieved by increased intestinal calcium and phosphorus absorption; increased resorption and decreased formation of bone; and decreased calcium with increased phosphorus excretion by the kidneys. Calcium deficiency in the diet may be absolute or relative, where there is an excess of phosphorus in relation to calcium. The calcium:phosphorus ratio should be of the order of 1:1.

Growing kittens are most sensitive to mineral imbalances and, classically, the condition is produced by feeding an all- or predominantly-meat diet. Muscle and organ meats are notoriously deficient in calcium and organ meats contain relatively high levels of phosphorus. Clinical signs are associated with the abnormal mineralisation of bone and its replacement with fibrous tissue, and include lameness due to joint pain and deformities, bone deformities, generalised myopathy and occasionally pathological fractures of the long bones or vertebrae. A loss of bone density is detectable on radiographic examination (see Chapter 17). Constipation and abdominal distension may be observed in relation to the generalised myopathy but these signs may also be associated with pathological fractures of the pelvis, resulting in a narrowing of the pelvic canal.

Treatment is aimed at correction of the dietary imbalances and the provision of a nutritionally balanced diet for the cat's needs. In advanced cases, calcium supplementation may be required in the initial stages to provide a Ca:P ratio of 2:1, but this should revert to a normal ratio of 1:1 once an improvement is noted. Affected cats should be confined to prevent the occurrence of pathological fractures and, if necessary, non-steroidal analgesics may be used although pain is rapidly alleviated following dietary correction. The prognosis in most cases is good but an affected kitten may be left with skeletal deformities and a retarded growth rate; prevention of the condition is therefore preferable to cure.

Obesity

In general, cats will restrict their food intake to their energy requirement but a significant proportion of the cat population (6–12% in the UK; a suggested 40–50% in the USA) can be considered overweight. Although cats may not suffer the complications of obesity to the same extent as dogs and humans, links have been made between obesity and the occurrence of feline lower urinary tract disease, diabetes mellitus and hepatic lipidosis. Furthermore, the condition may reduce the cat's quality of life and presents difficulties in grooming which can result in skin problems.

Two stages are apparent in the development of obesity: an initial 'dynamic' phase in which the cat's energy intake exceeds its requirements, resulting in the deposition of fat; and a subsequent 'static' phase in which body-weight remains fairly stable and appetite is controlled by various biofeedback mechanisms. During the static phase, owners may be confused as food intake may be normal or even reduced, although the cat remains fat.

In cats, fat deposition commonly occurs in an area just anterior to the inguinal region to form an 'apron'. There is usually a large accumulation in the abdominal cavity, but this must be distinguished from other causes of abdominal enlargement such as ascites, pregnancy or abdominal organ enlargement.

Weight loss can be achieved by a programme of controlled calorie reduction and a target weight should be set initially which should either be the ideal weight or, if the cat is more than 15% overweight, should represent a 15% loss in weight. Using a diet which provides 60% of the calculated daily maintenance energy requirements for the cat's target weight, a weight loss of approximately 15% can realistically be achieved in 18 weeks.[17]

An obese cat requires approximately 60kcal/kg/day.[4] In some cases, it is sufficient to feed less of the normal diet, but this may lead to a relative deficiency of other nutrients and to increased demands for food owing to the reduced volume being fed. Commercially prepared low calorie diets address these issues and provide a convenient and effective means of achieving weight loss in cats. Owners should be encouraged in their efforts, and cats on a weight loss programme should be weighed and re-assessed every two weeks. Client education is important in preventing future recurrence of the condition.

Essential fatty acid deficiency

The cat has only a limited ability to convert linoleic acid to the more complex 'derived' essential fatty acids such as arachidonic acid. As arachidonic acid is almost entirely absent from plant tissues, the cat must be provided with a source of animal fat in the diet. Clinical manifestations of essential fatty acid deficiency in cats are slow to appear but may be evident as listlessness and a dry, scaly, staring coat which is greasy to the touch. Slow wound healing, retarded growth, increased susceptibility to infection and fatty infiltration of the liver have also been reported. There may be reproductive failure as males may develop flaccid testes and queens fail to come into oestrus. The condition responds well to supplementation and correction of the diet.

Calcium oxalate urolithiasis

The development of calcium oxalate urolithiasis in cats may be the paradoxical result of dietary correction for another urinary problem, struvite urolithiasis. Hypercalciuria may be induced by the urinary acidifying effect and reduced magnesium content (magnesium inhibits calcium oxalate crystal formation) of the modified diets which reduce struvite formation.

DIET-RESPONSIVE CONDITIONS

It is important to distinguish between these and diet-induced conditions in order to eliminate confusion among owners who may interpret the introduction of therapeutic dietary modifications as evidence that the illness was caused by diet.

Chronic renal failure

Many signs associated with chronic renal failure are related to azotaemia, which develops as the kidneys become progressively less efficient in their excretion of the products of protein metabolism. Dietary management of the condition is usually aimed at limiting protein catabolism by restricting dietary protein to the animal's requirement and providing alternative sources of energy (see Chapter 14). In the cat, dietary protein and phosphorus restriction may delay the progression of existing renal disease. Protein restriction also helps to reduce the intake of phosphate and hence the risk of developing hyperphosphataemia, which would contribute to the production of renal secondary hyperparathyroidism.

However, cats have a relatively high dietary requirement for protein (adults need 25 g/400 kcal diet) and they are unable to adapt to very low levels of protein intake. Excessive protein restriction would therefore result in a negative nitrogen balance and lead to weight loss, muscle wasting, hypoalbuminaemia and immunosuppression. Furthermore, low protein diets are not palatable to cats and this problem is exacerbated when the cat is already inappetent, as in cases of chronic renal failure.

Energy needs of affected cats are assumed to be similar to normal maintenance requirements (60–80 kcal/kg/day) and it is recommended that dietary protein should provide 20–30% of the calorie intake for cats with chronic renal failure. This is equivalent to 3.3–3.5 g of high quality protein per kg BW/day. Fat is a useful non-protein source of energy and corn oil or strips of bacon fat may be added to the basal diet and will also help to augment its palatability. Water-soluble vitamins may be lost in polyuric cats and the diet should be supplemented with these at about twice the normal amounts required for maintenance.

Feline Lower Urinary Tract Disease

Feline Lower Urinary Tract Disease, FLUTD (previously known as FUS), is a complex condition with a multiple aetiology (see Chapter 14). Although early studies implicated diet as a cause of the condition, it is now thought more appropriate to view diet as merely one of a number of different contributory factors, which may include viruses or bacteria as well as individual susceptibility to the condition. However, manipulation of dietary factors have been shown to be important in the management of FLUTD, particularly where struvite urolithiasis is involved. The most important factor in the development of struvite urolithiasis appears to be the acidity of the urine, and crystallisation out of solution is more likely to occur when the urinary pH is higher than 6.5. Precipitation of struvite crystals is also more likely when there is a low volume of concentrated urine. The crystals are composed of magnesium ammonium phosphate, and very high levels of magnesium (higher than those in commercial cat foods) can also promote struvite urolithiasis. However, this is probably dependent on the form in which it is given, as this can also affect urinary pH.

Cats which are fed dry diets tend to have a lower water intake than those on canned or semi-moist foods. Furthermore, high fibre diets of low digestibility produce bulkier faeces with a resultant increase in water loss via this route. Dietary management of cases of FLUTD will help to prevent recurrence. Moist foods should be provided and extra water may be added to make them even wetter; drinking water should be freely available; excessive dietary magnesium should be avoided; oral urinary acidifiers may be administered and if these are given at the time of feeding, the effects of the post prandial 'alkaline tide' will be minimised. Urinary acidifiers should be used with care to avoid the development of acidosis; overacidification can result in depressed growth, increased urinary excretion of calcium and potassium, hypokalaemia and possibly bone demineralisation. They should not be given in conjunction with an already acidified diet, or one formulated to produce an acidic urine.

Hypokalaemic polymyopathy

Low plasma potassium levels may be a complication of a number of chronic disease conditions including chronic renal and hepatic failure, systemic infections, thyrotoxicosis, hyperaldosteronism and neuromuscular or CNS disease. Recently, the use of diets containing urinary acidifiers with a marginal potassium content has also been associated with hypokalaemia (see Chapter 17).

A myopathy attributed to hypokalaemia has now been described which mimics the signs of thiamin deficiency in some respects. Affected cats show a generalised weakness and muscle pain with a persistent ventroflexion of the neck. Renal disease may be present, often as a predisposing factor, but it appears that hypokalaemia can exacerbate an existing nephropathy and potassium supplementation in such cases can improve renal function. Muscle strength is improved within days of potassium supplementation. For treatment regimes, see Chapter 17.

Food intolerance and food allergy

Adverse reactions to a particular food (dietary sensitivity) can be classified as either food intolerance, where inappropriate metabolic or biochemical interactions occur between the body and the food, or food allergy (hypersensitivity) in which the reaction is immunologically mediated. A classic example of food intolerance in the cat is that of lactose intolerance. Lactase activity is progressively reduced post-weaning and in some cats the ability to digest lactose is lost completely. Even if able to digest some lactose in milk, most cats are unable to cope when presented with an excessive substrate load or when enzyme levels are reduced due to inflammatory changes in the intestine. Undigested lactose in the intestines exerts an osmotic effect and also allows the pro-liferation of lactose-fermenting bacteria which produces a local inflammatory response. The combined effect is to generate a profuse, watery diarrhoea. Cases of lactose intolerance resolve spontaneously within 2–3 days of eliminating all forms of milk from the diet and this strategy is likely to prove beneficial in the treatment of all cases of enteritis and other forms of diarrhoea. Another area of food intolerance is reaction to drug-like substances, such as histamine, in certain foods, but their effects in cats have not been assessed.

Food allergies generally manifest as intensely pruritic skin lesions (see Chapter 22), particularly around the face and neck, or as gastro-intestinal disturbances but diagnosis may be complicated by the presence of other factors which contribute to the overall clinical picture. Many basic food ingredients are potential allergens in cats and proteins in cow's milk, beef and fish have been implicated in over half the reported cases.[16]

Elimination diets can be formulated by studying the cat's dietary history, which may reveal some foods that the cat has never eaten and from which a 'hypoallergenic' diet can be formulated. If this is not possible, a restriction diet may be prepared which contains only one or two sources of protein, preferably ones which have not been consumed within the preceding month. Chicken has proved to be particularly useful in cats, although lamb and rabbit are also suitable but any diet must be complete and balanced in all the essential nutrients. A diet of 100 g chicken with 100 g rice per day is adequate for the average adult cat.

Feeding an elimination or restriction diet should result in a dramatic improvement in clinical signs and should be continued for at least 21 days. All other sources of allergen must be avoided during this time and so the cat should be confined indoors. Diagnosis may be confirmed by reintroducing the original diet, and looking for a recurrence of clinical signs.

Diabetes mellitus

Cases of diabetes mellitus in the cat generally respond well to insulin therapy in conjunction with careful dietary regulation (see Chapter 16). By providing a consistent and regular calorie intake and controlling the cat's energy output, the dosage of insulin can be adjusted easily to the animal's requirement for the control of hyperglycaemia. Carbohydrate levels need not be restricted, as long as they are kept constant, but simple sugars (as are often used as humectants in semi-moist foods) may provoke hyperglycaemic peaks in diabetics and are best avoided.

Both type I (insulin-dependent) and type II (non-insulin-dependent) diabetes mellitus occur in cats and there is evidence that obesity predisposes a cat to type II diabetes, in which there is an insensitivity of the peripheral tissues to the effects of insulin. Obese diabetic cats may therefore benefit from a diet which is formulated to produce a degree of weight loss, at least in the initial stages.

Furthermore, the use of high fibre diets in the control of obesity in cats with type II diabetes mellitus may result in the discontinuation of insulin in some cases. Fibre, particularly soluble fibre, has been shown to be beneficial in the control of post-prandial hyperglycaemia in both types of diabetes mellitus, although the mechanism responsible for this effect is still unclear. Extrapolation from studies in other species suggests that a fibre content of 16% of dry matter is required but this may present a palatability problem in cats. High fibre diets should not be used for thin cats until a normal weight has been achieved. If the fibre content of a diet is increased by the addition of, for example, vegetables or grains, care must be taken to ensure that the levels of other essential nutrients remain within the acceptable range for the cat.

Idiopathic feline hepatic lipidosis

Hepatic lipidosis is a problem which typically (though not always) affects obese, mature cats which have undergone a preceding period of stress such as boarding, moving house, surgery or transient illness (see Chapter 13). The stressful event induces a period of anorexia which promotes lipolysis and the mobilisation of free fatty acids from peripheral fat depots to the liver. Hepatocytes metabolise fatty acids to provide energy, but excessive rates of mobilisation result in triglyceride accumulation and lipidosis in the liver. The condition may also be inadvertently induced by deliberate starvation designed to promote weight loss in obese cats.

Clinically affected cats become anorectic and weak with progressive weight loss and muscle wastage. Jaundice may be observed in the latter stages, and laboratory analysis generally reveals raised serum levels of ammonia, liver-specific enzymes, bilirubin and triglycerides. Spontaneous recovery is unlikely and about 50% of treated cases may still die despite intensive therapeutic measures.

Therapy is aimed at providing profound nutritional support. In the earlier stages, attempts to stimulate the appetite may prove worthwhile. Forced feeding is almost always required and in severe cases the use of naso-gastric, pharyngostomy or gastrostomy tubes may be necessary. High quality meat-based foods may be used but should be homogenised to allow passage through the feeding tube. Commercial cat foods and meat-based baby foods are suitable although the latter may require supplementation to meet the cat's special requirements for taurine, essential fatty acids and B-vitamins. Cats which survive may take 6–8 weeks before starting to eat voluntarily, but the response to therapy is probably dependent on the initial severity of the condition.

FEEDING INAPPETENT CATS

Cats are notoriously fastidious feeders even when healthy and this problem is exacerbated when the cat is inappetent through illness. Consideration of their known preferences and natural feeding habits can provide clues for ways in which dietary manipulation may tempt a sick cat to eat. The following strategies may be attempted:

- Ensure that food is palatable and fresh with a strong odour.
- Remove uneaten food after 10–15 minutes.
- Warm the food to around 35°C but not over 40°C.
- Offer frequent, small meals which repeatedly expose the cat's senses to fresh stimuli.
- Feed wet foods, which tend to be more palatable than dry foods.
- Introduce a new or veterinary diet gradually until it becomes familiar to the cat.
- Appetite may be improved if the utensils, attendant, diet and feeding time are all familiar.
- Some cats respond to being fed by hand.
- Unless contra-indicated, group feeding may encourage an inappetent cat by providing competition for food.

If the cat refuses to eat despite these measures, syringe or tube feeding may become necessary. In any event, it is preferable to offer foods which are nutrient dense, low in bulk and of high digestibility to obtain maximum benefit from the small amount of food that may be accepted.

REFERENCES

1. Beliveau G.P., Morris J.G., Rogers Q.R., Freedland R.A. (1981) Metabolism of serine, threonine and glycine in isolated cat hepatocytes. *Fed. Proc.* **40**: 807, abstract number 3504.
2. Boudreau J.C., White T.D. (1978) Flavour chemistry of carnivore taste systems. ASC Symposium No. 67 *Flavour Chemistry of Animal Foods.* pp 102–128.
3. Deady J.E., Anderson B., O'Donnell J.A., Morris J.G., Rogers Q.R. (1981) Effects of level of dietary glutamic acid and thiamin on food intake, weight gain, plasma amino-acids and thiamin status of growing kittens. *J. Nutr.*, **111**: 1568.
4. Earle K.E., Smith P.M. (1991a) Digestible energy requirements of adult cats at maintenance. *J. Nutr.*, **121**, 545.
5. Earle K.E., Smith P.M. (1991b) The effect of dietary taurine content on the plasma taurine concentration of the cat. *Brit. J. Nutr.*, **66**: 227–235.
6. Everett G.M. (1944) Observations on the behaviour and neurophysiology of acute thiamin deficient cats. *Am. J. Physiol.*, **141**: 439.
7. Gershoff S.N., Andrus S.B., Hegsted D.M., Lentini E.A. (1957) Vitamin A deficiency in cats. *Laboratory Investigation*, **6**: 227–240.
8. Hassam A.G., Rivers J.P.W., Crawford M.A. (1977) The failure of the cat to desaturate linoleic acid: Its nutritional implications. *Nutrient Metabolism*, **21**: 321–328.
9. Kendall P.T., Holme D.W., Smith P.M. (1982) Comparative evaluation of net digestive and absorption efficiency in dogs and cats fed a variety of contrasting diet types. *J.S.A.P.*, **23**: 577–587.
10. MacDonald M.L., Anderson B.C., Rogers Q.R., Buffington C.A., Morris J.G. (1984) Essential fatty acid requirements of cats: Pathology of essential fatty acid deficiency. *Am. J. Vet. Res.* **45**: 1310–1317.
11. Mugford R.A., Thorne C.J. (1980) Comparative studies of meal patterns in pet and laboratory housed dogs and cats. In: Anderson R.S. (ed.) *Nutrition of the Dog and Cat*, Pergamon Press, Oxford.
12. Rivers J.P.W., Sinclair A.J., Crawford M.A. (1975) Inability of the cat to de-saturate essential fatty acids. *Nature*, **258**: 171–173.
13. Rogers Q.R., Morris J.G., Freedland R.F. (1977) Lack of hepatic enzyme adaptation to low and high levels of dietary protein in the adult cat. *Enzyme*, **22**: 348–356.
14. Seawright A.A., English P.B. (1967) Hypervitaminosis A and deforming cervical spondylosis of the cat. *J. Comp.Path.* **77**: 29–39.
15. White T.D., Boudreau J.C. (1975) Taste preference of the cat for neurophysiologically active compounds. *Physiol. Psychol.*, **3**: 405–410.
16. Wills J.M. (1991) Dietary hypersensitivity in cats. *In Practice*, **13**: 87–91.
17. Wills J.M., Butterwick R., Sloth C.J., Gettinby G. (1993) A study of obese cats on a calorie-controlled weight reduction programme. Veterinary Record (submitted for publication).

FURTHER READING

Armstrong P.J., Hand M.S. (1989) Nutritional Disorders. In: Sherding R.G. (ed.) *The Cat – Diseases and Clinical Management*, Ch 7, pp 141–161, Churchill Livingstone.

Baines F.M. (1981) Milk substitutes and the hand rearing of orphaned puppies and kittens. *J.S.A.P.*, **22**: 555–578.

Buffington C.A. (1991) Nutrition and Nutritional Disorders. In Pedersen N.C. (ed.) *Feline Husbandry – Diseases and Management in the multiple-cat environment*, Ch 6, pp 325–356, American Veterinary Publications Inc.

Earle K.E. (1990) Feeding for Health. *J.S.A.P.*, **31**: 477–481.

Edney A.T.B. (1985) Feline Nutrition and Disease. In: Chandler E.A., Gaskell C.J., Hilbery A.D.R. (eds) *Feline Medicine and Therapeutics* pp 339–351. Blackwell Scientific Publications.

Markwell P.J. (1988) Clinical Small Animal Nutrition. In: Edney A.T.B. (ed.) *The Waltham Book of Dog and Cat Nutrition*, pp 97–115. Pergamon Press.

O'Donnell J.A., Hayes K.C. (1987) Nutrition and Nutritional Disorders. In: Holzworth J. (ed.) *Diseases of the Cat*, Ch. 2, pp 15–42. W.B. Saunders Company.

4

Feeding the Hospitalised Cat

SUSAN DONOGHUE and DAVID S. KRONFELD

The care of hospitalised cats requires knowledge of their husbandry and physiology, including (and perhaps most importantly) feeding management and nutrition. Good feeding management, which is the mainstay of the responsible care of hospitalised cats, involves more than simply sound nutritional science. By providing appropriate diets, it meets the cat's fluid, nutritional and energy requirements for specific purposes, but in addition it takes full account of the animal's instincts and emotions and delivers the diet with as little stress to the patient as possible. Even healthy feline boarders are stressed by strange surroundings.

Some hospitalised cats have diseases that adversely affect their metabolism and nutritional requirements; others are recovering from surgery or are suffering from trauma-induced wounds and fractures. Their environment should provide comfort by means of optimal temperature and humidity, shelter and security. The task of those responsible for feeding hospitalised cats is to accomplish the work quickly and efficiently, whilst identifying the problem case suffering from anorexia or digestive upset. An understanding of nutrient requirements, energy needs, the kinds of foods available for patients, and each food's advantages and less desirable characteristics, will help in formulating a feeding plan.

ANOREXIA

Anorexia of cats that are sick or injured is a major frustration for veterinary health care providers. In the past these patients, perhaps with a long convalescence or with a chronic debilitating disease, literally starved to death. The most intricate surgical procedure or advanced chemotherapeutics are of little benefit if the patient is not receiving the fuels and nutrients that permit its body to heal. Injected appetite stimulants are of short-term advantage only, having minimal influence on the patient's nitrogen balance. The challenge of feline anorexia has been met by nutrition support, through the provision of nutrients and energy by enteral and parenteral routes. To succeed, however, hospital nutrition must be integrated into sound patient management.

GENERAL PLAN

Hospital nutrition tends to become dominated by the nutritional support of selected patients. Cases which need tube feeding or intravenous glucose attract everyone's attention. However, one should never overlook the general feeding programme in the wards, where it may be regarded as a treatment adjunct.

Our examination of the ward feeding programme for a large veterinary teaching hospital revealed several areas of hospital nutrition that required special attention. These included gathering the patient's feeding history, the inclusion of appropriate information in the medical record, assessment of the patient's body condition, and discrimination between available ward diets.

Diet history

It is important to learn about the cat's usual and recent diets, which may differ. Knowing the patient's feeding history provides useful information about food preferences (which influence intake), usual appetite and body condition. Although it might be decided not to feed the same or even a similar type of pet food, owners should be asked about brands and varieties fed at home, free choice foods and meals, snacks, treats and table foods, and hunting activity. They should also be asked who is responsible for the purchase of cat foods and the actual feeding, for household members may have different perceptions about feeding management.

Body condition

The medical record of each hospitalised cat should include body weight and body condition as well as feeding history. About 25% of the 4,000 case records we examined lacked information on body condition. Although body weights of cats do not show the range of weights for dogs, there is still a significant distribution and it is important to note body condition as well as weight. For example, a 2.5 kg cat may be a young Siamese in good condition or an emaciated Norwegian Forest tom. Cats can lose or gain body condition with less than a kilogram lost or added and, while clinic scales are not always accurate enough to note significant changes in body weight, physical examination usually picks up changes in condition.

We use a simple 5-point body condition scoring system:

Score	Condition
1	Cachetic; no obvious body fat.
2	Thin; limited body fat evident.
3	Optimal; ribs palpated easily but not observed readily.
4	Overweight; ribs difficult to palpate.
5	Obese; large amounts of subcutaneous fat, obvious incapacity.

A system of diagrams to select body condition is currently under development in a study with veterinary practitioners. The system – quick, efficient, and able to be utilised by cat owners and lay staff – simply requires selection of the silhouette most closely resembling the patient (see Fig. 4.1).

The implications of a cat losing 20% of its body weight seem obvious, but the small size of cats tends to mask the clinical significance of small absolute weight changes. A decrease on the clinic scales from 4.5 kg to 3.5 kg indicates a significant loss of tissue protein and usually fluids, as well as fat. An acute loss of 10% body weight signals the need for nutrition support in humans, but a 10% loss in a cat (say, from 4.5 kg to 4.1 kg) may be missed entirely. Failure to observe weight loss contributes to the overall difficulties in maintaining appetite and body condition of sick cats.

Surroundings

Most hospitalised cats are sick or injured, and virtually all are unsettled by the unfamiliar surroundings. Only the blood donors seem truly contented in a clinic atmosphere. Some healthy cats enjoy company but many, sick or otherwise, prefer solitude. We often provide a sick cat with a cardboard box in which to hide at its own option. The box is placed in the cage with its open side facing the back wall. The presence of a hide box, however, reinforces the need for astute observation by nursing staff to ensure that a patient with a deteriorating condition is identified readily.

The wards should be well-ventilated and clean, and cleaning should be completed before feeding. More controversial are noise levels (e.g. background radio) and temperature ranges in wards. Ward conditions should be examined if food intake is a problem.

Critically ill animals need a warm environment. A general guide is that if the ambient temperature is comfortable for the humans working in a ward or intensive care unit, then the environment is probably too cold for the animals. The issue is complex, however, because there is likely to be a mix of house pets and outside animals and short- and long-haired dogs and cats. There may also be patients with fevers and those which are chilled. Ambient temperature affects energy needs: cats in cool or very hot environments need more energy.

Once the history is taken, body condition assessed, and comfortable surroundings assured, attention is turned to water, nutrients, and energy sources. Of these three, water is most critical.

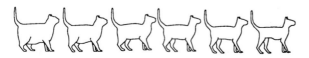

FIG. 4.1   Identifying body condition.

WATER BALANCE AND FLUID THERAPY

Water provides no energy but is the most crucial nutrient. Cats appear to tolerate mild dehydration better than dogs and maintain superior urine concentrating abilities, but we would prefer to test this desert heritage in healthy rather than sick cats.

Water output

Water is lost continually in urine, faeces, expired air, milk, saliva, and via the skin. Sick cats may lose large volumes of fluid from vomiting and diarrhoea. Water may also be lost in blood or exudates, or sequestered in haematomata or as oedema.

Water intake

Cats take in water as 'free water' from liquids and solid foods and also as 'oxidation water' from the metabolism of fuel sources.[14] The water yield after oxidation of each fuel is as follows:[3]

    100 g protein yields 40 g water.
    100 g fat yields 107 g water.
    100 g carbohydrate yields 55 g water.

When expressed as a ratio to dry matter intake, water intake averages almost 2:1 for dry foods (which contain 10% water) and about 3.5:1 for canned food (about 75% water). Thus, more water is available from canned foods than from dry foods. On average, cats fed dry foods drink water as frequently as they eat meals, i.e. about 16 times daily.[14]

For cats, maintenance intake approximates 60 ml/kg, and a 4.0 kg healthy cat at maintenance needs about 240 ml water daily, as well as 7.5 mEq sodium, 6.6 mEq potassium, and 5.4 mEq chloride.[5] Losses from respiration and faeces approximate 20 ml/kg daily in cool environments, and increase with warmer ambient and body temperatures. Losses from urination approximate 20–40 ml/kg daily.

While experimental data on the water balance of average healthy cats are useful in understanding a sick cat, we focus on the individual patient, and extremes may appear to be the rule. Some cats seemingly never drink in health; they receive adequate water from canned foods and fresh prey. Some cats drink only fresh water, others prefer water that has 'settled' for a few hours. A few cats are sensitive to changes in water taste and odour, and in veterinary hospitals they will reject water that is chlorinated or served in plastic containers.

Fluid deficits

Before feeding the hospitalised cat, and especially in critically ill individuals, attention is given to the correction of fluid deficits. For many patients, fluid needs are met by voluntary intake of water, coupled with water intake via moist foods. Water should be offered continually in clean, stainless steel bowls and should be replaced at least once a day.

Hospitalised cats often suffer from disorders that lead to dehydration. Water loss is clinically evident when greater than 5%. Signs become more obvious as dehydration worsens and include loss of skin elasticity, shrunken eyes and dry mucous membranes. Dehydration over 12% leads to shock and risks death. Laboratory values include elevated packed cell volume and total solids. Electrolyte and acid-base abnormalities are common but variable, depending on the patient's disease, history, metabolic state and prior treatment.

Fluid therapy is usually provided by subcutaneous and intravenous routes. Intraosseous routes may be employed and intraperitoneal injections are often more convenient in small kittens.

Subcutaneous routes are reserved for mild dehydration and for at-home fluid therapy. Fluids are given two or three times a day; complications are rare. Subcutaneous fluids are unsatisfactory in cats with moderate to severe dehydration, vasoconstriction, extreme fluid shifts or skin trauma. Examples include cats in shock and those with hypothermia, severe burns and generalised pyoderma.[5] Fluids can be administered by gravity flow using an administration set and an 18- or 20-gauge needle, or by injection using a syringe and needle. Multiple sites with the application of 50 to 100 ml per site are recommended, as is massage of the fluid pocket following injection of larger volumes.[5]

Intravenous fluid therapy can be provided via catheterisation of jugular and cephalic veins, and, less commonly, femoral and lateral saphenous veins. Advantages and drawbacks of each site, equipment and placement techniques have been detailed.[2,5] In general, strict aseptic techniques are employed to place indwelling catheters for administration of fluids and electrolytes via administration sets at drip volumes approximating 60 drops/ml.[5] Complications include infection (local or generalised), phlebitis and thrombosis, and from mismanagement, fluid overload and electrolyte abnormalities.

Fluid volumes are calculated and adjusted every 12 to 24 hours. The estimated per cent dehydration multiplied by the cat's weight in kilograms provides the fluid replacement volume in litres. Haematocrit, plasma total protein, urine specific gravity and serum electrolytes are usually monitored. Measuring body weight will be useful only if scales are sensitive to 0.1 kg changes.

Multiple electrolyte fluids are formulated for replacement and maintenance. Generally, replacement fluids contain more sodium and less potassium than maintenance fluids.[2] Reviews providing detailed information on formulas should be consulted when selecting appropriate fluids for feline patients.[2,5]

Fluid therapy in nutrition support

Enterals and canned products contain over 75% water. Once nutritional needs are met, additional water may be given to maintain adequate hydration if needed. In most cases, water from the diets and from voluntary intake maintain hydration but occasionally these sources must be supplemented with intravenous maintenance fluids to meet the cat's full needs. A guideline is to provide 1 ml water/kcal. Though water is important, its routine use to dilute slurries is not recommended, for it defeats specific goals for calories and nutrients in most cases and fails to meet hydration needs during critical illness.

NUTRIENT REQUIREMENTS

The nutrient requirements of cats, which are unique among our domestic animals but characteristic of strict carnivores, resemble the nutrient contents of small mammals, their usual prey – high protein levels and high nutrient bioavailabilities. Feline biochemistry, however, can play a secondary role when nutrition support is provided to sick cats. When relying on voluntary food intake, feline behaviour influences the achievement of nutritional goals and affects food prefer-ences and meal patterns. Accordingly, feeding management of hospitalised cats concerns both biochemistry and behaviour.

Cats relish foods with high levels of animal-based protein and fat. Throughout the life cycle, they thrive on 30–40% protein (ME basis) of the quality found in most commercial foods. Minimum requirements are lower than this range but still higher than in dogs. Cats are unable to down-regulate hepatic metabolism of amino-acids and have specific requirements for arginine, taurine, retinol, niacin and arachidonic acid.[3,14]

ENERGY

The patient's energy requirement is usually the first hurdle for the clinician who aspires to provide adequate nutrition support. As an alternative to calculations, we can use a table (see Fig. 4.2). It saves time but to use it properly, one needs to understand the calculations.

Energy requirements

Energy expenditure is measured in terms of respired gases (indirect calorimetry) in many human hospitals. Patients are categorised as hypo-, normo-, or hypermetabolic. These terms relate to energy metabolism and estimate whether a patient is burning calories below, equal to, or above the number of calories expended when healthy. Measurement of energy expenditure is not yet available in animal hospitals, however, so estimates must be made by analogy with human conditions and from the animal's history and clinical condition.

An abandoned cat, for example, which has suffered from several weeks of inadequate food intake is likely to be hypometabolic and may exhibit low heart and respiratory rates and low body temperature. A cat with clinical hyperthyroidism is usually hypermetabolic and may exhibit elevated heart and respiratory rates. Categorisation of energy status is an indispensible step in feeding hospitalised cats.

The number of calories needed by a sick cat is estimated in two steps. First, the average metabolisable energy (ME) requirement for maintenance (M), is calculated from body weight.[14]

ENERGY NEEDS OF HYPOMETABOLIC, NORMOMETABOLIC AND HYPERMETABOLIC CATS[a]							
Body Weight		Percentage of maintenance (kcal ME/day)					
lb	kg	50	80	100	110	125	150
2	0.9	32	51	**64**	70	80	96
3	1.4	48	76	**95**	104	119	142
4	1.8	64	102	**127**	140	159	190
5	2.3	80	127	**159**	175	199	239
6	2.7	96	153	**191**	210	239	286
7	3.2	112	178	**223**	245	279	334
8	3.6	127	204	**254**	280	318	382
9	4.1	143	229	**286**	315	358	429
10	4.5	159	254	**318**	350	394	477
11	5.0	175	280	**350**	385	438	525
12	5.4	191	306	**382**	420	479	573
13	5.9	207	331	**414**	455	518	621
14	6.4	222	356	**445**	490	556	668

[a] $M = 70(BW_{kg})$ where M=maintenance energy requirement of metabolizable energy, kcal/day, and BW=body weight in kg. This is an average for healthy cats; one cat in seven needs 20% more, and another cat from the same seven needs 20% less.

FIG. 4.2 Average daily energy required by hypometabolic, normometabolic and hypermetabolic cats. Calories were calculated as percentages of maintenance (M) energy. Clinical conditions appropriate for each feeding level are described in the text. Maintenance energy intakes are shown in bold type in the 100 column.

Second, the individual goal is adjusted downward or upward according to the degree of hypo- or hyper-metabolism (estimated during nutritional assessment).

The average requirement varies from $M = 60(BW_{kg})$ for inactive cats housed in metabolic cages, to $M = 80(BW_{kg})$ for active cats spending much time outdoors, where M = ME for maintenance (kcal/day) and BW = body weight in kg.[14] In our Nutrition Support Service, we use the first equation for all critically ill cats and the common formula $M = 70 (BW_{kg})$ for most hospitalised cats.[14] This is 1.4 times the mean interspecies basal metabolic rate.

Hypo- and hypermetabolism

For the sick individual, a second step is necessary for estimating daily energy requirements. The average maintenance ME requirement calculated above is modified downward or upward, depending on the degree of estimated hypo- or hypermetabolism, respectively. The hypometabolic cat may receive from about 40% to 90% of M, the normometabolic cat from 85% to 115% of M, and the hypermetabolic cat from 90% to perhaps as high as 200% of M. Wide ranges are provided because actual recommendations will depend on clinical evaluation of patient responses to the food and to the total amount of calories. Calories for hypo- and hypermetabolic cats are given in Fig. 4.2.

Protein balance and fuel sources

Illness and injury affect the patient's needs for total calories, and for one particular source of calories – protein. The patient needs amino-acids, from dietary protein or from tissue protein, for anabolic processes such as antibody production and wound healing, and for conversion to glucose, which is an essential energy source for brain, erythrocytes, renal medulla and repairing tissues.

Cats may be categorised as catabolic, i.e. in negative nitrogen balance, but normo- or even hypometabolic. We have recognised such catabolic states in cats suffering from advanced malignancies. These cats are mobilising protein but not burning excessive calories overall. They can be supported nutritionally with high protein, energy- and nutrient-dense diets fed at levels below or approximating calorie requirements for maintenance.

Our concerns with feeding hospitalised cats are to meet their needs for protein and calories. Proprietary pet foods are examined for their protein and calorie contents to compare them with the patient's protein and calorie needs.

COMMERCIAL CAT FOODS FOR HOSPITALISATION

The selection of a particular type or brand of pet food is based in large part on the food's percentages of protein, fat and carbohydrate, for these provide the calories needed by animals. Protein and carbohydrate provide between 3 and 4 kcal/g of food; the exact number varies with the type of food. Fat provides between 8 and 9 kcal/g. Because fat is so calorie-dense and so variable in pet foods, the percentages of protein, fat and carbohydrate are often expressed on an energy (ME) basis instead of a dry matter (DM) basis. Unfortunately, the percentages of protein and fat found on pet food labels are neither ME nor DM; the basis is moist, also called 'as-fed'.

Labels

For hospital use, the first six ingredients on a pet food label should include at least three, preferably four or five, meat-based ingredients. Only one or two should be plant-based. Meat-based ingredients are generally more digestible than plant-based ingredients in pet foods. Foods of animal origin are digested efficiently by enzymes in the small intestine. In contrast, the galactosides in soybeans and the fibres in fillers undergo relatively inefficient fermentative digestion in the large intestine. The byproducts of fermentation are gases, short-chain fatty acids and lactic acid. The latter accumulates during rapid fermentation and attracts water; this process leads to bowel distension, loose stools and, if extreme, osmotic diarrhoea.

The percentages of protein, fat, and fibre on the label depend in part on the amount of water in the food. Within a type of pet food (dry or canned) look for the highest levels of protein and fat, and, in most instances, the lowest levels of fibre. Fibre may be beneficial in certain cases of large bowel disease. The role of fibre in management of diabetes mellitus in cats is far from clear. Many high fibre products are so low in calories that their use may possibly precipitate hepatic lipidosis in cats.

The guaranteed values on the label are not identical with average values. They are close to them in most dry foods but in canned products fat tends to vary in the ingredients, and it may exceed the guaranteed minimum by a sufficient amount to influence calculations.

Selection of appropriate proportions of fuel sources thus requires calculations with data provided on labels as well as an understanding of the metabolic changes likely to be occurring in the sick cat. Amounts and proportions of dietary protein, fat and carbohydrate are selected that will be used by the cat with maximal efficiency and minimal metabolic stress. These levels depend on the cat's physiological state – its degree of starvation and level of stress.

Cat foods for starvation

When fasting, mammals use first glycogen, then endogenous fat and protein for energy. Fatty acids are oxidised as the primary energy source. Branched chain amino-acids are oxidised in muscle, and other amino-acids are mobilised for gluconeogenesis. Uncomplicated fasting, like that observed in some weight reduction programmes, results in a loss of about 1 gram protein per 3 grams of fat in omnivorous species.[16] Mammals that are strictly carnivorous, like cats, already have high rates of protein utilisation for gluconeogenesis when in a fed state.[13] Fasting a carnivore, at least for a few days, causes minimal metabolic disturbance, compared with omnivores. Blood glucose levels remain constant and the high rates of gluconeogenesis continue.[10,13] However, starvation can induce hepatic lipidosis in cats (Chapter 13).

Thus, foods for cats with long-standing anorexia should contain relatively high levels of protein and fat, as well as all essential nutrients. Digestibility, nutrient bioavailability and palatability should be high.

Cat foods for stress

Hospitalised cats may be assumed to be stressed to some degree. Thus the routine hospital diet should have a stress profile, that is, contain certain nutrients (those affected by stress) at higher levels relative to energy. These nutrients include protein, ascorbic acid, vitamin A, vitamin E, zinc, copper, iron, perhaps carnitine and choline. We achieve best results by mixing different foods to fit different needs of individual patients.

When metabolically stressed from disease or surgery, animals mobilise amino-acids and fatty acids. Stress overrides the protein-sparing mechanisms that operate during fasting; much nitrogen is lost. Peripheral insulin resistance is an additional response to stress which is distinct from fasting. When the metabolically stressed patient is re-fed, protein catabolism, fat oxidation, gluconeogenesis and insulin resistance continue.

These general stress responses have not been confirmed in sick cats but may be inferred from clinical observations. The cat may exhibit loss of skeletal muscle mass, malfunction of organ systems (because protein is lost from organs), and hyperglycaemia (from insulin resistance). Thus, foods for stressed cats should contain minimal carbohydrate.

Fuel sources in cat foods

While both cats and dogs that are fasted or medically stressed use fat and protein for energy, the species differ in that cats require high protein and use relatively more of the same fuels (protein and fat) when healthy. Carbohydrates play a minor role in the energy metabolism of wild and feral cats eating small mammals, and of domestic cats eating high quality commercial canned cat foods. Similarly, carbohydrates play a small role in the energy metabolism of sick and post-operative cats, and the goals of dietary management reflect this principle.

Cats lack hepatic glucokinase, an enzyme with a high affinity for glucose which removes glucose from blood during alimentary hyperglycaemia in most mammals.[13] Cats apparently lost this adaptation to starchy meals during evolution. Large intakes of carbohydrate are alien to cats from the points of view of evolution, enzymes and preferences. They may be tolerated better by healthy cats than sick cats, but have little role in the feeding of hospitalised cats.

Guides to levels of protein, fat and carbohydrate for sick cats are provided in Fig. 4.3. Estimating the nutrient and calorie contents of ward diets for comparison with Figs 4.2 and 4.3 will be difficult if the only information comes from labels. Generally, one cupful (capacity 8 fluid ounces/227 ml) of dry premium food contains about 100 g or 400–450 kcal, and an equal volume of the lower calorie dry food contains about 250–350 kcal. A 13 oz (370 g) can of pet food contains about 400 kcal, while the 6 oz (170 g) can contains about 200 kcal. These are approximations. For more precise numbers, contact the manufacturers and request information on the calorie contents and average levels from proximate analyses for protein, fat and fibre, and data on digestibilities.

Contraindicated diets

Cat foods with substantial levels of carbohydrate, usually from plant ingredients, are unsuitable for hospitalised cats for reasons detailed above. Such foods provide the wrong proportions of fuel sources and tend to have lower digestibilities and palatability.

Cat foods containing propylene glycol are contraindicated. Propylene glycol fed to cats induced Heinz bodies in red blood cells, shortened erythrocyte life span, and induced anaemia.[6] The response is dose dependent and is present even at 6%.[1] The threshold is at or below the amounts of propylene glycol found in commercial semi-moist cat foods.

Feeding management

Healthy cats are commonly offered food once a day, but twice is better. They are often offered foods ad libitum, but food intake is difficult to ascertain. Hospitalised cats accommodate smaller meals better than larger ones and we usually recommend routine feeding of two main meals a day, at least 6 hours apart, at about the same times

FIG. 4.3 Tentative optimal ranges of fuel sources in diets for sick and postoperative cats, and the ranges found in selected commercial products. Values for cat food are presented on an 'as fed' basis, as they appear on labels. All other values are presented on a metabolisable energy basis.

FUEL SOURCES IN DIETS			
	Protein	**Fat**	**Carbohydrate**
Optimal Ranges Per cent kcalME			
Hypometabolic	30 – 48	35 – 55	5 – 20
Normometabolic	30 – 48	35 – 55	5 – 20
Hypermetabolic	40 – 50	40 – 55	5 – 20
Protein restricted	20 – 28	40 – 60	10 – 40
Fat restricted	40 – 50	5 – 20	10 – 40
Product Ranges Per cent as fed, Canned product[a,b]	8 – 13	4 – 7	–
Per cent as fed, Dry product[a,c]	27 – 33	9 – 20	–
Per cent kcal ME, Enteral products			
Low carbohydrate	>15	>39	<40
High carbohydrate	<20	<39	>40
Low fat	<20	<10	>70

[a] Assumptions include 4.5 kcal/g diet dry matter, 4 kcal/g protein, 9 kcal/g fat. Product estimates are intended to serve simply as guidelines for clinicians.
[b] 78% moisture
[c] 12% moisture

each day. Meal times are an opportunity for social interactions and for careful observation of the animal's demeanour and responses to the feeders as well as the food. The offering of two meals doubles this opportunity.

When a cat is first admitted to the veterinary hospital, abrupt changes in diet should be avoided if possible because they often aggravate inappetence in sick animals or lead to digestive upsets, such as anorexia and diarrhoea. If the cat's previous diet is unknown, or if the same type of food cannot be fed, then a mixture of dry and canned food is prudent, at least initially. For most cases, a diet change becomes necessary when protein and energy intake must be increased.

SPECIAL DIETS AND ROUTES OF ADMINISTRATION

Clinical experience assures us that cats are less likely than dogs to eat or drink voluntarily when sick or stressed. Of 260 cats provided with nutrition support, 32% (compared with 16% of dogs) were fed by involuntary methods.[9]

Liquid enterals

Of cats supported by involuntary feeding, 21% were fed blends of commercial canned products diluted with liquid enterals.[9] Enterals provide calories, protein, vitamins and minerals with partially hydrolysed and elemental ingredients. Because they pass easily through the smallest tubes, enterals became the diets of choice for feeding cats via nasogastric or jejunostomy tubes.

Protein modules, such as dehydrated cottage cheese and casein, are included in blends to meet protein goals. Most (but not all) enterals made for humans lack selenium, taurine and arachidonate, but these deficiencies are overcome if high quality commercial cat foods are included in blends for gastrostomy feeding. If fed alone, human enteral products provide sub-optimal but life-saving and usually adequate calories and nutrients. Human enteral products supplemented with dehydrated cottage cheese have been fed to sick hospitalised feline patients for as long as 64 days using nasogastric and jejunostomy tubes with no signs of nutrient deficiencies.[9]

Three types of enterals are recommended for use in cat clinics. In brief:

(i) **low carbohydrate enterals** (less than 40% of kcal ME) provide adequate protein and fat for most sick cats;

(ii) **high carbohydrate enterals** are useful when protein restriction is required;

(iii) **low fat enterals** are recommended for cats with severe hypometabolism or malabsorption, requiring fat restriction.

Enteral product labels

Human enteral products are freely available, and their labels provide valuable details on all nutrients, fuel sources and calories. Most data are presented on an energy basis and no calculations are required. Most have telephone numbers for queries and company personnel are willing to provide ready assistance.

Labels on most commercial pet foods contain only a guaranteed analysis of minimum protein and fat, and maximum fibre and water. Data are presented on an 'as fed', moist, or wet weight basis, so that calculations and assumptions must be made when using the food to provide nutrition support. Although the list of ingredients is of some help, there are no indications of digestibility or nutrient bioavailability.

Most commercial pet food ingredients consist of complex molecules. In contrast, enterals are made up of simpler molecules, such as partially hydrolysed and elemental ingredients. Digestibility and nutrient bioavailability are higher than for commercial pet foods. Thus recommended percentages of protein, for example, can be lower when feeding enterals than when feeding pet food. In this situation, 'protein' also refers to peptides and amino-acids.

In order to compare the suggested intakes of protein, fat and carbohydrate in Fig. 4.3 with those available in enteral products, one simply reads the label. To compare with commercial pet foods,

energy values must be calculated from the label, after assumptions have been made about digestibility.

Involuntary feeding

Feeding by force or by repeated daily orogastric or nasogastric intubations always causes discomfort, often increases patient stress markedly, and rarely meets the patient's need for calories. For these reasons, the two methods are rarely recommended. Feeding by indwelling tube is relatively safe and simple. Details and key references on tubes and placements have been reviewed.[8]

Indwelling nasogastric tubes

Indwelling nasogastric tubes can be placed without sedation and are tolerated well by most cats.[7] Compliant tubes allow animals to eat and drink, preserving attitude, appetite and enterocytes. Liquid enterals are the diets of choice. Slurries of commercial foods and water are less convenient, are not sterile, and tend to clog small-bore tubes unless filtered, the act of which removes calories and nutrients. Indwelling nasogastric tubes are recommended when involuntary feeding is to be used as an adjunct to voluntary intake for only a few days, and when a patient's condition is too critical to risk anaesthesia for placement of a gastrostomy tube.

Feeding via gastrostomy tube

Feeding via gastrostomy tube is another excellent method in cases that require involuntary nutrition support. The tubes are relatively easy to place, manage and remove.[4] They are wide-bore and hence able to accommodate most types of diets, including slurries. Owners can maintain their cat with a gastrostomy tube, administering medication as well as diets. The tubes are especially useful when a cat has head trauma, tumours or abscesses in the head or neck, or oesophageal disease.

Jejunostomy tube feeding

Jejunostomy tube feeding is restricted to those cats with serious disease involving the upper gastrointestinal tract. Examples include massive gastric resection and severe duodenal disease. Only liquid enteral diets are fed. As these contain partially hydrolysed ingredients, they are readily absorbed from the jejunum and ileum.

Diets for tube feeding

Diets for tube feeding demand selection as critical as that for voluntary intake. Concerns centre on ingredients, digestibility and bioavailability of nutrients. Factors that improve digestibility and bioavailability also favour palatability. The diet selected for a slurry is used also for voluntary intake when making feeding transitions during convalescence.

Commercial diets used for slurries are mostly meat-based, with relatively high protein and fat, limited carbohydrate, low fibre, no soy, and with high nutrient content. Nutritional goals for most cats require that diluents for slurries should be the liquid enteral products. Water should rarely be used as a diluent, for it usually dilutes the calories and nutrients below nutritional goals, though it may be added to enterals to lower osmolality for the first meals.

HOMEMADE DIETS

Some cats do not care to eat commercial pet foods, and some owners indulge these pets. At other times, a sick cat requires restriction of protein or fat, additions of fibre or special ingredients. We have developed a simple system for cooking for dogs and cats in the home or hospital.[11] It consists of a basal recipe and variations. The main ingredients in the basal recipe (Fig. 4.4) are

BASAL RECIPE		
Rice, dry	1/3 cupful	70g
Meat (20% fat)	2/3 cupful	140g
Liver	1/8 cupful	30g
Bone meal	3 teasp	11g
Corn oil	2 teasp	5g
Iodized salt	1/2 teasp	2g

FIG. 4.4   Basal recipe for a homemade diet for a 4.0 kg adult cat.

ground meat and rice supplemented with liver (for vitamins and trace minerals), bone meal (for calcium and phosphorus), corn oil (for essential fatty acids and vitamin E) and iodised salt (for iodine). Arachidonic acid and taurine are derived from meat.

All ingredients should be wholesome and fit for human consumption. The rice should be long- or medium-grain (not instant). The meat (lean beef, chicken, lean lamb or pork) should be ground, minced or cubed. Bone meal is found in many health food stores; tablets can be crushed.

To cook, simmer the rice in 2 cups of water for 15 minutes. Stir in ground meat, chopped liver and other items. Simmer for another 5–10 minutes until thoroughly cooked. Cool before serving. Refrigerate or freeze.

When limited amounts of a highly digestible carbohydrate source, such as rice, are added to meat and meat by-products, a degree of digestive adaptability is attained. Such blends tend to mitigate gastrointestinal upsets during abrupt dietary changes. Thus highly digestible diets, which combine rice with meat, poultry and their byproducts, are well suited to nearly all cats. Less rice can be used for cats that reject carbohydrates.

The basal recipe provides about 800 kcal, using medium fatty meat; it also supplies 31% protein on an ME basis, 1.3% calcium on a dry basis, 1.1% phosphorus, 0.45% sodium and 0.15% magnesium. It provides enough food for a healthy 4.0 kg cat for about 3 days.

Many recipe variations are possible, to suit the needs of most patients.

(i) **Low fat:** Use very lean meat, with 1 teasp sunflower or safflower oil. About 700 kcal.

(ii) **Low salt:** (a) Use 'Lite' salt, half potassium chloride, thus reducing sodium to 0.2%; or (b) leave out iodized salt, reducing sodium to 0.05%, but add a source of iodine such as kelp or dilute tincture of iodine.

(iii) **Elimination:** Start with unusual sources of carbohydrate and protein, such as tapioca and turkey, or sago and sole. Or use rice with lamb, venison, rabbit or horsemeat. Add iodized salt, multiple vitamin-mineral supplement manufactured for humans, safflower or sunflower oil, and dicalcium phosphate (2 teasp) to achieve a balanced diet.

(iv) **Anti-struvite:** Lower phosphorus and magnesium by replacing bone meal with calcium carbonate (2 teasp) or ground limestone ($\frac{1}{2}$ teasp), which reduces phosphorus to 0.3% and magnesium to 0.08%. Acidifying agents, such as ammonium chloride, ascorbic acid or methionine, could be added with care. The high meat content of the basal recipe should yield a naturally acidic urine, especially if offered in at least three meals daily instead of one large meal.

DIETARY SUPPLEMENTS FOR HOSPITALISED CATS

After the diet and feeding management are selected, are supplements beneficial? Most supplements contain vitamins and minerals. Practical guides for other essential nutrients are needed occasionally. We usually use values for essential nutrients (including those in commercial foods) that are 1.2–2.0 times the National Research Council's (NRC) minima, depending on the animal's condition and the nature of ingredients in the diet. Even higher values, up to 3 times NRC minima, may be used for stress and for diets with ingredients that reduce the bioavailabilities of nutrients. High quality pet foods often supply adequate or optimal levels of vitamins and minerals. Adding just one or two nutrients imbalances the diet and may be dangerous, and a broad-spectrum vitamin-mineral supplement is preferred. Use according to maker's recommendations.

FEEDING SCHEDULES AND PATIENT MONITORING

Feeding schedules are amended as patient responses indicate. In general, sick cats are fed frequent small meals. Schedules range from 4 to 12 meals daily, depending on the severity of the illness. Also, meals proceed from isosmolar to hyperosmolar, from simple (elemental) ingredients to complex.

For hospitalised cats that are less critically ill,

the feeding programme is simpler. The variation among cat foods is not especially large, and the nutrient requirements of cats are strict. One key point to remember is that cats need high protein intakes throughout their lives, for behavioural as well as biochemical reasons. A second key point is that cats cannot be forced to eat a food they reject. Simply 'waiting out' the cat will not work. It is far healthier for the cat to be given a food it likes.

Immediate weight gain is often a part, but not a goal, of feeding during nutrition support. The first weight gained following re-feeding is primarily water and fat, not protein. Because water and fat stores do not aid immune function, wound repair or homeostasis, early weight gain should not be interpreted as a sign that the patient is out of danger from malnutrition. Other signs and laboratory data are monitored to assess the cat's functional responses to feeding.

Overfeeding, intended to increase weight rapidly, will not help cats and may overburden digestive and metabolic systems. Overfeeding in sick humans has been associated with respiratory and cardiac failures, even death. High carbohydrate formulae produce excessively high respiratory CO_2. Ventilatory load is decreased by feeding high fat formulae, which lower carbon dioxide production and respiratory quotient. Meal feeding, rather than continuous feeding, is used as well to decrease the metabolic load.

DISCHARGE FROM HOSPITAL

Cat behaviour continues its profound influence on feeding programmes during recovery in hospital and convalescence at home. Some feline behaviours that we recognise and ways we accommodate them in nutrition support are outlined in Fig. 4.5. We urge you to reflect on each point summarised in Fig. 4.5, especially when counselling owners about their cat's convalescence. Note that most of the behaviour patterns described are different from those exhibited by dogs.

Feeding schedules for cats with adequate voluntary intake follow the same principles. Most cats seem comfortable eating frequent small meals of meat-based ingredients, high in animal protein and fat, and eating alone. Food intakes are noted

FELINE BEHAVIOUR AND NUTRITION SUPPORT	
Behaviour pattern	**Application**
Solitary carnivore	Feed in an area protected from noise and animals. In a clinic, place a cardboard box in the cage or drape a cloth to give privacy.
Strict carnivore	Offer meat-based diets or enterals. Offer meat, fish, poultry or cheese as snacks. Use protein modules.
Many meals daily	Feed a minimum of 4 times daily, 6 to 12 times daily is better.
Refuses diets with low palatability	Never assume that the cat will eat when it gets hungry enough. Offer a variety of high-quality diets until one is consumed readily, or feed involuntarily.
Prefers dense diets, animal protein, fat	Try mixing a teaspoon of canned cat food into an enteral product for voluntary consumption.
Consumes a new diet for 1–3 days, then refuses to eat	When changing a diet, forewarn the owner that the cat may refuse a previously accepted diet. Follow up patients 5–7 days after diet change.

FIG. 4.5   Applications of feline behaviour in the practice of nutritional support.

in the medical record, and written instructions are provided upon discharge. Hypometabolic conditions usually return to normal within two to seven days of re-feeding. However, hypermetabolic conditions may persist for weeks.

Owners are counselled about diet selection. We describe types of commercial products, usually naming two or three brands that fit our recommended feeding regime and patient management. Procedures outlined in Fig. 4.5 are discussed with the owner.

During the recovery period, owners are encouraged to keep written diaries of their cat's food, meal size and frequency, and drinking. We review these records by telephone every day for debilitated cats, and every four or five days for simple recoveries. We re-evaluate the case if the cat fails to maintain 85% of our goal.

TOTAL PARENTERAL NUTRITION

Although the convenience and effectiveness of enteral tube feeding has diminished the need for parenteral nutrition in hospitalised cats, the latter may be preferred in certain conditions such as gut failure, or cases with uncontrolled vomiting when anaesthesia or sedation for tube placement are a risk.

Calories are delivered as amino-acids (from 2% to 10% solutions), dextrose (25% or 50% solutions), and fatty acids (10% or 20% emulsions) into large central veins. Generally, total daily calorie delivery does not exceed maintenance, and fuel sources approximate 20–25% protein, 40–50% carbohydrate and 40–50% fat. Rarely is *total* nutrition provided intravenously; vitamins and trace elements are frequently excluded.

Intravenous amino-acids are utilised with low efficiency in omnivores and we expect that nitrogen losses may be even more critical for carnivores. Calculations should account accurately for protein as an energy source especially for cats. The practice of assigning zero calories to protein given intravenously is unsound in theory and leads to erroneous and undesirable lower protein:calorie ratios in practice.[12]

Complications of intravenous nutrition include sepsis, phlebitis and thrombosis, fatty liver, hyperglycaemia and hypokalaemia. Intravenous nutrition is expensive, starves enterocytes, and requires intensive nursing care and attention to detail, coupled with thorough patient evaluation and monitoring.

THE FUTURE OF HOSPITALISED CAT CARE

As clinical medicine and nutrition support for cats proceeds, innovative additions to patient care will develop. Special enterals for cats are now marketed and more products specifically for cats are likely to appear. These should contain the essential dietary nutrients, such as taurine and arachidonate, needed by cats.

Techniques for nutritional assessment will

be improved, perhaps including ultrasound, calorimetry, labelled water or potassium, and bioelectrical impedance.[15]

Appetite stimulants for cats bring only short-term effects of limited value. Developments in drug therapies should enable us to provide long-term chemotherapeutic assistance to improve voluntary food intake in sick cats. The use of such products as blocking antibodies to specific cytokines will prevent the nausea and malaise of sepsis and associated with certain cancer treatments. The antibodies will thus promote appetite, anabolism and more effective nutrition support. Therapeutics may be directed towards control of circulating levels of cachectin in cats. Other substances to be addressed may be the small bowel fuel glutamine, the large bowel fuels such as beta-hydroxybutyrate, and growth hormone and other growth factors as promotors of healing and anabolism.

REFERENCES

1. Bauer M.C., Weiss D.J., Perman V. (1991) Hematologic alterations in adult cats fed 6 or 12% propylene glycol. *Am. J. Vet. Res.* **53**: 69–72.
2. Bell F.W., Osborne C.A. (1989) Maintenance fluid therapy. In: Current Veterinary Therapy **X**, (ed. Kirk R.W.). W.B. Saunders, Philadelphia.
3. Burger I.H. Blaza S.E. (1988) Digestion, absorption and dietary balance. In: *Dog and Cat Nutrition*, 2nd ed. (ed. Edney A.T.B.) Pergamon Press, Oxford.
4. Bright R.M., Okransji E.B., Pardo A.D. (1991) Percutaneous tube gastrostomy for enteral alimentation in small animals. *Compend. Cont. Educ. Pract. Vet.* **13**: 15–22.
5. Chew D.J. (1989) Parenteral fluid therapy. In: *The Cat, Diseases and Clinical Management* (ed. Sherding R.G.). Churchill Livingstone, New York.
6. Christopher M.M., Perman V., Eaton J.W. (1989) Contribution of propylene glycol-induced Heinz body formation to anemia in cats. *J. Amer. Vet. Med. Assoc.* **194**: 1045–1056.
7. Crowe D.T. (1986) Clinical use of an indwelling nasogastric tube for enteral nutrition and fluid therapy in the dog and cat. *J. Amer. Anim. Hosp. Assoc.* **22**: 675.
8. Donoghue S. (1989) Nutritional support of hospitalized patients. *Vet. Clin. N. Amer.: Small Anim. Pract.* **19**(3): 475–495.
9. Donoghue S. (1991) A quantitative summary of nutrition support services in a veterinary teaching hospital. *Cornell Vet.* **81**: 109–128.
10. Kettlehut I.C., Foss M.C., Migliorini, R.H. (1980) Glucose homeostasis in a carnivorous animal (cat) and in rats fed a high-protein diet. *Am. J. Physiol.* **239**: R437–R444.
11. Kronfeld D.S. (1986) Therapeutic diets for dogs and cats including a simple system of recipes. *Tijdschrift voor Diergeneeskunde* **111**: 37S–46S.
12. Kronfeld D.S. (1991) Protein and energy estimates for hospitalized dogs and cats. *Proceedings of Purina Internat. Nutr. Symp., Orlando* pp 5–11.
13. Morris J.G., Rogers Q.R. (1989) Comparative aspects of nutrition and metabolism of dogs and cats. In: *Nutrition of the Dog and Cat. Waltham Symposium Number 7* (ed. Burger I.H., Rivers J.P.W.) pp 35–66. Cambridge University Press, Cambridge.
14. National Research Council (1986) *Nutrient requirements of cats*. National Academy, Washington DC.
15. Stanton C.A., Hamar D.W., Johnson D.E. Fettman M.J. (1992) Bioelectrical impedance and zoometry for body composition analysis in domestic cats. *Amer. J. Vet. Res.* **53**: 251–257.
16. Stunkard A.J. (1987) Conservative treatments for obesity. *Am. J. Clin. Nutr.* **45**: 1142–1154.

5

Paediatrics

JOHNNY D. HOSKINS

Clinical evaluation of the kitten from birth to young adulthood is often complicated by age-related changes in body systems, the development of which continue after birth. Thorough clinical evaluation of the young kitten should include the case history, physical examination and routine laboratory tests, ultrasound, electrocardiography and radiography where appropriate.[7]

PHYSICAL EXAMINATION

The physical examination of a kitten should be conducted in a systematic manner.[7] The first phase is careful observation of the animal's responses, specifically noting the kitten's general condition, mental activity, posture, locomotion and breathing pattern. Next, the body temperature, respiratory and heart rates, capillary refill time and body weight should be recorded. The third phase is the assessment of the function of specific body systems (Fig. 5.1).

Clinicians often use a commercial laboratory for such routine tests as haemograms, serum chemistry profiles and urine analyses. Reference intervals for interpretation of laboratory data for kittens are presented in Fig. 5.2. Samples collected from kittens younger than 8 weeks old, however, are often inadequate for testing by these laboratories. As an alternative, the clinician can use in-house laboratory tests, including microhaematocrit for the packed cell volume (PCV), blood film examination for erythrocyte and leucocyte morphology, feline leukaemia virus antigen and feline immunodeficiency virus antibody tests, blood glucose and urea nitrogen (BUN) by reagent strip for whole blood, urine evaluation by reagent strip for urinalysis and a urine sediment examination, and total plasma solids and urine specific gravity by refractometer. The results of these few tests may be sufficient to confirm illness or assist in the case management of an illness.[7]

Routine radiography

Kilovoltage should be greatly reduced for routine radiography of young kittens because of minimal absorption of X-rays by partially mineralised bones, the thinness of soft tissue body parts and a lack of body fat. Therefore, most radiography of young kittens is performed in the 40–60 kVp range; increasing or decreasing the kVp by 4 to 6 kVp doubles or halves the film exposure, respectively.[15] An additional step that can be helpful in producing maximum quality radiographs for young kittens is to use a single high-detail intensifying screen (rare-earth high-detail type) within the cassette. The single screen should be adhered to the back inner surface of the cassette, which is then loaded with single-emulsion radiographic film to take advantage of the increased detail that such a film can produce. The emulsion side of the film must be positioned toward the screen. This cassette/film combination can be used for radiographing all body parts of the young kitten.

SEPTICAEMIA IN THE KITTEN

Kittens are born into a microbiologically and virologically complex world. They are exposed to organisms that establish one of the most complex ecological systems, referred to as the 'natural microflora'. In many clinical situations, the natural microflora can be life-threatening to the young kitten.

Of the life-threatening illnesses that can affect kittens, noenatal septicaemia is common. Bacterial invasion of the bloodstream occurs frequently in cats but is rarely of consequence in healthy adults. When overwhelming bacteraemia develops, the severity of the cat's predisposing illness is the single most important factor influencing survival. Kittens are commonly predisposed to natural microflora-induced septicaemic conditions by the coexistence of inadequate

PHYSICAL EXAMINATION OF KITTENS	
Head and oral cavity	Check for malformations of the skull, cleft lip, stenotic nares, or cleft palate. The mucous membranes should be light pink and moist. The teeth, if present, should be examined for early occlusion.
Ears	External ear canals open between 6 and 14 days after birth and should be completely open by 17 days. When ear canals first open, cytological examination shows an abundance of desquamative cells and some oil droplets. A thorough otoscopic examination can be made in kittens older than 4 weeks.
Eyes and eyelids	The eyelids separate into upper and lower eyelids at 5 - 14 days after birth. Menace reflex may not appear until 3 - 4 weeks of age. Reflex lacrimation begins when the eyelids separate; evaluation of tear production by Schirmer's tear test can be done thereafter. Pupillary light responses are present after the eyelids open but may not be evident until 21 days of age.
Nose	Check appearance and patency of the nostrils and the presence of fluids (mucus, pus, blood, milk, clear discharges).
Thorax	Check the thoracic wall, for symmetry or deformity, and auscultate the thorax using a stethoscope with a paediatric chest piece (2 cm bell; 3 cm diaphragm). The normal heart rate is approximately 220 beats/min, and the respiratory rate is 15 - 35 breaths/min during the first 4 weeks of life, thereafter becoming similar to the adult rate (Fig. 11.3). The normal heart rhythm of kittens is a regular sinus rhythm. Heart sounds are localized to the left cardiac apex (left 5th to 6th intercostal space, ventral third of thorax), the left cardiac base (left 3rd to 4th intercostal space above the costochondral junction) or the right cardiac apex (right 4th to 5th intercostal space opposite the mitral valve area). Heart murmurs are the most common type of abnormal sound heard, frequently being a functional murmur and not a murmur associated with congenital heart disease. Absence of lung sounds or audible asymmetry may indicate abnormalities within the thorax or lungs.
Abdomen	Unless the liver margins extend beyond the ribs, the liver is not enlarged. The spleen is not normally palpable unless it is enlarged. Both kidneys are palpable in all kittens. The stomach may feel like a large, fluid-filled sac if it is full. The intestines can be palpated as soft, slightly fluid or gas-filled structures that are freely movable and are not painful. The urinary bladder can be gently squeezed to determine resistance to urine outflow.
Skin and umbilicus	The skin should be inspected for wounds, state of hydration and condition of foot pads. The skin and haircoat should also be examined for evidence of bacterial infection, external parasites, or dermatophytosis. The umbilicus should be carefully inspected for evidence of inflammation, infection or abnormalities of the abdominal wall. The umbilical cord normally drops off by 2 - 3 days of age.
Limbs, tail, anus and genitalia	Check the limbs for deformities or absence of long bones, number and position of toes and pads, position of limbs at rest and during movement, presence of soft tissue injury (bruises, swelling, wounds) and condition of joints (deformities, range of mobility). The tail is inspected for length, mobility and deformities. The anus should be evaluated for patency, redness and signs of diarrhoea; and the genitalia should be checked for position and appearance.
Nervous system	The sucking reflex is present at birth and disappears by 3 weeks of age. Eliminative behaviours are controlled for the first 3 - 4 weeks of life by anogenital reflex.

Fig. 5.1 Physical examination of kittens.

LABORATORY REFERENCE INTERVALS FOR HEALTHY KITTENS				
	Age			
Parameter	**2 Weeks**	**4 Weeks**	**6 Weeks**	**8 Weeks**
Red blood cell count (x10^6/µl)	5.05 – 5.53	4.57 – 4.77	5.66 – 6.12	6.31 – 6.83
Haemoglobin (g/dl)	11.5 – 12.7	8.5 – 8.9	8.3 – 8.9	8.8 – 9.4
Packed cell volume (%)	33.6 – 37.0	25.7 – 27.3	26.2 – 27.9	28.5 – 31.1
Mean corpuscular volume (fl)	66.5 – 69.3	52.7 – 55.1	44.3 – 46.9	44.6 – 46.6
Mean corpuscular haemoglobin (pg)	22.4 – 23.6	18.0 – 19.6	14.2 – 15.4	13.6 – 14.2
Mean corpuscular haemoglobin concentration (%)	33.7 – 35.3	32.5 – 33.5	31.3 – 32.5	30.4 – 31.4
Total white blood cell count (x10^3/µl)	9.10 – 10.24	14.10 – 16.52	16.08 – 18.82	16.13 – 20.01
Band neutrophils	0.04 – 0.08	0.07 – 0.15	0.14 – 0.26	0.14 – 0.30
Segmented neutrophils	5.28 – 6.64	6.15 – 7.69	7.92 – 11.22	5.72 – 7.78
Lymphocytes	3.21 – 4.25	5.97 – 7.15	5.64 – 7.18	8.01 – 11.16
Monocytes	0.00 – 0.02	0.00 – 0.04	0	0.00 – 0.02
Eosinophils	0.53 – 1.39	1.24 – 1.56	1.22 – 1.72	0.88 – 1.28
Basophils	0.01 – 0.03	0	0	0.00 – 0.04
Plasma sodium (mmol/l)	n.d.	149 – 153	151 – 156	150 – 152
Plasma potassium (mmol/l)	n.d.	4.0 – 4.8	4.5 – 5.5	4.1 – 5.3
Plasma chloride (mmol/l)	n.d.	120 – 124	119 – 125	119 – 125
Plasma calcium (mg/dl)	n.d.	9.4 – 10.6	9.5 – 10.7	9.4 – 10.0
Plasma phosphorus (mg/dl)	n.d.	6.3 – 7.5	6.9 – 9.3	7.3 – 9.1
Plasma osmolality (mOsm/kg)	n.d.	293 – 321	287 – 319	309 – 327
Blood urea nitrogen (mg/dl)	<30	<30	<30	<30
Plasma creatinine (mg/dl)	n.d.	0.4 – 0.6	0.5 – 0.7	0.6 – 0.8
Glucose (mg/dl)	76 – 129	99 – 112	<120	<120
Total protein (g/dl)	4.0 – 5.2	4.6 – 5.2	4.4 – 5.0	4.5 – 5.3
Albumin (g/dl)	2.0 – 2.4	2.2 – 2.4	2.2 – 2.5	2.3 – 2.4
Bile acids (µmol/l)	<10	<10	<10	<10
Total bilirubin (mg/dl)	0.1 – 1.0	0.1 – 0.2	n.d.	n.d.
Alanine aminotransferase (IU/l)	11 – 24	14 – 26	n.d.	n.d.
Aspartate aminotransferase (IU/l)	8 – 48	12 – 24	n.d.	n.d.
Alkaline phosphatase (IU/l)	68 – 269	90 – 135	n.d.	n.d.
Cholesterol (mg/dl)	164 – 443	22 – 434	n.d.	n.d.
Endogenous creatinine clearance (ml/min/kg)	n.d.	0.54 – 2.24	2.09 – 3.41	2.72 – 3.94
24-hour urine protein excretion (mg/kg/day)	n.d.	0.73 – 4.35	1.87 – 10.29	5.57 – 13.15
Urine protein-to-creatinine ratio	n.d.	0.16 – 0.36	0.14 – 0.40	0.19 – 0.41
Urine specific gravity	n.d.	1.020 – 1.038	1.024 – 1.026	1.047 – 1.080
Urine osmolality (mOsm/kg)	n.d.	748 – 1374	896 – 2238	1697 – 2903

n.d. = not determined

FIG. 5.2 Laboratory reference intervals for some common parameters in healthy kittens.

nutrition and thermoregulation, viral infections, parasitism, genetic disorders and congenital or acquired immunodeficiency diseases. Consequently, bloodstream invasion is usually by the more common bacteria – *Staphylococcus*, *Escherichia coli*, *Klebsiella*, *Enterobacter*, *Streptococcus*, *Enterococcus*, *Pseudomonas*, *Clostridium perfringens*, *Bacteroides*, *Fusobacterium* and *Salmonella*

FIG. 5.3 Medical management of the septicaemic kitten.

MEDICAL MANAGEMENT OF THE SEPTICAEMIC KITTEN

I. External warming procedure
(a) Use circulating hot water blanket and hot water bottle
(b) Take at least 20-30 minutes for gradual warming of the patient
(c) Turn the patient every hour
(d) Record rectal temperature every hour

II. Parenteral fluid therapy
(a) Use multiple electrolyte solution supplemented with 5% dextrose solution
(b) Supplement the fluids with potassium chloride solution if plasma potassium concentration is less than 2.5 mmol/l
(c) Administer warm fluids slowly by intravenous or intraosseous route

III. Glucose replacement therapy
(a) Administer 5% dextrose solution intravenously or intraosseously, to effect
(b) Administer 1-2 ml/kg of body-weight of a 10-25% dextrose solution if the patient is profoundly depressed or having seizures
(c) Maintain plasma glucose concentration at 80-200 mg/dl for euglycaemia

IV. Antimicrobial therapy
(a) Collect bacterial culture samples (whole blood, urine, exudate, faeces) before initiation of antimicrobial therapy
    1. For blood culture, collect 1 ml of whole blood aseptically and inoculate blood directly into enriched tryptic or trypticase soy broth, dilute the whole blood 1:5 to 1:10 in enriched broth, and examine broth for bacterial growth 6-18 hours later
    2. For urine culture, collect urine by cystocentesis and culture it by the standard methods
    3. For exudate and faecal cultures, collect and culture by standard methods
(b) Empirical treatment with an antimicrobial agent begins immediately after collection of appropriate bacterial culture samples
(c) Adjust the dosage and dosing interval of antimicrobial agent selected
(d) Administer the antimicrobial agent by the intravenous or intraosseous route

V. Provide oxygen and nutritional therapy
(a) Administer oxygen by mask or intranasally to counter tissue hypoxaemia
(b) Encourage food intake once patient is normothermic and adequately hydrated

VI. Monitor the effectiveness of medical management
(a) Observe for improvement in the patient's general demeanour
(b) Regularly assess the cardiopulmonary status (It is extremely easy to overhydrate the septicaemic patient and attentive monitoring of breathing pattern is helpful for recognition of overhydration)
(c) Weigh the patient 3-4 times a day to assess gain in weight
(d) Observe for moistness of mucous membranes in assessing for adequate hydration

species – and of these, Gram-negative bacilli occur most often.[2] Common sources from which Gram-negative bacilli enter the bloodstream include gastrointestinal tract and peritoneum, respiratory tract, skin, wound, and urinary tract infections. Clinical signs resulting from bacteraemia in kittens may vary. Death may be so sudden that noticeable signs are virtually absent. Typically, kittens will cry a lot and show restlessness, poor muscle tone, hypothermia, diarrhoea, respiratory signs, haematuria, failure to thrive, cyanosis and sloughing of extremities.

Because septicaemic conditions may result in sudden death, kittens suspected of having septicaemia should be treated immediately (Fig. 5.3). In most instances, initial antimicrobial therapy is selected empirically. Kittens should also be given fluid therapy for dehydration, oxygen to counter tissue hypoxaemia, and glucose if hypoglycaemia is present. In addition, it is imperative to conduct a thorough search for the source of infection and collect appropriate bacterial culture samples prior to initiating antimicrobial therapy.

Unfortunately, the information necessary for accurate dosing of the antimicrobial agents in young kittens is incomplete. Drug distribution, especially for kittens younger than 5 weeks old, differs from that of adults because of differences in body composition, such as lower total body fat, higher percentage of total body water, lower concentrations of albumin and poorly developed blood-brain barrier; therefore, modifications of the adult dose (which should be reduced by as much as 30–50%) or dosing frequency may be necessary when most antimicrobial agents are administered. Furthermore, all antimicrobial agents should be administered intravenously or intraosseously for potentially life-threatening septicaemia, as systemic absorption following oral, subcutaneous or intramuscular administration is not always reliable. Most drugs ingested by the nursing queen appear in the milk but the amount is generally only 1–2% of the mother's dose, so that treating the nursing queen will never be effective in treating kittens with life-threatening septicaemia.

Antimicrobial agents for septicaemia

Aminoglycosides

The risks of using aminoglycosides (neomycin, streptomycin, kanamycin, amikacin, gentamicin, tobramycin and netilmicin) in young kittens may outweigh the benefits of these agents. The spectrum of activity of aminoglycosides includes many aerobic Gram-negative bacteria, especially *Escherichia coli*, *Klebsiella pneumoniae*, *Pseudomonas aeruginosa*, *Proteus* sp., and *Serratia* sp.. Aminoglycosides frequently cause nephrotoxicity, which can be minimised by:[1]

1. using the least nephrotoxic drug, i.e., amikacin rather than gentamicin;
2. ensuring the kitten's hydration status is normal;
3. increasing the dosing interval;
4. using combination therapy with synergistic antimicrobial agents when indicated for serious infections;

5. avoiding use of other nephrotoxic or nephroactive drugs including antiprostaglandins and furosemide.

Beta-lactam antimicrobials

The beta-lactam antimicrobial agents are generally the drugs of choice for septicaemic kittens whenever possible. They include penicillins, cephalosporins, and the combination beta-lactam antimicrobials and beta-lactamase inhibitors. Bacteria capable of producing beta-lactamase enzymes include many of the Gram-negative organisms such as *Escherichia*, *Haemophilus*, *Klebsiella*, *Pasteurella*, *Proteus*, *Pseudomonas* and *Salmonella* species. Most often, beta-lactamase enzymes produced by Gram-negative bacteria are effective against both penicillins and cephalosporins. The combination of beta-lactam antimicrobial agents with lactamase inhibitors, such as clavulanic acid and sulbactam, will increase the effective spectrum of these drugs.

The spectrum of activity of beta-lactam antimicrobial agents varies widely (Fig. 5.4).

The major disadvantages of the cephalosporins include the lack of specific dosing regimens in young kittens and the necessity of intravenous or intraosseous administration in most cases. Cephalosporins are a relatively non-toxic group of antimicrobial agents. Adverse effects reported include coagulopathies and bleeding (vitamin K-responsive), urticaria, anaphylaxis, immune-mediated reactions such as haemolytic anaemia, leukopenia, thrombocytopenia, and positive Coombs' antiglobulin tests, gastrointestinal side effects (vomiting, diarrhoea, anorexia) and abnormal liver and renal function tests.[3]

Potentiated sulphonamides

The Gram-positive and Gram-negative spectrum of the combination of a sulphonamide with trimethoprim or ormetoprim is broad, including *E. coli*, some *Salmonella* species, and other Gram-negative bacteria. Most potentiated sulphonamides have a wide margin of safety, but their dosage and dosing interval should be modified in young kittens because of a prolonged half-life, resulting from decreased metabolism by the liver and decreased renal excretion.[1]

Fɪɢ. 5.4 Activity of
beta-lactam antimicro-
bial agents for use in
kittens.

ACTIVITY OF BETA-LACTAM ANTIMICROBIAL AGENTS	
Amoxicillin **Ampicillin**	Broad-spectrum drugs, although beta-lactamase sensitive. Combination products improve their effectiveness towards *E. coli, Klebsiella* and some *Proteus* species but not towards *Pseudomonas* species
	Amoxicillin-clavulanic acid: especially useful for an amoxicillin-resistant *E. coli* urinary tract infection
	Ampicillin-sulbactam: effective against many ampicillin-resistant isolates of *Pasteurella multocida* and *P. haemolytica*
Penicillins	Broad-spectrum pencillins with extended spectra towards *Pseudomonas, Proteus* and some *Klebsiella, Shigella* and *Enterobacter* species include:
	carbenicillin and its indanyl ester form (can be administered orally)
	ticarcillin (2-4 times greater activity towards *Pseudomonas* species than carbenicillin)
	piperacillin (the highest antipseudomonal activity)
Cephalosporins First generation	Active against many Gram-positive bacteria and some Gram-negative bacteria such as *E. coli, Klebsiella* sp and *Proteus* sp. Include: cephalothin (10-30mg/kg tid) cephalexin cephapirin (10-30mg/kg tid) cephradine cefadroxil cefazolin (10-30mg/kg tid, somewhat more efficacious)
Second generation	Improved activity towards *Enterobacter,* some *Proteus sp, E. coli, Klebsiella* sp and some anaerobic bacteria. Include: cefamandole cefaclor cefoxitin (10-20 mg/kg tid)
Third generation	Reduced activity against Gram-positive organisms. Generally reserved for serious Gram-negative bacteria such as *Pseudomonas aeruginosa, Haemophilus influenzae, Neisseria, Enterobacter, Serratia, Citrobacter* and *Bacteroides* sp. Therapeutic levels in the cerebrospinal fluid are achieved, therefore they are preferred for treating most life-threatening septicaemias

FADING KITTEN SYNDROME

Kitten losses during the first 12 weeks of life usually approximate 15–40%, although precise figures may vary.[9,10,13] Most kitten losses will occur during specific periods: *in utero* (abortions, foetal resorptions); at the time of birth (stillbirths); immediately after the birth period (0–2 weeks of age); or in the immediate post-weaning period (5–12 weeks of age). Losses after these periods are generally low.

Kittens that die during the time period immediately after birth are often referred to as part of the 'fading kitten syndrome' with the 'fader' being a kitten apparently healthy at birth but failing to survive beyond 2 weeks of age. This age distinctness is arbitrary, however, and it might be considered more valuable to encompass the period from birth to 12 weeks of age.

Causes

Kitten losses up to 12 weeks of age usually result from problems acquired *in utero*, during the birth process (0–2 weeks of age), or in the post-weaning period.[11] Death losses during the latter period are primarily attributed to infectious diseases potentiated by weaning stress, exposure to pathogenic organisms in the immediate environment, and diminished local or systemic immunity. In general, most kitten losses occur because of congenital anomalies, nutritional diseases resulting from improper diets fed to the dam or her young, abnormally low birth weights, traumatic insults during or after the birth process (dystocia, cannibalism, maternal neglect), neonatal isoerythrolysis, infectious diseases, and other miscellaneous factors.[11]

Congenital anomalies

Congenital anomalies are those present at birth with their cause unspecified. In many situations, they are of genetic origin, but teratogenic factors could be responsible. Some congenital anomalies (particularly those involving the central nervous, cardiovascular, and respiratory systems) may be immediately incompatible with life, resulting in death at birth or within 2 weeks of a normal birth, while other anomalies might remain unnoticed until the animal is fully ambulatory. Often, these congenital anomalies are first diagnosed during the initial clinical examination prior to vaccination, or as the result of obviously limited exercise tolerance or failure to thrive. Anatomic anomalies may include cleft palates, cranial deformities, agenesis of the small or large intestines, cardiac anomalies, extensive umbilical or diaphragmatic hernias, anomalies of the kidneys and lower urinary tract, and musculoskeletal anomalies. Congenital anomalies of a microanatomic or biochemical type probably account for an equal number of kitten losses.[11] Such defects go unreported and are usually included under the general heading of stillbirths, 'faders', or undetermined causes of death.

Teratogenic effects

To what extent kitten losses may be attributed to teratogenic effects in unclear. There are well-authenticated reports of the teratogenic potential of some drugs and chemicals that are believed to contribute to congenital anomalies or 'faders'. As a general rule, it is best to avoid the administration or application of any drug or chemical during pregnancy. Although specific information for canine and feline species may be lacking, it is certainly advisable to avoid the use of any drug or chemical, such as corticosteroids and griseofulvin, with known adverse teratologic effects in animal species.

Nutrition

Queens fed inadequate diets during pregnancy may produce diseased or weak kittens. The most serious dietary problem documented in the last decade has been taurine deficiency, which is known to cause foetal resorptions, abortions, stillbirths, and poor growing kittens.[14] Malnutrition of a kitten may also occur as a result of severe maternal malnutrition or due to lack of adequate maternal blood supply, possibly because of competition for placental space.

Low birth weight

Low birth weights are associated with higher kitten losses. The birth weight of kittens is not affected by their sex, litter size, or weight of the dam.[4,9] The causes of abnormally low birth weights have not been determined but probably involve several factors. Though low birth weight is often attributed to prematurity, most abnormally small kittens are born at term. Their small stature is probably caused by congenital anomalies or nutritional origins.

Not only is low birth weight associated with greater likelihood of stillbirths and deaths during the first 6 weeks of life,[9] but there is also a tendency for a disproportionate number of underweight kittens to be chronic poor doers and to die at a young age. Many 'faders' that die in the first weeks of life are of normal size, but their growth is slow and they are well below normal weight at the time of death. It is important to weigh kittens at birth and also at frequent intervals until they are at least 6 weeks old.

Traumatic insult

Kitten losses from traumatic insults during birth or the first 5 days of life are usually associated with dystocia, cannibalism, or maternal neglect. Cannibalism often occurs in nervous or high-strung mothers. In addition, cannibalism of sickly kittens is common, so that it is not always correct to incriminate trauma as the direct cause of death. It may not be possible to differentiate maternal neglect of otherwise normal kittens from maternal neglect of sickly kittens, the latter being a programmed response of mothers that is akin to cannibalism.

Neonatal isoerythrolysis

Neonatal isoerythrolysis occurs infrequently among domestic kittens but may be relatively common in certain purebred kittens.[5] In contrast to puppies, kittens have naturally occurring antibodies (commonly referred to as alloantibodies) against the other blood types in their plasma. Kittens acquire maternal alloantibodies of the IgG class and to a lesser extent of the IgM class via colostrum.

Blood type A kittens have weak anti-B alloantibodies, whereas blood type B kittens have strong anti-A alloantibodies with haemagglutinin and haemolysin titres of 1:64 or higher. At 6–10 weeks of age, kittens begin to produce their own alloantibodies, and these titres may reach their maximal levels by a few months of age. Prior blood transfusion or pregnancy therefore, is not necessary for the production of alloantibodies in kittens. These alloantibodies, particularly anti-A alloantibodies, are responsible for the major incompatibility reactions: colostral anti-A alloantibodies from blood type B queens may cause neonatal isoerythrolysis in blood type A (or blood type AB) kittens; and

blood type AB mismatched blood transfusions have a short half-life and are thus inefficacious and cause life-threatening transfusion reactions in blood type B cats.

During the first 24 hours of life, maternal antibodies are normally transferred to the kitten via colostrum. If the kitten has blood type A (or blood type AB) and the queen has blood type B, these colostral alloantibodies will bind to and lyse erythrocytes in the kitten. The haemolysis may be intravascular as well as extravascular and cause severe anaemia, chromoproteinuric nephropathy, and other organ failures as well as disseminated intravascular coagulopathy. Because all blood type B cats have high alloantibody titres, even primiparous queens can have litters with neonatal isoerythrolysis.

Clinical signs of neonatal isoerythrolysis often develop in blood type A (or blood type AB) kittens born to blood type B queens. Because the feline foetus is protected from maternal antibodies, kittens at risk are born healthy and usually start nursing vigorously. However, after colostrum intake, which contains high titres of maternal alloantibodies, these kittens show the first clinical signs within hours or days. The clinical course may vary but often includes kittens that die suddenly during the first day of life without showing any clinical signs; kittens that stop nursing during the first three days of life and fail to thrive (clinical findings include dark, brown-red urine caused by severe haemoglobinuria and affected kittens may develop icterus and severe anaemia, continue to fade and may die during the first week of life or surviving kittens may rarely develop a tail-tip necrosis between first and second week of life as part of this syndrome); or kittens that continue to nurse, thrive, and show no obvious signs of clinical illness except for the tail-tip necrosis, but may exhibit laboratory abnormalities such as a positive direct Coombs' test and a moderately responsive anaemia.

Infectious diseases

Infectious diseases account for a substantial proportion of kitten losses, especially to bacterial infections during the post-weaning period of 5–12 weeks of age. During this time, most deaths are attributed to a primary infection of either the respiratory tract or gastrointestinal tract and peritoneal cavity. When kittens are exposed to bacteria under nonstressful conditions, mild self-limiting or clinically inapparent infections usually occur. When host and environmental factors are unfavourable, immediate illnesses are more apt to be severe and kitten losses high. When bacterial infections exceed the ability of the kitten's immune system to protect against infectious agents, neonatal sepsis occurs.

When overwhelming sepsis develops in kittens 5–12 weeks of age, the severity of their illnesses usually influences survival. Factors predisposing kittens of this age group to septicaemic conditions include coexistence of inadequate nutrition and thermoregulation, viral infections, parasitism, and developmental and heritable defects of the immune system.

Neonatal sepsis is usually caused by the more common bacteria and has been discussed earlier.

Several viral groups, i.e., parvovirus, coronavirus, herpesvirus, calicivirus, and retrovirus, are implicated in kitten losses. Clinical signs of viral infections vary according to the route and time of infection and the degree of passively derived antibody protection in the individual kitten. Even against a background of routine vaccinal protection of breeding stock, situations exist in which passive immunity protection is not acquired, possibly because of colostral deprivation, and in which kittens are susceptible to viral infections normally considered to be well controlled.

Miscellaneous factors

Roundworm and hookworm infections have also been implicated in kitten losses, in which the intestinal worm burden was detrimental to the kitten's growth. Deaths attributable to ectoparasitism are not, however, common, although newly weaned kittens are not infrequently presented exhibiting well-established flea or tick burdens.

Although poorly understood, other causes of kitten losses are known to exist. Kitten loss is lowest in fifth litters; first litters and litters after the fifth parity have higher losses.[9] Middle-size queens tend to have lower losses than large or small queens. Losses are twice as high in one-kitten litters as in larger litters; the lowest losses occur in litters with 5 kittens.

Diagnosis

Kitten loss appears to be a common and often unavoidable problem within breeding establishments. Pre-weaning losses (live-born deaths and stillbirths) more than 20% and post-weaning losses (weaning to 7 months of age) more than 10% are reasons for major concern.[11] Disproportional losses to any one cause, such as congenital anomaly or specific infectious disease, at greater percentages than described above are additional reasons for major concern regardless of the overall percentage number.

The clinical approach to identifying the cause of 'fading kitten syndrome' should be based on thorough clinical evaluation of the kitten, which includes history, physical examination, routine laboratory tests, lead II rhythm strip, and possibly radiography/ultrasonography.[7] A complete physical examination should always be performed. Ideally, a complete blood count, plasma chemistry profile, urinalysis, urine and/or blood culture, and culture of suspected sources of infection should also be obtained. It is imperative to conduct a thorough search for the primary source of the 'fader' and collect appropriate bacterial culture samples prior to initiating antimicrobial therapy.

The haemograms are particularly helpful in septicaemic kittens. Normochromic normocytic anaemia, thrombocytopenia, and mild to moderate neutrophilia with a left shift may be present. Another laboratory finding that is consistent with, but by no means specific for, septicaemic 'fader' is hypoglycaemia. The remaining laboratory values from the plasma chemistry profile and urinalysis may reflect a specific organ failure.

Obtaining complete and accurate necropsies is the most expensive and crucial aspects of identifying the cause of 'fading kitten syndrome' in breeding establishments.[11] It is preferable to sacrifice the kitten and perform a fresh necropsy as soon as it becomes apparent that death is inevitable. Kittens that die before they are euthanised should be refrigerated immediately; freezing ruins tissues for gross and histopathological examination and should be avoided. Necropsies should be done by competent people. Gross abnormalities are often subtle and may go unnoticed by untrained eyes. Representative tissues should be taken as aseptically as possible and frozen for microbiological (viral, bacterial, and fungal cultures) or toxicological studies, should they prove to be necessary. A wide sampling of tissues should also be preserved in formalin for histopathological examination. Formalin-fixed tissues, along with detailed descriptions of gross lesions and clinical histories, should then be forwarded to veterinary pathologists for microscopic examination. If tissues indicate an infectious or toxic disease as the cause of death, samples of frozen tissues can then be submitted to competent microbiologists or toxicologists for further study.

Management

As previously indicated, a certain number of kitten losses is unavoidable. However, it may be possible to identify the specific cause of a 'fading kitten syndrome' and initiate the most appropriate management measures. Once the primary cause is determined, a concerted effort must be made to eliminate the causative factors before the next breeding or purchase.

RAISING THE ORPHAN KITTEN

If the queen is healthy and well-nourished, the nutritional needs of the kitten for the first four weeks of life should be provided completely by her. Kittens not receiving adequate milk cry constantly, are restless or extremely inactive, and may fail to attain weight gains of 10–15 g/day.[6]

A homemade recipe for rearing orphan kittens is shown in Fig. 5.5. Commercially prepared milk replacement formulas are preferred for raising motherless kittens, because they compare more closely to queen's milk (see Chapter 3). They

---

HOME-MADE RECIPE FOR ORPHAN KITTENS

3 ounces condensed milk
3 ounces water
4 ounces plain yogurt
3 large or 4 small egg yolks

FIG. 5.5   Homemade diet for orphan kittens.

usually provide 1–1.24 kcal of metabolisable energy per ml of formula. Based on typical energy needs of 22–26 kcal per 100 g of body weight, most kittens should receive the following daily amounts of formula per 100 g body weight:[6]

Up to 1 week old:	13 ml
1–2 weeks old:	17 ml
2–3 weeks old:	20 ml
3–4 weeks old:	22 ml

These amounts are fed in equal portions three or four times daily.

When preparing the formula, always follow the manufacturer's directions on the label and keep all feeding equipment scrupulously clean. Before each feeding, the formula should be warmed to about 100 F (37.8°C), or near body temperature for the first 3 weeks of life. For each of the first feedings, the amount of formula should be less than that prescribed; it should be increased gradually to the recommended level by the second or third day, and then increased accordingly as a favourable response to feeding occurs and the kitten gains weight.

WEANING

Weaning from queen's milk to other foods should be a gradual process. Kittens should be encouraged to begin eating solid food at 4 weeks of age. At the beginning of weaning, the kitten can be offered a mixture of a good quality food designed for growth, mixed with milk or water to form a thick gruel (1 part dry food blended with 3 parts water or milk, or 2 parts canned food blended with 1 part water or milk). The kitten should be encouraged to eat by smearing some of the gruel on its lips, being careful not to get any in its nose; or the feeder can touch a finger into the gruel and then into the kitten's mouth. Once the kitten is eating the gruel well, gradually reduce the milk or water content until the animal is consuming only solid food. Most kittens are weaned successfully at 6–8 weeks of age. Early weaning and separation from litter-mates prior to 6 weeks can result in behavioural problems such as slowness to learn and more suspicious, cautious and aggressive actions.

The kitten's eating habits are still in the formative stage after weaning, therefore easily digested, high-quality, calorie-dense food should be fed daily. Plenty of fresh drinking water should be made available and cow's milk should never be fed in place of it. Ad libitum feeding, or feeding at least three times a day, is preferred during growth; and all supplementation should be avoided.

MALNUTRITION

Malnutrition occurs when basic nutritional requirements are not being met. It is especially common during the time when kittens depend entirely on the queen for their nutritional needs. Several factors can contribute to malnutrition in nursing kittens.[6] The kitten may ingest insufficient or inadequate milk because the queen dies or disowns her young, cannot adequately care for too large a litter, or there may be partial or complete lactation failure by the queen due to illness, mastitis, metritis or underdeveloped mammae. In addition, kittens may be born prematurely or underdeveloped; they may be so weak and sick that they cannot suckle normally, or may have congenital defects that preclude adequate milk intake. Failure to provide an adequate growth diet at 4 weeks of age can also result in inadequate nutrient intake to meet the demands of growth.

Immediate recognition of a malnourished kitten is usually based on its smaller, lighter appearance, feeble attempts to feed or inability to attain adequate weight gain for its age. High-pitched, constant crying or inactivity accompanied by a weak sucking reflex are advanced indications that the nursing kitten is receiving insufficient or inadequate milk. Reduced body tone and muscle strength may be evident on handling. Coexisting congenital defects that are not immediately life-threatening may be detected on physical examination as well.

The treatment of malnutrition in the nursing kitten generally requires that proper nourishment is provided. Complications that are frequently encountered during the management of malnutrition are diarrhoea, dehydration, hypoglycaemia and hypothermia.[6] If diarrhoea occurs during feeding of adequate amounts of a properly prepared commercial milk replacement formula, immediately reduce the amount of solid intake by one half. This can be done by diluting the formula 1 to 1 with water or, preferably, with a mixture of equal parts of multiple electrolyte solution and 5% dextrose/water solution. As the condition of the faeces improves, gradually increase the amount of solids to the recommended level.

Hypoglycaemia and dehydration occur quickly when a malnourished kitten is not fed adequately. To help alleviate or prevent dehydration and mild hypoglycaemia, offer an equal mixture of warm multiple electrolyte solution and 5% dextrose/water solution parenterally until the kitten responds. No type of milk replacement formula should be given to a weak and severely chilled kitten that displays a diminished sucking reflex or a rectal body temperature below 35°C (95°F).

REFERENCES

1. Boothe D.M., Tannert K. (1992) Special considerations for drug and fluid therapy in the pediatric patient. *Compend. Contin. Educ. Pract. Vet.* **14**: 313–329.
2. Dow S.W., Curtis C.R., Jones R.L., et al (1989) Results of blood culture from critically-ill dogs and cats: 100 cases (1985–1987). *J. Am. Vet. Med. Assoc.* **195**: 113–118.
3. Fekety F.R. (1990) Safety of parenteral third-generation cephalosporins. *Am. J. Med.* **88** (suppl 4A): 38S–44S.
4. Festing M.F.W., Bleby J. (1970) Breeding performance and growth of SPF cats (*Felis catus*). *J. Small Anim. Pract.* **11**: 533–542.
5. Giger U. (1992) The feline AB blood group system and incompatibility reactions. In: Kirk R.W., Bonagura J.D. (eds) *Current Veterinary Therapy XI* pp 470–474. W.B. Saunders Co., Philadelphia.
6. Hoskins J.D. (1990) Nutrition and nutritional disorders. In: Hoskins J.D. (ed.) *Veterinary Pediatrics: Dogs and Cats from Birth to Six Months*; pp 473–486. W.B. Saunders Co., Philadelphia.
7. Hoskins J.D. (1990) Clinical evaluation of the kitten: From birth to eight weeks of age. *Compend. Contin. Educ. Pract. Vet.* **12**(9): 1215–1225.
8. Kilgore W.R. (1989) Clavulanate-potentiated antibiotics. In Kirk R.W. (ed.) *Current Veterinary Therapy X*, pp 78–81. W.B. Saunders Co., Philadelphia.
9. Lawler D.F., Monti K.L. (1984) Morbidity and mortality in neonatal kittens. *Am. J. Vet. Res.* **45**: 1455–1459.
10. Norsworthy G.D. (1979) Kitten mortality complex. *Feline Pract.* **9**: 57–60.
11. Pedersen N.C. (1991) Common infectious diseases of multiple-cat environments. In: Pedersen N.C. (ed.) *Feline Husbandry: Diseases and Management*

in the Multiple-Cat Environment, pp 177–183. American Veterinary Publications, Inc., Goleta, California.

12. Riviere J.E. (1989) Cephalosporins. In: Kirk R.W. (ed.) *Current Veterinary Therapy X*, pp 74–77. W.B. Saunders Co., Philadelphia.

13. Scott F.W., Geissinger C., et al. (1978) Kitten mortality survey. *Feline Pract.* **8**: 31–34.

14. Sturman J.A., Gargano A.D., et al. (1986) Feline maternal taurine deficiency effects on mother and offspring. *J. Nutr.* **116**: 655–667.

15. Watters J.W. (1990) Radiography. In: Hoskins J.D. (ed.) *Veterinary Pediatrics: Dogs and Cats from Birth to Six Months*, pp 7–17. W.B. Saunders Co., Philadelphia.

6

Geriatrics

CARMEL T. MOONEY

Improved veterinary care and more advanced preventive measures, balanced nutrition and responsible ownership mean that pets, on average, live longer. Therefore, an expanding proportion of the cats seen by the veterinarian will be middle-aged and ageing.

Ageing itself is not a disease but is a normal and complex biological process resulting in progressive reduction of an individual's ability to maintain homeostasis under internal physiological and external environmental stresses. This decreases the subject's viability, increases its vulnerability to disease and eventually causes its death.[2] As such, ageing results in a loss of organ reserve, regenerative powers of organ function and adaptability.[6]

Clearly, the effects of ageing bring their own specific problems which tend to be irreversible, progressive and often subclinical. Geriatric health care programmes must recognise the changes and loss of function associated with ageing and attempt to minimise the rate of progression and thereby improve the quality of life for the older cat. In addition, certain diseases have an age bias and even if there is no age predisposition, the older animal exhibits a decreased ability to compensate for disturbances and diseases that would be tolerated well by a younger patient. Another complicating factor in the older patient is that once a problem arises in one organ system it is relatively easy for serious disturbances to develop in both related and unrelated organ systems as a result of the primary problem itself or because of therapy. The multitude of problems, both clinical and subclinical, that can co-exist in the older patient and the ramifications and repercussions of any one single problem in that individual must be recognised.

It is not easy to define accurately when a cat is 'geriatric'. In a recent survey, cats were considered to be geriatric at a mean (± sd) age of 11.88 (± 1.94) years.[2] Mixed breeds appear to live longer than pure breeds, presumably as a result of hybrid vigour. Exceptions include Siamese cats, which live longer, and Chinchillas, which have shorter life spans. Neutered animals appear to live longer. Obese pets have a decreased longevity, and animals maintained strictly on balanced commercial diets live longer than animals fed table scraps. The survey also suggested that indoor cats live longer than outdoor cats and that rural animals have a greater life-expectancy than those in an urban environment. However, despite this survey it is usually more practical to consider any cat over the age of 6 years to be geriatric, because it is from this age that subtle changes in organ function are first noted. In addition, those diseases that generally occur in the older animal become prominent in the differential diagnoses in animals over 6 years.

EFFECTS OF AGEING

Little information is available regarding the normal physiological changes that occur in the aged cat. Our knowledge has therefore been extrapolated from other species, including man and the dog. It is important to differentiate those changes which are intrinsic to the ageing process from those which are pathological. Understanding the effect of ageing on each individual body system enhances the ability to develop diagnostic criteria, establish health and therapeutic programmes and predict the response of the patient. Thus, it seems pertinent to review those changes noted particularly in the last third of an animal's life span. These changes have been reviewed in more detail.[6]

General effects

In the aged animal the metabolic rate declines slowly and this, together with a lack of activity,

61

decreases the energy need by some 30–40%. The capacity for thermoregulation decreases, leading to intolerance of heat and cold. This is due in part to decreased heat production and in part to slow or less pronounced peripheral vasomotor reactions. A decrease in the number of osmoreceptors in the lateral and superior hypothalamus and the development of arteriocapillary fibrosis contributes to reduced sensitivity to thirst. Sleep becomes more intermittent with increased restlessness and less rapid eye movement sleep patterns. The proportion of body fat to lean body mass increases. The skin loses elasticity and the coat becomes dull. Grooming and excretory habits become less fastidious and there is a decrease in mental alertness. Immunological competence diminishes with less efficient phagocytosis and chemotaxis. There is greater susceptibility to infectious diseases and neoplasia and the occurrence of immune-mediated diseases increases.

Alimentary system

The prevalence of dental disease increases with age. There is a build-up of dental calculus, which may be accompanied by gingivitis and gingival hyperplasia or periodontitis with gingival retraction, gingival atrophy and bone loss. The subsequent loss of teeth may also reflect a calcium deficit with alveolar demineralisation.[5] Periodontitis can result in absorption of bacterial toxins causing airway constriction ultimately leading to pulmonary problems, or periodic bacteraemia causing conditions such as endocarditis or nephritis. The incidence of neck lesions of teeth, a problem often overlooked in cats, increases with age.

Oesophageal function is altered by a reduction in the number of neurons in the sympathetic ganglia and the myenteric and Auerbach's plexus resulting in a loss of muscle tone and hypomotility. The gastric mucosa becomes atrophic and fibrotic. The incidence of idiopathic megacolon increases and may be related to degeneration or a relative paucity of myenteric ganglia.

Hepatocyte numbers decrease and an increased percentage are binucleate. The percentage of fat in the liver increases and mild hepatic fibrosis develops. Subsequently liver function decreases and may have important consequences for drug metabolism in these patients. Biliary and intestinal secretions decrease and pancreatic enzyme output diminishes. There is a reduction in the height and breadth of intestinal villi and diminished epithelial cell renewal. These changes can result in reduced absorption of calcium and lipids and therefore those vitamins that are lipid-soluble.

Respiratory system

Atrophy of secretory structures occurs in the aged patient together with an increase in the viscosity of secretions and a decrease in the function of the mucociliary apparatus. There is a general loss of lung elasticity, an increase in pulmonary fibrosis and a decrease in alveolar number and diffusion capacity. Atrophy and weakening of respiratory muscles, with calcification of costal cartilages, decrease the cough reflex and expiratory ability.

Circulatory system

There are few data on age-related cardiac changes in the cat. It is likely that, as in the dog, cardiac output decreases as the animal reaches old age. This is most obvious at times of stress, since the maximal heart rate and maximal oxygen consumption decrease, limiting reserve capacity. If general anaesthesia is induced, it is advisable to institute intravenous fluid therapy in order to minimise cardiovascular dysfunction.

The bone marrow becomes pale and fatty with advancing age. The red cell count and haemoglobin concentrations decrease. The erythropoietic response may become dampened; red cell regeneration as a response to haemorrhage may take twice as long in the older patient.[6]

Urinary system

Kidney function gradually declines with age. Kidney weight decreases as a result of a reduction in the total number of glomeruli and nephron mass. Glomerular filtration rate and renal plasma flow decline. This has been attributed to glomerular hyperfiltration resulting from increased pressure across the glomerular capillary basement membrane, a response to the reduction in the number of nephrons or linked to a high dietary protein intake. Tubular changes include atrophy, decreased tubular diameter, tubular disruption and tubular hypertrophy. These changes result in a reduction in renal reserve capacity. Stresses handled well by the younger animal, such as periods of water deprivation or the effects of general anaesthesia, may precipitate a renal crisis.

Nervous system

As age advances there is a general slowing of the nervous system and a decrease in the number of cells in the cerebrum and cerebellum. Reflexes may become more sluggish and their absence loses diagnostic significance on neurological examination. Owners may report an unwillingness in their cats to respond to external stimuli, and they may be irritable when disturbed. The progression to senility may be noted by inappropriate soiling in a previously house-trained animal.

Special senses

Vision acuity decreases. The viscosity of tears increases and this may result in an increased susceptibility to ocular infections. The number of endothelial cells of the cornea decreases, so that there is greater susceptibility to damage. Iris atrophy can occur and pupillary light reflexes become sluggish. Wax accumulates in the ear, which may require frequent cleansing. The sense of smell (particularly important in the cat) becomes less acute as a result of atrophy of the mucosa, neural degeneration, cell dehydration and alterations in blood supply. Presumably, as in man, there is a similar decline in the perception of taste.

Musculoskeletal system

There is a gradual loss of muscle and bone mass. Muscle cell number and size decrease, and there is increased fibrosis and atrophy, with a reduced sensitivity to (and regeneration of) adenosine triphosphate. Bone cortices become thinner, more dense and brittle. Osteoblast activity is decreased. The amount of cartilage and its regeneration are reduced and there is increased susceptibility to trauma.

Endocrine system

Changes in the endocrine system are poorly documented. Considering the prevalence of endocrine disease in the geriatric cat population, information on these changes would be useful. Growth hormone concentrations decrease and may be related to the diminished protein synthesis and muscle mass in the aged cat. The thymus atrophies and is replaced with connective and adipose tissue once sexual maturity has been attained. Adrenal changes have not been studied but in other species involution of adrenal tissue occurs and there is reduced adrenal reserve, which may adversely affect the stress response. Adrenal calcification is not an unusual radiographic finding in the aged cat, but it is not, as in the dog, an indicator of adrenal neoplasia. The thyroid response to thyroid stimulating hormone (TSH) is apparently depressed in geriatric dogs, but this has not been studied in cats. Reduced tolerance to glucose loading has been reported in old dogs and they may require a longer period for blood glucose concentrations to fall post-prandially but, again, such studies have not been reported for cats.

Females continue to cycle into old age and males continue to remain fertile. However, there may be a progressive increase in the interoestrus interval, a reduction in litter size and an increase in congenital defects and difficulties during parturition.[7]

MANAGEMENT OF THE HEALTHY GERIATRIC CAT

The management of the healthy geriatric cat owes as much to the owner as to the veterinarian. Many owners fail to recognise that their cat is ageing and are unaware of the changes expected with advancing years. The role of the veterinarian is to advise on the normal facets of ageing, and to discuss the implementation of simple management changes which may significantly alter the progression of ageing.

Nutrition

The lowered metabolic rate of the geriatric reduces energy requirements. Obesity may result if this is not accommodated. In addition, geriatrics may have a reduced ability to metabolise and excrete excess protein waste. The fat content of the diet should be reduced in order to restrict energy, but the fat present should be highly digestible and rich in essential fatty acids to compensate for reduced digestive function and to aid the absorption of fat soluble vitamins. A small amount of fibre in the diet will aid calorie restriction and will also enhance intestinal function. Moderately increased intakes of vitamins A, B_1, B_6, B_{12} and E are indicated. Mild phosphorus restriction is recommended to decrease renal excretory workload and glomerular hyperfiltration.

Taking all factors into consideration, simply feeding smaller amounts of a maintenance diet is often inadequate.[4] Diets specifically designed with the aged patient in mind may increase well-being and longevity. However, the diminished perception of smell and taste may significantly reduce appetite. A compromise is to find the highest quality diet, fulfilling most requirements, but which is palatable for the cat. Whatever is fed, it is advisable to decrease the amount offered per meal while increasing the frequency of feeding, thereby compensating for reduced digestive function and decreasing the time available for catabolic processes to commence. Abrupt changes in diet are rarely tolerated and may lead to episodes of vomiting and diarrhoea. Water must be available *ad libitum*.

General care

Dental care is extremely important in older animals. Cats are particularly intolerant of oral pain and a mild problem, well tolerated in another species, may lead to anorexia, adipsia, dehydration and lethargy.[8] Once the appropriate dental treatment has been instituted, home-care by the owner may be effective in preventing recurrence, or at least controlling it. With persistence, cats may tolerate brushing with a soft toothbrush or cotton bud coated with 0.1% chlorhexidine and hard dry foods will promote dental health.[8] Regular grooming, particularly in the long-haired varieties, should be encouraged. Immune competence diminishes and therefore annual booster vaccinations should be maintained.

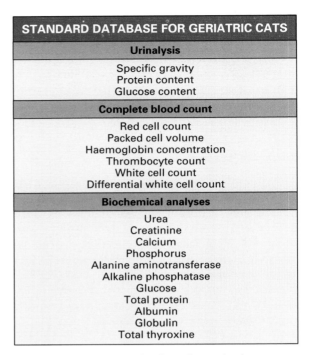

STANDARD DATABASE FOR GERIATRIC CATS
Urinalysis
Specific gravity
Protein content
Glucose content
Complete blood count
Red cell count
Packed cell volume
Haemoglobin concentration
Thrombocyte count
White cell count
Differential white cell count
Biochemical analyses
Urea
Creatinine
Calcium
Phosphorus
Alanine aminotransferase
Alkaline phosphatase
Glucose
Total protein
Albumin
Globulin
Total thyroxine

FIG. 6.1   Standard database for geriatric cats.

DISEASES OF THE GERIATRIC CAT

When dealing with the sick geriatric cat, the veterinary clinician must be aware of the complexity of problems that can exist and the potential for disease in one organ system to lead to dysfunction of other systems in the aged patient. To define adequately the primary disease process and to identify secondary problems (the presence of which may be masked by the primary problem or which may be subclinical, it is usually necessary to carry out a complete history, thorough physical examination, urinalysis, complete blood count, biochemical profile and, where indicated, thoracic and abdominal radiographs. Without this 'standard data base' (Fig. 6.1), unrecognised problems will progress, leading to a frustratingly inadequate response to therapy.

Certain diseases require special attention in the geriatric cat – see chapters dealing with chronic renal failure, hyperthyroidism, diabetes mellitus, hepatic disease and chronic bronchial disease.

The incidence of neoplasia in the older cat requires special mention. Haemolymphatic neoplasms represent the most common group and

COMMON NEOPLASMS OF THE GERIATRIC CAT	
Type	**% of all tumours**
Skin and subcutis	15 – 47
Epithelial (55%)	
Basal cell tumour	
Squamous cell carcinoma	
Adnexal tumours	
Mesenchymal (45%)	
Fibrosarcoma	
Mast cell tumour	
Digestive System	5 – 20
Oropharynx (20-54%)	
Squamous cell carcinoma	
Fibrosarcoma	
Gastrointestinal (60-80%)	
Adenocarcinoma	
Lymphosarcoma	
Hepatic neoplasms (9-24%)	
Hepatocellular carcinoma	
Bile duct adenocarcinoma/	
adenoma	
Pancreatic neoplasms (8-18%)	
Adenocarcinomas	
Mammary neoplasms	5 – 15
Adenocarcinomas (> 75%)	
Respiratory system	1 – 9
Intranasal/paranasal (73%)	
Squamous cell carcinoma	
Adenocarcinomas	
Bronchial/pulmonary (25%)	
Adenocarcinoma	
Bronchoalveolar carcinoma	
Squamous cell carcinoma	

FIG. 6.2   Common neoplasms of the geriatric cat.

generally occur in younger cats as a consequence of feline leukaemia virus infection. In general, the incidence of all other tumours increases with age, with most cats affected being more than 5 years old.[1,3] While tumours are more common in dogs than in the cat, the frequency of malignant tumours is considerably higher in cats. In older cats, neoplasia should always form part of a differential list and any 'lump' should be presumed malignant unless proven otherwise. Figure 6.2 lists the more common types of tumours seen in the older cat. For further information see Couto (1989).

PHARMACOLOGY, THERAPEUTICS AND AGEING

Many of the normal changes associated with ageing can affect the distribution, metabolism, clearance, effectiveness and potential toxicity of therapeutic drugs. These alterations may require modifications of drug dosage or regimen in older patients.

The effect of ageing on the absorption of drugs administered *per os* is probably minimal. Although there is a decrease in mucosal absorptive surface area, this is probably cancelled by a decrease in gastrointestinal transit time. The rate of subcutaneous absorption is probably reduced because of less interstitial fluid and vascularity, and the susceptibility of an aged patient to dehydration. Intramuscular injections tend to be more painful and are best avoided because of the decreased muscle mass and increased adiposity.

The increased total body fat and decreased lean body mass of the geriatric patient adversely affect drug distribution. Highly lipophilic drugs will be distributed into fat, resulting in decreased plasma concentrations and therefore lower efficacy. However, plasma half-life will be increased as the fat stores will act as a drug reservoir. Highly polar drugs will remain in the plasma compartment and be distributed poorly in body tissues, producing higher concentrations and increasing the potential for toxicity. Decreased hepatic metabolism, biliary excretion, renal blood flow and glomerular filtration rate increase the half-life of drugs in the geriatric patient.

Specific guidelines for adjusting each drug's dosage and dosing frequency are inadequately reported. In general, the lowest dosage and longest duration between dosing should be used. Caution should always be employed, with frequent assessments of efficacy and prompt withdrawal if any untoward effects are noted.

REFERENCES

1. Couto C.G. (1989) Oncology. In: Sherding R.G. (ed.) *The Cat. Diseases and Clinical Management*, Vol. 1, 589–647. Churchill Livingstone, New York.
2. Goldston R.T. (1990) Special considerations for the geriatric patient. *Proc. 8th Am. Coll. Vet. Int. Med. Forum*, 635–643.

3. Kitchell B.E. (1989) Feline geriatric oncology. *Comp. Cont. Educ. Pract. Vet.* **11**: 1079–1084.
4. Markham R.W., Hodgkins E.M. (1989) Geriatric nutrition. *Vet. Clin. N. Am.: Small Animal Practice* **19**: 165–185.
5. Mosier J.E. (1981) Canine geriatrics. *Proc. Am. Anim. Hosp. Assoc.* 137–145.
6. Mosier J.E. (1989) Effect of aging on body systems of the dog. *Vet. Clin. N. Am.: Small Animal Practice* **19**: 1–12.
7. Ross L.A. (1989) Healthy geriatric cats. *Comp. Cont. Educ. Pract. Vet.* **11**: 1041–1045.
8. Sams D.L., Harvey C.E. (1989) Oral and dental diseases. In Sherding R.G. (ed.) *The Cat. Diseases and Clinical Management*, Vol. 2, 875–906. Churchill Livingstone, New York.

7

Behavioural Problems

PETER NEVILLE

The human/cat relationship is based on many, often contrasting factors. Indoors the cat is valued for its cleanliness, affection and playfulness, and admired for its highly evolved play behaviour. Although not a group hunter, the cat retains an enormous capacity to be sociable and accepts the benefits of living in the human family and den without compromising its self-determining and independent behaviour. Outdoors the lack of compromise in the domestication of the cat is reflected in its ability and desire to hunt, even when well fed: the motivation to hunt is governed by instinctive behavioural patterns, triggered by the movement or sound of prey, and is independent from the immediate demands of hunger and appetite.

The cat views the members of its human family largely as maternal figures. In their company, the adult cat continues much of its kitten behaviour, such as relaxed purring, initiation of playful and affectionate encounters and willingness to respond to vocal and tactile cues. The frequent demonstration of affectionate responses of an infantile character helps to build an extremely strong bond between owner and cat, and it is essential to bear this bond in mind when treating a cat's medical or behavioural problems. Most cat owners will tolerate a much higher level of disruption to their social life and household hygiene than dog owners and are far less likely to apportion blame to a cat for its actions. They are often very sensitive to their cat's emotions and, being used to the idea that cats are not easily trained to perform set tasks, accept that their cat may not be causing problems deliberately; instead, they often blame themselves for any difficulties.

A breakdown of cases referred by veterinarians to clinics held by the author in veterinary hospitals in the United Kingdom and the Republic of Ireland and at the Dept of Veterinary Medicine at Bristol University Veterinary School is shown

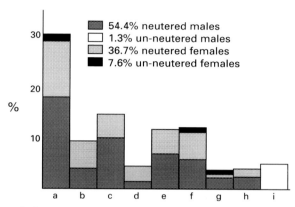

54.4% neutered males
1.3% un-neutered males
36.7% neutered females
7.6% un-neutered females

a: Indoor spraying
b: Other indoor marking (scratching, urination, middening)
c: House-training (loss of)   d: Nervous urination
e: Nervous conditions, eg. fear of visitors, agoraphobia
f: Aggression to other cats   g: Aggression to people
h: Self-mutilation   i: Other

FIG. 7.1   Author's practice caseload 1990–91.

in Fig. 7.1. Pro rata, owners of high-value breeds were more likely to seek help than owners of crossbred cats. While only 8% of British cats are of recognised breeds, 44% of the caseload involved pedigree strains, 14% first-cross pedigree strains and 42% domestic short-haired and long-haired cats. Most of the cats seen were between 1 and 5 years old, divided thus: 1–2 yr (26%), 2–3 yr (21%), 3–4 yr (18%) and 4–5 yr (11%). The most common case profile is a 1–2 year old neutered male domestic short-haired or Siamese cat which lives with one other cat and which sprays or soils inappropriately indoors.

Pedigree strains are more likely to be housed permanently indoors and so are more likely to present noticeable problems due to being sensitive to change within the home. The most popular breeds such as Siamese and Burmese are often reported by owners and breeders as being generally more 'sensitive', reactive or emotional, but this may be biased because owners observe and interact more with these cats compared with those that have access to the outdoors.

INDOOR MARKING (SCRATCHING, SPRAYING, MIDDENING)

Chin, head and flank rubbing are normal forms of scent marking and social communication which are encouraged by most owners but other types of marking behaviour may not be tolerated indoors. Scratching to strop claws can usually be transferred from furniture to an acceptable alternative (such as a post or board covered with sisal, hessian or bark) placed in front of the scratched furniture for a few days and then steadily moved away to a more convenient location once the cat has adopted it. When found scratching on any other surface indoors, the cat should gently be lifted away and placed at the new scratching post as quickly as possible and encouraged manually to continue there. Such training also usually works well with kittens and younger cats to prevent the problem from arising.

Scratching as a marking behaviour in the home often appears to be performed as a dominance gesture in the presence of other house cats. It should be treated in the same light as other forms of marking such as urine spraying, associative urination and defecation away from the litter tray. The latter two actions are often performed on beds or chairs, where the owner's smell is most concentrated and from which the cat presumably perceives the benefit of associating its smell with that of a protecting influence against challenges, real or imagined. The scenario most commonly cited by owners is defaecation on their bed or armchairs when they go on holiday and leave friends or minders to care for their cats. Associative marking can also occur on door mats, where challenging smells from the outside may be brought in on the owner's shoes.

In contrast, urine spraying is a more normal and frequent act of marking practised outdoors by most cats, both male and female, entire and neutered. Spraying is carried out from a standing position and usually a small volume of urine is directed backwards against a vertical post. Such marks help the perpetrators to feel more confident by surrounding themselves with their own familiar smell. The response of other cats to a spray mark is often to investigate it but then to continue normally rather than run away or exhibit fear. It does not necessarily present a challenge to other cats, though most cats are clearly able to distinguish between urine marks deposited by either sex.

When such marking occurs indoors (often against chairlegs, curtains etc.) it is usually a sign that the cat's lair is under some challenge. The cat, perhaps upset by strange smells or objects or new inhabitants, may be trying to repair 'scent holes' created in the security of its own protective surroundings by the change or intrusion. Most cats have no need to spray indoors because their lair is already perceived as secure and requires no further endorsement.

The challenge perceived by the cat may be an obvious one such as the recent arrival of another cat, a dog or, commonly, a new baby; it may be an increased challenge from a cat outdoors, or it may result from furniture being moved or changed, redecoration of the house, a family bereavement, unfamiliar guests staying, the introduction of novel items (especially plastic bags) or objects anointed by other cats, or even the loss of a contributor to the familiar communal smell that helps identify every member of the den.

The most commonly troublesome challenge is the installation of a cat flap, which can totally destroy the cat's sense of indoor security even without any rival cat or small local dog using the flap to enter the inner sanctum of the home. Spraying in this case probably occurs because the outdoors is suddenly perceived as continuous with the indoors and hence more susceptible to change or challenge. The home therefore needs to be re-anointed in a similar manner to the outdoors to identify occupancy and ensure that the resident encounters its own smell frequently.

Spraying by at least one cat is more common where increasing numbers of cats are expected to share a home base. However, this does not mean that the greater the number of cats in a household, the more likely it is that one or more will spray. It seems that there is a variable threshold in numbers, beyond which spraying and other attention-seeking behaviour is often suppressed. This suggests that acquiring one or more acceptable, confident, non-spraying companion cats might alleviate the problem for some animals.

It has been suggested that cats which spray indoors may be more restless generally and more active nocturnally than non-spraying cats, and may also be relatively more aggressive towards the owner. Protest spraying is observed particularly in some oriental breeds (which tend to have close attachments to their owners) when frustrated or denied their attention.

Treatment

The cause should be identified if possible and the cat's exposure to any physical challenges controlled. Local rival cats should be chased out of the garden; cat flaps should be boarded up to define den security; sprayed or middened areas should be cleaned as outlined in the 'House Soiling' section and baited similarly with dry food. The cat should never be punished either at the time or, worse, after the event, as this furthers indoor insecurity and increases the need to mark. However, confining the cat to one room when unsupervised can create a new safe 'core' which needs no further identification by spraying and this can be expanded gradually by one cleaned, baited room at a time, initially under the supervision of the owner. Despite the frustrations of owning an indoor sprayer, increased affection from the owner should be offered in frequent short doses, and frequent small meals of the cat's favourite food will also help the cat view its owner as a secure, maternal influence and help it relax indoors. Establishing routines of contact, feeding, grooming and play can also help the cat find security with its owners and in its home den and so reduce its feelings of vulnerability and negate the need to spray. Protest sprayers, however, should be ignored and the whole relationship between owner and cat restructured so that the cat only receives contact, food and affection at the owners initiation, in a manner similar to the treatment of over-demanding or dominant dogs. (This type of spraying may worsen initially before responding positively to treatment.) Drug support is very much case-dependent but a gradually

reducing dose of oral progestins (e.g. megestrol acetate at 2.5 mg bid orally for week 1, dropping by one-third over successive weeks while management and relationship changes are introduced) or sedatives (e.g. diazepam, up to 1 mg tid orally for 2–3 weeks) may assist treatment. However, the potential side-effects of megestrol acetate should be considered (see page 000).

HOUSE SOILING

Inappropriate urination and defaecation, as acts of normal elimination or as a result of nervousness, should first be distinguished from deliberate acts of marking by urine spraying described earlier or associative marking by urination and middening. Most cats instinctively tend to use loose substrate such as cat litter as their latrine when first venturing from the maternal nest, and learn by experimentation and perhaps some observation of their mother that litter is a surface on and in which to excrete. Prior to this they are unable to excrete without physical stimulation from the mother. Initially this is carried out in the nest and the action enables the mother to clean all waste and prevent the kittens from soiling the nest. This process is developed when the mother carries the kittens out of the nest and licks them to stimulate excretion with the result that the majority of cats are taught early never to soil their own bed. The house is often seen as an extension of the bed and a feeding lair in adulthood. Excretion therefore normally takes place away from it, or remains specifically targeted into a litter tray.

Poor maternal care can disrupt this latrine-association learning process and occasionally kittens are weaned without becoming house-trained, especially some Persian strains. For others, medical or emotional trauma, especially during the cat's adolescence, decreases the security of home and an initial breakdown in hygiene may then continue long after the source of the problem has disappeared or been treated. Cats that are generally nervous or incompetent may excrete repeatedly indoors rather than venture outside.

The siting and nature of the litter tray can affect toileting behaviour. Being offered food too close to the tray will deter many cats from using it, and positioning of the tray in a site that is too busy, open or otherwise vulnerable may also cause cats to seek safer places. Some cats that are normally fastidious in their personal hygiene are reluctant to use soiled or damp trays, or to share with other cats. Trays may need to be cleaned more frequently or more trays may need to be provided.

The type of litter offered is another important factor. Certain compressed wood pellet litters appear to be less comfortable for cats to stand on, especially for cats living permanently indoors which may have more sensitive pads than cats whose feet are toughened by an outdoor lifestyle. Litter which releases deodorizing scents when damp has also been implicated in deterring cats from urinating in the tray, possibly because it may irritate the pads when it is damp. Inflammation and cornification of the pads should be looked for in such cases. Litter containing chlorophyll is also reported as being unattractive to some cats and should be changed when problems arise.

Cats may also associate pain and discomfort with their tray if they are suffering from cystitis, feline lower urinary tract disease, colitis or constipation. They may then seek alternative surfaces and continue to find carpets or beds more attractive as latrines. Other cats simply forget where the tray is, get 'caught short', or become lazy or less mobile in old age and need more trays or easier access to them.

Treatment

It is often worth trying a finer grain commercial litter or fine sterile sand which cats, perhaps because of their desert ancestry, seem to find more attractive than woodchip pellets or coarse grain litters. Some litters clump when wet, and these can be more convenient to remove when cleaning the litter tray. The position of the tray should be checked, especially relative to the position of food bowls and for security. Placing the tray in a corner or offering a covered tray or, if the cat is unwilling to be enclosed, at least a tray with sides but no roof, may help to improve the security of the latrine. The tray should be cleaned less frequently to allow the smell of cat's urine to accumulate (which improves identification and association and the smell itself may stimulate animals to urinate) but the cat may be deterred if the whole litter surface is allowed to get too dirty or too damp. Once-per-day cleansing per cat is usually adequate. For vaccinated outdoor cats, up to 50% garden soil can be added to the litter or sand. Transfer to using the outdoors can be achieved over a period of 2–3 weeks by moving the indoor tray progressively nearer the door and then out on to the step and finally into the garden.

For serious cases, confinement in a small room for a few days may help to reduce the opportunity for mistakes. Confinement in a pen where a simple choice between tray and bed can be provided may ensure that any early learning is reinforced. The cat can steadily be allowed more freedom indoors, one room at a time, when able to target excretion into the tray. Previously soiled areas in the house must be cleaned thoroughly but never with an agent that contains ammonia as this is a constituent of urine and may endorse the idea of the cleaned area being a latrine. Many proprietary agents and cleaners only mask the smell to the human nose and may not be effective for the cat. Instead, the use of a warm solution of a biological detergent may be followed by a wipe or scrub down with surgical spirit or other alcohol. (Certain dyes in fabrics may be affected and so should be checked first for fastness under this cleaning system.) Cleaned areas should be thoroughly dry before the cat is allowed supervised access. Bowls of dry cat food may act as a deterrent to toileting at cleaned sites.

The cat should never be punished, even if caught in the act. Punishment makes cats more nervous and more likely to excrete in the house, even in the presence of the owner. Instead, the cat should be calmly placed on its tray or outside the house to continue. Timing of feeding can help to make faecal passage time more predictable in kittens and young cats and enable the cat to be put in the right place at the right time. Drug support is usually only helpful in cases of inappropriate excretion caused by nervousness, when oral sedatives for 1–2 weeks in addition to management may be beneficial.

ATTACHMENT/BONDING DIFFICULTIES

The critical time for socialising kittens with humans, other cats, dogs and a normal household environment, is at 2–7 weeks of age. Most problems of nervousness and social incompetence in adult cats would never have arisen had they been handled intensively during this period and exposed to a wide range of stimuli and experiences. At 4–12 weeks (prior to completion of vaccination courses) they should be subjected to as complex and active a home environment as possible. Though kittens are blind and deaf at birth, imprinting on the mother cat probably occurs in the few hours after birth through smell, and so handling a new-born kitten may also help produce a friendlier, more tractable pet later.

It has been suggested that there are two distinct character types in cats: one with a high requirement for social contact and one for which such contact may be tolerated but not seen as an essential feature of the quality of life. Cats in the latter group seem to have a higher requirement for play and predatory activity rather than affectionate interactions. A cat may therefore need to live with other cats and be socially less competent on its own, or need to lead a solitary life and be less able to be sociable with other cats. In its relations with humans it is suggested that a cat will either have a high requirement for physical contact and petting from the owner, or will never appreciate it even if the owner is very insistent at trying to provide it. Cats more typical of this second category may well prove less rewarding as pets, especially to those owners seeking a very affectionate relationship based on physical contact with the cat. However, these categorisations take little account of a cat's temperament changes in adulthood, or resulting from personality differences between one owner and the next. Furthermore, improvements may also result from trying to treat individual aggressive or nervous conditions.

Under-attachment

Cats perceived by their owners to be 'under-attached' are often intolerant of the owner's proximity or approach; they especially dislike handling and fail to relax when held. Causes may include a lack of early socialization, over-enthusiasm on the part of the owner, trauma or necessarily invasive handling during illness, leading to fear of the owner's subsequent approach.

Treatment

Treatment involves increasing the cat's bond with and dependence on the owner. A major feature is feeding frequent, small, attractive meals preceded by much vocal communication and encouraging the cat to follow the owner for its food. Feeding while attempting gentle handling along the cat's back only is the next step. Actions that may improve the cat's perception of the owner as rewarding include steadily increasing the frequency and intensity of handling, offering treats at other times, and occupying favoured resting positions on the floor by the fire or radiator so that the cat comes to sit on the owner to gain access. Owners should discontinue all efforts to chase the cat with a view to handling, especially if the cat seems to fit the second, less sociable categorisation of temperament and is of a more predatory and less affectionate nature generally. The more an owner tries to initiate contact with this type of cat, the less time it will actually spend in voluntary contact with the owner. If, however, owners make themselves more attractive to their under-attached cats by offering food, titbits and toys or by lying passively by favourite resting places and allowing the cat to initiate the interaction, then the total time spent with the cat will increase. In severe cases the cat can be penned for a short time to accustom it to close human presence and owners can try to approach the cat carefully, head first, to simulate the greeting behaviour observed between friendly cats; hands (perhaps otherwise viewed as threatening weapons) should only be introduced slowly afterwards. It is essential that owners always respond positively with an affectionate touch and a calm, gentle voice to any initiating gesture the cat may make in approaching them in the home, especially for cats which are allowed outdoors. Drug support is usually not necessary except with severely traumatised cats or those unhandled before about 8 weeks of age, but tapered prescription of progestins may help if they can be administered without causing distress.

Over-attachment

The over-attached cat may be agitated or nervous when isolated, and such cats often demonstrate prolonged infantile behaviour, sucking their owner's clothes or skin. Owners may then feel guilty about rejecting the cat's affection, or fear loss of contact if they do not respond, and are often at fault themselves in encouraging close association so that a very young cat fails to lose sucking and other nursing responses after weaning. Over-attachment may also occur after intensive nursing during illness, or during old age when the cat becomes increasingly dependent and may follow its owner constantly, perhaps crying regularly in an effort to attract physical contact, especially when it has been left alone or feels insecure during the night. Once the owner has responded to the cat's distress calls by getting up (perhaps because they suspect some medical problem in their ageing pet), the reassured cat often simply settles down to sleep.

Treatment

Treatment involves detachment by non-punishing rejection of the cat's advances, together with periodic physical separation and replacement by alternative forms of affectionate contact for short periods of time, initiated by the owner. Provision of novel objects helps the cat to learn to explore. Aversion therapy using loud startling noises, or a jet of water, can be used in severe cases. Old cats can be offered a secure, warm bed in the owner's bedroom and will usually then remain reassured and quiet through the night without needing to cry out to gain their immediate physical attention.

NERVOUSNESS, PHOBIAS AND SEPARATION ANXIETIES

Nervousness, phobias and separation anxieties are presented as a range of problems that vary from the cat failing to adapt to 'normal' household events (such as noise and visitors) to lack of confidence in individual family members, failure to cope when away from the owner, and agoraphobia. Cats may be shy and fearful if not exposed to a range of experiences and handling during the 'sensitive period' at 2–7 weeks of age. This is particularly likely if they are the type with play/predatory temperaments and they are pursued too frequently or handled too roughly at any stage. Behaviour includes becoming withdrawn and secretive, moving fearfully with a low crouching gait and dilated pupils, reluctance to enter open spaces or go outdoors, inappetence, or psychogenic vomiting in very severe cases. Low-threshold flight reactions and defensive (fear) aggression may occur if the cat is unable to avoid the challenge. Cats with such fears may have suffered a lack of early social experience or a trauma; agoraphobia, for example, can be based upon fear of attack by cats outdoors. Indeed, agoraphobia is the only recognised genuine phobia reported in cats. Old age and its associated loss of competence may also be a factor in the development of nervous conditions.

Treatment

Systematic desensitization involving controlled exposure to known problem stimuli can be presented in low but increasing doses, while denying the opportunity to escape and so providing the possibility for habituation. With general nervousness or incompetence this is best achieved by penning the cat indoors (or outdoors for agoraphobic cats) and forcing it to experience 'normal' household events – such as the sound of everyday kitchen utensils and machines, proximity of visitors, the family and other pets – while protected. The cat may thus come to learn that their presence is not threatening, though care must be exercised to avoid exposing the cat to too much too soon. Frequent short meals should be offered by an increasing number of people, including visitors. Detachment from an over-favoured member will encourage the cat to spread its loyalties to more people. Drug support is often helpful. Oral progestins and sedatives can be administered as before, during desensitization.

OVER-GROOMING AND SELF-MUTILATION

Most cats groom their flanks or back when confused, immediately after some mild upset or when unable to avoid general threatening stimuli. The behaviour seems to have little effect on layering or quality of the coat but apparently serves to relieve stress. This function may be mediated, as in social monkeys, by the release of opiates from grooming and repetitive self-interested behaviour patterns. The behaviour is usually harmless but occasionally a cat will over-groom in response to continued stress such as the presence of too many cats in the house, the introduction of a dog, an emotional disturbance between family members, isolation from its owner, physical punishment or harassment by the owner for other behaviours such as house-soiling. Grooming may progress to the point of breaking hairshafts and producing a balding appearance on the flanks, the base of the tail, the abdominal area or the legs. In severe cases of unresolved stress or in particularly sensitive or incompetent individuals, the cat may actually pluck out large quantities of fur and cause large bald patches. In its initial stages this is often secretive behaviour, as the cat may feel more comfortable in the owner's presence and so refrain from the activity, but in the later stages the cat may mutilate itself in their presence as well. This is an area where behaviourists and dermatologists are now conferring as it is thought that these reactions can also be triggered by flea allergy or sensitivity to diet, and occasionally by allergy to household dust, but then go far past the normal groom or scratch behaviour because of some underlying 'stress' (see Chapter 22).

Actual self-mutilation of body tissue is extremely rare and severe self-inflicted damage is usually directed at itchy infected plucked areas or, less explicably but typically, at the tail or mouth. In these cases the behaviour is usually manic and occurs in frequent or occasional episodes, which may be self-reinforcing because of the euphoria engendered by the release of opiates. Many cases, such as sporadic clawing at the tongue presented approximately every six months by one Burmese cat in the UK, have no obvious clinical, environmental or psychological cause. Other obsessive compulsive disorders which have been described in cats include air-licking, prolonged staring, air-batting, jaw-snapping, pacing, head-shaking, freezing, paw-shaking and aggressive attacks at the tail or feet accompanied sometimes by yowling.

Treatment

Any dermatosis should initially be investigated for medical disorders (for example, flea sensitivity, atopy or dietary allergy) and treated accordingly (see Chapter 22). Behaviour therapy can only be considered when such disorders have been ruled out, or as an associative treatment. If separation anxiety is suspected, building up the competence of a cat to cope alone by restructuring its relations with the owner is required. Stimulation with novel objects and situations, and controlled change of husbandry patterns, can also be offered. Generally increased levels of contact initiated by the owner may also help to define relations better and to offer more security in the home without the cat becoming over-dependent on the owner's presence. Self-mutilation can sometimes be resolved in single cats by the acquisition of another cat. The use of an Elizabethan collar for a short time may also help healing and perhaps break any learned behaviour patterns. During severe episodes of mutilation, the cat may also be distracted with sudden movement, loud noises or jets of water.

The sedative diazepam may be given as immediate treatment to control severe episodes of self-mutilation and on a lower dose during lifestyle modification lasting several weeks. Some cats become hyper-excitable as a result of this treatment, though this is not dose-related and disappears after above five days of treatment without loss of beneficial effects. Anti-convulsants such as phenobarbital and anti-depressant and anti-anxiety drugs such as amitriptyline, clomipramine and fluoxetine have been employed with some success in cats and dogs in Canada, although they are not approved for use in these species. Morphine antagonists such as naloxone may inhibit the behaviour, perhaps by enabling the animal to feel the pain of its self-mutilation. Unfortunately, this drug is only active for 20 minutes or so, but longer acting versions such as nalmefene have shown promising results. The effectiveness of any drugs at treating such problems is believed to be influenced by the length of time the behaviour has been expressed and the presence and ability of the owner to control conflicts and stresses in the cat's lifestyle and home environment.

AGGRESSION

Aggression towards other cats

Aggression towards other cats may vary from occasional or frequent hissing or scuffling between two individuals in multi-cat households to serious physical attacks against all cats on sight, indoors or out. Despotic aggression, victimisation and, most commonly, persistent intolerance of new feline arrivals to the household are all quite common. Behaviour may include physical attack, low threshold arousal in response to the sight or movement of other cats, or a total lack of initial investigatory or greeting behaviour. The cat may also be generally hyperactive and territorial. Nape-biting and mounting of younger or passive cats may also be observed. Aggression rarely seems to be a defensive reaction, but occasionally attack becomes a learned policy to avoid investigation by other cats.

Depending on its early experiences, a cat may have an emotional need to share a home base with other cats or to be more solitary. In the latter case, the cat may be able to tolerate other house cats but never forms close social ties based on mutual grooming and resource sharing. Causes may include individual dislike or intolerance of one or more individual cats, or lack of social learning or contact with other cats when young. There may be marked territorial defence reactions with failure to recognise and respond to friendly or neutral reactions from other cats, which may compound the success of early assertive or rough play with siblings. Territorial defence reactions and mutual intolerance of entire male cats, and defence of kittening areas by fertile and oestrous queens or kitten defence by mothers are normal and expected forms of aggression and not regarded as treatable. Finally, medical conditions such as hyperthyroidism, brain lesions and diet sensitivity may also lead to aggressive behaviour and diagnosis and treatment of any underlying clinical problem should be tackled wherever possible by the veterinary practitioner prior to attempts to modify what may be only a behavioural sign of the condition.

Treatment

Treatment is highly variable. Controlled frequent exposure to new arrivals by housing the original cat and the new arrival alternately in an individual pen allows protected introductions and establishes the occupancy of the new cat physically in terms of incorporating its scent in the resident's home territory. Distraction techniques such as bringing cats together when feeding, initially with one cat in the pen and the other outside but fed progressively closer to the pen, modification of owner relations (especially with more 'rank-conscious' oriental breeds) and instilling a hierarchy favouring the top cat in all greeting and play have all been known to help. Rubbing catnip essence on to the fur of both cats or intensive alternate grooming to transfer respective body scent can further the acceptability of one cat to the other during controlled introductions and subsequent freer encounters. For the sake of safety, however, only when the protagonists cease to become aroused at the sight of each other on introductions should unsupervised free contact be allowed. In severe cases, the only safe option may be the rehoming of one of the cats, usually the one most recently acquired.

Drug support includes tapered doses of progestins, anti-androgenic injectables which may calm the aggressor (even if neutered), and sedatives. Some 'complementary' treatments may also help a traumatised victim relax more during controlled introductions.

Aggression towards visitors and owners

Cats may attack people, grabbing them with claws and biting, though this is rarely accompanied by vocalisation. The behaviour is often sudden and unpredictable; it may be predatory in origin and triggered by sudden movement such as passing feet, or occasionally by certain high-pitched sounds. Defensive aggression to prevent handling is often caused by a lack of either early socialization or gentle human contact. Predatory chasing of feet and other moving body targets, territorial defence, especially in narrow or confined areas (only seen so far in oriental breeds), hyper-excitement during play, dominant aggression towards people when vulnerable (e.g. lying or sitting down), occasionally food guarding and kitten defence against owners by nursing mothers have all been recorded. Most problematic is redirected aggression by very territorial cats agitated by the sight of rivals through a window: the movement of owners who approach to pacify their cat may inadvertently stimulate an attack. 'Petting and biting syndrome' also occurs in many cats but this is usually tolerated or avoided by the owner. Initially the cat accepts affection but it may then suddenly lash out, grab and bite the owner, and then leap away to effect escape. The threshold of reaction is usually high and injury slight.

Treatment

Treatment must always be considered in relation to the member of the family most at risk, especially those with jerky or unpredictable movement patterns (such as children and elderly relatives). Controlled exposure to habituate the cat to normal family movements and activities can help. However, stimulation in the form of another carefully introduced cat (preferably a kitten, which may be less threatening than a more socially, territorially or sexually competitive adult) together with the opportunity to go outdoors (free-ranging where possible, or perhaps on a harness and lead in urban areas), frequent presentation of novel objects and concentrated play sessions (predatory chase, capture) of half an hour per day can be highly therapeutic. The use of a moving target such as a ball or string to attract the release of aggression will help an excited or frustrated cat more safely and facilitate owner intervention afterwards with less risk.

Diet sensitivity and its effects on feline behaviour are little understood but may be investigated by providing a home-prepared diet of chicken and rice for two weeks. Once the effect of diet on behaviour has been established, the cat can then often be managed on a different complete dry or canned food to the one used before and its behaviour monitored carefully. Access to catnip toys should be denied during assessment, to preclude concomitant excitability in sensitive cats.

Drug support using progestins for 3–6 weeks may help and some 'complementary' medicinal approaches have produced excellent responses in easily agitated oriental breeds in particular, especially Burmese cats.

PICA

Pica is the depraved ingestion of non-nutritional items. The disposition is usually thought to be inherited though is otherwise unexplained. The eating of house plants may be due to the desire to obtain roughage or a source of minerals and vitamins and is regarded as a normal feature of ingestive behaviour which only becomes a problem if excessive or targeted onto toxic or valuable house plants. Occasional cases are reported of cats eating rubber and electric cables but the main problem concerns the ingestion of wool and other fabric. Wool eating was first documented in the 1950s and was thought to be limited to Siamese strains, but a recent survey of 152 fabric-eating cats shows the behaviour to be more widespread. Responses to the survey showed that fabric eating was presented most often by Siamese (55% of responders) and Burmese (28%) cats, occasionally by other oriental strains and, more rarely, by crossbred cats (11%). Males are as likely culprits as females and the majority of responders were neutered. The typical age of onset for fabric eating is 2–8 months. Most cats (93% in the survey) start by consuming wool, perhaps attracted by the smell of lanolin, but later transfer to other fabrics: 64% in the survey ate cotton and 54% consumed synthetic fabric as well as wool.

While some fabric eaters chew or eat material on a regular basis, others act in sporadic bursts. Many consume large amounts of material such as woollen jumpers and cotton towels, underwear, furniture covers etc, without apparent harm, although surgery is required in a few cases to clear gastric obstructions and impaction of material. Some have caused such a high level of economic damage to property that they have been euthanased, but most owners of fabric-eating cats seem remarkably tolerant of their cat's behaviour.

The exact cause of the behaviour is unknown but a variety of factors have been considered, including genetic ones. Wool eating is suggested to be a largely inherited trait, though rarely expressed, caused by a physiologically based hyperactivity of the autonomic nervous system. Such neuronal disturbances could affect the control of the digestive tract and thereby produce unusual food cravings and inappropriate appetite stimulation, although the exact mechanism is unclear.

Another suggestion is that the desire to suck and knead fabric is a redirected form of suckling behaviour that results from the failure of the cat to mature fully. Some cats grow out of the behaviour at maturity but others will continue to eat fabric despite good nutrition and husbandry. The behaviour is usually more prevalent in cats housed permanently indoors. Fabric eating is sometimes secretive but it is usually blatant and unaffected by punishment. While most cats will consume fabric at any time, some will take a woollen item to the food bowl and eat this alternately with their usual diet and only at meal-times.

Fabric eating may sometimes be triggered by some form of stress, perhaps in the form of medical treatment, or the introduction of another cat to the household. A significant number of cats in the survey first exhibited fabric eating within one month of acquisition. Insufficient handling of kittens before adoption or separation from the mother at too early an age may also lead to stress and trigger the behaviour.

Continuing infantile traits such as over-dependence on the physical presence of the owner can lead to separation anxiety when the owner departs and cause the cat to start to eat fabric. The behaviour may then be triggered during subsequent stressful experiences as a learned pattern, even in response to previously tolerated influences. The best hope for treatment of fabric eating probably rests with such cases, where the relationship between owner and cat can be modified so that the cat is made less dependent on its owner for emotional security and the need to eat fabric as a form of anxiety-relieving displacement behaviour can be reduced.

Fabric eating also seems to form part of a prey catching/ingestion sequence usually unexpressed in the day-to-day repertoires of a pet cat which is fed prepared and easily digested food. Indeed, 40% of the cats reported in the survey had little or no access to the outdoors and hence restricted or no opportunity to develop exploratory and hunting behaviour, including ingestion of small prey.

Treatment

Treatment currently involves a combination approach of social restructuring with the owner (see Over-attachment) and increasing the level of stimulation for the cat through play, increased activity at home, opportunity to investigate novel stimuli and, where possible, the opportunity for indoor cats to lead an outdoor life. This can mean allowing free outdoor access or housing in a secure outdoor pen or accustoming the cat to being walked on a lead and harness.

Increasing the fibre content of the diet has also brought improvements in many, and even a few total cures, in the form of bran or tissue paper and gristly meat chunks blended in with their usual wet canned diet. Aromatic taste deterrents such as eucalyptus oil or mentol applied to woollen clothes may be employed, though traditional deterrents using pepper or chilli powder seem only to broaden the cat's normal taste preferences! Remote aversion tactics using touch-sensitive cap exploders under clothes deliberately made available can deter some cats and some may be safely channelled into chewing only acceptable items at meal and resting times. Owners have found that such cats need to be kept supplied with a cheap stock of the favourite fabric in order to preserve other clothes and household items. No drugs are as yet recognised as being helpful with treatment.

COUNSELLING OWNERS AND TREATING BEHAVIOUR PROBLEMS IN CATS

Counselling owners of cats with behavioural problems involves patience, understanding and, most of all, time. Owners will often be distressed not only because of a soiled house or scratched furniture but because they feel that the cat itself is upset. Many problems occur as a result of lack of awareness of the cat's requirements, poor or changed indoor facilities, unrealistic owner expectations or inappropriate interactive behaviour between the owner and cat or cats. The initial aim of treatment is therefore to establish communication with the owner so that a full history can be given and all concerns expressed without fear of ridicule or rejection. This is usually assisted by the presence of the cat itself, even if only in a basket in the surgery. The initial phases of consultation at least should be held in private and the process should not be disturbed. After consultation it is essential that the consultant remains available and contactable by telephone to receive progress reports and deal with continuing concerns.

Very few problems have simple answers and most necessitate the recording of a complete problem history, relevant medical history, lifestyle and relationship data within the family. The nature of the home environment is crucial both to the cause of many problems and, through modification of access, in the treatment of most.

PSYCHOACTIVE DRUGS

Treatment of many cases may be facilitated in the short term by supportive drug therapy, though this can rarely be recommended in the long term. Progestins, in decreasing doses over a few weeks, are most frequently used as 'calming agents' to assist behavioural modification techniques rather than for any identifiable hormonal influence. Anti-androgenic injectables are employed for the same reasons, most frequently on a single dose basis. Sedatives and other compounds such as anti-depressants and morphine antagonists may be used as required in the treatment of obsessive compulsive disorders such as self-mutilation.

Occasionally, homoeopathic and other 'complementary' treatments have been employed under the guidance of a veterinary surgeon with a special interest in that area. With many cases of aggression or indoor spraying by oriental breeds, these alternative approaches were found to be more helpful than traditional medicine and, although this cannot be explained, it should not be overlooked.

In all cases, drug support of any kind is rarely curative and usually inhibits learning. The use of drugs often has to be based on a trial-and-error approach as there are marked variations in response between breeds and individuals. Where used, drugs are offered as a short-term vehicle to facilitate the application and acceptance by the cat of management, husbandry or behaviour modification techniques and to facilitate learning by degree during systematic desensitisation. The use of psychoactive drugs, especially progestins, without any behaviour modification advice has often been tried by veterinarians prior to referral and found to be ineffective, or only effective in modifying the cat's behaviour for the period of dosage. Progestins especially are usually best offered only after a failed period of treatment without drug support and only on a reducing dose for no more than 3–4 weeks and in support of behaviour modification advice.

After consultation, the owner should receive a letter summarizing the analysis and cause(s) of the problem, suggestions for treatment, rationale behind any accompanying supportive drug therapy, and perhaps the likelihood and timescale for successful treatment.

FURTHER READING

Association of Pet Behaviour Counsellors (1990). *Annual Report 1990*. London.

Hart B.L. and Hart L.A. (1985) *Canine and Feline Behavioural Therapy*. Lea and Febiger, Philadelphia.

Luescher U.A., McKeown D.B. and Halip J. (1991) Stereotypic or obsessive compulsive disorders in dogs and cats. In *Advances in Companion Animal Behaviour. Veterinary Clinics of North America* **21**(2). W.B. Saunders Company. Philadelphia.

Neville P.F. (1990) *Do Cats Need Shrinks?* Sidgwick and Jackson Pan MacMillan, London.

Neville P.F. (1992) *CLAWS . . . and purrs. Understanding both sides of your cat*. Sidgwick and Jackson Pan MacMillan, London.

Turner D.C. and Bateson P. (eds) (1988) *The Domestic Cat – the biology of its behaviour*. Cambridge University Press, Cambridge.

Turner D.C. and Stammbach-Geering M.K. (1990) Owner assessment and the ethology of human-cat relationships. In *Pets, Benefits and Practice*. British Veterinary Association Publications, London. Waltham Symposium 20, Ed. I.H. Burger. pp 25–30.

8

Pharmacology and Toxicology

SUE MAYER

DRUG METABOLISM

Most of the process of drug metabolism takes place in the liver and tends to fall into two phases. In Phase I, the drug is broken down by oxidation, reduction or hydrolysis. This may make the compound either less or more active. In Phase II the product of Phase I or the original drug is joined, or conjugated with compounds such as amino-acids, carbohydrates, acetic acid or inorganic sulphate. The resulting product can then be excreted.

The production of glucuronide is one of the major conjugation reactions in most species. In the cat, however, conjugation with glucuronic acid is deficient. The reaction may be up to 100 times slower than in other species. This is thought to be because of a relatively low level of glucuronyl transferase. This metabolic deficiency has particular implications, for both therapy and toxicology in the cat, which will emerge later. A large number of drugs are conjugated with sulphate rather than glucuronic acid for the cat.

Pharmacokinetic studies are particularly important, as the cat's impaired ability to conjugate with glucuronic acid may result in a reduced rate of excretion and thus there is a danger of drug accumulation and resultant toxicity. For instance, it has been determined that a drug such as acetyl salicylic acid (aspirin), which is only very slowly metabolised and excreted by cats, could be given on a 24 hour or longer protocol without causing accumulation.

THERAPEUTIC AGENTS

Sedatives and anticonvulsants

Diazepam

Diazepam is a benzodiazapine which has anxiolytic, sedative and anticonvulsant properties. It is also reported to be useful in briefly increasing appetite in anorexic cats.[9] It has a short half-life of 5.5 h which tends to restrict its clinical usefulness as a general tranquilliser. However, it is very valuable and safe in the acute treatment of convulsions and excitement.

Phenobarbitone

Phenobarbitone is probably the most useful long-term anticonvulsant available for cats. Initial dose rate is 2–4 mg/kg divided between two doses. This may have to be increased as tolerance develops with the induction of hepatic microsomal enzymes involved in metabolising the drug.

Primidone

Some authors consider primidone too toxic for use in the cat but some studies contradict this view.[5] Therefore it is probably wise to avoid this drug routinely but to be aware that it may be found to be useful in feline medicine in the future. Such conflicts merely serve to illustrate the paucity of pharmacokinetics and clinical pharmacology studies undertaken in the cat.

Phenothiazines

Acetylpromazine is the most widely used phenothiazine in cats, largely for anaesthetic premedication and as a sedative for travel. Although some reports suggest it may cause aberrant behaviour, this is disputed. Acetylpromazine should not normally be used as an anticonvulsant: it is well recognised that it may lower the threshold at which a convulsion will occur. Nor should it be used in situations where an animal is in either hypovolaemic or normovolaemic shock, because its hypotensive effects can be life threatening.

FIG. 8.1 The classification of non-steroidal anti-inflammatory drugs, their plasma half lives in dogs and cats (when available), and their relative safety in the cat.

NON-STEROIDAL ANTI-INFLAMMATORY DRUGS				
		Half life (hours)		
Class	**Examples**	**Cat**	**Dog**	**Safety**
Carboxylic acids				
Salicylates	Acetylsalicylic acid	22	9	C
Quinolones	Cinchophen		8	C
Aminonicotinic acids	Flunixin	4	3	P
	Clonixin			N
Propionic acids	Naproxen			N
	Ibuprofen			N
	Flurbiprofen			N
	Carprofen			N
Anthranilic acids	Meclofenamic acid			N
	Mefanamic acid			N
	Tolfenamic acid	7	8	P
Indolines	Indomethacin			N
Enolic acids				
Pyrazolones	Phenylbutazone			C
	Oxybutazone			C
Oxicams	Piroxicam			N
	Miloxicam			N
	Tenoxicam			N

Key
C = can be used with care
P = shows potential for use in cats
N = not enough data available to determine safety

Anti-inflammatory drugs

The pharmacology and therapeutics of the non-steroidal anti-inflammatory drugs (NSAIDs) have been reviewed recently.[3,4] The two broad classifications of NSAIDs as carboxylic or enolic acids can be further subdivided as shown in Fig. 8.1. The main therapeutic effects of NSAIDs are central analgesia and antipyrexia, plus peripheral anti-inflammatory action as well as anti-thrombotic and antiendotoxaemic effects. All these effects are considered to be mediated by the prevention of prostaglandin production by inhibition of cyclo-oxygenase. The differential spectrum of effects of the different NSAIDs probably reflects differences in their activity against cyclo-oxygenases in different tissues.

Prolonged half-lives and acute toxicity are not seen with all the NSAIDS and an indication of half-lives and safety (where available) is indicated in Fig. 8.1. Better tolerated NSAIDs may become available with further study. The more general toxic effects of NSAIDs in terms of gastrointestinal damage, (particularly following prolonged administration) are also seen in the cat.

Aspirin

Relatively little is known of the pharmacokinetics of the majority of NSAIDs in cats. Best described is the fate of acetylsalicyclic acid, which has a half-life of 22 hours in the cat compared with 9 hours in the dog.[3] Suggested dose rates of aspirin in the cat range from 25 mg/kg every 24 hours to 42 mg/kg every 77 hours. Signs of aspirin toxicity are given in Fig. 8.2, and the treatment of such poisoning is aimed at restoring acid-base balance through intravenous fluid therapy with Ringer's lactate or glucose saline supplemented with bicarbonate, alkalinising the urine to increase excretion (see later).

TOXICITY FROM ASPIRIN AND PHENYLBUTAZONE	
Aspirin	**Phenylbutazone**
Clinical signs	
Depression	Depression
Inappetence	Inappetence
Inco-ordination	Vomiting
Vomiting	Weight loss
Diarrhoea	
Jaundice	
Coma	
Death	
Diagnostic findings	
Aciduria	Anaemia
Anaemia	Haemorrhagic gastroenteritis
Heinz body formation	Hepatitis
Increased WBC count	Renal damage
Toxic hepatitis	
Haemorrhagic gastroenteritis	
Reduced platelet function	
Ecchymotic haemorrhages	

FIG. 8.2 The clinical signs and diagnostic findings of toxicity from aspirin (acetyl salicylic acid) and phenylbutazone in the cat.

Phenylbutazone

The use of phenylbutazone in the cat has to be undertaken cautiously. Dosage should be less than that for dogs. A dose of 5–12 mg/kg bid PO should not result in toxicity. However, courses should be short and administration stopped if there is any sign of inappetence or depression. Signs of toxicity are given in Fig. 8.2.

Steroidal anti-inflammatory drugs

The use of corticosteroids in cats is broadly similar to their use in other species and no special considerations apply. Megestrol acetate, a synthetic analogue of progesterone which also has glucocorticoid activity, is widely used as an anti-inflammatory as well as for behaviour modification and reproductive control. Prolonged treatment can result in adverse side effects such as endometritis, pyometra, diabetes, mammary hyperplasia and adenocarcinoma.

Analgesics

Morphine

Cats have a greater sensitivity to several opiate analgesics and morphine at the dose rates used in other species. Apprehension, excitement and even mania can develop at very high dosage. However, at low dose rates of 0.1–0.2 mg/kg SC, morphine produces good analgesia without excitement.

Pethidine

Pethidine can be used at levels of 2.5–10 mg/kg SC to give analgesia without depression or excitement. The usefulness of the analgesia and its duration of action are widely debated.

Codeine

Opinions vary on the safety of codeine in the cat and there is little specific information available. Dose rates of 0.25–1.0 mg/kg PO appear safe but the preparation used should be chosen carefully as many proprietary brands combine codeine with aspirin or paracetamol.

Diphenoxylate

Diphenoxylate is found in antidiarrhoeal preparations but is toxic and should be avoided. Excitement and mydriasis progressing to blindness and ataxia have been reported. It is probably safer to use loperamide in these situations.

Paracetamol

Paracetamol (acetaminophen) is extremely toxic for cats and should never be used. Because conjugation with glucuronic acid is so limited, paracetamol is oxidised to a highly reactive intermediary compound which is hepatotoxic and mediates the conversion of haemoglobin to methaemoglobin. Clinical signs include a characteristic facial oedema, pulmonary oedema, cyanosis, depression, hypothermia and vomiting. Haematological examination reveals chocolate-coloured blood, due to methaemoglobin formation, and Heinz bodies are found in blood smears.

Treatment is aimed at supplying glutathione precursors to increase the availability of glutathione which is conjugated to the toxic metabolite and then excreted. To do this, N-acetylcysteine is given orally at an initial dose rate of 140 mg/kg followed by maintenance doses of 70 mg/kg every six hours for a 36-hour period. Adjunctive therapy with cimetidine can also be given orally at a dose of 10 mg/kg bid to slow the production of toxic intermediate compounds. Symptomatic and supportive care is also given: for instance, oxygen if cyanosis is severe and fluids to correct acidosis.

Antimicrobial agents

The use of antibiotics in the cat has been reviewed recently.[7] Antimicrobial agents against septicaemia in kittens are reviewed in Chapter 5.

Penicillins and cephalosporins

Relevant general pharmacological and therapeutic principles should be applied.

Aminoglycosides

Mainly used to treat Gram-negative infections, these antibiotics can cause nephrotoxicity, neurotoxicity and ototoxicity. The cat appears particularly sensitive to ototoxicity. Streptomycin and dihydrostreptomycin are the aminoglycosides most widely used in veterinary practice. The others include gentamycin, neomycin and kanamycin.

There are two important drug interactions that should be remembered:

1. The ototoxic effects of aminoglycosides are potentiated by concurrent administration of frusemide.
2. Aminoglycosides cause a degree of muscle relaxation which can potentiate that caused by ether, halothane or methoxyflurane during anaesthesia and may cause respiratory failure.

Chloramphenicol

Chloramphenicol is a broad spectrum bacteriostatic agent, also active against rickettsia and some mycoplasma. Its clinical pharmacology has been reviewed recently.[8] Prolonged high dosage can lead to haematological abnormalities and there is a reversible suppression of bone marrow function resulting in anaemia and leucopenia. The length of the administration is as important as the dose level in the appearance of toxicity.

However, chloramphenicol can be used safely. Although a dose rate of 50 mg per cat bid would be ideal, the lack of a tablet of less than 125 mg makes this difficult. If 125 mg is given bid, this dosage should not be continued for longer than one week or haematological changes will be seen. In most situations an alternative will be readily available and it is preferable to reserve chloramphenicol for severe intracellular or central nervous system infections.

Sulphonamides

No particular considerations apply in the use of these antibiotics.

Tetracyclines

Tetracyclines are valuable in the treatment of chlamydial and *Haemobartonella felis* infections. Common side-effects of tetracycline compounds in cats include gastrointestinal disturbances, anorexia, and drug-induced fever. The usual precautions taken for other species should be followed. For instance milk will lower the absorption of tetracyclines. Administration to kittens or to queens in the last weeks of pregnancy may result in staining and imperfections in the enamel of the deciduous or permanent teeth respectively. Doxycycline, a tetracycline derivative, can be given with food, once daily, and there is no evidence that it can adversely affect teeth.

Griseofulvin

The antifungal agent griseofulvin should be avoided in the treatment of pregnant cats as it may cause foetal abnormalities when used in the first third of pregnancy. Idiosyncratic reactions to griseofulvin have been reported and include neurological disturbances and bone marrow suppression.

Cardiovascular therapy

Digoxin

Although digoxin therapy for cardiac disease is feasible, it should be undertaken with care. Cats do seem to have an increased sensitivity to the toxic side effects of digoxin and there is also great variation in absorption of digoxin depending on the preparation used.[2] Cats should be digitalised using the estimated maintenance dose in the range 0.004–0.01 mg/kg bid. Liquid, alcohol-based preparations are not well-tolerated by cats. The signs of digoxin toxicity in the cat are depression, anorexia, vomiting and salivation.

Propanolol

Propanolol is a non-selective beta-adrenergic antagonist which reduces heart rate and the force of contraction and improves myocardial relaxation. A dose rate of 2.5–5.0 mg/kg two or three times a day may be useful in the management of hypertrophic cardiomyopathy.

Propanolol must be withheld until pulmonary oedema has been resolved and should be used with caution in congestive myopathy. It is also contraindicated in diabetes mellitus, asthma, atrioventricular block, sinoatrial block and acute systemic thromboembolism.

Anthelmintics

Piperazine

Piperazine has been used extensively as an anthelmintic to treat round worms in cats and kittens. Although generally safe it has been associated with toxicity. Affected cats have vomiting, diarrhoea, depression and nervous signs including muscle weakness, hindlimb ataxia, head-pressing and ataxia. Dyspnoea and muscle twitching have also been reported. Symptomatic and supportive care is indicated and recovery occurs in 3–4 days.

Ivermectin

Owner administration of ivermectin intended for horses has resulted in poisoning of cats. Cats become agitated and vocal, and have central nervous system symptoms including blindness. Recovery may take 3–4 weeks and supportive care is needed.

TOXICOLOGY

Sensitivity of cats to poisoning

There are both behavioural and biochemical features which may protect the cat from or render the cat sensitive to poisoning. Generally cats are less commonly poisoned than dogs.

Behavioural

Cats are fastidious eaters, which reduces their susceptibility to ingesting contaminated feed, but they are curious by nature and may chew toxic house plants. They are also predators and are susceptible to secondary poisoning following ingestion of poisoned rodents.

During grooming, cats may ingest toxins which contaminate the coat – in particular, wood preservatives such as phenols, oil or coal tar.

Biochemistry

In comparison with other domestic species, cats have a reduced capacity for drug biotransformation. This seems to be in large part due to

FIG. 8.3 The major systems affected by poisons recorded in the cat. The predominant clinical signs are often associated with the system indicated but this is not invariably the case – many poisons have a variety of effects.

MAJOR SYSTEMS AFFECTED BY POISONS
I. Poisons reducing oxygen supply to or utilisation by tissues
(a) Reduced uptake of oxygen from alveoli 　　Paraquat 　　Diquat 　　Gases - NH_3; N_2O (b) Reduced oxygen carriage by blood 　　Paracetamol 　　Carbon monoxide 　　Coumarins (c) Inhibition of oxygen utilisation by tissues 　　Cyanide (d) Increasing tissue oxygen demand 　　Chlorophenols 　　Nitrophenols
II. Poisons causing CNS stimulation or depression
(a) Direct damage to nervous tissue 　　Organic mercury (b) Having a specific action on the nervous system 　　Organophosphates 　　Carbamates 　　Strychnine (c) Having a mixed or unknown action 　　Organochlorine compounds 　　Lead 　　Metaldehyde 　　Bromethalin 　　Cannabis 　　Benzoic acid 　　Alpha-chloralose
III. Poisons causing abdominal distress
Corrosive/concentrated chemicals Arsenic
IV. Poisons causing severe liver damage
Aspirin Phenylbutazone
III. Poisons causing severe kidney damage
Cholecalciferol Ethylene glycol

the low levels of glucuronyl transferase, which results in a lowered capacity to detoxify certain environmental contaminants and drugs. In particular phenol and other aromatic compounds are only poorly detoxified. Perhaps the most practically important compounds in this group are aspirin and paracetamol. Cats show unusual receptor sensitivity to some compounds, the best example being the effect of morphine in cats.

It has also been suggested that cats' red blood cells are more sensitive to Heinz body formation, methaemoglobin formation and haemolytic anaemia following exposure to oxidants.

Diagnosis

Diagnosis of poisoning in any species depends on a particularly careful history taking. As an aid to diagnosis, Fig. 8.3 classifies poisons according to the major system affected. Specific toxins and treatments are as follows.

Insecticides

Organophosphates and carbamates

Organophosphates and carbamates are widely used as insecticides. Organophosphates cause an irreversible inhibition of acetylcholine esterase (AChE); carbamates cause a reversible inhibition. Signs of poisoning are related to overstimulation of nerve endings by acetylcholine (ACh) which is normally removed by AChE. ACh is a neurotransmitter at parasympathetic, nicotinic cholinergic and central nervous system sites. The clinical signs associated with each of these are shown in Fig. 8.4. The signs of organophosphate toxicity are more severe and prolonged than those of carbamate toxicity. The cat is also susceptible to delayed neurotoxicity caused by organophosphates which manifest as a progressive hind limb weakness and ataxia.

Treatment of organophosphate and carbamate poisoning is by administration of atropine at 0.25–0.5 mg/kg. One quarter is given IV and the remainder SC. Repeat at intervals of 3–6 hours for organophosphate poisoning. Carbamates usually require less prolonged treatment. In organophosphate poisoning it is also possible to try to reactivate AChE by use of pralidoxime. The dose is 20–50 mg/kg IV or IM as a 10% solution.

The main situations where toxicity arises are when two sources combine to produce toxicity. For instance, a cat may be wearing a flea collar impregnated with a carbamate and is then sprayed with a flea spray containing organophosphate, or an organophosphate insecticide is used in the home.

Organochlorine compounds

Organochlorine compounds are used as pesticides in a wide variety of situations. They are particularly persistent in the environment and therefore clinical signs may not be seen for considerable periods after the initial use. Organochlorines may be absorbed percutaneously from dry material as well as orally or by inhalation (a particular problem immediately after use). They may also bioaccumulate over periods of time. Therefore they pose well documented risks to cats when used as preservatives in paints and as woodworm treatments (such as dieldrin, eldrin, DDT and lindane). Many have been withdrawn from use in different parts of the world but illegal use is likely to continue.

Cats show a wide range of clinical signs, mainly associated with CNS stimulation, including muscle tremors, twitching, ataxia, hypersalivation, hyperaesthesia, depression, weight loss and pyrexia. Treatment is purely symptomatic and supportive, and the prognosis is often poor. Signs of excitation can be controlled with phenobarbitone.

Rodenticides

Coumarin and derivatives

These are the most widely used rodenticides and comprise anti-coagulants of the first generation

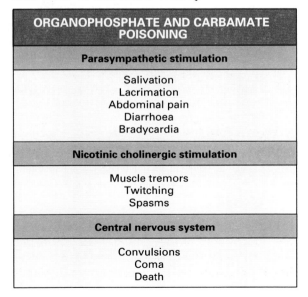

ORGANOPHOSPHATE AND CARBAMATE POISONING
Parasympathetic stimulation
Salivation
Lacrimation
Abdominal pain
Diarrhoea
Bradycardia
Nicotinic cholinergic stimulation
Muscle tremors
Twitching
Spasms
Central nervous system
Convulsions
Coma
Death

FIG. 8.4   Clinical signs associated with organophosphate and carbamate poisoning in the cat.

(e.g. warfarin, coumarin) and second generation (e.g. bromadilone, brodifacoum). They act by inhibiting the enzyme epoxide reductase which converts Vitamin K epoxide to Vitamin K. Therefore levels of Vitamin K decline and there is a reduction in the coagulation factors (II, VII, IX and X) which require Vitamin K in their activation. There is also interference with prothrombin synthesis. The second generation anticoagulants are more persistent (less rapidly metabolised in rodents) and have been developed in response to emerging resistance in rodent populations.

Cats are susceptible to secondary poisoning following ingestion of poisoned rodents. The second generation compounds are more toxic in this manner. Clinical signs are delayed for two to three days and their severity depends on the amount ingested. Haemorrhage may be internal or external leading to haemothorax, abdominal bleeding, melaena, or blood from the mouth or other orifices. There will be consequent anaemia, weakness, rapid weak pulse, dyspnoea and possibly collapse. Affected cats may also have swollen joints and haematomas.

Treatment consists of administering the specific antidote – Vitamin K. Phytomenadione, a Vitamin K_1 analogue available as injection or tablets, is given at a dose of 2.5 mg PO tid for five days. This should be continued for 3–4 weeks if a second generation anticoagulant was responsible. If signs are very severe it is possible to give up to 5 mg IV but this should be over 6–8 hours and adverse reactions may be seen. The intramuscular route is therefore preferable. Menadiol is a synthetic Vitamin K_3 but is *not* as effective in treatment. Whole blood transfusion may also be indicated to compensate for loss of blood and Vitamin K.

Cholecalciferol

Cholecalciferol (Vitamin D_3) toxicoses have increased in domestic species in recent years in parallel with the introduction of rodenticides based on these products.[1,6] Juvenile cats (under one year) seem more susceptible than adults, possibly because of their less discriminatory feeding habits, higher relative dose ingested due to their small body size or greater sensitivity to cholecalciferol or its toxic metabolites. Concern is also being raised because the levels causing toxicity are often 10–20 times lower than the quoted LD_{50} of 88 mg/kg in dogs.

Cholecalciferol and its active metabolites act to increase intestinal absorption of calcium, stimulate bone resorption and increase the renal tubular reabsorption of calcium. Cholecalciferol is metabolised by the liver to 25-hydroxycholecalciferol which is further metabolised in the kidney to calcitrol. Calcitrol is the most potent metabolite in terms of bone resorption and calcium uptake from the intestine.

Clinical signs, which result from hypercalcaemia and dystrophic calcification, include weakness, anorexia, vomiting, polydipsia, polyuria and diarrhoea. There may be signs of bradycardia and cardiac arrhythmias. Clinical examination may show firm plaques on the oral mucosa and there will be marked hypercalcaemia.

Treatment is largely symptomatic and supportive. Fluid therapy and diuresis with frusemide can be given to encourage excretion, with the administration of oral prednisolone (2 mg/kg bid) and, if there has been no response, salmon calcitonin (4–6 IU/kg SC every 2–3 hours). Diuretics and corticosteroids should be maintained for at least 2 weeks and withdrawn slowly.

Bromethalin-based rodenticides

Introduced in the mid-1980s, these compounds may increase in their importance as poisons for cats. They cause vomiting, ataxia, seizures, depression, coma and mydriasis. Clinical signs are thought to be associated with an elevation in cerebrospinal fluid pressure and treatment involves the careful use of osmotic diuresis and corticosteroids.

α-Chloralose

α-Chloralose is both a rodenticide and a laboratory anaesthetic. Toxicity is manifested as hyperexcitability and aggression followed by weakness, convulsions and respiratory depression. Treatment consists of preventing further absorption and controlling convulsions and maintenance of body temperature.

Fungicides

Pentachlorophenol

Pentachlorophenol and other fungicides may be used in wood preservatives and thus pose a threat to cats. Pentachlorophenol uncouples oxidative phosphorylation. Despite evidence of adequate oxygenation of blood as evidenced by red mucous membranes, the animal shows signs of oxygen starvation. There is an increased respiratory rate and tachycardia as well as hyperpyrexia. Treatment is symptomatic, with ice baths to reduce temperature and sedatives to control nervous symptoms.

Molluscicides

Metaldehyde

Metaldehyde is one of the most widely used slug and snail baits and it is in this form that it poses a threat to cats. Its formulation to make it palatable to the snail also results in its increased palatability to domestic species. It causes both autonomic and central nervous signs, including tachycardia and tachypnoea, panting and dyspnoea, salivation and vomiting, muscle tremors, tonic seizures, opisthotonos, generalised convulsions and a marked hyperpyrexia.

There is no specific antidote. Treatment is aimed at reducing absorption and using diazepam or pentobarbitone to control nervous signs. Since acidosis is a feature, fluid therapy is essential with Ringer's lactate or normal saline with bicarbonate supplementation.

Toxic plants

Toxic plants are a minor cause of toxicity in the cat and are mainly associated with the chewing of house plants. It is sometimes difficult to determine which of several chewed plants is implicated and it can also be difficult to identify the exact species of plant from its common name. Some of those implicated include *Euphorbia* (such as poinsettias and the castor oil plant), hyacinth or narcissus bulbs, the Rubber plant and *Araceae* (such as philodendrons and the Swiss Cheese plant). Many of these may cause a localised irritation with ulceration of the buccal mucosa and salivation, possibly accompanied by gastroenteritis.

Metals

Lead

Lead is a relatively uncommon cause of poisoning in the cat but lead-contaminated water, soil or food may be eaten, or ingested while grooming a contaminated coat. Clinical signs are gastrointestinal or nervous: they include depression, anorexia, vomiting, diarrhoea, hyperexcitability, hyperaesthesia, and convulsions. Blood lead levels are not always elevated to a diagnostic level.

Treatment involves chelation of lead using calcium disodium ethylenediamine tetra-acetate (CaEDTA) at 75–100 mg/kg in three divided doses, IV or SC, as a 1–4% solution in normal saline. It is important to use the calcium salt to avoid chelation of calcium and hypocalcaemia. D-penicillamine (12.5 mg/kg PO qid) has been used successfully in the dog.

Mercury

Mercury poisoning is well described in cats, particularly where fish containing high concentrations are ingested. Acute effects are manifested in changes to lung vasculature, whereas chronic poisoning causes neurological defects. Loss of balance, muscle weakness and changes in temperament are seen. Treatment involves chelation of mercury with dimercaprol (3 mg/kg IM every four hours for 1–2 days); the dose is then reduced to every 6 hours for one day then twice daily until clinical signs resolve for up to a maximum of 10 days. Supportive care will also be needed.

Phenols, coal and wood tar derivatives

These compounds may be found in a variety of wood preservatives. The cat's poor ability to metabolise them results in toxicity, especially following contamination of the coat. Signs of poisoning include salivation, abdominal pain, diarrhoea, vomiting, convulsions and collapse.

Treatment is supportive and symptomatic. Contaminated coat should be removed with clippers followed by washing with a mild detergent.

Principles of treatment of poisoning

There are five basic principles of treatment of poisoning cases:

1. Prevent further exposure and absorption of toxin.
2. Use specific antidotes.
3. Increase the rate of elimination of the toxin.
4. Give supportive care.
5. Educate the owner.

1. Preventing further exposure or absorption

This essentially involves moving the animal from the source of the toxin and either physically washing to remove coat contamination or hastening removal of the toxin from the intestinal tract if ingested. This is either by the administration of emetics (with care, and syrup of ipecac at 3–6 ml/kg is the emetic of choice), the use of gastric lavage (under general anaesthesia and with a cuffed endotracheal tube in position), or the administration of laxatives or adsorbents.

The administration by stomach tube of activated charcoal (1 g in 5–10 ml of water and given at a rate of 2–8 mg/kg) will bind organic compounds such as alkaloids, barbiturates and ethylene glycol but not heavy metals. It should be followed 30–40 minutes later by a cathartic such as mineral oil. Avoid vegetable oils as these are absorbed by the intestines.

2. The use of specific antidotes

This is given in the sections above considering specific poisons.

3. Increasing the rate of elimination of the toxin

Once absorbed, this may be achieved in one of three ways:

- Using fluid therapy to ensure adequate renal function. Diuretics such as mannitol (2 g/kg/h) and frusemide (5 mg/kg) can be very helpful.

- Altering urine pH to ionise polar compounds in urine and thereby prevent their reabsorption. Acidic compounds such as aspirin and barbiturates can be ionised by the alkalinisation of urine with sodium bicarbonate (5 mEq/kg/h). Ammonium chloride (200 mg/kg/day in divided doses) can be used to acidify urine and increase the rate of excretion of basic compounds such as amphetamines.

- Peritoneal dialysis with normal saline particularly if animals are oliguric.

4. Supportive and symptomatic care

Includes the following:

- Maintenance of a patent airway and ventilation. Provision of an oxygen enriched atmosphere when needed.
- Maintenance of an effective circulating blood volume. This involves the provision of appropriate parenteral fluid therapy.
- Control of body temperature.
- Control of pain.
- Control of nervous system excitation or depression.

5. Education of clients

Education of clients is particularly important to avoid a recurrence of poisoning or the exposure of other animals to the same source.

REFERENCES

1. Dorman D.C. (1990) Anticoagulant, cholecalciferol and bromethalin-based rodenticides. *Vet. Clin. N. America. Small Anim. Pract.* **20**: 339–385.
2. Erichsen D.F., Harris S.G., Upson D.W. (1980) Therapeutic and toxic plasma concentrations of digoxin in the cat. *Am. J. Vet. Res.* **41**: 2049–2058.
3. Lees P., May S.A. McKellar Q.A. (1991) Pharmacology and therapeutics of non-steroidal anti-inflammatory drugs in the dog and cat: 1. General Pharmacology. *J. Small Anim. Prac.* **32**: 183–193.
4. McKellar Q.A., May S.A., Lees P. (1991) Pharmacology and therapeutics of non-steroidal anti-inflammatory drugs in the dog and cat: 2. Individual agents. *J. Small Anim. Prac.* **32**: 225–235.
5. Sawchuk S.A., Parker A.J., Neff-Davis C., Dais L.E. (1985) Primidone in the cat. *J. Am. Animal Hosp. Assoc.* **21**: 647.

6. Thomas J.B., Hood J.C., Gaschk F. (1990) Chole-calciferol rodenticide toxicity in a domestic cat. *Aust. Vet. J.* **67**: 274–275.

7. Watson A.D.J. (1991,a) Systemic anti-microbial drug therapy in cats. *In Practice* **13**: 73–79.

8. Watson A.D.J. (1991,b) Chloramphenicol 2. Clinical pharmacology in dogs and cats. *Aust. Vet. J.* **68**: 2–5.

9. Wickle J.R. (1989) Principles of drug therapy. In: Sherding R.G. (ed.) *The Cat. Diseases and Clinical Management* Churchill Livingstone, New York. pp 23–34.

9

Laboratory Diagnostic Aids

ANDREW H. SPARKES and TIMOTHY J. GRUFFYDD-JONES

Adoption of a systematic approach is an integral part in the development of effective clinical skills. However, various factors inherent in feline medicine may complicate the use of the problem-orientated approach in this species. The lifestyle and nature of their pets are such that cat owners may fail to notice certain clinical signs such as polyuria/polydipsia, exercise intolerance or diarrhoea which might be readily recognised by the dog owner, and which may be important early indicators of disease. The ability of cats to adapt their lifestyle to compensate for many disease processes and therefore mask clinical signs is well recognised. For these reasons the history may be of limited value in helping to define the clinical problem. Many cats are presented simply as sick cats, and the wide range of conditions to be considered may limit the value of the problem-orientated approach. Diagnostic aids, and especially laboratory testing, may play a crucial role in the investigation of such feline cases – particularly viral screening, since viral infections are such an important factor in many feline disease conditions. In the past this has led to over-enthusiastic adoption and unrealistic expectations of certain diagnostic tests for some problem feline conditions – such as coronavirus serology for the diagnosis of FIP. The purpose of this chapter is to provide a realistic appraisal of the commonly used diagnostic tests, underlining pitfalls and limitations in their application. In addition, the particular value of different tests for certain clinical syndromes are outlined in Figs 9.5 to 9.14.

HAEMATOLOGY

Haematology is one of the laboratory tests most often used as a diagnostic aid. It frequently reveals abnormalities, particularly in the form of changes in the distribution of the white blood cells (WBCs) and the presence of anaemia. However, it is important to appreciate the limitations of those features. Whilst changes may be quite sensitive indicators of disease, their specificity for particular disease conditions is usually poor, which limits their diagnostic value. Interpretation of changes in the haematological picture is also complicated by the very wide normal range for some of these parameters in cats. An important contributory factor is the pronounced effect that any stress associated with the collection of blood samples (restraint, examination, transport to a veterinarian, unfamiliar surroundings, etc) may have on some parameters. Nevertheless, changes in haematological parameters can be particularly florid in this species, such as very high WBC counts and very low packed cell volumes (PCVs) and haemoglobin concentration (Hb).

Red blood cells (RBC)

Red cell parameters

Haematocrit (HCT)/Packed Cell Volume (PCV), Haemoglobin Concentration (Hb) and Red Blood Cell (RBC) Count.

Technical factors

Great care is necessary in the assessment of the RBC count. This is generally determined by an automated cell counter or, in a practice laboratory, by means of a haemocytometer. RBC counts determined by means of a haemocytometer suffer from the technical limitation that applies to RBC counts in any species – that this is a technically demanding technique with a high degree of variability (up to 30%) which is inherent in the technique itself and can readily exceed changes of clinical significance. Automated cell counters work on the principle of discriminating between particles of varying size. However, feline

RBCs show a particular tendency to deform and to clump, an effect due possibly to their haemoglobin internal structure or the nature of the RBC membrane. This will occur with all standard anticoagulants and may confuse the particle size discriminator. In addition, platelet clumping and the appearance of macrothrombocytes are common in cats and may overlap with the size of the smaller RBCs leading to further inaccuracies in the RBC count.

There are no particular technical considerations relevant to determination of HCT/PCV and Hb in cats. As in any species, HCT and PCV will vary slightly due to the different methods by which they are determined, and also (as with other species) collection and handling of blood samples is important to avoid distortion of RBCs, particularly haemolysis or swelling due to delay in processing. Any inaccuracies in the RBC count will be reflected in the derived red cell indices, particularly the mean cell volume (MCV).

Interpretation

Increased red cell parameters (RBC, Hb, PCV, HCT): polycythaemia

Stress can readily increase RBC parameters in cats and this possibility must always be considered in interpretation. Unfortunately there are no reliable, simple blood changes which can provide corroborative evidence of stress or that will quantify the degree of stress. The expression of stress probably varies considerably between individual cats and therefore attempts at assessing stress on the basis of behavioural changes may be misleading.

Apart from stress, dehydration is the most common cause of polycythaemia. Cats readily become anorexic and adipsic in many illnesses, and therefore dehydration is a common complicating factor. There will usually be a corresponding increase in some blood biochemical parameters, such as urea and proteins.

Polycythaemia as a specific feature of an underlying disease process is uncommon in cats and the major causes are summarised in Fig. 9.1. In some of these conditions other clinical signs

MAJOR CAUSES OF POLYCYTHAEMIA

Relative polycythaemia (haemoconcentration)
  Dehydration/hypovolaemia
 	
Absolute polycythaemia (increased RBC production)
  Chronic hypoxia
    Pulmonary disease
    Right to left cardiac shunts
    Erythropoietin-producing tumours
  Polycythaemia vera

FIG. 9.1   Major causes of polycythaemia in the cat.

may be evident. Severe polycythaemia leads to increased viscosity of blood and hence the 'hyperviscosity syndrome' may develop, with lethargy and depression, and dilated tortuous retinal blood vessels will be evident on ophthalmoscopic examination.

Decreased red cell parameters (RBC, Hb, PCV HCT): anaemia

The major indication for assessing red cell parameters is usually to check for the presence of anaemia, which is particularly common in cats. Clinical assessment of anaemia can be difficult in any species and haematological examination is essential to confirm its presence, to assess its degree and to help to characterise the type of anaemia. This assumes particular importance in cats for two reasons. Firstly, the clinical signs associated with anaemia are rather non-specific, and therefore of limited help in alerting the owner and clinician to its presence. Exercise intolerance is the most important early sign of anaemia in other species but is rarely noted in cats. Secondly, assessment of mucous membrane colour, which is one of the most useful clinical indicators of anaemia, can be very misleading in cats. Anaemic cats are frequently anorexic and associated dehydration will influence red cell parameters, so that the degree of anaemia may be readily underestimated.

Anaemia is a very common feature of many disease processes, particularly the major infectious diseases. An important priority in the diagnostic evaluation of anaemic cats is, therefore, to attempt to establish whether the anaemia results from a primary haematopoietic disorder or is secondary to some systemic disease. Other clinical and laboratory diagnostic investigations are crucial to making this distinction. The general approach to the investigation of anaemia is covered in detail in Chapter 19, and this section will be restricted to consideration of factors which specifically relate to the interpretation of red cell haematological parameters in the assessment of anaemia.

It is essential to establish whether or not a regenerative response is present. This is of major importance in differentiating between the blood loss/haemolytic anaemias, and those involving disordered haematopoiesis. Unfortunately this distinction may be difficult to make, as in many cases the signs of regeneration are equivocal. Assessment of the derived red cell indices, especially MCV, should provide an indication of the presence of any regeneration, but frequently this is increased only marginally in cats with other evidence of a brisk regenerative response. Red cell morphology may provide useful indicators for characterising the type of anaemia.

Assessment of red cell morphology

A major difficulty in assessment of red cell morphology of cats is that unusual forms of RBCs are occasionally encountered in the normal individual and interpretation of their significance may be difficult. For example, Heinz Bodies or erythrocyte refractile bodies are found in 'normal' cats affecting up to 10% of RBCs – but are considered significant if seen in greater numbers.

Red cell morphology plays an important part in the assessment of regeneration. Young, immature polychromatic cells are readily recognisable in blood smears prepared for differential counting using stains such as Leishman's and May-Grunwald. Such cells are larger than normal, indicating the presence of anisocytosis.

Assessment of reticulocytes presents particular difficulties in cats. Suitable blood smears are prepared by prediluting the blood with a supravital stain, such as new methylene blue or Romanowsky, before making the smear. However, two major forms of reticulocyte occur and their differentiation can be difficult. The mature punctate form contains numerous tiny accumulations of reticular material. These reticulocytes can survive in the peripheral circulation for several weeks and up to 10% of RBCs may show this feature in normal cats. The aggregate reticulocytes are the more immature form and contain clumps of reticular material. These equate with the polychromatic cells seen on differential smears, and are uncommon (<0.5%) in normal cats. Only the aggregate form should be counted in assessing reticulocyte counts. Nucleated red blood cells may be recognised on the differential smear, indicating a brisk regenerative response. Occasionally, and particularly in cats, early nucleated RBCs may be recognised, with no concurrent significant increase in reticulocytes. These contradictory indicators of whether or not a regenerative response is present suggest a dyshaematopoietic anaemia with disorganised RBC production. Such cases may involve myelophthisis and are frequently associated with FeLV.

The other major morphological abnormalities seen in feline RBCs are summarised in Fig. 9.2. Heinz Bodies are considered to represent denatured haemoglobin. A proportion of RBCs may show Heinz Bodies in normal cats, but in cats with a Heinz Body anaemia associated with some oxidative insult to the RBCs, such as exposure to an oxidative toxin or autointoxication, a high proportion of RBCs is affected. The Heinz Bodies may be identifiable in differential smears or unstained smears as refractile bodies, but can be readily demonstrated using supravital stains. In extreme cases extruded Heinz Bodies may be seen outside the RBCs.

Howell-Jolly bodies are thought to represent

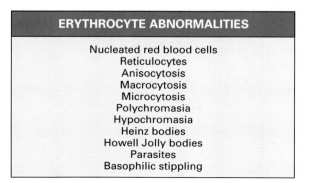

ERYTHROCYTE ABNORMALITIES

Nucleated red blood cells
Reticulocytes
Anisocytosis
Macrocytosis
Microcytosis
Polychromasia
Hypochromasia
Heinz bodies
Howell Jolly bodies
Parasites
Basophilic stippling

FIG. 9.2   Erythrocyte abnormalities in the cat.

nuclear remnants. These small, intensely staining, round inclusions are visible in differential smears. They may be found in the RBCs in normal cats, but an increased number reflects recent regeneration.

Autoagglutination, whilst not pathognomonic, is strongly suggestive of autoimmune haemolytic anaemia (AIHA) in dogs. Feline RBCs seem to autoagglutinate much more readily and this is sometimes seen in cats anaemic for reasons other than AIHA or in cats sick for other reasons. Other useful indicators of AIHA in dogs are also less helpful in cats. The normal morphology of feline RBCs precludes the recognition of spherocytes, and schistocytosis is a rare finding in cats. Indeed, the diagnosis of AIHA is much more difficult in cats (see also Coombs' tests) and AIHA is much more likely to be secondary.

RBC examination in anaemic cats should include a check for protozoal RBC parasites, particularly *Haemobartonella felis* and this technique with its many inherent technical and interpretative problems is covered in Chapter 23.

Coombs' tests

Coombs' reagents for screening for AIHA in cats are now readily obtainable. However, it is important to ensure that any activity against blood group determinants has been absorbed with feline RBCs representing the major blood groups prior to their use in order to avoid false positives.

White blood cells (WBC)

Total WBC count: technical factors

The WBC count is usually determined in the same way as the RBC count using either an automated cell counter or a haemocytometer, after first lysing the RBCs in the sample by addition of a detergent agent. Immature RBCs release their nuclei when lysed and these will be included in the WBC count by an automated cell counter. The WBC count should therefore be corrected by determining the ratio of nucleated RBCs to WBCs whilst assessing the WBC differential. If a marked regenerative response is present, this may introduce a significant error in the uncorrected WBC count. Two

other factors may also lead to inaccuracies – clumping of the WBCs and clumping of the platelets.

Interpretation

The feline WBC count is subject to marked changes induced by stress. This contributes to the very wide normal range for WBC counts seen in cats. Abnormal WBC counts and differentials are common in feline conditions, particularly the major viral infections. They are not specific to certain diseases and may be of limited value in identifying the underlying cause of illness.

Changes in neutrophils

The most common WBC change is a neutrophilia which may indicate any infections or inflammatory disorder and may be accompanied by a left shift with increased numbers of immature band forms. Some of the more important causes are listed in Fig. 9.3. These are so varied that a neutrophilia is of limited diagnostic value. If a particularly vigorous neutrophilic response is present, myelocytes and metamyelocytes may also be identified on blood smears. Other features of the neutrophils are occasionally identified. Döhle bodies are intensely staining intracytoplasmic inclusions which are sometimes seen following viral infections. Toxic vacuolation appears as numerous, round

CAUSES OF NEUTROPHILIA
Stress-induced
Inflammation
Suppurative
Non-suppurative
Infection
Bacterial
Viral
Parasitic
Fungal
Others
Physiological leukocytosis (excitement)
Exogenous glucocorticoids
Myeloproliferative disorders

FIG. 9.3   Causes of neutrophilia in the cat.

intracytoplasmic darkly staining vacuoles. It indicates a toxic degenerative change which may occur in particularly severe infections and is often associated with a neutropenia rather than a neutrophilia.

A degenerative left shift with neutropenia, the presence of bands possibly with earlier forms such as myelocytes and metamyelocytes and with toxic vacuolation, is an indication of a severe infectious process. Neutropenia may also reflect inadequate production due to primary myeloid disease or some toxic or metabolic suppression of marrow. It may also be an important feature of some of the major viral infections, particularly FIV and FeLV. Neutropenic cats are predisposed to persistent or recurrent infections and this is an important consideration in cats presented for investigation of pyrexia of unknown origin. In some individuals the neutropenia appears to be cyclical in nature with periods of clinical normality and pyrexia interspersed. A compensatory monocytosis is a common feature in neutropenic cats.

Changes in lymphocytes

Both lymphocytosis and lymphopenia are common but non-specific changes which occur in many feline diseases. They are frequently seen in cats infected with the major feline viruses – FIP, FIV and FeLV. Thus lymphocyte changes may prove a helpful indicator of viral infection, although they do not help to differentiate between these. The absence of lymphopenia may be useful for ruling out viral infections and we have found that lymphopenia is present in about 75% of FIP cases.

Changes in lymphocytes are also a common feature in lymphosarcoma, most often appearing as a lymphopenia. Lymphoblasts may also be identifiable in peripheral blood smears, although this has been an unusual finding in cats with lymphosarcoma seen at our clinic. Lymphopenia in response to either corticosteroid treatment or hyperadrenocorticism is a much less predictable finding than in dogs.

Changes in monocytes

A monocytosis is common in infective processes, particularly of a chronic nature, but is of limited diagnostic value.

Changes in eosinophils and basophils

The eosinophil plays an important role in parasitic infections and allergy. Endoparasitism and infection with ectoparasites, particularly fleas, are remarkably common in cats, and therefore an eosinophilia is frequently seen. The priority on finding an eosinophilia is to discount parasitism as a possible cause before considering investigation of other, less common, causes. Eosinophil counts in cats are very labile and in our clinic we attempt to verify that an eosinophilia is persistent in two further samples, taken on consecutive days at different times of day, before ascribing significance to this.

Eosinophilia may indicate allergic disease, particularly if associated with basophilia. With the exception of hypersensitivity linked with parasitic infections, eosinophilia associated with suspected allergic disease is most often encountered in coughing cats. A peripheral eosinophilia is also an inconsistent feature of the diseases of cats characterised by eosinophilic infiltration of tissues – eosinophilic granuloma complex, eosinophilic pneumonia and eosinophilic gastritis/enteritis. The relationship, if any, of these conditions to the hypereosinophilic syndrome is unclear, but in the latter condition an eosinophilia is much more consistently observed and may reach extraordinarily high levels. Eosinopenia is not a consistent feature of hyperadrenocorticism.

BLOOD BIOCHEMISTRY

Serum proteins

Serum proteins comprise two fractions – albumin and the globulins. Fibrinogen (a precursor of fibrin) is also found in plasma, accounting for the slightly higher protein levels in plasma compared with serum. Little information can be gained from measurement of total serum protein, and it is usual to obtain albumin and globulin values, and in some cases further analysis by serum protein electrophoresis.

Albumin

The liver is responsible for the production of albumin, which has an important role in the maintenance of plasma oncotic pressure, and thereby maintenance of blood volume. Hypoalbuminaemic states will usually result in hypovolaemia.

Hypoalbuminaemia

Hypoalbuminaemia may be associated with reduced protein intake (inadequate nutrition is a *very* rare cause, but malassimilation may contribute to hypoalbuminaemia) or reduced synthesis due to generalised liver disease, or it may result from excessive loss of albumin. The latter is the most common cause of moderate to severe hypoalbuminaemia, and underlying aetiologies may include protein-losing nephropathy (e.g. glomerulonephritis, renal amyloidosis), protein-losing enteropathy (e.g. severe inflammatory bowel disease), haemorrhage, and exudates. Protein-losing nephropathies are usually accompanied by a normal or increased serum globulin level, whereas hypoglobulinaemia normally accompanies hypoalbuminaemia to a greater or lesser extent in most other protein wasting diseases.

Hyperalbuminaemia

Hyperalbuminaemia is usually accompanied by hyperglobulinaemia and indicates dehydration or shock.

Globulins

The liver is also responsible for the synthesis of the majority of globulins. The alpha- and betaglobulin fractions comprise a variety of proteins, glycoproteins and lipoproteins, many of which are present in elevated concentrations in serum in response to inflammation (e.g. 'acute phase proteins'). Immunoglobulins are the major serum protein not synthesised by the liver, and these form most of the gamma- and part of the betaglobulin fraction.

Hyperglobulinaemia

Hyperglobulinaemia may be associated with dehydration, infections, immune-mediated disorders, neoplasia, and other inflammatory diseases.

Serum protein electrophoresis is commonly employed to gain further information about abnormalities of serum globulins. A polyclonal gammopathy suggests increased immunoglobulin production in response to an infectious agent or in an immune-mediated condition, whilst a monoclonal gammopathy is usually associated with lymphoma or multiple myeloma. Occasionally a monoclonal gammopathy has been seen in response to infectious agents (e.g. FIP). Specific increases in alpha- and betaglobulins are usually seen in association with acute or chronic inflammatory disorders. Care should be taken not to over-interpret results of protein analysis, including protein electrophoresis. For example, much has been made of the hyperproteinaemia and hyperglobulinaemia seen in association with FIP, and in this disease serum protein electrophoresis often shows elevations of alpha2- and gammaglobulins. However, critical assessment of this and other laboratory tests for FIP has shown that they have poor sensitivity and specificity for the disease.

Hypoglobulinaemia

Hypoglobulinaemia may be seen in protein-losing disorders such as haemorrhage and protein-losing enteropathies/nephropathies, in severe liver disease, or in B-lymphocyte disorders resulting in hypo- or agammaglobulinaemia.

Urea and creatinine

Urea

Measurement of serum/plasma urea is probably the most commonly used test of renal function. Urea synthesis occurs primarily in the liver where it arises from catabolism of endogenous or exogenous (dietary) amino-acids and proteins. Urea is excreted primarily through the kidneys (although some may occur via the gastrointestinal tract), where it is freely filtered at the glomerulus. As urea freely crosses cell membranes, some is re-absorbed from the glomerular filtrate in the tubules, therefore renal clearance of urea cannot be used as a means of estimating glomerular filtration rate (GFR).

Creatinine

Creatinine is formed by the spontaneous dephosphorylation of phosphocreatine in muscle cells. Creatinine is released into the blood at a fairly constant rate for any individual but there is variation between individuals. Blood creatinine concentration is primarily dependent on muscle mass and renal excretion, and normal values correlate well with body weight. Creatinine is eliminated by renal excretion where filtration at the glomerulus is followed by no significant tubular resorption or secretion in the cat, and creatinine concentrations are therefore more highly correlated with the GFR.

Interpretation of raised urea or creatinine levels (azotaemia)

As the kidneys are responsible for the excretion of both urea and creatinine, it follows that elevations in serum/plasma levels can occur with any disease lowering the glomerular filtration rate (GFR). Prerenal azotaemia can arise from many conditions including dehydration, shock, and decreased cardiac output, whilst postrenal azotaemia is usually associated with urethral obstruction or a ruptured bladder. Primary renal azotaemia may arise from acute or chronic disease, but significant elevations of urea and creatinine generally are not detectable until there is loss of around 75% of functioning nephrons. Furthermore, as urea and creatinine have a non-linear relationship to renal function, care needs to be exercised in interpreting levels in the high-normal to mildly elevated range, where even quite marked deteriorations in renal function will result in only relatively small elevations of urea and creatinine levels. In prerenal azotaemia, the proportional elevation in urea is often greater than that with creatinine.

Non-renal causes of elevated urea and creatinine

Serum urea levels may be raised for a number of reasons other than decreased GFR, including dietary intake of protein (it takes 10–18 hours following ingestion of a meal for urea levels to fall to baseline, and higher protein diets result in higher baseline levels), the use of catabolic drugs (e.g. corticosteroids, cytotoxic agents), gastro-intestinal haemorrhage, and increased catabolism associated with pyrexia and infections. With creatinine, in addition to the considerations of body weight (lean body mass), transient elevations may also occur with acute muscle necrosis. There is minimal post-prandial change in creatinine levels, but non-creatinine chromogens in blood may interfere with many creatinine assays resulting in a margin of error in interpretation of results.

If non-renal factors are eliminated, azotaemia implies functional loss of at least 75% of nephrons through either renal, prerenal or postrenal causes (see earlier). In renal failure, therefore, both urea and creatinine are relatively insensitive markers until very advanced disease is present. As they suffer from different limitations, it is generally recommended that both are measured together on a routine basis. The insensitivity of urea and creatinine in the diagnosis of renal insufficiency has led to the evaluation of other more precise measurements of GFR to detect early deterioration in renal function and monitor progress. Although methods have been validated for measurement of GFR in the cat (e.g. exogenous creatinine clearance, inulin clearance), these tests are technically demanding and there is currently no reliable test that can be recommended for general clinical use.

Phosphate

Phosphorus absorption from the small intestine is enhanced by vitamin D, but serum phosphate levels are regulated primarily through modifications of renal excretion. Phosphate is filtered at the glomerulus and then undergoes variable resorption from the tubules where parathyroid hormone (PTH) and calcitonin both inhibit resorption. Serum phosphate levels may thus be altered by renal disease, parathyroid gland diseases, and dietary intake (Fig. 9.4).

Hyperphosphataemia

Hyperphosphataemia is most frequently seen as a consequence of compromised renal function

FIG. 9.4 Common causes of calcium and phosphate abnormalities in the cat.

COMMON CAUSES OF CALCIUM AND PHOSPHATE ABNORMALITIES						
	Calcium			Phosphate		
	High	Normal	Low	High	Normal	Low
Hypoparathyroidism			+	+	+	
Renal failure		+	+	+	+	
Primary hyperparathyroidism	+				+	+
Nutritional hyperparathyroidism	+	+	+	+	+	
Hypervitaminosis D	+	+		+	+	

(decreased GFR), and therefore may accompany any of the causes of azotaemia listed above. Other potential causes of hyperphosphataemia include hypoparathyroidism (idiopathic or iatrogenic following thyroid surgery), hypervitaminosis D, hyperthyroidism, nutritional secondary hyperparathyroidism and administration of phosphate enemas. Pseudohyperphosphataemia can be seen with haemolysis.

Hypophosphataemia

This is seen much less commonly than hyperphosphataemia, but can be seen with hyperparathyroidism and hypercalcaemia of malignancy amongst other disorders.

Calcium

Nerve conduction, neuromuscular transmission, muscle contraction and blood coagulation are amongst the many processes that depend on accurate calcium homeostasis. Important indications for the measurement of serum calcium include weakness, muscle tremors/fasciculations, tetanic spasms, seizures, azotaemia, and polyuria/polydipsia (signs associated with hypercalcaemia).

Serum calcium is present in three forms – protein bound (approximately 40%) mainly to albumin, chelated (approximately 10%) and ionised (approximately 50%). Only the ionised form is metabolically active, but total serum calcium is measured routinely. The ionised serum calcium concentration is controlled closely by the actions of PTH, calcitonin and vitamin D. Total serum calcium may be increased or decreased in association with hyper- and hypo-proteinaemia respectively because of the protein binding that occurs, but this does not necessarily reflect changes in the ionised (active) calcium levels. In man and dogs, formulas are available to correct for this, e.g.:

Adjusted Ca (mg/dl) =
total Ca (mg/dl) − albumin (g/dl) + 3.5

Unfortunately, although serum calcium levels are highly correlated with albumin concentrations in cats, adjustment factors have not proved reliable in use.

Hypercalcaemia

Important causes of hypercalcaemia include hypervitaminosis D (toxicosis), primary hyperparathyroidism (usually parathyroid neoplasia), hypoadrenocorticism and hyperproteinaemia (Fig. 9.4). Hypercalcaemia of malignancy is a well recognised syndrome in dogs, seen in association with a number of tumours, but the prevalence in cats with malignancies is much lower. Where present, it is almost invariably associated with lymphosarcoma or myeloproliferative disorders.

Hypocalcaemia

Hypocalcaemia is encountered most frequently with hypoalbuminaemia or hypoparathyroidism (idiopathic or iatrogenic following thyroid surgery). With hypoparathyroidism the hypocalcaemia can rapidly become fatal. Other causes of hypocalcaemia include lactational tetany, ethylene glycol intoxication, renal failure, nutritional secondary hyperparathyroidism, hyperthyroidism and malabsorption.

Glucose

Glucose estimations are readily available and simple to perform. Home glucose monitors used by human diabetic patients provide satisfactory results if used carefully. The major interest in glucose estimation is to check for hyperglycaemia, particularly in cats presented with polydipsia in which diabetes mellitus is a differential diagnosis requiring consideration. An important complication in the interpretation of hyperglycaemia in cats is the influence of stress. Cats show a particularly marked hyperglycaemic response to stress induced by both catecholamine and corticosteroid release, which may exceed the renal threshold (of around 12 mmol/l) and may persist for several days. A diagnosis of diabetes mellitus must not therefore be based solely on demonstration of hyperglycaemia in a single blood sample – it requires presence of clinical signs compatible with diabetes mellitus. Repeat blood glucose estimations may be necessary for diagnosis. In equivocal cases a glucose tolerance test (GTT) may be considered, but we have found the IV GTT to have a poor reproducibility in cats. Results must be interpreted cautiously as the test itself is probably affected by stress hormones.

If diabetes mellitus is diagnosed, further investigations may be indicated to determine whether the diabetes is secondary to some other underlying factor such as hyperadrenocorticism, acromegaly or progestagen administration. Hypoglycaemia is much less common in cats. Irrespective of the underlying cause, hypoglycaemia will lead to disorientation, behavioural changes, ataxia and, if severe, seizures. Hypoglycaemia probably occurs in neonatal kittens that are not receiving adequate food intake but is seldom confirmed by blood estimation. Functional insulinomas have been reported as a rare condition in cats and there have also been occasional reports of hypoglycaemia associated with other forms of neoplasia such as hepatic tumours.

Bilirubin

Bilirubin estimations are of limited value in feline medicine and probably over-used and over-interpreted. Total bilirubin estimation is frequently used to confirm the presence of jaundice. Clinical assessment of mucous membrane colour is not a sensitive means of identifying mild jaundice but

POLYPHAGIA		
Test	**Value**	**Comments**
T_4	++	Reliable test for hyperthyroidism.
Serum biochemistry		
Liver enzymes	+/–	Non-specific, but elevations may be found with hyperthyroidism or lymphocytic cholangitis.
Glucose	+	Hyperglycaemia may indicate diabetes mellitus, but care must be taken to differentiate this from 'stress hyperglycaemia.'
Haematology		
White cell count	+/–	Inflammatory bowel disease may be accompanied by neutrophilia and/or eosinophilia, but these are non-specific changes, seen with many other conditions including parasitic diseases. Occasionally a very high neutrophilia may be seen in association with inflammatory bowel disease.
Faecal trypsin/BT-PABA	–	Exocrine pancreatic insufficiency is extremely rare in cats, and assessment of faecal trypsin is neither a sensitive nor a specific test. Insufficient cases have been seen to evaluate the BT-PABA test, but other small intestinal diseases are known to give false positive results.

FIG. 9.5 Diagnostic tests for use in polyphagia.

VOMITING AND DIARRHOEA		
Test	**Value**	**Comments**
Haematology		
Anaemia	–	This is a non-specific finding but may be seen in association with blood loss from the GIT (e.g. tumour), or secondary to a chronic infectious/ inflammatory disorder.
Leukocytosis/ neutrophilia	+/–	Another non-specific finding, but may accompany GIT neoplasia or inflammatory bowel disease (IBD). Sometimes marked neutrophilia (e.g. > 30 x 10^6) seen with IBD.
Eosinophilia	+/–	May be seen with intestinal parasitic infestations or IBD, but extra-intestinal parasitic diseases and other hypersensitivity disorders must be considered.
Leukopenia	+	May be seen with panleukopenia virus infection, or accompanying infection with FeLV or FIV.
Serum biochemistry	+/–	Only helpful in a small proportion of cases.
Renal function	+/–	To rule out uraemic gastrointestinal disturbances.
Liver function	+/–	May be indicated to investigate possible biliary stasis in cases of steatorrhoea. Elevations of liver enzymes are non-specific but can be seen in association with diabetes mellitus, hyperthyroidism and primary liver disease.
Albumin	+/–	Hypoalbuminaemia may be due to a protein-losing enteropathy (e.g. severe IBD) or protein-losing nephropathy. Severe hypoalbuminaemia may lead to oedema of the intestinal wall inducing malabsorption.
Amylase/lipase	–	Acute pancreatitis is very rare in cats. These tests, and especially amylase, have poor sensitivity and specificity.
T$_4$	+	Hyperthyroidism is frequently associated with gastrointestinal signs, but other signs usually dominate.
Faecal tests	+/–	Of limited value.
Parasites	+	Screening for *Giardia* (3 faecal samples on sequential days) is perhaps most valuable, but this is relatively insensitive, and many healthy cats may also shed the parasite. Other parasites are rarely important.
Culture	–	Bacterial enteropathogens are rarely important in cats with chronic diarrhoea.
Microscopy/faecal trypsin	–	EPI is very rare in cats, and these are unreliable diagnostic tests.
Serum B$_{12}$/folate	+/–	The value of these tests in cats is not fully established, but they are probably less useful than in dogs.

FIG. 9.6   Diagnostic tests for use in vomiting and diarrhoea.

this can be identified readily by checking for yellow discoloration of the plasma or serum in a spun blood sample, or by urinary bilirubin estimations which can be easily and reliably performed using commercial urinalysis test strips. Estimation of the total bilirubin concentration may give some indication of the likely type of jaundice. If the jaundice is severe, with total bilirubin in excess of around 100–150 mmol/l, it is more likely to be hepatic or obstructive in origin, rather than pre-hepatic associated with haemolyis. The premise that differential bilirubin estimations reliably differentiate between conjugated and unconjugated forms is now questioned and therefore their diagnostic relevance is dubious.

Bile acids

Bile acid measurement is used as an indicator of hepatobiliary function. Increased levels occur with hepatic dysfunction, particularly if this is obstructive in nature. Prior fasting for twelve hours is essential before collecting blood samples for bile acid estimation since feeding stimulates their release. Assessment of the increment in bile acid concentrations in samples collected before and $\frac{1}{2}$–2 hours after feeding may be more sensitive in identifying impaired entero-hepatic circulation. This procedure is particularly useful for investigating cases of suspected porto-systemic shunts. It had been hoped that bile acid estimations would obviate the need for dye retention tests, which have disadvantages for use in practice; however, the sensitivity of bile acids for assessing liver dysfunction has not matched original expectations.

Dye clearance tests

Dye clearance tests assess the excretory mechanism of the liver which provides an indication of hepatic function. Special considerations are required for their use in cats. Bromosulphthalein (BSP) is excreted more rapidly in cats than other species and therefore the test procedure requires modification to maintain sensitivity of the test. The dosage of BSP is based on the weight of the cat (0.5 mg/kg) from which the circulating volume is surmised. A blood sample is collected just prior to intravenous administration of BSP to provide a plasma blank, and a second sample collected 15 minutes after injection from another vein. In normal cats less than 5% will be retained at this time, whereas retention of over 10% is considered abnormal. As in other species, special care is required in the performance and interpretation of this test. Severe reactions occur with perivascular injection in man and whilst this may be a less serious risk in cats, it will render the results inaccurate. Anaphylactic reactions to BSP have also been reported in man but have not been documented in cats. Any factor which affects circulatory function will impair BSP excretion and this should be taken into account in interpreting results. BSP is bound to plasma albumin and therefore low albumin levels will also influence BSP excretion. Since BSP and bilirubin are excreted by similar mechanisms, BSP retention does not provide any useful additional information in jaundiced animals. Although BSP has been widely used for dye clearance tests, other dyes can be used, particularly indocyanine green, for which

excretion in cats is more comparable with excretion in other species.

Ammonia

Blood ammonia is an important test for the diagnosis of hepatic encephalopathy. In the UK this is almost invariably indicative of congenital porto-systemic shunts and is therefore seen primarily in young cats. However, in the USA hepatic encephalopathy is reported as a complication of idiopathic hepatic lipidosis, although this is rare in the UK. Ammonia is a particularly important test for congenital porto-systemic shunts since other blood biochemical changes (apart from bile acids) are inconsistent in this condition in cats.

Ammonia testing does present some practical difficulties. EDTA plasma must be separated within around 30 minutes of collection of the blood sample, and unless the plasma is stored frozen, the ammonia estimation should be performed within a few hours. This usually precludes the use of commercial diagnostic laboratories but blood ammonia can now be reliably determined in practice laboratories using some of the more recent dry chemistry system analysers. Prior fasting for 12 hours is important before collection of blood samples. An ammonia tolerance test involving monitoring of blood ammonia following ammonium chloride loading can be used if starved blood ammonia concentrations are equivocal, though the indications for this procedure are infrequent and it does carry risk of side effects.

Cholesterol

Blood cholesterol estimation is of limited value in cats and we do not believe its inclusion in routine feline profiles is justifiable. The most common cause of hypercholesterolaemia is probably glomerulonephropathy, but in this and the other diseases which may lead to changes in cholesterol, such as endocrine and hepatic disorders, other tests are of much greater value in diagnosis.

Sodium

Sodium is the principal inorganic cation of extracellular fluid, and together with chloride constitutes

POLYURIA/POLYDIPSIA		
Test	**Value**	**Comments**
Serum biochemistry		
Urea/creatinine/PO$_4$	++	To assess renal function, but non-renal factors may also cause azotaemia.
Na/K	+	Disturbances may occur secondary to renal disease, especially hypokalaemia, but hypokalaemia may also induce or contribute to renal dysfunction.
Glucose	++	Hyperglycaemia may indicate diabetes mellitus, but care must be taken to exclude "stress hyperglycaemia".
Ca	+	Hypercalcaemic nephropathy is uncommon in cats, and if present is usually secondary to lymphosarcoma.
Albumin/cholesterol	+/−	Glomerulonephritis may result in hypoalbuminaemia with or without hypercholesterolaemia, and may lead to renal failure.
Urinalysis		
Specific gravity	+	Loss of concentrating ability is not a sensitive indicator of renal disease in cats, and isosthenuria does not occur until renal failure is advanced.
Deposit	+/−	Examination of urine deposit may help identify the cause of a nephropathy (e.g. pyelonephritis).
Protein: creatinine ratio	+	Useful in assessing significance of proteinuria (e.g. suspected glomerulonephritis), correlates well with 24 hour protein excretion.
Haematology	−	Generally not diagnostically helpful.
Anaemia	−	Non-specific, but may see non-regenerative anaemia associated with chronic renal failure.
WBC	+/−	Leukocytosis/neutrophilia may be seen with pyelonephritis.
Cortisol/ACTH Stim/ DXM screening tests	+	Indicated in cats with insulin-resistant diabetes mellitus.
FIV/FeLV	+	Some studies have linked FIV with renal disease, and FeLV infection may lead to renal lymphosarcoma.

FIG. 9.7 Diagnostic tests for use in polyuria/polydipsia.

a major part of the oncotic pressure of blood and extracellular fluid.

Hypernatraemia

Hypernatraemia is most often found with dehydration, but may rarely be associated with other diseases such as hyperaldosteronism and CNS disease.

Hyponatraemia

Important causes of hyponatraemia include hypoadrenocorticism, vomiting and diarrhoea. Natriuresis (renal failure, natriuretic diuretics), haemorrhage and diabetes mellitus may also lead to hyponatraemia.

Chloride

Chloride concentrations are generally affected by the same disease processes that affect sodium, but additionally acid-base disturbances will also frequently alter chloride levels. Bicarbonate is the other major anion in extracellular fluid, and to maintain a normal anion gap alterations in bicarbonate concentrations are normally accompanied by opposite changes in chloride concentrations.

Hyperchloraemia

Major causes of hyperchloraemia are dehydration and acidosis.

PYREXIA OF UNKNOWN ORIGIN		
Test	**Value**	**Comments**
Haematology	++	Important part of diagnostic evaluation.
Neutrophilia/ monocytosis	+	May suggest a focus of infection, but may also be observed in other non-infectious inflammatory disorders or associated with stress.
Lymphopenia	+/–	Commonly seen with many viral infections (e.g. FIP), but also frequently accompanies stress.
Neutropenia/leukopenia	++	A relatively common finding in cases of PUO, may indicate a viral infection (e.g.FeLV/FIV), or bone marrow disorder.
Anaemia	+	Non-specific finding, but may occur for example secondary to chronic inflammation or infection, with FIV or FeLV infection, with bone marrow disorders with immune-mediated haemolysis or FIA infection.
FIA	+	Diagnosis is problematic (poor sensitivity), and significance of a positive finding is not always clear. Underlying diseases should be considered.
FIV/FeLV	++	Important priorities, tests are generally sensitive and specific but note a proportion of FIV-infected cats are antibody-negative and will therefore test negative.
Serum biochemistry		
Serum proteins/SPE	+	Globulins are frequently elevated in PUO cases reflecting either an inflammatory and/or immunoglobulin response. Findings are usually non-specific but SPE may reveal a paraproteinaemia suggesting a myeloma although occasionally other diseases (e.g. FIP) may also show this change.
Liver enzymes	+/–	Rule out liver or renal disease.
Renal function	+/–	Limited value, may help to localise infection e.g. cholangiohepatitis, pyelonephritis
Urinalysis	+	Important, especially for suspected pyelonephritis which is often difficult to diagnose and may easily be overlooked.
Marrow biopsy	+	Important in the further investigation of cases showing unexplained myeloid/erythroid disorders e.g. abnormal cells in the circulation or unexplained cytopenias. Also valuable in any persistent undiagnosed PUO (? aleukaemic leukaemias).
Blood cultures	+/–	Rarely of diagnostic value in the cat
Coronavirus serology	+/–	Poor specificity - high prevalence of healthy seropositive cats. Other supportive tests mandatory (haematology, biochemistry, fluid analysis). Diagnosis can only be confirmed by histopathology.
Toxoplasma serology	+/–	Poor specificity, high prevalence of healthy seropositive cats. IgM serology more specific for recent/active infection but diagnosis based on this is very presumptive.
ANA titre	–	Autoimmune diseases are relatively infrequent causes of PUO in cats. ANA has poor sensitivity and specificity in this species.
Pyrexia is a very non-specific sign of feline disease, commonly seen in a number of disorders including stress. Due to the many potential underlying diseases and the difficulty in diagnosing these on the basis of routine laboratory tests, a large number of tests must be considered but many of these have poor sensitivity and specificity.		

FIG. 9.8   Diagnostic tests for use in pyrexia.

SEIZURES AND ATAXIA		
Test	**Value**	**Comments**
Serum biochemistry		
Ammonia/bile acids	+	Valuable tests for hepatic encephalopathy. Ammonia is more specific than bile acids.
Urea/creatinine	–	Rule out uraemic encephalopathy.
Serum proteins/SPE	+/–	Globulins may be increased with some CNS infections (e.g. FIP) but non-specific.
CPK	+	Valuable to check for possible myopathies (may sometimes be difficult to distinguish from neuropathies).
Ca/glucose	+/–	Rule out possible hypoglycaemic or hypocalcaemic syndromes -rare in cats other than iatrogenic.
Urinalysis	+/–	Presence of ammonium biurate crystals may suggest hepatic encephalopathy.
FeLV/FIV	+	Both may be primary causes of CNS disease or may lead to secondary CNS infections.
CSF analysis		
Cell counts	+	Elevated counts indicate infection, inflammation or trauma.
Culture	+/–	May be valuable for rare fungal or bacterial meningitis.
CPK	+	Elevated levels may indicate infection, inflammation or trauma.
Haematology	+/–	Changes may be found in association with CNS infection or inflammation but poor sensitivity and specificity.
Coronavirus serology	+/–	Poor specificity - see under PUO.
Toxoplasma serology	+/–	Poor specificity - see under PUO.
Toxicology	+/–	Only practical to investigate if suspicion of exposure to a specific toxic agent.

FIG. 9.9 Diagnostic tests for use in seizures and ataxia.

Hypochloraemia

Causes of hyponatraemia will also result in hypochloraemia, and additionally it may be seen in association with alkalosis. Selective chloride loss may be seen with gastric vomiting.

Total CO$_2$ (TCO$_2$)

Due to technical difficulties in performing blood gas analyses, measurement of TCO$_2$ in venous blood is often the only practical method of assessing acid-base status. Bicarbonate forms most of the TCO$_2$ in blood, and therefore this measurement generally reflects levels of bicarbonate. TCO$_2$ levels accompanied by appropriate clinical signs and ancillary tests will usually be sufficient to diagnose metabolic acidosis or alkalosis, but provides less information on respiratory acidosis or alkalosis. Increased TCO$_2$ may be caused by metabolic alkalosis (e.g. gastric vomiting), or compensated respiratory acidosis (due to hypoventilation). Decreased TCO$_2$ may be due to metabolic acidosis (shock/decreased tissue perfusion, diabetic ketoacidosis, ethylene glycol intoxication, severe diarrhoea, administration of ammonium chloride, renal tubular acidosis), or compensated respiratory alkalosis (due to hyperventilation).

Potassium

Potassium is the major intracellular cation, with a low concentration being maintained in extracellular fluid/serum (around 4.0–4.5 mmol/l). Hypokalaemia alters the resting membrane potential of myocytes and induces muscle weakness progressing to rhabdomyolysis in severe cases. Feline hypokalaemic polymyopathy syndromes have become well recognised over recent years and are the most frequent cause of generalised muscle weakness, being characterised by hypokalaemia and elevations in serum creatine kinase which may be profound. Hypokalaemia may also induce bradycardia and may adversely affect the renal capacity to concentrate urine. Hyperkalaemia can induce a severe life-threatening bradyarrhythmia with concomitant signs of weakness and collapse.

Hypokalaemia

Common hypokalaemic polymyopathy syndromes recognised in the cat are (1) associated with chronic renal failure (kaliuresis has been proposed as the mechanism underlying the hypokalaemia but this has yet to be confirmed), (2) an apparently familial episodic hypokalaemia seen in Burmese kittens in several countries, (3) associated with hyperaldosteronism (aldosterone secreting adrenocortical tumour). Hypokalaemia may also be seen in association with hyperthyroidism, alkalosis, vomiting or diarrhoea, renal tubular acidosis, and with the use of potassium depleting diuretics and insulin.

Hyperkalaemia

This is much less common than hypokalaemia, but may occur with urethral obstruction/bladder rupture, hypoadrenocorticism, excessive potassium supplementation, acidosis, and severe tissue injury. As in certain breeds of dog (e.g. Akita) it

MUSCLE WEAKNESS AND COLLAPSE		
Test	**Value**	**Comments**
Serum biochemistry		
CPK/K	++	CPK levels usually increase dramatically with polymyopathies. Hypokalaemic polymyopathy is the most common cause of generalised muscle weakness, and is usually associated with chronic renal failure, hyperaldosteronism, or a familial disease in Burmese kittens.
Urea/creatinine	+	Chronic renal failure is the disease most commonly associated with hypokalaemia and secondary polymyopathy.
Ca/glucose	+/–	Rule out possible hypoglycaemic or hypocalcaemic syndromes - rare in cats other than iatrogenic.
Blood gases/urine pH	–	Renal tubular acidosis is a rare cause of hypokalaemia and secondary polymyopathy.
Na	–	Hypernatraemia has been reported as a cause of polymyopathy in cats.
Urinalysis		
24 hour K clearance	+/–	Kaliuresis may indicate hyperaldosteronism. It is unclear at present whether the hypokalaemia associated with chronic renal failure is characterised by kaliuresis.
pH/blood gases	–	See above under blood gases.
T$_4$	+/–	Muscle weakness or collapse are occasional features of hyperthyroidism but other signs usually dominate.
Aldosterone	+/–	To check for hyperaldosteronism (Conns' syndrome) - valuable if other causes of hypokalaemia excluded or if kaliuresis confirmed.
ACTH stim test	–	Hypoadrenocorticism may cause muscle weakness but is rare in cats.
Anti-ACh receptor antibodies	–	May help confirm suspected acquired myasthenia gravis.

Fɪɢ. 9.10   Diagnostic tests for use in muscle weakness and collapse.

appears that some cats may have high levels of potassium in their erythrocytes leading to pseudo-hyperkalaemia which may occur with thrombo-cytosis or leucocytosis, where potassium is released from platelets or leucocytes after the blood is collected. Pseudohyperkalaemia may be differentiated from true hyperkalaemia by immediate separation of plasma after blood has been collected.

ENZYMES

The enzyme tests are largely used to investigate liver disease in cats.

Alanine aminotransferase (ALT)

An increase in ALT is very specific for liver disease in cats. Since this enzyme is found in the cytoplasm of hepatocytes as well as within the mitochondria, cellular death and destruction are not essential for its release and fatty infiltration with resulting increase in cell membrane permeability may lead to leakage of enzyme into the circulation. Increases in ALT are therefore not very specific to primary liver disease, and moderate increases are found in many conditions in which secondary liver pathology occurs, e.g. fatty infiltration secondary to diabetes mellitus. A common cause of elevated ALT concentrations in old cats is hyperthyroidism, although the explanation for this increase is not clear. Marked increases in serum ALT concentrations generally indicate hepatocellular damage.

Aspartate aminotransferase (AST)

This is a transaminase with a similar function to ALT. However, it is also found in other tissues, most notably muscle. It is therefore less specific than ALT and there is little indication for its use in testing for liver disease.

Alkaline phosphatase (ALP or SAP)

This enzyme has a wide tissue distribution, particularly in bone and as a brushborder enzyme in the biliary tract, kidney and intestine. However, increases in serum ALP are generally specific for biliary tract disease, as an indicator of cholestasis.

Enzyme leaking from the kidneys and intestine is lost through urine and intestinal contents, with no consequent increase in circulating concentrations. Severe bone disease may cause rises in serum concentrations, which may also be higher in young animals with active bone growth, but associated increases are generally small and not diagnostically helpful.

The half-life of SAP is short in cats and therefore cholestasis must be quite pronounced to result in a significant increase in serum concentrations. SAP estimations are extremely useful in assessing liver disease since increases usually indicate cholestasis. (Increases in SAP in dogs are much less specific, and therefore less useful diagnostically. The pronounced increases in SAP in dogs induced by corticosteroids are not seen in cats as they lack the steroid-induced isoenzyme.)

Gamma glutamyl transferase (Gamma GT)

The tissue distribution of Gamma GT is similar to that of SAP with the exception of bone. Intestinal or renal damage, as with SAP, leads to loss of enzyme without increase in serum concentrations, and a rise in Gamma GT is specific for cholestasis.

Creatinine phosphokinase (CPK)

CPK is found in muscle and nervous tissue. Nervous disorders do not generally result in a significant rise in serum CPK although increases in CSF concentrations of CPK may be detectable, e.g. in FIP. Serum concentrations may increase in cardiomyopathy but the most dramatic increases are seen in skeletal muscle damage, particularly with polymyopathy associated with hypokalaemia. The half-life of CPK is short and therefore serum concentrations may fall back to normal rapidly, and the enzyme is labile necessitating prompt assay after collection of serum. Different iso-enzymes of CPK occur but their relative distribution and clinical value in cats have not been evaluated.

LDH

As this enzyme is found in a wide range of tissues (muscle, liver, kidney, nervous tissue) any increase

JAUNDICE		
Test	**Value**	**Comments**
Serum biochemistry		
Bilirubin	++	Confirm presence of hyperbilirubinaemia. Differentiation of direct and indirect bilirubin often of very limited value.
Liver enzymes/ bile acids	++	May help identify hepatic or obstructive causes of jaundice. If hepatopathy present, tests will not identify the aetiology e.g. lymphocytic cholangitis, cholangiohepatitis, toxic hepatopathy, hyperthyroidism, neoplasia etc.
BSP/ICG clearance tests	–	Generally of no value if jaundice present.
Serum proteins/SPE	+/–	Elevated alpha-and gammaglobulins are often seen with FIP and lymphocytic cholangitis but are non-specific findings. Hypoalbuminaemia is rarely seen with liver disease in cats.
Haematology:		
Anaemia	+	Acute haemolysis may result in pre-hepatic jaundice, but in many diseases the presence of anaemia may not be directly related to the jaundice.
FIA	+	Rarely a severe parasitaemia may cause acute haemolysis resulting in jaundice. See also FIA under PUO section.
Neutrophilia/ leukocytosis/ lymphopenia	+/–	Non-specific changes that may be seen with neoplasia, cholangiohepatitis, lymphocytic cholangitis, FIP etc.
Bilirubinuria	+	This is always a significant finding in the cat, suggesting hyperbilirubinaemia.
Coronavirus serology	+/–	Poor specificity - see under PUO.
FeLV	+	May be associated with haemolysis or rarely hepatic neoplasia.
Bacterial culture of liver biopsy/aspirated bile	+	To confirm cholangiohepatitis and assist selection of appropriate antibiotic therapy.
T4	+/–	Hyperthyroidism may result in jaundice but other signs usually evident to assist diagnosis.
Toxicology	–	Hepatotoxins are a common cause of jaundice in the cat but toxicological investigations are only practical if exposure to a specific toxin is suspected.

FIG. 9.11   Diagnostic tests for use in jaundice.

is non-specific and of limited diagnostic value. LDH is not recommended for inclusion in standard feline biochemical profiles.

Amylase

Amylase is found in the salivary glands and pancreas. For dogs, the major diagnostic value of increased serum amylase concentrations is in the assessment of pancreatic disease, although the test has poor sensitivity and specificity. The value of amylase is even more questionable in cats, and serum concentrations fell in an experimental study of pancreatitis. In addition, acute pancreatic disease is rare except as a complication of injury associated with the high rise syndrome. Amylase is excreted in the urine and increased serum concentrations may occur in renal disease. We have seen persistent marked increases in serum amylase in a number of Siamese cats, though there has been no evidence of pancreatic or renal disease and we have been unable to associate this with any specific clinical problem. Enzyme studies have indicated that the increased levels are not salivary in origin.

ASCITES		
Test	**Value**	**Comments**
Fluid analysis Protein, A:G ratio, cytology	++	Confirm nature of fluid - i.e transudate, modified transudate or exudate. An exudate with globulins > albumin is consistent with FIP, but can also be seen with lymphocytic cholangitis and occasionally other conditions.
Culture	+	Important if bacterial peritonitis suspected.
Serum biochemistry Serum proteins/SPE	+	Elevated alpha-and gammaglobulins are often seen with FIP, but also occur with lymphocytic cholangitis and other conditions. Marked hypoalbuminaemia may lead to accumulation of abdominal transudate, but fluid usually present at other sites also.
Urea/creatinine/ cholesterol	+/–	Azotaemia and hypercholesterolaemia may accompany glomerulonephritis, but both may be normal.
Urinalysis Urine protein: creatinine ratio	+	Accurate assessment of urine protein losses, important if hypoalbuminaemia demonstrated or suspected.
Haematology Neutrophilia/ lymphopenia/anaemia	+/–	Non-specific changes. May reflect infectious or inflammatory process e.g. bacterial peritonitis, FIP etc.
Coronavirus serology	+/–	Poor specificity, other supporting evidence of FIP must be sought. See comments under PUO.

FIG. 9.12 Diagnostic tests for use in ascites.

Lipase

Concurrent estimation of lipase with amylase is recommended for assessing pancreatitis. The indications for lipase estimation are therefore infrequent, although lipase may be of particular value in view of the limitations of amylase.

URINALYSIS

Obtaining the sample

Urinalysis forms an integral part of the investigation of many diseases, but is probably an underused diagnostic aid, perhaps in part due to perceived difficulties in collection of urine samples. Urine may be collected in a number of different ways including cystocentesis, manual expression of the bladder, litter tray collection (after replacing litter with an inert product such as aquarium gravel), and catheterisation under anaesthesia or sedation. For reasons of practicality and quality of the specimen, cystocentesis is the preferred collection method for diagnostic urinalysis in most circumstances.

Cystocentesis

Cystocentesis is a rapid and simple technique, very well tolerated by almost all cats with a minimal level of restraint. A handler providing gentle manual restraint is generally all that is required. The bladder should be grasped gently near the neck and drawn cranially and toward the body wall so that the size, shape and location can be appreciated. After minimal skin preparation with alcohol, a 1″ 23 g needle attached to a 5–20 ml syringe is passed into the lumen of the bladder. The angle of the needle should not be altered once the bladder is entered. Cats may be restrained either standing, or in dorsal or lateral recumbency, with the needle introduced through either the flank or the ventral abdomen. Chemical restraint for cystocentesis is rarely required. Cats with LUTD tend to urinate spontaneously with even minor manipulation of the bladder, so that

DYSPNOEA/COUGH		
Test	**Value**	**Comments**
Haematology Leukocytosis/ neutrophilia	+/–	Non-specific changes, may reflect infectious or inflammatory process such as pyothorax, FIP, neoplasia, pneumonia, suppurative bronchitis.
Eosinophilia/ basophilia	+/–	Non-specific, but may occur with eosinophilic bronchitis or pulmonary infiltrates with eosinophils. May suggest hypersensitivity disorder especially if eosinophilia accompanied by basophilia. Other (non-respiratory) causes should also be considered, e.g. parasitic infections.
Anaemia	++	Important to rule out hypoxia as a cause or contributing to dyspnoea.
Cytology/culture of broncho-alveolar lavage fluid	+	May help to distinguish infectious from non-infectious or allergic causes of cough. The presence of even high numbers of eosinophils is normal in some cats so care must be taken in interpreting this finding.
Blood gas analysis	+/–	See Anaemia above.

FIG. 9.13   Diagnostic tests for use in dyspnoea/cough.

collection of urine by cystocentesis can be difficult. These cats should be placed in a cage without a litter tray for 4 hours prior to handling. The penis or vulval area should be grasped to occlude the urethra and prevent urination while bladder manipulation and cystocentesis is performed.

Catheterisation

Sedation is required for catheterisation of both male and female cats. In male cats, the penis should be exteriorised and grasped by the preputial mucosa then drawn caudally and slightly ventral to the plane of the vertebral column. This manoeuvre straightens the urethra and facilitates passage of the catheter. In female cats, passing the catheter along the ventral midline vulva can achieve catheterisation in many instances. Direct visualisation of the urethral opening is facilitated by gentle caudoventral tension on the ventral tip of the vulva. A short otoscope or fine-bladed vaginal speculum can be used. Good lighting is essential and catheters should be well lubricated.

Analysing the sample

Urine should be evaluated for colour and turbidity. Discoloration may indicate haematuria (red, red/brown) or bilirubinuria (brown), whilst turbidity normally suggests a high cellular content (e.g. pyuria). Semi-quantitative chemical analysis of the sample can be performed rapidly with commercial urinalysis test strips, but in some circumstances further quantitative tests may be indicated, and additionally microscopic examination of urine sediment may be valuable.

Specific gravity (SG)

Some urine test strips contain pads for SG analysis, but these are very unreliable, and SG should be determined by standard methods (e.g. refractometer).

The SG of glomerular filtrate is 1.007–1.015, which may be modified as it passes down through the tubules and loop of Henle. Urine classifications by SG range are: hyposthenuric (<1.007), isosthenuric (1.007–1.015), and hypersthenuric (>1.015). Typical values for urine SG in normal cats are in the mild to moderately hypersthenuric range (1.015–1.050), but this will depend largely on the hydration status and water intake.

Urine SG may be useful in the diagnosis of a range of diseases. Contrary to the situation in dogs and other species where renal concentrating ability is lost when function is reduced by around 65%, in cats concentrating ability may be retained even with advanced (azotaemic/uraemic) renal failure. The presence of hypersthenuric urine, therefore, cannot be taken to imply adequate renal function, although isosthenuria in the face of dehydration would imply serious renal damage. Persistent hyposthenuria may indicate diabetes insipidus.

Urine chemistry

pH

Feline urine is normally acidic. Its pH value ranges from 5.0 to 7.5 but will vary according to diet and time of collection in relation to feeding. A pH persistently greater than 7.5 may indicate urinary tract infection (UTI) or renal tubular acidosis.

Glucosuria

The finding of glucosuria warrants further investigation to determine the cause. Diabetes mellitus cannot be assumed, and other causes of hyperglycaemia must be eliminated (stress-induced, or drug-induced, e.g. xylazine) as well as causes other than hyperglycaemia, such as urinary tract haemorrhage and renal tubular anomalies. False positive results may occasionally occur with some test strips due to cross-reactivity with other reducing substances.

Ketonuria

The presence of ketonuria is almost always due to diabetes mellitus, although it may be found in association with starvation.

Bilirubin

The renal threshold for bilirubin is higher in cats than dogs, and therefore any amount of bilirubin in feline urine must be regarded as significant and warrants further investigation to determine the underlying cause (e.g. hepatopathy, bile duct obstruction, haemolysis).

Haemoglobin

Haemoglobinuria may be secondary to lysis of erythrocytes in haematuria, or may be due to haemoglobinaemia (haemolysis). Test-strips will not distinguish haemoglobinuria from myoglobinuria (myositis, extensive muscle trauma).

Nitrite

Many test strips will detect nitrituria which may be formed by UTI with nitrate-splitting bacteria. This is an insensitive screening test for UTI and has little value in the cat.

Protein

Test strips provide a semi-quantitative estimation of urinary protein that must be determined in the light of the urine SG (amount of urine produced). The test strips are also much more sensitive to albumin than to other proteins. In healthy cats, urine protein levels are usually below 100 mg/dl, and values above 200 mg/dl may be regarded as abnormal. Accurate assessment of significant proteinuria requires 24-hour urine collection or, more practically, calculation of the urine protein:creatinine ratio (UPC) on a single sample, as this is highly correlated with 24-hour urinary protein excretion values.

$$UPC = \frac{\text{Urinary total protein (mg/dl)}}{\text{Urinary creatinine (mg/dl)}}$$

In healthy cats the UPC is <1, and a value >2 suggests significant proteinuria that requires further investigation. Values between 1 and 2 should be reassessed and should be investigated again if persistently >1. Potential causes of proteinuria include prerenal (haemoglobinuria, myoglobinuria, Bence-Jones proteins), renal (glomerulonephritis, amyloidosis, renal failure, pyelonephritis) and post-renal (lower UTI or inflammation). If proteinuria is severe (UPC >4) then glomerulonephritis (or rarely amyloidosis) is highly likely.

Urine sediment analysis

To gain maximum benefit from urine sediment analysis, it should be performed as soon as possible on a fresh sample. Delay in examination, or in sending the sample to a commercial laboratory, may significantly decrease the diagnostic value. Samples should be centrifuged for 5–10 minutes, with the resulting pellet being resuspended and examined microscopically.

Epithelial cells

These are normally found in urine, but may be increased in numbers in inflammatory conditions.

Erythrocytes (haematuria)

The presence of haematuria might suggest lower urinary tract disease (LUTD, sterile cystitis), UTI, inflammation, necrosis, trauma, or neoplasia.

Leukocytes (pyuria)

Pyuria will commonly accompany LUTD/sterile cystitis, UTI, neoplasia, and urinary tract inflammation.

Bacteria

Cystocentesis samples are normally sterile, and the presence of bacteria indicates UTI. Where

ANAEMIA		
Test	**Value**	**Comments**
Haematology		
RBC indices	++	Confirm clinical suspicion of anaemia, determine if anaemia regenerative (may be difficult in cats - see Chapter 19), and characterise type of anaemia (e.g. microcytic, hypochromic).
WBC indices	+	Non-specific but may suggest underlying inflammatory or infectious disease, or may reveal presence of pancytopenia which may suggest a bone marrow disorder.
Thrombocytes	+/–	Non-specific and accurate measurement difficult but decreases may be associated with coagulopathies leading to anaemia, infectious diseases (e.g. FIV) or bone marrow disorders; while increases may reflect the rare primary thrombocythaemia or may occur following recent haemorrhage.
FIA	++	Important to assess in anaemia cases but tests are not sensitive, and a positive finding can sometimes be difficult to interpret. Predisposing disease(s) should be sought.
FeLV/FIV	++	Important priorities, both these viruses are major causes of anaemia.
Serum biochemistry		
Hyperbilirubinaemia	+	Occasionally seen with severe, acute haemolysis.
Serum proteins/SPE	+	Hypoproteinaemia may be seen following haemorrhage. Elevations in globulins are a non-specific finding but may occur in association with some diseases associated with anaemia such as FIV and FIP.
Urea/creatinine/PO$_4$	+	Chronic renal failure commonly causes a non-regenerative anaemia due to lack of erythropoietin.
Marrow biopsy	+	Indicated if haematology shows unexplained non-regenerative anaemia or pancytopenia, if abnormal cells are seen in blood smears or if there is persistent undiagnosed anaemia.
Urinalysis		
Haematuria/ haemoglobinuria	+	Valuable in detecting direct blood loss from the urinary tract.
Bilirubinuria	+	Always a significant finding in cats, see under hyperbilirubinaemia above.
Coagulation screening	+	Indicated if evidence of unexplained haemorrhage.
Coombs' test	–	Primary autoimmune haemolytic anaemia is rare in the cat, and the Coombs' test carries poor specificity in this species.
ANA	–	This test has poor specificity in cats.
Occult faecal blood	–	This test is used to detect gastrointestinal haemorrhage, but its value is limited due to very poor specificity.

Fig. 9.14   Diagnostic tests for use in anaemia.

bacteriuria is a significant finding it will normally be accompanied by pyuria or haematuria.

Casts

Casts are primarily formed from mucoproteins secreted by epithelial cells lining the tubules and collecting ducts. Their presence may indicate involvement of these structures in a disease process, and their contents may suggest an aetiology.

Hyaline casts – may be present in normal urine, increased numbers often accompany proteinuria.

Erythrocyte casts – may be seen with glomerular or tubular haemorrhage (e.g. severe glomerulonephritis).

Leukocyte casts – seen with renal infection or inflammation.

Granular casts – contain degenerate tubular cells and may be seen with a number of conditions including nephritis or tubular hypoxia.

Waxy casts – seen in various disorders.

Fatty casts – more common in cats than dogs, and may accompany a variety of conditions (i.e. non-specific).

Crystalluria

Crystalluria is a common finding, and in many cases is normal. The presence and type of crystal is in part dependent on urine pH, temperature and specific gravity. Struvite ($MgNH_4PO_4$, 'triple phosphate') crystals are the most common to be found in feline urine, and may be considered normal. Oxalate and amorphous phosphate crystals are also considered normal findings. Large numbers or the presence of other crystals may be significant, though care is necessary in interpreting such findings. Ammonium biurate crystals may be seen in urine from cats with porto-systemic shunts.

FAECES

Faecal testing is relatively unimportant in cats. The endoparasites which can be readily diagnosed by faecal testing are generally of minor clinical importance, but faecal screening is unreliable for clinically important endoparasites such as giardia and toxoplasma. Interpretation of faecal bacteriology is complicated by the frequent occurrence of bacteria which are considered as potential enteropathogens in normal cats, such as *Campylobacter* spp. Tests for occult faecal blood are unreliable, frequently giving positives in normal cats, irrespective of diet. Faecal fat estimations are potentially of value in assessing malassimilation but are not popular with diagnostic laboratories and create problems for timed faecal collections. Faecal trypsin estimations are notoriously unreliable. If they are undertaken, several consecutive faecal samples should be assessed and one of the more reliable analytical methods should be used, such as the azo-casein test. However, pancreatic insufficiency is an exceedingly rare clinical problem in cats.

10

Disorders of the Respiratory System

ALICE M. WOLF

NASAL CAVITY DISORDERS

Clinical signs

The most common clinical signs associated with disorders of the nasal cavity include obstructed or noisy breathing, sneezing, nasal discharge, and destruction or distortion of the nasal or facial anatomy. Obstructed or noisy breathing (stertor, stridor) occurs because of disruption of the normal airflow pattern through the sinuses, nasal cavity, or nasopharynx. Stridor may be the only clinical sign noticed in cats with nasopharyngeal polyps. Sneezing is caused by intranasal irritation, particularly in the rostral half of the nasal cavity. Inhaled foreign bodies (e.g., grass awns) often cause acute paroxysms of sneezing until the foreign body is dislodged or becomes settled deeper in the nasal cavity. Sneezing caused by a chronic foreign body or other nasal disorder is less frequent and is accompanied by other signs of nasal cavity disease (e.g. stertor, discharge).

Serous discharge is produced in the initial stages of viral upper respiratory infections in cats and in patients with early parasitic or allergic rhinitis. Chronic primary or secondary bacterial rhinosinusitis, primary ciliary dyskinesia, or lymphoplasmacytic rhinitis usually cause mucopurulent discharge. Frank haemorrhage from the nasal cavity (epistaxis) is most often caused by acute foreign body inhalation, direct trauma, or a systemic coagulation disorder. Fungal infections and neoplasia usually cause mucoid to mucopurulent nasal discharge that may intermittently contain fresh blood.

Most patients with allergic, immunologic, parasitic, and primary or secondary bacterial rhinitis will have bilateral nasal discharge throughout the course of the disease. Patients with fungal and neoplastic disorders will usually have unilateral nasal discharge initially, but both sides often become involved as these lesions progress. Foreign bodies and dental disease may cause unilateral or bilateral discharge.

Chronic bacterial rhinosinusitis may cause internal destruction of the turbinates and erosion of the nasal mucosa but should not erode or distort the nasal or facial bones. Significant internal destruction of the nasal cavity or overlying bones, or obvious facial distortion, is usually caused by erosive or expansile neoplastic or fungal mass lesions.

Diseases that affect the nasal cavity may extend into the brain because of the communication to this structure through the olfactory apparatus via the cribriform plate. Although foreign body and parasitic penetration is possible, the brain is most commonly affected by invasive neoplastic or fungal diseases. Signs of central nervous system involvement (e.g. seizures, behavioural changes, depression, ataxia, gait abnormalities) sometimes occur without obvious evidence of nasal cavity disease.

Pain in the nasal cavity is usually caused by nasal trauma, or erosive or expanding mass lesions. A cat with a nasal foreign body or allergic rhinitis may rub or paw at its muzzle. Unilateral or bilateral exophthalmos can result from retrobulbar extension from the nasal cavity. Ocular discharge can be produced by blockage of the nasolacrimal drainage system. Gagging may occur if foreign bodies or mass lesions extend into the nasopharynx or if a large amount of discharge is draining from the posterior nasal cavity. Lesions that erode or disrupt the hard palate (e.g. neoplasia, trauma) may cause food to be expelled from the nares.

Diagnostic evaluation

History and physical examination

Obtain a complete history including the patient profile, current complaint (duration, progression, response to previous therapy), environment, travel, preventive health care, and previous medical and surgical problems. Further questions should be directed to evaluate all body systems.

Perform a thorough physical examination of all body systems. When attention is focused on the nasal cavity, assess the patient for the presence of nasal obstruction or stertor. Occlude the nostrils alternately to determine if the obstruction is unilateral or bilateral. Note the amount and type of nasal discharge draining from the nares and nasopharynx, and palpate the nasal cavity and sinuses for swelling, distortion, or pain. Manually repulse the globes of the eyes gently back in the orbits to detect retrobulbar extension of an expanding mass lesion. A fundic examination may reveal retinal lesions suggestive of cryptococcosis or other granulomatous diseases.

Clinical pathological evaluation

Routine haematological and biochemical tests in patients with nasal cavity and sinus disease are often normal. An inflammatory leukogram may be found in some patients but is a nonspecific finding. Anaemia or thrombocytopenia might indicate a bleeding disorder (e.g., coagulopathy, immune-mediated thrombocytopenia) but could also result from acute or chronic epistaxis. Coagulation studies should be performed if an hereditary coagulopathy or exposure to anticoagulant rodenticide is suggested by the patient's history.

Test cats for feline leukaemia virus and feline immunodeficiency virus infection because these immunosuppressive diseases will predispose the cat to some disorders and worsen the severity of others. Other than the latex agglutination test for *Cryptococcus*, fungal serology is not a useful screening test for systemic mycoses and because false negative test results are common. In addition, *Cryptococcus*, *Histoplasma* and *Aspergillus* are usually readily discovered in cytological or histological specimens.

Radiographic evaluation

Perform nasal and sinus radiographic studies with the patient under general anaesthesia to facilitate proper positioning. Use nonscreen film or high detail screens and film to enhance visualisation of intranasal structures. Take at least three views including a lateral, an open mouth ventrodorsal, and a frontal sinus view. Obtain oblique studies of the maxilla to detect the presence of apical abscesses in patients with dental disease.

Increased fluid density in the air spaces of the nasal cavity or sinuses indicates the presence of a noninvasive soft tissue mass (e.g. inflammation, fungal ball, early neoplasia) or fluid (blood, mucus). Destruction or distortion of the nasal turbinate structures can occur with chronic inflammation but is more likely the result of a more invasive process such as neoplasia or fungal rhinitis. Destruction or distortion of the nasal or facial bones is highly suggestive of neoplasia but can occur with fungal infections. If computed tomography is available it can be used to differentiate among the causes of nasal disease and determine the extent of nasal cavity and sinus involvement.

Bacteriological culture

Routine and guarded swabs can be used to obtain material from the nasal cavity for bacteriological culture and sensitivity testing. However, regardless of the culture technique, interpretation of bacterial culture results is difficult because of the variety of potential pathogens that reside as normal commensal organisms in the nasal cavity. Bacterial secondary infections are common in all types of nasal disorders but true primary bacterial rhinitis and sinusitis is rare. Fungal cultures taken from nasal swabs are often falsely positive for *Aspergillus* or *Penicillium* because of the ubiquity of these organisms in the environment. Fungal cultures taken from surgical biopsy specimens are more likely to produce reliable results.

Rhinoscopy

Care must be taken during all intranasal procedures to avoid accidental penetration of the cribriform plate. Measure the distance from the external nares to the medial canthus of the eye, mark all instruments with this measurement, and do not insert them into the dorsal portion of the nasal cavity beyond this point.

Examination of the nasal cavity must be performed with the patient under a surgical plane of anaesthesia with a cuffed endotracheal tube in place because of the sneeze reflex and the danger of aspiration during the procedure. A paediatric otoscope can be used to examine the anterior portion of the nasal cavity in most cats. Retrieval of foreign bodies and biopsy specimens is easier if an operating head is used. An arthroscope can also be used for rhinoscopy in larger patients but it is often difficult to keep the lens clear of secretions and blood. If intranasal debris prevents good visualisation of the nasal cavity, normal saline solution can be flushed through a cannula around the arthroscope to wash material from the lens. Before flushing, position several gauze sponges in the nasopharynx to absorb fluid and recover debris for examination. If excessive bleeding occurs during rhinoscopy, apply cotton-tipped swabs soaked in 1:10,000 epinephrine solution to the bleeding area and leave them in place for several minutes.

To evaluate the posterior portion of the nasal cavity and nasopharynx, retract the soft palate cranially with a spay hook and examine the area with a penlight and dental mirror. If available, a flexible fibre optic endoscope provides even better access to and visualisation of this area.

Cytological examination and biopsy

Specimens for cytological examination can be taken during rhinoscopy with cotton swabs, by suction with a feline side hole urinary catheter or canine polyethylene urinary catheter with the tip cut off at an angle, and by pinch or punch biopsy.[4] Apply cytology specimens to a clean glass slide, make horizontal pull-apart smears, and stain them with Wright's Giemsa type haematological and fungal stains (e.g. methenamine silver stain, periodic acid Schiff).

If cytological specimens are not diagnostic, larger biopsy specimens for histological examination can be collected with alligator forceps, clamshell biopsy forceps, catheters, or needlepunch techniques.[1] To avoid loss during handling and to facilitate histological processing, small tissue specimens should be placed on a piece of paper towel or absorbable gelatin foam surgical sponge before being immersed in formalin. Stain biopsy specimens with haematoxylin eosin and fungal stains.

Exploratory surgery

If biopsies obtained by rhinoscopy are not diagnostic, exploratory surgery of the nasal cavity may be required to evaluate the disease process further and obtain sufficient tissue for definitive diagnosis. Mass removal, curettage of the nasal cavity or sinus(es), and implantation of drainage or flush tubes can be performed during the same procedure.

SPECIFIC NASAL CAVITY DISORDERS

Feline upper respiratory disease complex
(See Chapter 23)

Herpesvirus or calicivirus is the primary agent in 90% of cats with upper respiratory infection (URI). Other agents (*Chlamydia*, *Mycoplasma*, reovirus, coronavirus, bacteria) may be primarily or concurrently involved. The severity of clinical signs seen with these diseases is dependent on the age of the cat at infection, the level of maternal or acquired immunity, the general health status of the cat including the presence of concurrent diseases (particularly FeLV and FIV), and the duration of exposure and challenge dose of the virus. Clinical signs usually include fever, malaise, anorexia, and oculonasal discharge. Tongue and nasal ulcers and herpes keratitis occur in some cats. Treatment consists of good nursing care by avoiding stress, providing fluid and caloric support, and frequent removal of discharge from the eyes and nose. Specific treatment with bronchodilators, antibiotics and humidification is given to cats with lower airway involvement. Cats with herpes keratitis should receive antiviral ophthalmic medication (idoxuridine, vidarabine, trifluorothymidine). Chronic sequelae to infection by herpesvirus and calicivirus include a chronic carrier state, chronic rhinosinusitis, chronic gingivitis and stomatitis, and chronic conjunctivitis or keratitis.

Chronic rhinitis/sinusitis (chronic 'snufflers')

Most cats develop chronic rhinitis and sinusitis following infection with one of the feline viral URI agents (usually herpesvirus) early in life. The virus causes permanent damage to the turbinate structures of the nasal passages, prediposing the cat to secondary bacterial infection. This disorder can occur in any cat but cattery cats in general have a higher incidence of chronic rhinosinusitis because of endemic URI in these populations, stress, and early exposure of kittens to the disease. Persian, Himalayan and Siamese cats have an increased incidence of the problem.

Clinical signs include periodic sneezing, nasal discharge and noisy breathing. There are usually no systemic signs of disease. The nasal discharge is mucopurulent and is usually bilateral although unilateral disease occurs in some cats.

The diagnosis of chronic bacterial rhinosinusitis is made by ruling out more serious disorders. The laboratory data base (CBC, biochemistry panel, urinalysis) is usually normal. Serology for FeLV and FIV should be performed because the presence of these diseases makes treatment more difficult. Nasal cavity radiographs usually reveal diffuse increased density in the nasal passages or frontal sinuses; evidence of bone lysis is unusual. Nasal cavity cytology and biopsy reveals only chronic, purulent inflammation associated with bacteria. Bacteriological culture of the nasal cavity is rarely helpful because a mixed bacterial population is usually present and because the normal flora may contain potential pathogens.

Treatment of chronic rhinosinusitis often results in only temporal remission of clinical signs. The owner should be warned that recurrences are likely and intermittent treatment may be needed for the life of the cat. A broad-spectrum antibiotic (amoxicillin, cephalosporin, trimethoprim-sulpha, enrofloxacin) is given to reduce bacterial numbers. Paediatric strength topical nasal decongestants can be used in alternate nostrils once or twice daily for 4–5 days to reduce intranasal swelling and improve breathing. Intranasal EDTA Tris buffer seems to help some cats with pure culture *Pseudomonas* infection. Antihistamines (e.g. diphenhydramine 1.1 mg/kg PO bid) may be helpful in some cats. Humidification with a vaporiser or nebuliser improves clearing of secretions. Some clinicians have reported improvement in cats with chronic rhinosinusitis following intranasal vaccination with modified live virus intranasal

herpesvirus and calicivirus vaccine. Several surgical procedures have been developed to remove damaged turbinate bones or implant fat grafts in the frontal sinuses. In my experience, surgical procedures are very traumatic and do not result in long term improvement. The overall prognosis for control of the symptoms of rhinosinusitis is fair to poor and complete resolution of signs is unlikely.

Fungal rhinitis

Cryptococcus neoformans is the most common fungal agent infecting the nasal cavity of the cat. *Blastomyces*, *Histoplasma*, *Aspergillus*, *Penicillium* and *Sporothrix* are rarely found in this location. These diseases are acquired by inhalation of fungal organisms from organic matter in the environment. Pathological changes are usually limited to one side of the nasal cavity initially; however, the infection can spread to the other side over time. Enlarging granulomatous inflammatory masses associated with fungal infection can destroy the bones overlying the nasal cavity resulting in swelling or discharging lesions on the face. Fungal infections may occasionally involve the regional lymph nodes.

Cryptococcal rhinitis is relatively uncommon. There is no age, breed or sex predilection for this disease. Clinical signs include sneezing and nasal discharge that is usually unilateral (at least initially) and mucoid, and may contain fresh blood. Nasal cavity radiographs may reveal unilateral or bilateral increased density; bone destruction is present in some cats (Fig. 10.1). Rhinoscopic examination often reveals a friable, granulomatous mass in the nasal passage(s). Nasal cytology or biopsy usually demonstrates numerous *Cryptococcus* organisms with variable numbers of inflammatory cells (Fig. 10.2). A serum cryptococcal antigen titre (LCAT) is available from some diagnostic laboratories and is useful for confirming the diagnosis and to monitor the response to antifungal therapy.

The treatment of choice for cryptococcal rhinitis at this time is ketoconazole (KTZ) at a dose of 10–15 mg/kg PO bid. Early side effects of treatment include anorexia and vomition. If this occurs, stop drug administration for several days, then resume at a lower dose. Full dose therapy can

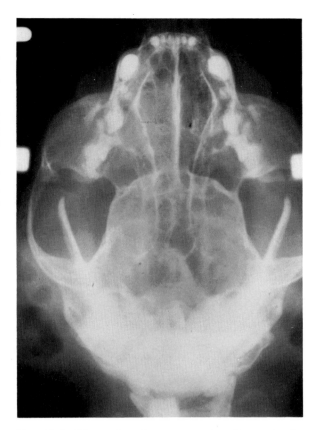

FIG. 10.1 Ventrodorsal, open-mouth radiograph of a cat with nasal cryptococcosis. There is increased density of the right side of the nasal passage and the nasal septum is intact.

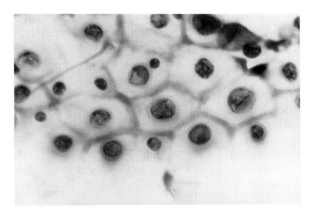

FIG. 10.2 Cytological specimen from a cat with nasal cryptococcosis. The specimen contains numerous small budding yeasts with a wide non-staining capsule. Wright's Giemsa stain.

Parasitic rhinitis

Cuterebra larvae have been recovered from the nasal passage of kittens and adult cats. Manual removal results in prompt resolution of all signs of sneezing and nasal obstruction.

Nasopharyngeal polyps

Nasopharyngeal polyps are non-neoplastic, inflammatory masses that originate in the middle ear, traverse the eustachian tube and emerge in the nasopharynx. These masses may also grow in the opposite direction and occlude the external ear canal. The cause underlying the development of these inflammatory lesions is unknown but feline calicivirus has been isolated from some of these patients. Most affected cats are less than 6 years of age; there is no breed or sex predilection. Clinical signs are usually those of chronic upper respiratory obstruction, stridor and gagging or sneezing. Owners may also notice a change in voice or dysphagia. There are generally no signs of systemic illness.

The diagnosis requires thorough examination of the nasopharynx with the cat under anaesthesia. A spay hook or Allis tissue forceps is used to pull the soft palate forward and a dental mirror or flexible endoscope is used to visualise the posterior nasopharyngeal wall. Radiographs should be taken of the tympanic bullae because these are often involved in the disease process.

often be resumed in 7–10 days. Long-term effects of KTZ include liver dysfunction, alopecia and lightening of the hair coat colour. These changes are reversible when KTZ therapy is discontinued. The response to treatment should be monitored by following the clinical response of the patient and evaluation of decreasing LCAT levels. Treatment should be continued for at least one month following apparent resolution of clinical signs. Relapses have occurred but resistance to this drug has not been reported. Newer azole antifungals, itraconazole (10 mg/kg PO sid) and fluconazole (5.0–10 mg/kg PO sid or bid) are also effective against *Cryptococcus* but have not yet been fully evaluated for efficacy or safety in the cat. Amphotericin B and flucytosine can be used for cats with severe disease or those unresponsive to azole therapy.

Treatment consists of surgical removal of the polyp. Fortunately, these have a relatively avascular, narrow stalk and can be easily twisted free or excised. Bulla osteotomy is recommended by some clinicians if radiographs reveal bulla involvement. Failure to remove inflammatory tissue in the bulla may result in recurrence of the polyp.

Nasal neoplasia

Nasal tumours are unusual in the cat. The most common tumour types are lymphosarcoma, adenocarcinoma, and squamous cell carcinoma. Mesenchymal tumours (fibrosarcoma, osteosarcoma) are very rare. Nasal lymphosarcoma most often affects middle-aged cats; the other tumours are seen most often in aged animals.

The clinical signs, laboratory test results and radiographic findings in cats with nasal neoplasia are similar to those previously described for fungal rhinitis (Fig. 10.3). Cytology or biopsy of the nasal mass is most important to differentiate between these two disorders. In cats with confirmed neoplasia, thoracic radiography and aspiration cytology or biopsy of regional lymph nodes should be performed to detect local or distant tumour metastasis.

The recommended treatment for nasal neoplasia depends on the type of tumour and extent of the lesion. Lymphosarcoma is the most responsive tumour type. Cobalt radiotherapy or chemotherapy have produced long-term remissions in some cats. Squamous cell carcinoma may be radiosensitive but is poorly responsive if bone invasion has already occurred. The other tumours are usually radio-resistant and do not respond to chemotherapy. Surgical intervention is traumatic, cannot be expected to be curative, and may not significantly prolong the life of the cat.

Traumatic disorders

Nasal cavity trauma occurs most commonly from vehicular trauma or falling from a height ('high rise syndrome'). Associated problems often include midline hard palate maxillary fractures, mandibular fractures, and localised or generalised subcutaneous emphysema. Most nasal bleeding stops spontaneously. Treatment should be directed at care of the fractures and other concurrent injuries.

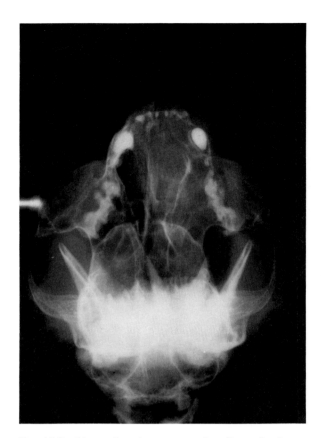

FIG. 10.3   Ventrodorsal, open-mouth radiograph of a cat with a nasal adenocarcinoma. There is considerable destruction and distortion of the anterior portion of the left nasal cavity. The soft tissue density mass lesion has destroyed the nasal septum and has invaded the right nasal cavity.

The majority of nasal foreign bodies are grass and cereal awns or other plant materials. These usually cause signs of acute, dramatic nasal irritation with paroxysmal sneezing with or without epistaxis. If not recognised acutely, chronic rhinitis will develop. At this time the signs may appear similar to bacterial rhinosinusitis. A thorough diagnostic evaluation and nasal cavity examination should reveal the cause of the problem in most cats. Removal of the foreign body is curative.

DISORDERS OF THE LARYNX AND TRACHEA

Laryngeal paralysis

Laryngeal paralysis is usually an acquired disorder that occurs secondary to accidental or surgical trauma. Failure of one or both sides of the larynx to open during inspiration causes dyspnoea, dysphonia, and respiratory stridor. Diagnosis is based on history, physical examination, and laryngeal examination. Laryngeal examination should be performed under a light plane of injectable anaesthesia. An endotracheal tube, oxygen, and supplies necessary to perform a tracheostomy should be available in the event that hypoxia occurs during the examination. Possible approaches to the treatment of laryngeal paralysis include laryngeal cartilage resection or tieback, and permanent tracheostomy. Complications of laryngeal surgery include laryngeal oedema acutely and aspiration pneumonia. Problems associated with permanent tracheostomy include difficulties in maintaining tube patency and aspiration pneumonia. The prognosis for cats with laryngeal paralysis is fair.

Tracheal stenosis/ruptured trachea

Tracheal stenosis and rupture usually occur secondary to trauma. Tracheal stenosis most often results from overinflation of the endotracheal tube cuff during anaesthetic intubation. Scarring and stenosis usually develop slowly and signs of respiratory stridor and dyspnoea may not appear for several weeks after the traumatic event. Tracheal rupture can also occur secondary to endotracheal intubation but most commonly results from severe blunt trauma to the thorax (e.g. vehicular trauma, falling from a tree). Tracheal rupture usually causes acute inspiratory and expiratory dyspnoea; pneumomediastinum, pneumothorax, or subcutaneous emphysema are common accompanying findings. Occasionally, signs of dyspnoea do not appear for some time after the traumatic event. The diagnosis of tracheal stenosis or rupture is made on the basis of history (trauma or intubation), localisation of stridor and dyspnoea, physical examination, and radiographic findings. Plain film radiographs of the cervical and thoracic trachea may demonstrate the tracheal narrowing or discontinuity. Tracheal endoscopy with a rigid or fibre optic endoscope is performed using the anaesthetic technique and with the precautions described for laryngeal examination. Tracheal stenosis can sometimes be corrected with progressive mechanical dilatation techniques (bouginage).

Surgical resection of the damaged segment is necessary in some patients. Small tracheal tears may heal without surgical intervention. Anastomosis of the severed tracheal segments is required to correct complete tracheal rupture. The major complication of tracheal surgery is post-surgical stricture.

Laryngeal/tracheal neoplasia

Neoplasia of the larynx and trachea is rare in the cat. Clinical signs associated with laryngeal and tracheal neoplasia are similar to those seen with laryngeal paralysis or tracheal stenosis. Examination of the affected structure will reveal the neoplastic mass. Definitive diagnosis can be made on the basis of tissue cytology or biopsy. Reported tumours of the larynx in their order of frequency include lymphosarcoma, squamous cell carcinoma, and adenocarcinoma. Tumours of the trachea include adenocarcinoma, lymphosarcoma, and squamous cell carcinoma. Lymphosarcoma is potentially responsive to chemotherapy or radiation therapy and the prognosis for short-time survival with appropriate treatment is fair to good. Laryngeal and tracheal carcinomas are usually locally invasive, often metastatic, and are poorly responsive to any treatment modality. Surgical resection may be palliative but the prognosis for cats with these tumours is grave.

Tracheal collapse

Tracheal collapse is a rare condition in the cat. Most reported cases have occurred secondary to an obstructive intratracheal mass lesion.

PLEURAL EFFUSION

Pleural effusion results from an imbalance between the rate of production and the rate of reabsorption of fluid in the pleural space. Clinical signs associated with pleural fluid result from mechanical restriction of lung expansion during respiration and the toxic products associated with lysosomal enzymes or bacteria. Signs vary depending on the underlying cause of the effusion, the rate at which the fluid accumulates, and secondary complications that may occur.

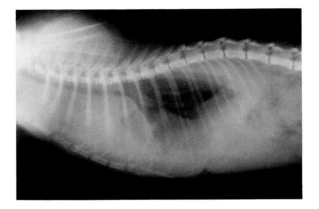

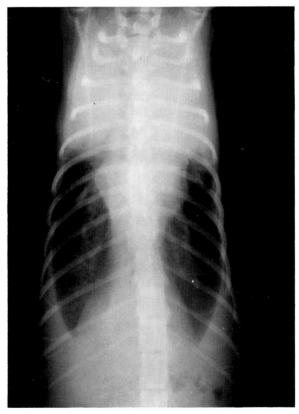

FIG. 10.4 Lateral and ventrodorsal thoracic radiographs of a cat with pleural effusion.

Physical findings include laboured breathing with an abdominal 'lift', a sternal recumbent position with elbows abducted, open-mouth breathing and, rarely, coughing. Thoracic auscultation will reveal muffled heart and lung sounds in the ventral

thorax. Radiographic findings include loss of intrathoracic detail, blurring of the cardiac silhouette, widening of the mediastinum, scalloped lung margins, pleural fissure lines, and rounded costophrenic angles (Fig. 10.4).

Thoracentesis is used to improve ventilation, to obtain diagnostic radiographs unobscured by fluid, and to collect fluid samples for cytological examination and bacteriological culture. Fluid is used to prepare direct smears immediately and is placed in EDTA and sterile 'clot' tubes for further analysis or culture. The character of any effusion will change as it remains in the pleural space over time.

Septic inflammatory exudate (pyothorax)

This fluid may be yellow, red or brown in colour, and is turbid with a high protein content and specific gravity. There may be large amounts of fibrin and debris, and the fluid is often foul-smelling. Cytology reveals high cell counts; the predominant cell type is the neutrophil (PMN) in varying stages of degeneration (Fig. 10.5). Bacteria may or may not be seen within PMN or free in the exudate.

The most common agents associated with feline pyothorax include *Pasteurella*, *Bacteroides* and *Fusobacterium*. Physical findings include fever (variable, may be subnormal late in the course),

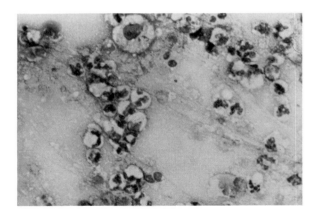

FIG. 10.5 Cytological specimen from a cat with pyothorax. The effusion contains degenerate and toxic neutrophils and occasional macrophages. The grainy background material is proteinaceous debris and degenerated cellular material. Wright's Giemsa stain.

anorexia, depression, dehydration and cough. The complete blood count often reveals an inflammatory leukogram; the presence of a degenerative left shift is a poor prognostic sign. Tests should be performed for FeLV antigen and FIV antibody because the presence of these diseases will make successful treatment more difficult. An aerobic and anaerobic bacteriological culture and sensitivity test should be performed on the pleural fluid.

Treatment of feline pyothorax includes closed chest tube drainage and pleural lavage for 3–5 days, with supportive nursing care, fluid therapy to maintain hydration, and nutritional support. Systemic antibiotics should be selected on the basis of culture and sensitivity testing of the pleural fluid and are given for a minimum of 4–6 weeks. Complications of pyothorax include fibrinous pleuritis, walled off abscesses in the lung, mediastinum and pleura, pneumothorax resulting from thoracentesis or tearing of lung adhesions, chronic lung lobe atelectasis, and lung lobe torsion.

Pyogranulomatous effusion

Pyogranulomatous effusion is usually straw to yellow in colour, clear to slightly cloudy, and has a high protein content and specific gravity. The aetiology of this type of effusion is feline infectious peritonitis (FIP). Electrophoresis of FIP effusion fluid demonstrates a high level of globulins. Cellularity is moderate with a mixed pattern of macrophages, PMNs and lymphocytes. Bacteria are not seen and bacteriological cultures of the fluid are negative.

Associated physical findings can be quite variable and include fluctuating, antibiotic-unresponsive fever, abdominal effusion, anorexia, depression, weight loss, and dehydration. The haemogram may reveal neutrophilic leukocytosis. Serum biochemistry profiles may demonstrate increased serum globulin and total protein levels, and evidence of internal organ dysfunction. Some FIP-affected patients have concurrent FeLV infection; the association with FIV is currently being investigated. Coronavirus serology ('FIP test') is not specific for FIP and cannot be used to validate this diagnosis. This disease is ultimately fatal in most cats. Combined chemotherapy with immunosuppressive drugs may slow the course of the disease in some patients.

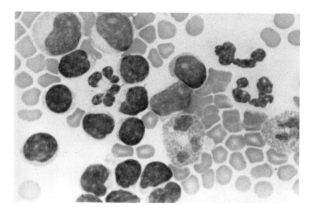

FIG. 10.6   Cytological specimen from a cat with chylothorax of several months duration. The effusion in this patient contains mostly small lymphocytes, occasional large lymphocytes, neutrophils, eosinophils, and RBCs. The inflammatory cells have appeared in response to chronic irritation of the pleura. Wright's Giemsa stain.

Chylous effusion

Chylous effusion has a characteristic opaque, milky white appearance with a moderate protein content and specific gravity. Initially, the fluid contains a moderate number of cells that are predominantly small lymphocytes with some RBCs, macrophages, and mesothelial cells that may contain fat vacuoles (Fig. 10.6). Because chyle is irritating to the pleura, more PMN will be present in the fluid in chronic cases. If chylous fluid is refrigerated or centrifuged, a 'cream layer' will rise to the surface of the sample. A Sudan III stained sample specimen may demonstrate chylomicra. Triglyceride levels are very high in this fluid. Ether treatment may cause the milky appearance of chyle to clear. The usual cause of chylous effusion in cats is traumatic rupture of the thoracic duct. Other causes include congenital malformations, neoplasia with lymphatic invasion, complication of thoracic surgery, and dirofilariasis.

Clinical signs usually develop gradually due to slow accumulation of the fluid. In addition to respiratory distress, cough is more likely to occur with this type of effusion than with others. Additional clinical signs associated with chylothorax include weight loss, fatigue and polydipsia. Fluid analysis will confirm the diagnosis; other laboratory findings include low circulating lymphocyte counts, low serum protein levels and a negative fat absorption test.

Conservative medical management consists of removal of the chylous fluid weekly for 4–6 weeks to improve respiration and allow for the spontaneous healing of the lymphatic leak. Pleurodesis with tetracycline has been used in treatment of chylothorax by some clinicians. Surgical approaches to therapy include ligation of the thoracic duct, cyanoacylate obstruction of the cysterna chyli, circumaortic ligation of the cysterna chyli, mesh fenestration of the diaphragm, or installation of a pleural-peritoneal shunt. Dietary management is an important adjunct to both medical and surgical treatment. A low-fat diet with medium chain triglyceride oil is recommended.

Pseudochylous effusion

This type of effusion has been described in the veterinary literature. Newer techniques of measuring triglycerides and cholesterol in fluid have revealed that most effusions previously called pseudochylous are truly chylous.

Obstructive effusions

This type of effusion is caused by obstruction, constriction or congestion of intrathoracic venous or lymphatic channels. Early in the course the fluid is sero-sanguineous with a low protein content and specific gravity. Cellularity at this time is low with RBC and lymphocytes predominating; an occasional PMN and macrophage may also be present. As this fluid remains in the pleural space, it will become more cloudy, have an increased protein content and specific gravity, and contain more PMN and macrophages on cytological examination.

Feline cardiomyopathy is the most common cause of obstructive effusion. Other causes include pulmonary atelectasis or torsion, diaphragmatic hernia, pericarditis, pericardial effusion, peritoneal-pericardial hernia, and neoplasia. Treatment consists of management of the primary cause of the effusion and supportive care.

Neoplastic effusions

The character of neoplastic effusions is variable and they may appear to be an obstructive type of non-septic inflammatory type. The distinguishing feature of a neoplastic effusion is the presence of neoplastic cells. Interpretation of the fluid cytology must be performed carefully because reactive mesothelial cells can easily be confused with neoplastic cells.

The most common cause of neoplastic effusion is thoracic (thymic) lymphosarcoma. Other tumours associated with neoplastic effusion include primary and metastatic intrathoracic adenocarcinomas and carcinomas. Mesenchymal tumours such as sarcomas rarely exfoliate cells into effusion fluid. Associated physical findings are variable depending on the underlying cause of the effusion. Treatment should be directed at identifying and treating the specific inciting neoplastic process.

Pure transudates

Pure transudates are characteristically water clear with a very low specific gravity (< 1.013), low protein content, and low cell numbers. These findings will change over time if the effusion persists in the pleural space. The most common cause of a pure transudate is hypoalbuminaemia (usually $<1.0\,g/dl$). This may result from nephrotic syndrome, protein-losing enteropathy, or hepatic failure. Iatrogenic fluid overload can also cause accumulation of a pure transudate in the pleural space.

Associated physical findings may include peripheral oedema or ascites. Other physical and laboratory findings vary, depending on the underlying cause of hypoalbuminaemia, and treatment is directed at correcting that cause. Supportive measures include discontinuation of parenteral fluid therapy (if this is the cause), diuretics, and plasma transfusion.

Haemorrhagic effusions

Haemorrhagic effusion fluid is similar in character to peripheral blood including protein content, cell counts and specific gravity. However, because blood extravasated into the pleural space will initially clot, then rapidly defibrinate, haemorrhagic effusion fluid should not clot when removed nor contain platelets. The most common causes of haemorrhagic effusion are trauma and post-surgical complications from intrathoracic procedures. Haemorrhagic effusion may occasionally be caused by anticoagulant rodenticide intoxication, spontaneous clotting disorders, disseminated intravascular coagulation (DIC), neoplastic erosion of a blood vessel, and lung lobe torsion.

Clinical findings associated with haemorrhagic effusion often include tachycardia, hypothermia, pale mucous membranes, and a weak pulse. If the haemorrhage is acute, the peripheral packed cell volume (PCV) may be normal at the time of the initial examination. A reduction in the PCV will be seen 12–24 hours following the bleeding episode. Diagnosis is made on the basis of history, clinical findings, and the fluid characteristics.

Treatment is directed at stabilisation of the patient and treatment for shock if necessary. A minimum amount of fluid should be removed from the thorax to allow improved respiration. Blood is rapidly reabsorbed from the pleural space and fluid 'pressure' may limit continuing active haemorrhage. Transfusion may be required if hypovolaemia due to haemorrhage is life threatening. The patient should be monitored carefully for continuing haemorrhage and exploratory surgery should be considered if intrathoracic bleeding persists.

DISORDERS OF THE LUNG

Feline asthma

The aetiology of this disorder is unknown but is believed to be an allergic response to inhaled allergens. The allergic reaction initially causes bronchospasm, peribronchial oedema, and inflammatory cell infiltration. Over time, the disease will produce bronchial and bronchiolar intimal proliferation, fibrosis, and chronic obstructive lung disease (COLD).

Young and middle-aged cats are most frequently affected. Clinical signs often have an acute onset and include mild to severe dyspnoea, forced expiration with an expiratory wheeze, and a paroxysmal, gagging, nonproductive cough. Thoracic radiographic findings are extremely variable. Increased interstitial and peribronchial density may be the only change in the acute phase. Patchy interstitial infiltrates, thickened bronchial walls, hyperinflation

of the lung, and bronchiectasis occur with chronicity. The haemogram may reveal eosinophilia. A tracheal wash, bronchoalveolar lavage, or lung aspirate usually contains a high percentage of eosinophils.

In acute cases of asthma with severe dyspnoea, epinephrine (1:1000) may be given at a dose of 0.1 to 0.2 ml IV or SC. Shock doses of rapidly acting corticosteroids and oxygen therapy (if available) should be given to all acutely dyspnoeic asthmatic cats. Anti-inflammatory doses of corticosteroids are given for weeks to months in cats requiring long-term maintenance therapy. Some cats will require low level immunosuppressive drug therapy for life. Bronchodilators (aminophylline, theophylline, terbutaline: 1.25–1.5 mg PO q8–12h, albuterol: 0.03 mg/kg PO q8–12h) have been a useful adjunct to therapy in some cases. Human asthmatic drugs such as chromolyn sodium and calcium channel blockers have not been used in cats to date. Identification of the source of the allergen is difficult because skin test results in cats are unreliable. Dusty, clay-type cat litter may aggravate this condition and should be avoided. The prognosis for control of feline asthma is good in early cases, but poor in cases with COLD.

Bacterial pneumonia

Primary bacterial pneumonia is rare in the cat. Bacterial pneumonia may follow viral URI (usually calicivirus), trauma, or inhalation of toxins or irritants. Clinical signs include fever, dyspnoea, anorexia, and cough. The haemogram may be normal or reveal leukocytosis with neutrophilia. The biochemistry panel and urinalysis are usually normal. Thoracic radiographs demonstrate a mixed bronchial and interstitial pattern with alveolar involvement. Consolidation of the right middle lung lobe is a common finding in chronic cases.

Aspiration cytology of a consolidated area of lung may be diagnostic for bacterial infection. Transtracheal wash, bronchoalveolar lavage, or endoscopy with bronchial brushing will reveal septic, purulent inflammation. Material collected aseptically with guarded swabs or by transtracheal washing should be submitted for bacteriological culture and sensitivity testing.

Treatment consists of specific antibiotic therapy directed by bacterial culture and sensitivity results.

Antibiotic administration should continue for 4–6 weeks in most patients. Humidification of the airways and chest percussion may aid in the removal of tenacious exudates. Other adjunctive therapy includes bronchodilators or expectorants. If focal lung consolidation persists, surgical removal may be required to resolve clinical signs.

Fungal pneumonia

Fungal pneumonia in the cat is unusual. The relative susceptibility of cats to the systemic mycotic agents is as follows: *Histoplasma* > *Blastomyces* > *Coccidioides*. These fungi are endemic in specific environmental life zones in North and South America and Africa.

Clinical signs associated with fungal infection are often nonspecific and include weight loss, lethargy, fever, anorexia, pale mucous membranes, and dyspnoea. The haemogram often reveals anaemia due to chronic inflammation and fungal infection of bone marrow; leukocytosis and leukopenia have been reported. *Histoplasma* organisms are sometimes seen on peripheral blood smears. Biochemistry panels and urinalyses are usually normal. Thoracic radiographs reveal a spectrum of changes from mild interstitial to miliary and coalescing patchy pulmonary infiltrates. Fungal organisms and evidence of granulomatous inflammation can often be recovered on lung aspiration. Transtracheal wash or bronchial brushings may also be helpful. Lymph node aspiration and bone marrow cytology are useful in selected cases. Fungal serology is falsely negative in most cats.

The treatment of choice for systemic mycoses is ketoconazole or itraconazole alone or in combination with amphotericin B. Amphotericin B is nephrotoxic and must often be discontinued early in the course of treatment. Treatment with KTZ is continued for at least 2 months following resolution of clinical signs; and is often needed for a total of 6 months in most cats. The response to therapy is monitored by the resolution of clinical signs and radiographic lesions.

Parasitic pneumonia

The three major parasites of the feline lung are *Aleurostrongylus abstrusus*, *Capillaria aerophila*, and *Paragonimus kellicotti*. These are rare infections in most of the world. Cats of any age may be affected; young cats are more likely to show clinical signs of illness than older cats.

Most infections are probably subclinical and self-limiting. Clinical signs, if present, include mild to severe dyspnoea and coughing. The haemogram may reveal eosinophilia and mild anaemia, but the remainder of the laboratory findings are usually normal. The diagnosis of parasitic pneumonia is made by finding eosinophilia and parasite eggs or larva (*Aleurostrongylus*) on faecal flotations, bronchial brushings, bronchoalveolar lavage, or transtracheal wash specimens. Treatment with fenbendazole 50 mg/kg for 10–14 days has been recommended for cats with symptomatic infections.

Neoplastic disease – lung tumours

Primary lung tumours are rare in the cat. The most common tumour type is of epithelial origin (carcinoma). Most primary lung tumours occur in cats over 10 years of age. Clinical signs usually develop slowly and include dyspnoea, cough, anorexia and weight loss. Thoracic radiographs usually reveal a solitary lung mass, however, and multiple or diffuse primary tumours have also been reported. Approximately half of cats with primary lung tumours have pleural metastasis or neoplastic pleural effusion at the time their tumour is discovered.

Clinical pathology findings are often normal. Aspiration of the mass or pleural fluid may be diagnostic. Transtracheal washings, bronchoalveolar lavage, endoscopic biopsies, and bronchial brushings are useful diagnostic tools in some cases. Exploratory surgery with excisional biopsy may be required for diagnosis in a few cats.

The most appropriate treatment for solitary primary lung tumours is surgical removal of the affected lung lobe(s). Unfortunately, metastasis will have occurred prior to diagnosis in many cats. Radiation and chemotherapy have not been useful in the treatment of primary pulmonary neoplasia.

The lung is a common site for metastatic neoplasia in the cat. Gastrointestinal, pancreatic and mammary adenocarcinomas are the most common tumour types. Clinical signs are similar to primary pulmonary neoplasia. Treatment is usually palliative and supportive.

Feline heartworm disease (dirofilariasis)

Feline dirofilariasis is caused by the canine heartworm, *Dirofilaria immitis*. Cats are much less susceptible to infection, have a low adult worm burden (1–9 adults), a reduced adult worm lifespan (< 2 years), and are usually amicrofilaraemic. Any cat residing in a heartworm endemic area is at risk of infection.

The clinical presentation in this disease can be quite confusing because the signs of illness are so variable. Acute signs include dyspnoea, collapse, vomiting, diarrhoea, convulsions, syncope, and blindness. Chronic signs include lethargy, anorexia, coughing, dyspnoea, vomiting, and pleural effusion. Physical examination is often normal. Thoracic auscultation may reveal tachycardia, a systolic heart murmur, gallop rhythm, and harsh, dry lung sounds.

Laboratory findings are variable. The haemogram may reveal eosinophilia and a mild, nonregenerative anaemia. Basophilia is rare but is suggestive of dirofilariasis if present. Serum biochemical determinations are usually normal, hyperglobulinaemia has been found in a few cats. Although most cats are amicrofilaraemic, concentration techniques using a large volume of blood (5 ml) may be helpful if a few microfilaria are present. Serological testing with adult *Dirofilaria* antigen tests may confirm the diagnosis in some cases. Radiographic changes in feline dirofilariasis are nonspecific and variable, and fluctuate rapidly. Non-selective angiography can be used to delineate enlarged pulmonary arteries. Transtracheal wash or bronchoalveolar lavage cytology may reveal eosinophils. The major differential diagnoses for patients with these findings are asthma and parasitic pneumonia.

Treatment of feline confirmed dirofilariasis is difficult because of the apparent sensitivity of the cat to thiacetarsemide sodium. This drug has been shown to cause fulminating, fatal pulmonary oedema in normal adult cats given the recommended therapeutic dose of 2.2 mg/kg IV bid for 48h. Treatment at a reduced dose may be safer but may not be effective in eliminating the adult *Dirofilaria*. Aspirin can be given at a total dose of 80 mg (1.25 g) PO q48–72h to reduce thromboembolic pulmonary complications. Additional therapy for symptomatic cats includes furosemide to control pulmonary oedema, corticosteroids to reduce pulmonary inflammation, and antibiotics to combat secondary bacterial pneumonia.

RECOMMENDED READING

1. McCarthy T.C., McDermaid S.L. (1990) Rhinoscopy. *Vet. Clin. North Am.* **20**: 1265–1295.
2. Roudebush P. (1990) Tracheobronchoscopy. *Vet. Clin. North Am.* **20**: 1297–1314.
3. Sherding R.G. (ed.) (1989) *The Cat. Diseases and Clinical Management*. Churchill Livingstone, New York, New York pp 755–874.
4. Withrow S.J., Susaneck S.J., Macy D.W., Sheetz J. (1985) Aspiration and punch biopsy techniques for nasal tumours. *J. Am. Anim. Hosp. Assoc.* **21**: 551.

11

Disorders of the Cardiovascular System

WENDY A. WARE

THE CARDIOVASCULAR EXAMINATION

History

The cardiovascular evaluation includes a complete medical history. Important questions to ask the owner include the cat's origin, age, diet, and activity level, as well as whether the cat spends time out-of-doors, and has had changes in appetite, breathing pattern or behaviour. Information regarding previous medications prescribed for cardiopulmonary signs (e.g. drugs used, if they were helpful) is also valuable.

Physical examination

The cat's attitude, posture, body condition, level of anxiety and respiratory pattern should be observed while interviewing the owner. A careful general physical examination is important. The cardiovascular examination consists of evaluating the peripheral circulation (mucous membranes), systemic veins (especially the jugular vein), systemic arterial pulses (usually the femoral artery) and precordium (chest wall over the heart), as well as auscultating the heart and lungs, and palpating or percussing for abnormal fluid accumulation (ascites, subcutaneous oedema, pleural effusion).

Mucous membranes

The mucous membrane colour and refill time are used to estimate the adequacy of peripheral perfusion. After digital pressure is applied to blanch the membrane, colour should return within 2 seconds. Slower refill times suggest either dehydration or high peripheral sympathetic tone and vasoconstriction. Both are associated with decreased cardiac output. *Pale* mucous membranes may result from anaemia or peripheral vasoconstriction. Capillary refill time is normal in patients with anaemia, unless hypoperfusion is also present. *Injected* or *brick-red* membranes can be associated with polycythaemia, sepsis, excitement, or other causes of peripheral vasodilation. *Cyanotic* mucous membranes may be caused by severe pulmonary or pleural space disease, congestive heart failure, or right-to-left shunting congenital cardiac defects; occasionally cyanosis is secondary to shock, cold exposure, or methaemoglobinaemia. Icteric membranes are associated with acute haemolysis, hepatobiliary disease, or biliary obstruction.

Jugular veins

The jugular veins should not be distended when the cat is standing or sternal with its head in a normal position (jaw parallel to the floor). Jugular pulsations extending higher than one-third of the way up the neck are also abnormal. Sometimes the carotid pulse wave is transmitted through the adjacent soft tissues in thin or excited animals, mimicking a jugular pulse. To differentiate a true jugular pulse from carotid transmission, the jugular vein should be occluded lightly below the area of the visible pulse; if the pulse disappears it is a true jugular pulsation. If the pulse continues, it is being transmitted from the carotid artery. Jugular pulse waves are related to atrial contraction and filling. Visible pulsations occur with tricuspid insufficiency, conditions causing a stiff and hypertrophied right ventricle (e.g. pulmonic stenosis, heartworm disease), and arrhythmias which cause the atria to contract against closed atrioventricular (AV) valves (e.g. ventricular premature contractions, complete AV block). Persistent jugular vein distension occurs with right-sided congestive heart failure secondary to high right heart filling pressures (e.g. with dilated cardiomyopathy or pericardial disease), with external compression of the cranial vena cava (e.g. with a cranial mediastinal mass), or with jugular vein thrombosis.

Arterial pulses

Palpation of the femoral arteries allows assessment of the strength and regularity of the peripheral arterial pressure waves as well as the pulse rate. Both femoral pulses should be palpated and compared, as obstruction of one side can occur, especially with cardiomyopathy. The femoral arterial pulse should be evaluated simultaneously with the direct heart rate (obtained by chest wall palpation or auscultation). Various cardiac arrhythmias induce pulse deficits (fewer femoral pulses than heart beats) by causing the heart to contract before adequate filling of the ventricles has occurred. Consequently, minimal or even no blood is ejected for those beats and a palpable pulse is absent.

Subjective evaluation of pulse strength depends on the difference between the systolic and diastolic arterial pressures (pulse pressure); when the difference is wide the pulse feels strong on palpation. When the difference is small or the time to maximum systolic pressure is prolonged, the pulse feels weak. Weak pulses usually occur with dilated cardiomyopathy, ventricular outflow obstruction, or shock. Strong pulses are common with excitement, hyperthyroidism, hypertrophic cardiomyopathy, and fever or sepis. Very strong, bounding pulses are also characteristic of patent ductus arteriosus. Femoral pulses may be difficult to palpate in overweight cats, even when normal; the femoral artery can usually be found by gently working the fingers toward the proximal femur between the muscles on the medial thigh.

Precordium

The precordium is palpated by placing the palm and fingers of each hand on the corresponding side of the patient's chest wall over the heart. Normally, the strongest impulse during systole is felt over the area of the left apex (approximately the 5th intercostal space just below the costochondral junction). Space-occupying masses within the chest or cardiomegaly may displace the heart, causing the precordial impulse to be located abnormally. Reduction in the intensity of the precordial impulse can be caused by obesity, weak cardiac contractions, pericardial effusion, intrathoracic masses, pleural effusion, and pneumothorax. The precordial impulse should be stronger on the left chest wall than on the right. Stronger precordial impulses on the right can be caused by right ventricular hypertrophy, or displacement of the heart into the right hemithorax by a mass lesion, lung atelectasis, or chest deformity. Very loud cardiac murmurs cause vibrations palpable on the chest wall known as a 'precordial thrill'. This is usually localised to the area of maximal intensity of the murmur.

Evaluation for fluid accumulation

Right-sided congestive heart failure usually promotes abnormal fluid accumulation within the pleural cavity and causes lung sounds to be muffled ventrally. Fluid accumulation secondary to right-sided heart failure is usually accompanied by abnormal jugular vein distension or pulsations (if the animal is not dehydrated with respect to circulating volume). Hepatomegaly or splenomegaly may also occur. Ascites and subcutaneous oedema are uncommon manifestations of heart failure in cats.

Cardiac auscultation

Heart sounds are classified as transient sounds (those of short duration) and cardiac murmurs (longer sounds occurring during a normally silent part of the cardiac cycle). Since many heart sounds can be difficult to hear, patient co-operation and a quiet room are important during auscultation. If possible, the cat should be standing, so that the heart is in its normal position. Purring in cats can usually be stopped by holding a finger over one or both nostrils or by turning on a nearby water tap. Both sides of the chest should be auscultated carefully. The stethoscope is moved gradually to all areas of the chest, including the left and right sternal borders.

The stethoscope should have both a stiff, flat diaphragm and a bell on the chestpiece. The diaphragm should be applied firmly to the chest wall; this allows auscultation of most heart sounds, especially those of higher frequency. The bell, applied lightly to the chest wall, facilitates auscultation of lower frequency sounds such as S_3 and S_4 (see below).

Transient heart sounds

The heart sounds normally heard in cats are S_1 (associated with closure and tensing of the AV valves at the onset of systole) and S_2 (associated with closure of the aortic and pulmonic valves at the end of systole). Audible diastolic sounds (S_3 and S_4) are abnormal. The precordial impulse occurs just after S_1 (systole) and the arterial pulse is felt between S_1 and S_2.

Gallop sounds

The third (S_3) and fourth (S_4) heart sounds occur during *diastole*, and are not normally audible in cats. When an S_3 or S_4 sound is heard, the heart may sound like the galloping of a horse; hence, the term 'gallop rhythm' or 'gallop' sounds. Note, however, that the presence or absence of an audible S_3 or S_4 has nothing to do with the heart's rhythm, i.e. the origin of cardiac activation and the intracardiac conduction process. Gallop sounds are usually heard best with the bell of the stethoscope since they are of lower frequency than S_1 and S_2. At fast heart rates, differentiation of an S_3 from an S_4 is difficult; it is most important to determine whether the extra heart sound occurs in systole or diastole. In cats, extra transient sounds most often are diastolic gallop sounds.

The S_3, also known as an S_3 gallop or ventricular gallop, is associated with vibrations resulting from the end of the rapid ventricular

filling phase. An audible S_3 usually indicates ventricular dilation with myocardial failure. This may be the only abnormality detectable by auscultation in a cat with dilated cardiomyopathy. The extra sound can be fairly loud or very subtle, and is heard best over the cardiac apex.

The S_4 gallop, also called an atrial or presystolic gallop, is associated with vibrations induced by blood flow into the ventricles during atrial contraction; it occurs just after the P wave on the ECG. An audible S_4 in the cat is usually associated with hypertrophic cardiomyopathy or other conditions causing ventricular hypertrophy (e.g. hyperthyroidism). A transient S_4 gallop of unknown significance is sometimes heard in stressed cats.

Cardiac murmurs

Cardiac murmurs are described by their timing within the cardiac cycle (systolic or diastolic, or portions thereof), intensity, point of maximal intensity on the precordium, radiation over the chest wall, quality, and pitch. Clinically, the first three parameters are most important. The intensity of a murmur is arbitrarily graded on a scale of I to VI (Fig. 11.1). The point of maximal intensity (PMI) is usually indicated by the hemithorax and intercostal space or valve area where it is located, or by the terms apex or base.

Murmurs are also described by their shape as it appears on a phonocardiogram (graphic recording of cardiac sounds). The shape and description of different murmurs are illustrated in Fig. 11.2. A plateau or regurgitant (*holosystolic*) murmur begins at about the time of S_1 and has a fairly uniform intensity throughout systole. Loud

GRADING OF CARDIAC MURMURS	
Grade I	Very soft murmur; heard only with careful auscultation in a quiet patient and quiet room
Grade II	Soft murmur, but easily heard at its point of maximal intensity
Grade III	Moderate intensity murmur
Grade IV	Loud murmur, but without a palpable precordial thrill
Grade V	Loud murmur, with a precordial thrill
Grade VI	Very loud murmur, with a precordial thrill; can still be heard when the stethoscope is lifted off the chest

FIG. 11.1 Grading of cardiac murmurs.

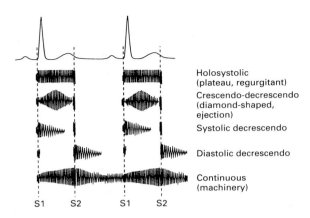

Holosystolic
(plateau, regurgitant)

Crescendo-decrescendo
(diamond-shaped,
ejection)

Systolic decrescendo

Diastolic decrescendo

Continuous
(machinery)

S1   S2   S1   S2

FIG. 11.2 Murmur shapes and descriptions. The phonocardiographic shapes and timing of different murmurs are depicted along with terms used to describe them. From Ware, W.A. Cardiovascular Disorders. In Nelson R. and Couto C.G. (eds), *Essentials of Internal Medicine in the Cat and Dog*, Malvern, PA, USA, 1992, Mosby-Yearbook Inc, with permission.

murmurs of this type may prevent distinction of S_1 and S_2 from the murmur. Atrioventricular valve insufficiency and interventricular septal defects commonly cause this type of murmur since turbulent movement of blood occurs throughout ventricular systole. A *crescendo–decrescendo* or diamond-shaped murmur starts softly, builds intensity in mid-systole, then diminishes. This murmur is also called an ejection murmur; it occurs with ventricular outflow obstructions during ejection. Physiological *systolic* murmurs (where the heart is normal but an altered physiological state exists) have been associated with anaemia, fever, high sympathetic tone, and hyperthyroidism.

Diastolic murmurs are rare in cats; causes include infective endocarditis of the aortic valve, or degeneration of this valve in some geriatric cats. A *continuous* murmur occurs throughout systole and diastole; it is characteristic of a congenital patent ductus arteriosus.

RECORDING AND INTERPRETING THE ELECTRO-CARDIOGRAM

When an ECG is being recorded, the cat should be placed on a nonconducting pad in right lateral recumbency, if possible. The proximal limbs should be parallel to each other and perpendicular to the torso. Front limb (arm) leads are placed at the elbows or slightly below, not touching the chest wall or each other. Rear limb electrodes are placed at the stifles or hocks. ECG paste or alcohol is used to ensure good contact. Communication between two electrodes via a bridge of paste or alcohol, or by physical contact, should be avoided. The animal is gently held in position to minimise movement.

Interpretation of the ECG includes calculation of the heart rate, evaluation of the heart rhythm and individual complexes, and estimation of the mean electrical axis. The entire ECG strip is scanned for irregularities and abnormal complexes. Measurement of waveforms and intervals is done using lead II. Amplitudes are recorded in millivolts and durations in seconds. Only one thickness of the inscribed pen line should be included for each measurement. At a paper speed of 25 mm/sec each small box on the ECG gridwork equals 0.04 seconds in duration from left

NORMAL ECG REFERENCE RANGES

Heart Rate (sinus rhythm): 160-240 beats/min
Mean electrical axis (frontal plane): 0 to + 160 degrees
Measurements (Lead II):
  P wave duration (maximum): 0.035 - 0.04 s
  P wave height (maximum): 0.2 mV
  P-R interval: 0.05 - 0.09 s
  QRS complex duration (maximum): 0.04 s
  R wave height (maximum): 0.9 mV; total QRS excursion should be less than 1.2 mV
  S-T segment deviation: no marked deviation
  T wave: maximum 0.3 mV; can be positive (most common), negative or biphasic
  Q-T interval duration: 0.12-0.18 (range 0.07-0.20) mV; varies inversely with heart rate

FIG. 11.3   Normal ECG reference ranges for cats.

to right. At a paper speed of 50 mm/sec each small box equals 0.02 seconds. At standard calibration, a deflection of the pen up or down 10 small boxes (1 cm) equals 1 mV. Fig. 11.3 shows normal ECG reference ranges for cats.

ECHOCARDIOGRAPHY (CARDIAC ULTRASONOGRAPHY)

Echocardiography is becoming widely available as a non-invasive tool for imaging the heart and surrounding structures. It allows evaluation of cardiac chamber size, wall thickness, valve configuration and motion. It is a sensitive method for detecting pericardial and pleural fluid accumulation, and can allow identification of mass lesions within and adjacent to the heart.

Three types of echocardiography are used clinically: M-mode, two-dimensional (2-D, real time) and Doppler. Each has important applications.

M-mode echocardiography

M-mode echocardiography provides a one-dimensional view (depth) into the heart (Figs 11.4 and 11.5). The M-mode images represent echoes from various tissue interfaces along the axis of the beam. These echoes, which move during the

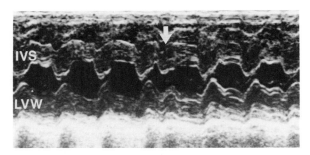

FIG. 11.4 M-mode echocardiogram from a cat with hypertrophic cardiomyopathy. Note the relatively small left ventricular lumen, thickened septum (IVS) and left ventricular posterior wall (LVW) – diastolic and systolic measurements of each were 7 and 11 mm, respectively. A ventricular premature contraction occurred during this recording (arrow). From Ware, W.A. Cardiovascular Disorders. In Nelson R. and Couto C.G. (eds), *Essentials of Internal Medicine in the Cat and Dog*, Malvern, PA, USA, 1992, Mosby-Yearbook Inc, with permission.

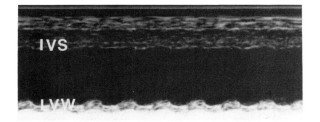

FIG. 11.5 M-mode echocardiogram from a cat with dilated cardiomyopathy depicting left ventricular dilation and poor left ventricular wall (LVW) and septal (IVS) motion. The fractional shortening was 10%.

cardiac cycle, are displayed across time. Thus, the lines which are seen on the recordings correspond to the positions of particular structures in relation to the transducer and other cardiac structures at any point in time. Measurements of cardiac dimensions and motion throughout the cardiac cycle are often obtained more accurately from M-mode tracings.

Two-dimensional echocardiography

Two-dimensional echocardiography images a plane of tissue (depth and width). A variety of planes through the heart can be viewed from several locations on the chest wall. Most standard views are obtained from either the right or left chest wall, over the heart and close to the sternum (parasternal) with the animal restrained gently in lateral recumbency. Valvular insufficiency and blood flow through cardiac shunts cannot usually be visualised using 2-D or M-mode images alone, although related anatomical changes or defects can be seen.

Doppler imaging

Doppler imaging allows evaluation of blood flow patterns and velocity, permitting documentation and quantification of valvular insufficiency or stenosis and cardiac shunts. Doppler echocardiography is based on detection of frequency changes occurring as ultrasound waves reflect off individual blood cells moving either away from or toward the transducer. Calculation of blood flow velocity is possible when the flow is parallel to the angle of the ultrasound beam. Colour flow mapping is a form of pulsed wave Doppler ultrasonography that combines the M-mode or 2-D modalities with blood flow imaging. The mean frequency shift obtained from many sample volumes is colour-coded for direction and velocity.

SIGNS OF HEART DISEASE AND HEART FAILURE

Clinical signs of heart disease

Signs of heart disease may be present without the cat being in a state of heart failure. Objective signs of heart disease include a cardiac murmur, gallop sound, rhythm disturbance, jugular pulsations, and cardiac enlargement. Other clinical signs suggestive of heart disease include syncope, excessively weak or strong arterial pulses, respiratory difficulty, exercise intolerance and cyanosis. Coughing is an uncommon manifestation of pulmonary oedema in cats. Heartworm disease frequently induces coughing as well as other respiratory signs in cats; pleural and pericardial effusions rarely cause coughing. Further evaluation of the patient by means of thoracic radiography, electrocardiography and cardiac ultrasonography is usually indicated when clinical signs suggestive of cardiovascular disease are present.

Clinical signs of heart failure

The clinical signs of heart failure are caused by a back-up of blood behind the heart (congestive signs) or inadequate blood flow out of the heart (low output signs). Congestive signs in cats with right ventricular failure relate to systemic venous hypertension and usually consist of pleural effusion, with ascites occurring rarely. Back-up of blood behind the left heart results in pulmonary venous hypertension and oedema. Chronic congestive left heart failure may lead to development of right heart failure in some cats. Biventricular failure may also be present. Low output signs include tiring, exertional weakness, syncope, prerenal azotaemia, and cardiac arrhythmias.

MYOCARDIAL DISEASES

Hypertrophic cardiomyopathy

Hypertrophic cardiomyopathy (HCM) is a primary myocardial disease characterised by excessive thickening of the left ventricular wall and interventricular septum. The aetiology of HCM is unknown. Another important cause of myocardial hypertrophy and secondary heart failure is thyrotoxicosis in cats with functional thyroid neoplasms (see Chapter 16). Compensatory hypertrophy can also result from a pressure overload on the left ventricle, as in systemic hypertension or congenital (sub)aortic stenosis.

The pathophysiology of HCM entails abnormal muscular hypertrophy, causing the left ventricle to become stiff and less distensible and impairing diastolic filling. Myocardial relaxation takes longer than normal and may be incomplete. An increasingly stiff left ventricle requires progressively higher filling pressures; thus, end diastolic pressures in both the left atrium and left ventricle rise. Left atrial size increases, sometimes dramatically, but left ventricular volume remains normal or decreased. Geometric changes of the left ventricle and papillary muscles or abnormal (anterior) systolic motion of the mitral valve may prevent the valve from coapting properly and cause mitral insufficiency, which exacerbates the rise in left atrial volume and pressure. This impedance to ventricular filling is referred to as diastolic dysfunction. Fast heart rates interfere further with left ventricular filling, exacerbate myocardial ischaemia and promote venous congestion by shortening the diastolic filling period. Contractility, or systolic function, is usually normal in these cats.

In a subset of cats with HCM, asymmetric hypertrophy of the interventricular septum causes left ventricular outflow obstruction during systole (functional subaortic stenosis) which contributes to systolic wall stress and myocardial oxygen demand; this in turn promotes the development of myocardial ischaemia, which further impedes relaxation. It may also cause an audible ejection murmur low on the left base. About 25 to 35% of cats with HCM are estimated to have asymmetrical septal hypertrophy.

Pulmonary venous congestion and oedema

result frequently from the increased left atrial pressures which accompany HCM. In some cats, secondary pulmonary arterial hypertension eventually may lead to right heart failure with pleural effusion. The effusion may be chylous, although a modified transudate is more common. Thrombi may form within the dilated left atrium; thromboembolic events result if portions dislodge and are released into the circulation.

Clinical features

Hypertrophic cardiomyopathy is most common in middle-aged cats, although the disease occurs in a wide age range; Persian cats may be predisposed. Respiratory distress or signs of thromboembolism may be the cause of presentation in cats with HCM. Recent onset of anorexia, lethargy, syncope and sometimes vomiting may occur. Clinical signs may be precipitated by stress, and sudden death can result. Early in the course of the disease clinical signs may be absent, with only a gallop sound (usually S_4) or systolic murmur (from mitral regurgitation or left ventricular outflow obstruction) heard on auscultation; arrhythmias are not uncommon. With the onset of heart failure, tachypnoea or acute dyspnoea, with or without cyanosis, occur secondary to pulmonary oedema, and some cats develop pleural effusion. Usually the femoral pulses are strong, unless thromboembolism of the distal aorta has occurred. A marked precordial impulse is often palpated in cats with HCM, and prominent lung sounds or pulmonary crackles accompany severe pulmonary oedema.

Diagnosis

Radiography often reveals a prominent left atrium, which sometimes confers a 'valentine-shaped' appearance to the heart on dorsoventral (DV) or ventrodorsal (VD) view. Usually the left ventricular apex point is maintained; there may be left ventricular enlargement (Fig. 11.6). Enlarged and tortuous pulmonary veins may be seen entering the left atrium, implying chronically high left atrial and pulmonary venous pressures. Left-sided heart failure is associated with variable degrees of patchy interstitial or alveolar pulmonary oedema.

The distribution of the oedema is also variable; diffuse or focal distribution throughout the lung fields is common, in contrast to the perihilar distribution characteristic of cardiogenic pulmonary oedema in dogs. The presence of significant pleural effusion suggests biventricular failure.

Electrocardiography sometimes reveals abnormalities in cats with HCM. A left axis deviation, left ventricular enlargement pattern, and possibly P wave or QRS prolongation are common findings; other conduction disturbances can occur, including complete AV block. Ventricular premature complexes also occur in cats with this disease. Atrial fibrillation or atrial premature beats may accompany marked atrial enlargement.

Echocardiography (or nonselective angiocardiography) is vital to establishing a definitive diagnosis, and differentiating HCM from the less common dilated cardiomyopathy. Characteristic findings on the echocardiogram are increased left ventricular and septal thicknesses (greater than 5.5 mm in diastole), reduced left ventricular lumen size, thickened papillary muscles, normal to increased left ventricular fractional shortening, and left atrial enlargement (Fig. 11.6). A thrombus is occasionally seen within the left atrium. Similar anatomical findings are demonstrated on angiocardiography.

Treatment and prognosis

Major goals in the treatment of HCM are to facilitate ventricular filling, to relieve signs of congestion, to optimise cardiac output, and to control arrhythmias. General principles of heart failure therapy apply in symptomatic patients (see Fig. 11.7). Minimising patient stress and activity are important. Ventricular filling is improved by slowing the heart rate and by enhancing relaxation; diuretics are used to reduce oedema and congestion.

The beta adrenergic blocker, propranolol, has traditionally been used to slow the heart rate and control tachyarrhythmias as well as to minimise any outflow obstruction (through its negative inotropic effects), thus reducing myocardial oxygen demand. The reduction in heart rate and myocardial ischaemia which result from beta-blocker therapy may indirectly improve filling.

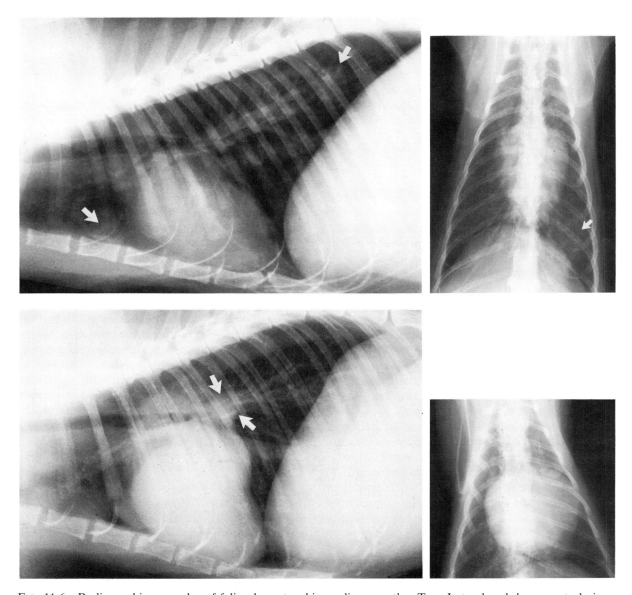

FIG. 11.6 Radiographic examples of feline hypertrophic cardiomyopathy. Top: Lateral and dorso-ventral views showing atrial and mild ventricular enlargement along with patchy interstitial pulmonary oedema (arrows) in a male domestic shorthair cat in left-sided congestive heart failure. Bottom: Lateral and dorso-ventral views of a male Siamese cat with marked atrial enlargement, dilated pulmonary veins (arrows) and atrial fibrillation. From Ware, W.A. Cardiovascular Disorders. In Nelson R. and Couto C.G. (eds), *Essentials of Internal Medicine in the Cat and Dog*, Malvern, PA, USA, 1992, Mosby-Yearbook Inc, with permission.

However, there is no direct enhancement of relaxation and some experimental evidence suggests that propranolol may slow the relaxation process. Although propranolol has historically been the backbone of therapy in cats with HCM, the calcium entry blocker diltiazem appears to be more effective and has fewer side effects. If propranolol is used, administration of the drug is usually delayed for 24 to 36 hours, until after the cat is stabilised and pulmonary oedema is largely

THERAPY OUTLINE – HYPERTROPHIC CARDIOMYOPATHY	
Initial therapy of acute failure:	
Diuretic agent	Frusemide (1-2 mg/kg bid, up to 4 mg/kg q8-12h, IV, IM SC, PO)
Supplemental oxygen	
Vasodilator	Nitroglycerin ointment (1/4 inch/0.75 cm q4-6h, cutaneously), (possibly captopril 0.5-2 mg/kg tid, PO)
Bronchodilator	Theophylline (4 mg/kg q8-12h) or aminophylline (5 mg/kg q8-12h)
Cage confinement	
Ca^{++} entry blocker	Diltiazem (1-2 mg/kg or 1/4 of 30 mg tab tid, PO)
or (+/–) Beta blocker	Propranolol (2.5-5 mg tid; avoid with pulmonary oedema or thromboembolism) or esmolol (500 µg/kg IV over 1 min, followed by infusion of 100 µg/kg/min)
+/– Anticlotting drugs	Aspirin (10 to 25 mg/kg, PO every 3rd day) Heparin (see text)
Other therapy	+/- Acepromazine (0.05 to 0.2 mg/kg SC) +/- Fluids +/- Supplemental heat +/- Thoracocentesis
Antiarrhythmic drugs	Propranolol (or other beta-blocker) +/- Lidocaine (0.25 mg/kg slowly IV, can repeat in 5-20 min) +/- Procainamide (25-50 mg total dose q6-8h, PO)
Chronic therapy:	
Diuretics (+/–)	Frusemide (lowest effective dose, see above) +/- Hydrochlorothiazide (1 to 2 mg/kg bid, PO)
Ca^{++} entry blocker	Diltiazem (see dose above)
or Beta blocker	Propranolol (see dose above)
Anticlotting drug	Aspirin (see dose above)
Exercise restriction	
Sodium restriction	
Antiarrhythmic (+/–)	Propranolol (see dose above)
See text for more information	

FIG. 11.7 Therapy outline for hypertrophic cardiomyopathy.

resolved. Because propranolol is a non-selective beta-blocker one of its adverse effects can be bronchoconstriction following antagonism of airway β_2 receptors. Exceptions to this guideline include cats with sinus tachycardia or ventricular arrhythmias, in which the advantages of slowing the heart rate and minimising the rhythm disturbance probably outweigh the risk of bronchospasm. Some cats do not tolerate propranolol well (e.g. lethargy, depressed appetite), in which case diltiazem should be used.

Calcium entry blocking drugs such as diltiazem or verapamil have been used effectively in humans with HCM and are currently being evaluated in cats. These agents also reduce heart rate, myocardial oxygen demand, systolic pressure gradients, and blood pressure. Additionally, they can directly facilitate ventricular relaxation and promote coronary vasodilation. Experimentally, diltiazem has been a more significantly effective therapeutic agent for long term use in cats than verapamil (or propranolol).

Supplemental oxygen, airway suctioning and possibly even mechanical ventilation with positive end expiratory pressure or continuous positive airway pressure may be useful, depending on the degree of pulmonary oedema. Rapid diuresis usually follows intravenous furosemide administration and is used for severely symptomatic cats; intramuscular injection can also be used initially

(Fig. 11.7). Once the oedema is controlled, furosemide is gradually reduced to the lowest effective dose and given orally. In some cats with a good response to diltiazem or propranolol, it may even be possible to discontinue furosemide therapy. Aminophylline, with its bronchodilating and mild diuretic effects, may also be helpful in cats with severe pulmonary oedema.

Acepromazine has been used to reduce anxiety as well as to promote peripheral redistribution of blood and impair platelet aggregation due to its alpha-adrenergic blocking effects. Caution is advised in cats with pre-existing hypothermia however, because peripheral vasodilation will exacerbate heat loss. Two percent nitroglycerine ointment applied cutaneously to hairless skin q4–6h for 1–2 days can also be used in cases of severe pulmonary oedema to increase venous capacitance and reduce pulmonary venous pressure. Captopril (an angiotensin converting enzyme inhibitor), in addition to furosemide, may be helpful for controlling signs of congestive heart failure. However, arteriolar vasodilators promote increased ventricular systolic shortening by reducing afterload, which could exacerbate any left ventricular outflow obstruction. Digoxin can also worsen left ventricular outflow obstruction and promote myocardial ischaemia by increasing contractility and muscle shortening. Digoxin (and other positive inotropic drugs) is relatively contraindicated, although it has been used in cats with refractory biventricular failure in which left ventricular outflow obstruction is absent.

Right-sided heart failure develops in some cats with chronic left heart failure. These cats may require higher doses of furosemide (up to 4 mg/kg tid) or, if that is not effective in controlling oedema and effusions, addition of another diuretic such as hydrochlorothiazide (1 to 2 mg/kg bid, PO). The patient should also be monitored for development of azotaemia or electrolyte disturbances. Refractory right heart failure in cats may also respond to digoxin or captopril.

Additional therapy for HCM includes aspirin to reduce platelet aggregation, although its effectiveness in preventing thromboembolism is still unknown. Some clinicians have recommended chronic warfarin therapy (0.08 to 0.1 mg/kg sid PO) for indoor cats only (because of their relative protection from trauma); this is of questionable efficacy and requires careful monitoring of coagulation times, because spontaneous bleeding may result. Exercise restriction is recommended, and a reduced sodium intake may be useful.

Complications of hypertrophic cardiomyopathy include arterial thromboembolism (see below). In addition, atrial fibrillation or other tachyarrhythmias may interfere with diastolic filling time and exacerbate venous congestion. Development of refractory heart failure is another potential complication.

Prognosis in any individual depends on several factors including the response to therapy, the occurrence of thromboembolic events, the progression of the disease, and the presence of arrhythmias. The prognosis in cases with atrial fibrillation or refractory right heart failure tends to be poor. In cats without thromboembolism the prognosis may be good (some cats survive for over 2 years), although future embolic events accompanied by decompensated heart failure or sudden death can occur. Cats with thromboembolic disease may do well if congestive signs can be controlled and vital organs have not been infarcted by the embolus. Recurrence of thromboembolism is not uncommon in these cases.

Dilated cardiomyopathy

A major cause of dilated cardiomyopathy (DCM) in cats is taurine deficiency. Since this was discovered, the taurine content of many commercial feline diets has been increased and DCM has become much less common. Plasma taurine measurement should be considered in cats diagnosed with DCM and is available through several research laboratories. Plasma taurine concentrations are influenced significantly by the amount of taurine in the diet, the type of diet, and the time of sampling in relation to eating; however, a plasma taurine concentration of 20 nmol/ml or less in a cat with DCM is considered diagnostic for taurine deficiency. Cats with a plasma taurine concentration under 60 nmol/ml should probably receive taurine supplementation or undergo a change in diet (see Chapter 3). In some cats, DCM may be the end-stage result of

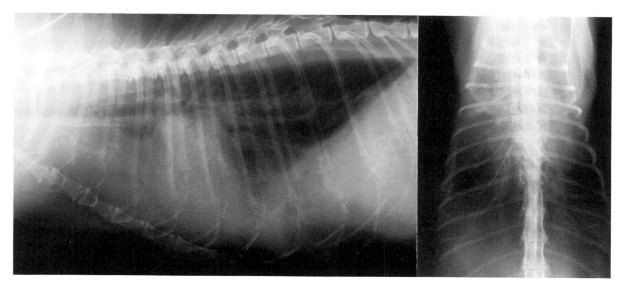

FIG. 11.8   Chest radiographs from a cat with dilated cardiomyopathy. Note generalised cardiac enlargement and pleural fluid accumulation.

other metabolic derangements, toxicities or infectious processes of the myocardium rather than taurine deficiency.

Pathophysiology

The major feature of DCM is poor myocardial contractility. Similarly to DCM in dogs, cardiac output falls and compensatory mechanisms are activated, leading to retention of salt and water, and vasoconstriction. Usually all cardiac chambers are dilated, and AV valve insufficiency can occur secondary to chamber enlargement and papillary muscle atrophy. This contributes to the increased cardiac volume, elevated atrial and venous pressures, formation of pulmonary oedema and pleural effusion, reduced forward cardiac output, and arrhythmias which accompany DCM. Biventricular failure with pleural effusion is common in cats.

Clinical features

Dilated cardiomyopathy occurs predominantly in young to middle-aged cats; there is no breed or sex predilection. Historical signs are frequently vague and often acute. They include anorexia, lethargy, and dyspnoea. Acute thromboembolism, usually of the distal abdominal aorta, may herald the presence of this disease or of other forms of cardiomyopathy.

Subtle evidence of poor ventricular function in conjunction with signs of respiratory compromise are usually present on physical examination. An attenuated precordial impulse, jugular venous distension and weak femoral pulses are common, as are a cardiac gallop sound (usually S_3) and a left or right apical systolic murmur. The heart rate can be normal, although bradycardia and arrhythmias are common. Increased respiratory effort, depression, dehydration and hypothermia are found frequently. Increased lung sounds and pulmonary crackles can be auscultated in some cats, while lung sounds are muffled if a large pleural effusion is present. Clinical signs of arterial thromboembolism may also be present (see below).

Diagnosis

Radiography commonly shows generalised cardiomegaly with rounding of the cardiac apex (Fig. 11.8). However, pleural effusion tends to obscure the heart shadow and any coexisting evidence of pulmonary oedema or venous congestion. Hepatomegaly and occasionally ascites might be detected.

Electrocardiography may reveal a left ventricular enlargement pattern, AV conduction disturbances or arrhythmias (either supraventricular or ventricular).

Echocardiography provides definitive diagnosis by allowing rapid and non-invasive assessment of chamber size, ventricular wall thickness, and contractile function (see Fig. 11.5). Non-selective angiocardiography constitutes an alternative to differentiate dilated cardiomyopathy from other diseases, especially hypertrophic cardiomyopathy. Characteristic angiocardiographic features include generalised chamber enlargement, atrophied papillary muscles, decreased aortic diameter, and

THERAPY OUTLINE – DILATED CARDIOMYOPATHY	
Initial therapy of acute failure:	
Positive inotrope	Digoxin (0.007 mg/kg q48h, PO; or: cats < 3 kg - 1/4 of 0.125 mg tab qod, cats 3-6 kg - 1/4 of 0.125 mg tab sid, cats > 6 kg - 1/4 of 0.125 mg tab q12-24h, PO; IV loading [use only with great caution]: (0.005 mg/kg give 1/2 of total, then 1 +/- 2hr later give 1/4 dose bolus(es), if needed) Dopamine (1-5 µg/kg/min IV infusion) or dobutamine (1-10 µg/kg/min IV infusion) +/- Amrinone (1-3 mg/kg initial IV bolus; 10 to 100 µg/kg/min IV infusion) *Note:* Digoxin, dopamine or dobutamine, and amrinone could be used simultaneously
Diuretic agent	Frusemide (1-2 mg/kg bid, up to 4 mg/kg q8-12h, IV, IM, SC, PO)
Supplemental oxygen Vasodilator	Nitroglycerin ointment (1/4 inch/0.75 cm q4-6h, cutaneously), (possibly captopril-0.5 to 2 mg/kg tid, PO; or hydralazine 2.5-5mg bid, PO)
Bronchodilator	Theophylline (4 mg/kg q8-12h) or aminophylline (5 mg/kg q8-12h)
Cage confinement +/– Anticlotting drugs	Aspirin (10-25 mg/kg, PO every 3rd day) Heparin (see text)
Other therapy	Thoracocentesis if needed +/- Acepromazine (0.05-0.2 mg/kg SC) +/- Fluids (20-35 ml/kg/day IV or SC, e.g. half strength saline and 2.5% dextrose) +/- Supplemental heat
Antiarrhythmic drugs	Propranolol (or other beta-blocker) +/- Lidocaine (0.25 mg/kg slowly IV, can repeat in 5-20 min) +/- Procainamide (25-50 mg total dose, q6-8h, PO)
Clinical therapy:	
Positive inotrope	Digoxin (see dose above)
Diuretics (+/–)	Frusemide (lowest effective dose, see above) +/- Hydrochlorothiazide (1-2 mg/kg bid, PO)
+/– Vasodilator	Captopril (see dose above)
Anticlotting drug	Aspirin (see dose above)
Taurine supplement	250-500 mg bid, PO
Exercise restriction	
Sodium restriction	
Antiarrhythmic (+/–)	Propranolol (2.5-5 mg q8-12h)
See text for more information	

FIG. 11.9 Therapy outline for dilated cardiomyopathy.

slow circulation time. Angiocardiography is not without risk, especially in cats with poor myocardial function or decompensated heart failure from any cause. Complications can include vomiting and aspiration, arrhythmias, and cardiac arrest.

The pleural fluid that accumulates with biventricular heart failure is usually a modified transudate, although true chylous effusions may occur. Prerenal azotaemia is a common associated abnormality; mild increases in liver enzyme activities and a stress leukogram may also be found. Elevations in serum muscle enzyme activities, abnormal blood clotting profiles and disseminated intravascular coagulation may be found in cats with thromboembolism.

Treatment

The goals of therapy are to increase cardiac output and improve pulmonary function (Fig. 11.9). Pleural fluid should be removed by thoracocentesis. Often this must be done to stabilise the patient before radiography and ancillary tests can be performed. Furosemide is used to promote diuresis; however, hydration status, renal function, electrolyte balance and peripheral perfusion should be monitored because cats are quite sensitive to the effects of this drug. Patients with dilated cardiomyopathy are especially dependent on high cardiac filling pressures to maintain cardiac output. If initial furosemide therapy is successful, the dose is reduced to the lowest effective dosage level and frequency.

Positive inotropic support is important. In critical cases, dobutamine or dopamine is given via intravenous constant rate infusion. Side effects of dobutamine can include seizures or tachycardia; if this occurs, the infusion rate should be decreased by 50% or the drug discontinued. Dopamine can be used as an alternative; its adverse effects usually occur at higher doses and include tachycardia and increased peripheral resistance due to the drug's alpha adrenergic effects. The beneficial dopaminergic effects which increase renal blood flow occur at low infusion rates. Intravenous digoxin has also been used initially in cats with decompensated dilated cardiomyopathy, but can be associated with serious toxicity.

Amrinone is another positive inotropic agent with peripheral vasodilating properties for intravenous use; however, the dose of amrinone is not well established for cats. Milrinone, the more potent relative of amrinone, shows promise for use in cats with dilated cardiomyopathy but is not yet available commercially. Oral digoxin is the positive inotropic drug of choice for maintenance therapy. Generally, digoxin tablets are used because cats frequently object to the taste of digoxin elixir. It has been shown that concurrent treatment with furosemide, aspirin and a low sodium diet alters digoxin's pharmacokinetics so that toxicity is more likely to occur at standard doses. Therefore, monitoring of serum digoxin concentration is recommended.

Cats in decompensated heart failure may need fluid therapy, since furosemide and vasodilating agents can reduce cardiac filling and predispose to cardiogenic shock. Half-strength saline with 2.5% dextrose or other low sodium fluids can be used intravenously at 20–35 ml/kg/day in several divided doses or by constant infusion; potassium supplementation is usually needed. Subcutaneous fluid administration could be used if necessary, although absorption of the fluids from the extravascular space may be impaired in severely hypoperfused patients.

Vasodilators can help maximise cardiac output, although the danger of inducing hypotension must be recognised and the cat should be monitored closely. In cats with significant pulmonary oedema, the venodilator nitroglycerin may be helpful. Hydralazine (an arteriolar vasodilator) or an angiotensin converting inhibitor such as captopril (with mixed vasodilating properties) can be used with caution.

Oral taurine supplementation, at a dose of 250–500 mg bid, should be instituted, because most cats with dilated cardiomyopathy appear to have low serum taurine concentrations. Because clinical improvement after taurine supplementation does not generally occur for 1–2 weeks, supportive cardiac treatment is vital in the initial phases. Hypothermia is common in cats with decompensated dilated cardiomyopathy and therefore external warming should be provided as needed. Aspirin is instituted to decrease platelet aggregation and thus decrease the risk of thromboembolism. The occurrence of a thromboembolic event in a cat with DCM constitutes a grave sign.

Chronic treatment for cats that survive the initial period includes oral furosemide, digoxin, aspirin, a vasodilator (possibly) and taurine supplementation or a high taurine diet. As many cats refuse to eat a low salt diet, they should be encouraged to eat any nutritionally-balanced diet. After 2–3 weeks of taurine supplementation, there may be significant improvement in cardiac function. After 6–12 weeks, drug therapy may become unnecessary for some cats, although echocardiographic improvement and radiographic confirmation of the resolution of pleural effusion is advised before discontinuing treatment. When echocardiographic measures of systolic function are at or near normal, taurine supplementation can be decreased and eventually discontinued, as long as the cat eats a diet known to support adequate plasma taurine concentrations (e.g. most brand-name commercial foods). It is thought that dry diets with 1000–1200 mg taurine/kg dry weight and canned diets with 2000–2500 mg taurine/kg dry weight will maintain normal plasma taurine concentrations in adult cats. Re-evaluation of the cat's plasma taurine level 2–4 weeks after discontinuation of taurine supplementation is advised.

Restrictive cardiomyopathy

Restrictive cardiomyopathy is a relatively uncommon problem that results from extensive endocardial, subendocardial or myocardial fibrosis or infiltrative disease. Restrictive cardiomyopathy causes diastolic dysfunction and thus has a similar clinical presentation to HCM. Systolic function is maintained in most cases, although high left ventricular filling pressures are required.

Clinical features and diagnosis

Restrictive cardiomyopathy appears to have no age, breed or sex predilection. Clinical signs are variable but usually reflect the presence of left or right-sided congestive heart failure. Signs are likely to develop or worsen suddenly, and thromboembolic events are common.

Diagnostic test results, often similar to those for HCM, include radiographical evidence of massive left atrial enlargement with tortuous proximal pulmonary veins, pulmonary oedema or pleural effusion and, rarely, hepatomegaly, ascites or pericardial effusion. The ECG most frequently shows a left heart enlargement pattern and ventricular or supraventricular arrhythmias. Echocardiographic features include left ventricular free wall and septal thickening, irregularity and narrowing of the left ventricular cavity, marked enlargement of the left atrium which may contain a thrombus, and normal to mildly decreased left ventricular fractional shortening. A hyperechoic endocardium and extraneous intraluminal echoes are occasionally seen; right ventricular dilation is frequently identified. Non-selective angiocardiography will reveal the same anatomical findings and highlight the distended and tortuous pulmonary veins.

Treatment

Treatment for cats with restrictive cardiomyopathy is similar to that for HCM (see Fig. 11.7). Cats with uncomplicated left heart failure have the best prognosis; however, thromboembolic events, serious arrhythmias and decompensated heart failure often develop.

Arterial thromboembolism

Thromboembolism can occur with any form of feline cardiomyopathy, although it appears to be more common with HCM. Intracardiac blood flow abnormalities, especially within the left atrium, as well as altered blood coagulability or local tissue or blood vessel injury may result in areas of blood stasis and clot formation. Hypercoagulability has been demonstrated in cats with thromboembolic disease, and feline platelets are known to be quite reactive. Disseminated intravascular coagulation (DIC) may occur in cats with a thromboembolus.

The most common site of embolisation is the distal aortic trifurcation ('saddle thrombus'), reported in over 90% of cats with thromboembolic disease. Other areas may be affected, including a brachial artery, various organs and the heart itself. Thromboemboli cause release of vasoactive

COMMON SIGNS OF ARTERIAL THROMBOEMBOLISM
Acute limb paresis
Posterior paresis Monoparesis
Vocalisation (pain and distress)
Characteristics of affected limb(s):
Painful Cool distal limbs Pale footpads Cyanotic nailbeds Absent arterial pulse Hard, contracted muscles
Signs of congestive heart failure
Tachypnoea/dyspnoea Lethargy/weakness Murmur or gallop sounds Arrhythmias Pulmonary oedema or pleural effusion Cardiomegaly
Haematological and biochemical abnormalities
Azotaemia Increased alanine aminotransferase, aspartate aminotransferase, lactate dehydrogenase, creatinine phosphokinase Hyperglycaemia Lymphopenia Disseminated intravascular coagulation

FIG. 11.10 Common signs of arterial thromboembolism.

Clinical features and diagnosis

Clinical signs depend on the area occluded; they occur acutely and are usually dramatic. Distal aortic embolisation is manifested by hind limb paresis. The cat is usually able to flex and extend the hips, but drags the lower legs. The femoral pulses are absent, the limbs cool, the nailbeds cyanotic and the affected muscles firm and painful. Sensation to the lower legs is poor. One side may have greater neurological deficits than the other; occasionally, only distal embolisation of one limb occurs resulting in paresis of the lower limb alone. Embolisation of a brachial artery causes forelimb monoparesis. Thromboembolism of the renal,

mesenteric or pulmonary arterial circulation may result in failure of those organs and death.

Respiratory distress and auscultatory signs of cardiomyopathy are often present. A summary of common clinical findings associated with thromboembolic disease is found in Fig. 11.10. Azotaemia may result from dehydration, poor cardiac output related to the cardiomyopathy or embolisation of the renal arteries. Widespread muscle injury causes increased lactate dehydrogenase and creatinine phosphokinase activities soon after the event; elevations in these enzymes may persist for weeks. Metabolic acidosis, DIC and hyperkalaemia may also be present, secondary to ischaemic muscle damage and reperfusion.

Echocardiography (or non-selective angiocardiography), in addition to delineating the type of myocardial disease, may reveal the presence of intracardiac thrombi. The absence of palpable femoral pulses in the cat with a distal aortic embolus, in conjunction with physical examination, auscultatory and radiographic findings, is usually diagnostic. However, other considerations for acute posterior paresis might include intervertebral disc disease, spinal neoplasia (e.g. lymphoma), trauma, fibrocartilaginous infarction, diabetic neuropathy and myasthaenia gravis.

Treatment and prognosis

The goals of treatment are to manage any congestive heart failure, provide supportive care (hydration, maintenance of body temperature) and attempt to prevent extension of the embolus and formation of additional thrombi. Treatment of heart failure is outlined above and in Figs 11.3 and 11.7. Propranolol is generally avoided because its beta-blocking effects may leave vascular alpha receptors unopposed and lead to peripheral vasoconstriction. In addition, propranolol has no antithrombotic effects at clinical dosages.

Heparin has been advocated for its inhibitory effects on coagulation, although existing thromboemboli are not affected. Heparin is given initially as an intravenous dose of 1,000 units (or approximately 220 u/kg), followed in 3 hours by 50 u/kg SC. The SC dose is repeated every 6–8 hours, with dosage adjustments made to prolong the patient's activated coagulation time from 1.5 to 2.5 times

The text "substances that impair development of collateral circulation and result in ischaemic damage to tissues served by the obstructed vessels." appears before "Clinical features and diagnosis".

Fig. 11.11 Dosage guidelines for protamine sulphate.

PROTAMINE SULPHATE DOSAGE	
Timing of previous administration of heparin	Dosage for protamine sulphate (per 100 u of heparin used)
Within preceding 60 minutes >1 but <2 hours More than 2 hours	1 mg 0.5 mg 0.25 mg

the pretreatment level. As expected, bleeding can be a major complication. If this occurs, protamine sulphate may be given; however, care must be taken as overdose of protamine can, paradoxically, cause irreversible haemorrhage. Dosage guidelines for protamine sulphate are given in Fig. 11.11.

Nonspecific thrombolytic agents such as streptokinase and urokinase have been used sporadically with inconsistent results. Tissue plasminogen activator (TPA) has higher specificity of action against fibrin within thrombi, but it has yielded variable results and is quite expensive. Surgical removal of the clot is not advised (except perhaps for a suprarenal thrombus). The surgical risk is high in most cases because of the presence of decompensated heart failure, arrhythmias, DIC and hypothermia. Furthermore, significant neuromuscular ischaemic injury has probably occurred by the time surgery could be performed. Clot removal via an embolectomy catheter has not been effective in cats.

The use of a vasodilating drug such as hydralazine or acetylpromazine maleate has been suggested to improve collateral circulation; however, it is not known whether these agents are effective in ameliorating vasoconstriction induced by serotonin and other vasoactive substances released by platelet activation. Furthermore, hydralazine has been shown to have little effect on skeletal muscle blood flow compared with its enhancement of splanchnic, coronary, cerebral and renal blood flow. Exacerbation of pre-existing hypothermia and hypotension are potential side effects of these agents.

Aspirin has been used to reduce further platelet aggregation after a thromboembolic event. The usual dose is 10–25 mg/kg (1.25 g per cat) orally every third day. However, the optimal dose of

aspirin to inhibit thromboxane A_2 production, but minimally affect prostacyclin synthesis by vascular endothelium, is not yet established. Additional chronic oral therapy using warfarin (coumarin 0.06–0.1 mg/kg/day, PO, initial dose) has been suggested for cats that survive an acute thromboembolic event. The dose is adjusted to maintain the prothrombin time at twice the baseline value at 8–10 hours post dosing. Up to 72 hours may be needed to see a clinical response. The clinical effectiveness of this therapy is not known and its potential for spontaneous bleeding is high.

If concurrent congestive heart failure can be controlled, return of function in the affected limbs should begin within 7–14 days. Many cats become clinically normal within 1–2 months, although residual deficits may persist for a variable length of time. In general, the prognosis is guarded. Some cats survive for several years after a thromboembolic event, although repeated events are common and worsen the long-term prognosis. Significant embolisation of the kidneys, intestines or other organs carries a grave prognosis.

OTHER ACQUIRED CARDIAC DISEASES

Cardiomyopathies are by far the most common of feline acquired heart diseases. This section provides a brief overview of other diseases, which occur with much less frequency.

Infectious endocarditis

Bacterial infection of the heart valves and endocardium is uncommon, although immuno-compromised cats are probably at greater risk.

The mitral valve is most often affected in cats as in dogs, followed in order of frequency by the aortic, tricuspid and pulmonic valves. Various aerobic and anaerobic organisms have been implicated. Bacteraemia, from infection elsewhere in the body or an infected intravenous catheter, exposes the heart valves to possible colonisation. Microbial colonisation results in ulceration of the valvular endothelium; subsequent exposure of subendothelial collagen stimulates platelet aggregation and activation of the coagulation cascade, which leads to the formation of vegetations. Vegetations consist mainly of aggregated platelets, fibrin and bacteria. Although vegetative lesions usually involve the valve leaflets, they may extend to the chordae tendineae, sinuses of Valsalva, mural endocardium or adjacent myocardium. The affected valve(s) will become deformed and incompetent.

Congestive heart failure may result from valve insufficiency. Cardiac function can also be compromised because of direct myocardial injury from bacterial infection. Embolisation of the coronary circulation or other organ systems can result when parts of the vegetative lesions break off. Septic thromboemboli result in local abscessation and inflammation and contribute to episodes of bacteraemia and persistent or recurrent fever. Infective endocarditis may also mimic immune-mediated disease.

Clinical signs

Clinical signs are generally related to valvular insufficiency, bacteraemia, infection in various body systems, congestive heart failure, or thromboembolism. Echocardiography is a useful diagnostic tool in some cases of endocarditis. Vegetative lesions may be imaged depending on the size and location of the lesion and the resolution capabilities of the ultrasound equipment. The sequelae of cardiac valve destruction can often be identified: corresponding chamber enlargement accompanying volume overload, and flail or otherwise abnormal valve leaflet motion.

Therapy

Therapy for bacterial endocarditis consists of aggressive treatment with appropriate antimicrobial agents as well as supportive care. The selection of antimicrobial agent is ideally based on blood culture and sensitivity results; however, the cultures are frequently negative despite a bacterial aetiology. Before culture results are known or in patients where cultures are negative but bacterial endocarditis is suspected, broad-spectrum bacteriocidal drugs that penetrate fibrin should be used. The recommended treatment consists of high doses of penicillin or a synthetic penicillin derivative (e.g. ampicillin or cephalothin), in combination with an aminoglycoside (e.g. gentamicin), if renal function is adequate. Supportive care includes treatment of congestive heart failure, arrhythmias, the predisposing cause of the endocarditis, and disease in other organ systems.

Degenerative valve disease

Degenerative lesions of the cardiac valves, as occur commonly in the AV valves of dogs, are rare in cats. However, some older cats have developed mitral or aortic valve insufficiency from degenerative changes, without evidence of myocardial disease. The clinical significance of this is minimal.

Myocarditis

Acute and chronic cases of suspected viral myocarditis have been described occasionally. Documentation of viral aetiology has been rare, although feline coronavirus has been shown to cause pericarditis/epicarditis. Therapy involves management of congestive signs and arrhythmias and other supportive care.

Bacterial myocarditis could result from sepsis or bacterial endocarditis or pericarditis, as in dogs. Myocarditis caused by *Toxoplasma gondii* occurs occasionally, usually in immunosuppressed cats as part of a generalised disease process.

Pericardial disease

Pericardial effusion occurs infrequently. The most common cause is feline infectious peritonitis. Other causes include effusions secondary to congestive heart failure (especially hypertrophic cardiomyopathy), lymphosarcoma of the heart, renal failure, and systemic infections. Pericardial mesotheliomas are uncommon, but have been reported in the dog and cat.

The presence of fluid within the pericardial space may not cause clinical signs unless intrapericardial pressure equals or exceeds cardiac filling pressures. The rate of fluid accumulation and the distensibility of the pericardial sac are important factors. Rapid accumulation of even small volumes of fluid can raise intrapericardial pressure significantly, because the pericardium can stretch only slowly. Cardiac tamponade results from progressive cardiac compression which reduces cardiac filling, cardiac output and arterial blood pressure, and leads to the development of congestive heart failure, myocardial ischaemia, and, eventually, cardiogenic shock.

Clinical findings

Clinical findings in cats with symptomatic pericardial disease usually reflect signs of right-sided congestive heart failure and poor cardiac output. Historical findings often include weakness, exercise intolerance, lethargy, abdominal enlargement, tachypnoea, syncope, and possibly coughing. Jugular vein distention, hepatomegaly, ascites, laboured respiration, weakened femoral pulses, sinus tachycardia, pale peripheral mucous membranes and prolonged capillary refill time are common signs. Heart sounds are muffled with moderate to large pericardial effusions, and lung sounds are attenuated ventrally with pleural effusion. Fever may be detected in cases of infectious pericarditis.

The 'classic' radiographic pattern is the globoid cardiac shadow seen on both views with massive pericardial effusion. However, in many cases this totally round heart shadow is not observed. Echocardiography is a highly sensitive technique for detecting pericardial fluid. Not only can the echofree pericardial space be identified, but abnormal pericardial thickness or motion, abnormal cardiac wall motion and chamber shape, and intrapericardial or intracardiac mass lesions may be imaged.

Pericardiocentesis is the therapeutic procedure of choice for cardiac tamponade, in addition to providing diagnostic information. It can be accomplished using a butterfly catheter, three-way stopcock and syringe. The cat should be tranquillised and the area over the right precordium shaved and prepared aseptically. The butterfly needle is inserted into the right precordium where the cardiac impulse is palpated best. The needle is slowly advanced with gentle negative pressure being applied to the syringe so that fluid is evident in the butterfly tubing as soon as the pericardium is entered. Continuous ECG monitoring is advised during the procedure. Pericardial fluid is saved for cytological examination and culture (if cytology suggests a bacterial agent).

Heartworm disease

The incidence of heartworm disease in cats is thought to parallel that in dogs in the same geographical area but at a lower rate. Infected cats generally have fewer adult worms than infected dogs. Because heartworms mature more slowly in cats, fewer numbers of infective larvae mature to adults and the adult lifespan is shorter. However, persistence of live worms for up to 2.5 years has been documented. Heartworm-infected cats usually have less than 8 adult worms in the right ventricle and pulmonary arteries. Most cats have no or only a brief period of microfilaraemia. Aberrant worm migration, predominantly to the lateral ventricles of the brain, is more common than in dogs.

Pathophysiological changes in the heart and lungs are similar to those of dogs. Vascular injury occurs, leading to myointimal proliferations and muscular hypertrophy in affected pulmonary arteries; increased vascular permeability, partial or complete lobar consolidation and, in some cats, allergic pulmonary reactions are also seen. Disease is most severe in the caudal lung lobes.

Clinical features

Most cats infected with *Dirofilaria immitis* are males; however, this may be related to an increased amount of time spent outdoors, where the risk of exposure to infected mosquitoes is higher. Primarily indoor cats have also been infected. Most cases reported have been in cats 3–6 years old but cats of any age are susceptible. In some individuals the infection is self-limiting.

Clinical signs of heartworm disease are variable. Historical complaints include lethargy, anorexia, vomiting, paroxysmal cough, dyspnoea, syncope and sudden death. Coughing is the most common pulmonary sign. Some cats experience syncope and right-sided congestive heart failure secondary to severe pulmonary arterial disease, but this appears to be less common than in dogs. Most patients exhibit chronic signs of disease, although pulmonary arterial obstruction can cause acute respiratory distress, shock and death. A sudden onset of neurological signs, often in association with anorexia and lethargy, is common with aberrant worm migration; these signs include seizures, dementia, apparent blindness, ataxia, circling, mydriasis and hypersalivation. Physical examination may be normal or it may reflect cardiopulmonary or neurological disease; only rarely do cardiopulmonary and neurological signs coexist. Cardiopulmonary signs are most common, including tachypnoea or dyspnoea, pulmonary crackles, muffled lung sounds (from pulmonary consolidation or pleural fluid accumulation), tachycardia, a cardiac gallop sound or murmur and occasionally ascites.

Diagnosis

Thoracic radiographs are a useful screening test in cats with heartworm disease. Characteristic radiographic changes include pulmonary artery enlargement with or without visible tortuosity and blunting, right ventricular enlargement, and diffuse or focal pulmonary infiltrates. The DV view is best for evaluating the caudal lobar arteries, which are more frequently abnormal on radiographs. The main pulmonary artery segment is not visible on DV or VD views in cats, as it is located more medially than in dogs. Appreciable right heart enlargement is not consistent; however, it is more likely when signs of right heart failure (e.g. pleural effusion) exist. Ascites, which is rare in heart failure secondary to cardiomyopathy, occurs in some cats with heartworm disease. Pulmonary infiltrates are associated with allergic pneumonitis as well as pulmonary thromboembolism; focal perivascular and interstitial changes are more common than diffuse infiltrates. Pulmonary arteriography via a large bore jugular vein catheter may confirm a suspected diagnosis of heartworm disease when serology is falsely negative. Morphological changes in the pulmonary arteries are outlined and worms appear as linear filling defects.

Approximately one-third of infected cats have eosinophilia at the time of diagnosis, and a similar proportion have mild nonregenerative anaemia; basophilia is rarely found. Advanced pulmonary arterial disease is associated with neutrophilia, which may be marked and accompanied by a left shift and monocytosis; thrombocytopaenia and DIC may accompany pulmonary thromboemboli. Hyperglobulinaemia is the most common biochemical abnormality; however, its occurrence is inconsistent.

Early in the disease course, tracheal wash cytology often yields an eosinophilic exudate suggestive of allergic or parasitic disease, that is similar to that found with feline asthma and pulmonary parasites. Later, tracheal wash cytology indicates chronic inflammation or is unremarkable. Pleural effusion from heartworm-induced right heart failure is usually a modified transudate, although it may be chyle.

The ECG is often normal, although most cats with secondary right heart failure have changes compatible with right ventricular enlargement. Arrhythmias appear to be uncommon, but are more likely with advanced pulmonary arterial disease and congestive heart failure.

Microfilaria concentration tests are usually negative. This results from a combination of factors including low numbers or absence of circulating microfilaria, a brief period of microfilaraemia, and an increased likelihood of unisex infections due to low adult worm burdens. Serological testing of cats with presumptive heartworm disease is helpful in confirming the diagnosis; an ELISA test for identification of adult *D. immitis* antigens in serum is recommended. This test does not depend on the presence of microfilaria or host immune response. However, low worm numbers may result in a false negative result. The IFA test for detecting feline antibodies to microfilarial cuticular antigens is useful in that false positive results do not occur; however, prepatent and unisex infections produce false negative results. Furthermore, few laboratories perform this test, which requires antifeline antiserum. Serological tests for antibodies directed at adult heartworm antigens are associated with a high rate of false positive reactions, although false negative results are not common.

Treatment of cats with uncomplicated heartworm disease

The decision to use adulticide therapy in a cat should be weighed carefully in light of the high prevalence of severe complications in this species, and the fact that cats are not significant reservoirs for transmitting heartworm disease to other animals. Cats with clinical signs of heartworm disease should probably be treated. However, therapy may be withheld from asymptomatic cats, which are monitored for development of clinical disease. Thiacetarsamide sodium (2.2 mg/kg IV), given twice a day for two days as for dogs, has been the recommended treatment, although the efficacy of this is still unknown. However, recent studies have shown that cats eliminate the drug more slowly than dogs, especially after multiple injections, and excessive drug concentrations may accumulate with this regimen. As in dogs, it is essential that extravasation of the drug be prevented. Some cats with microfilaraemia have required multiple courses of therapy, and young female worms appear to be the most resistant. Evaluation of successful therapy by microfilaria tests is obviously ineffective in most cats; serological tests to detect adult worm antigen are useful, since successful adulticide therapy should result in negative test results within three months.

Complications of adulticide therapy

Complications of adulticide therapy in cats can be severe. Some cats (3 of 14 in one study) experience a fatal respiratory distress syndrome consisting of acute, fulminant, non-cardiogenic pulmonary oedema and death within hours after the second dose of thiacetarsamide. Pulmonary thromboembolism was not evident in these cats. Other cats had increased respiratory effort and similar, but nonfatal, pulmonary oedema and emphysema on post-mortem examination. Arsenical toxicity is known to include arteriolar

dilation and loss of capillary integrity leading to protein exudation and oedema. Pretreatment with an antihistamine and soluble glucocorticoid has been suggested before thiacetarsamide in an attempt to prevent this reaction, although the efficacy of this is unknown. Anorexia, profound depression, nausea and vomiting frequently occur after each thiacetarsamide dose. If these signs are severe, discontinuation of thiacetarsamide, provision of supportive care as needed and repetition of adulticide therapy in 2–4 weeks can be tried.

The development of acute pulmonary thromboembolism after thiacetarsamide therapy is unpredictable. It appears to be more likely in cats with radiographical evidence of severe pulmonary arterial disease and is most likely to occur 5–14 days (possibly up to 4 weeks) after treatment. Clinical signs include fever, coughing, dyspnoea, haemoptysis, pallor, pulmonary crackles, tachycardia and hypotension. Supportive findings, such as poorly defined, rounded or wedge-shaped areas of interstitial +/− alveolar densities that obscure associated pulmonary vessels, are usually present on thoracic radiographs. A platelet count and assessment of the intrinsic clotting system (e.g. activated clotting time) should be evaluated, as well as a complete blood count (CBC) and a serum biochemical profile. Therapy involves cage rest and supplemental oxygen, intravenous fluids, a soluble glucocorticoid, and aminophylline, as needed. Mild cases may respond to aminophylline (4–6 mg/kg) and antiinflammatory dosages of a glucocorticoid. Cats with severe clinical signs should receive shock doses of a soluble glucocorticoid (e.g. 10 mg/kg prednisone sodium succinate), intravenous fluids, oxygen and aminophylline. Overhydration should be avoided. Sudden death or peracute respiratory distress may occur in these cats. Aspirin therapy does not appear to reduce the severity of pulmonary arterial disease in cats and is not recommended.

Treatment of cats with complicated heartworm disease

Complications such as allergic pneumonitis, pulmonary thromboembolism and congestive heart failure must be addressed prior to adulticide therapy. For allergic pneumonitis, corticosteroid therapy (prednisone, 2–4 mg/kg q8–24 h, depending on the severity of disease) for 3–5 days in conjunction with supportive treatment is usually effective. After resolution of radiographic signs, prednisone is discontinued and thiacetarsamide is given. If necessary, prednisone may be reinstituted 5 days after thiacetarsamide therapy.

Pulmonary thromboembolic events prior to adulticide therapy have similar clinical signs and are treated as described above for post-adulticide thromboembolism. Successful therapy is accompanied by haematological, clinical and radiographic improvement. After 1–2 weeks of cage confinement, adulticide therapy may be attempted.

Right-sided congestive heart failure develops in some cats with severe pulmonary arterial disease and is evidenced by pleural effusion with or without ascites. Coughing, pulmonary parenchymal disease or evidence of thromboembolic events may coexist inconsistently. Dyspnoea, related to pleural effusion, and jugular venous distension or pulsations are common. Right ventricular enlargement is usually suggested by radiographs and ECG. Therapy is directed initially at controlling signs of heart failure; thoracocentesis as needed, cage confinement and cautious frusemide therapy (e.g. 1 mg/kg q12–24 h) are recommended for at least 1–2 weeks before adulticide therapy is contemplated. Care must be taken to avoid dehydration. Digoxin is not generally recommended. A corticosteroid is indicated if pulmonary parenchymal disease coexists. Successful management may be followed by thiacetarsamide therapy; cage confinement and ancillary treatments should be continued for 6 weeks after adulticide therapy is given.

Microfilaricide and preventive therapy

Microfilaricide therapy should only be used in cats with circulating microfilaria. Both dithiazanine (6–10 mg/kg/day for 7 days) and levamisole (10 mg/kg/day for 7 days) have been used, although toxic reactions have occurred with the latter. Ivermectin may be an effective microfilaricide, but it has not been evaluated critically in cats. Preventive medication with diethylcarbamazine is rarely recommended because of the relatively low risk of reinfection and logistical problems with daily administration in cats. However, it has been used at doses similar to those for dogs with no apparent adverse effects. Ivermectin and milbemycin are not licensed for use in cats but may hold promise for feline heartworm prevention in the future.

CONGENITAL HEART DISEASES

Congenital malformations of the heart and related structures occur occasionally in cats. The most common is a ventricular septal defect. Other lesions include patent ductus ateriosus, isolated AV valve dysplasia, subaortic stenosis, tetralogy of Fallot and endocardial fibroelastosis (mainly in Burmese cats). Clinical and auscultatory features of these defects are similar in both dogs and cats. Ventricular septal defects cause a systolic murmur loudest at the right sternal border, with volume overload to the lungs, left atrium, left ventricle and right ventricular outflow tract. Moderate to large defects tend to cause dilation of the left heart, which does most of the work. Patent ductus ateriosus causes a volume overload to the pulmonary circulation, left atrium and left ventricle in both diastole and systole. Characteristic physical findings include a continuous murmur best heard high at the left base and hyperkinetic arterial pulses. Dysplasia of the mitral valve causes mitral insufficiency and secondary left heart enlargement. Chronic volume overload may lead to left-sided congestive failure with its associated signs in these three defects.

Various malformations of vessels arising from the embryonic aortic arches can occur; these may entrap the oesophagus, and sometimes the trachea, within a vascular ring over the heartbase. The most common vascular ring anomaly is the persistent right aortic arch. Clinical signs of regurgitation and stunted growth commonly develop soon after weaning, because the vascular ring prevents normal passage of solid food through the oesophagus. Dilation of the oesophagus cranial to the restriction occurs, where food may be retained. Respiratory signs such as coughing, wheezing, stridor and cyanosis occur in association with secondary aspiration pneumonia.

Peritoneopericardial diaphragmatic hernia is the most common pericardial malformation encountered in cats. It occurs when abnormal embryonic development allows persistent communication between the pericardial and peritoneal cavities at the ventral midline. The pleural space is not affected in these patients. The most common clinical signs relate to the gastrointestinal and respiratory systems. Physical examination findings may include muffled heart sounds on one or both sides of the chest, displacement or attenuation of the apical precordial impulse, an 'empty' feel on abdominal palpation (with herniation of many organs) and, rarely, signs of cardiac tamponade. Thoracic radiography shows enlargement of the cardiac silhouette, dorsal tracheal displacement, overlap of the diaphragmatic and caudal heart borders and, often, abnormal fat or gas densities within the cardiac silhouette. Ultrasonography or contrast radiographic procedures are useful for confirming the diagnosis in equivocal cases.

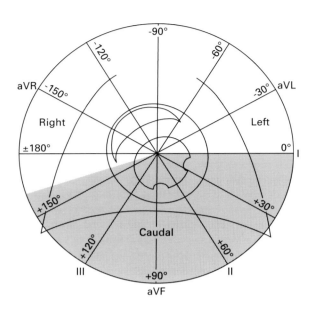

Fig. 11.12 Frontal lead system. Diagrams of the 6 frontal leads over a schematic of the left and right ventricles within the thorax. The circular field is used for determining the direction and magnitude of cardiac electrical activation. Each lead is labelled at its positive pole. The shaded area represents the normal range for mean electrical axis in the cat. From Ware, W.A. Cardiovascular Disorders. In Nelson R. and Couto C.G. (eds), *Essentials of Internal Medicine in the Cat and Dog*, Malvern, PA, USA, 1992, Mosby-Yearbook Inc, with permission.

CARDIAC ARRHYTHMIAS AND ELECTROCARDIOGRAPHY

Cardiac electrical activation and principles of electrocardiography in cats are similar to those in dogs. The normal cardiac rhythm originates in the sinoatrial node, then activates the atria, AV conduction system and ventricles in sequence. The ECG waveforms, P–QRS–T, are generated as the heart muscle is depolarised, then repolarised. Various 'leads' are used to evaluate the cardiac activation process. The bipolar and unipolar limb leads evaluate the heart's activation in the frontal plane; left–right and cranial–caudal currents are represented. Fig. 11.12 depicts the ventricles in the torso overlaid with the six frontal leads. Unipolar chest (precordial) leads which view the heart from the transverse plane are used sometimes.

The mean electrical axis (MEA) describes the 'average' orientation of the *ventricular* depolarisation wave. This is helpful for identifying major intraventricular conduction disturbances or ventricular enlargement patterns. The MEA is usually determined in the frontal plane; thus, only the six frontal leads are used. The MEA can usually be estimated by finding the lead with the largest R wave deflection. The positive electrode of this lead points to the approximate MEA.

Changes in the ECG waveforms can suggest enlargement or conduction disturbance of a particular cardiac chamber (Fig. 11.13). Widening of the P wave is often associated with left atrial enlargement; right atrial enlargement may be manifested as a tall, spiked P wave.

Right ventricular enlargement (due to dilation or hypertrophy) generally must be marked to be evident on the ECG. A right axis deviation and S wave in lead I are strong criteria for right sided enlargement (or right bundle branch block). Left ventricular dilation is usually manifested by greater than normal R wave voltages in the caudal leads. Left ventricular hypertrophy (as in hypertrophic cardiomyopathy) may cause a left axis deviation, but this is not consistent. Conduction blocks in the major ventricular conduction system also disturb the normal activation process.

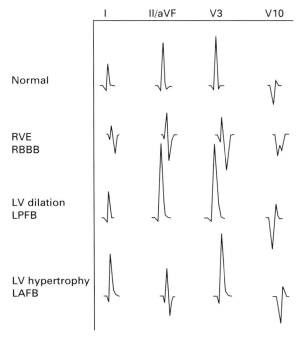

FIG. 11.13 Schematic of common ventricular enlargement patterns and conduction abnormalities. ECG leads are listed across the top. RVE = right ventricular enlargement, RBBB = right bundle branch block, LV = left ventricular, LPFB = left posterior fascicular block, LAFB = left anterior fascicular block. From Ware, W.A. Cardiovascular Disorders. In Nelson R. and Couto C.G. (eds), *Essentials of Internal Medicine in the Cat and Dog*, Malvern, PA, USA, 1992, Mosby-Yearbook Inc, with permission.

Sinus bradycardia

Regular sinus rhythm is normal in cats (Fig. 11.14). Sinus bradycardia has been associated with various drugs, trauma or diseases of the central nervous system, organic disease of the sinus node, hypothermia and hyperkalaemia, among other disorders. In most cases of sinus bradycardia, the heart rate increases in response to administration of atropine. Because sinus bradycardia and sinus arrhythmia are extremely rare in cats, a search for underlying cardiac or systemic disease is warranted in any cat with a slow or irregular rhythm.

Impulses originating from outside the sinus node are also abnormal and are described by their site of origin (supraventricular or ventricular). They are also characterised by whether they occur earlier than the next expected sinus impulse (premature) or whether they occur late (escape), as a rescue mechanism.

Supraventricular premature complexes

Supraventricular premature complexes originate above the AV node, in either the atrium or the AV junctional area. However, since they are conducted through the ventricles in the normal manner their QRS configuration is normal (unless an intraventricular conduction disturbance is also present). Atrial premature complexes are preceded by an abnormal P' wave; junctional complexes are usually not preceded by a P' wave. If the origin of the ectopic complex(es) is unclear, the more general terms 'supraventricular premature complex' or 'supraventricular tachycardia' (three or more complexes in sequence) are used. Atrial premature contractions and other atrial tachyarrhythmias are often associated with atrial enlargement in cats. Propranolol is the usual therapy for supraventricular tachyarrhythmias in cats with hypertrophic cardiomyopathy or hyperthyroidism. In cats with dilated cardiomyopathy, digoxin is the initial drug of choice.

Atrial fibrillation

Atrial fibrillation is associated with severe cardiac disease and atrial enlargement in cats. It is characterised by rapid, chaotic electrical activation of the atria; there are no P waves on the ECG (Fig. 11.14). The ventricular response rate is rapid and irregular, being determined by how quickly the AV node can conduct atrial impulses. Most often the QRS complexes appear normal in configuration. In cats with hypertrophic cardiomyopathy, atrial fibrillation is treated with propranolol or diltiazem (see Fig. 11.7).

Ventricular premature complexes

Ventricular premature complexes (VPCs or PVCs) and tachycardia originate below the AV node and do not activate the ventricles by the normal pathway; therefore they have an abnormal ECG configuration (wide and bizarre – Fig. 11.14). With ventricular tachycardia the R-R interval is

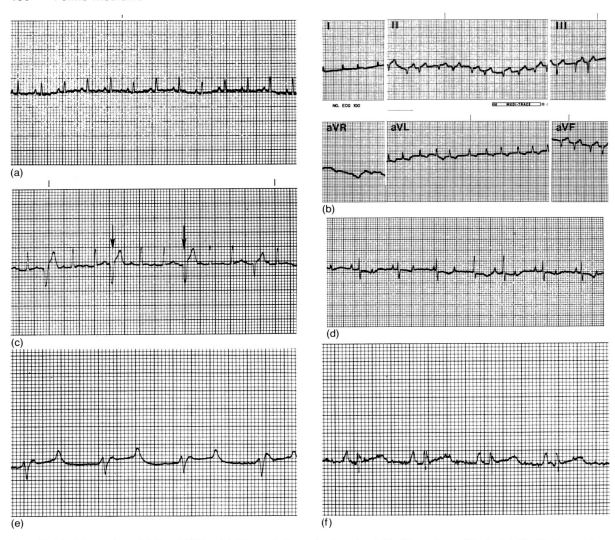

FIG. 11.14 Examples of feline ECGs. (a) Normal sinus rhythm, lead II, 25 mm/sec. (b) Atrial fibrillation with a left axis deviation (LAFB pattern) in a cat with hypertrophic cardiomyopathy, leads as marked, 25 mm/s. (c) Sinus rhythm with VPCs (arrows) in a cat with dilated cardiomyopathy, lead V_3, 25 mm/sec. (d) Complete A-V block in a 19-year-old cat with hypertrophic cardiomyopathy, lead II, 25 mm/s. (e) Effects of hyperkalaemia in a cat with urethral obstruction before treatment and (f) after, showing return of sinus P waves, lead II, 50 mm/s.

usually regular; unrelated sinus P waves may be superimposed on or between the ventricular complexes. VPCs have been associated with cardiac diseases as well as endocrine, metabolic and infectious diseases. In cats, propranolol is usually considered the drug of choice for the treatment of ventricular tachycardia. If this is ineffective, lidocaine can be used. Cats are quite sensitive to lidocaine's neurotoxic effects; therefore only tiny dosages are used (e.g. 0.25 mg/kg

slowly IV). Procainamide (e.g. 25–50 mg, q6–8 h, PO) and occasionally quinidine have also been used in this species.

Escape rhythms

Escape rhythms occur if there is cessation of sinus activity or prolonged AV conduction block. Escape rhythms are usually regular; they are of ventricular origin in the presence of complete

AV block. Ventricular escape rhythms (idio-ventricular rhythms) usually have a rate less than 100 beats/minute in the cat. It is important to differentiate escape from premature complexes. Escape activity should *never* be suppressed with antiarrhythmic drugs.

Conduction disturbances within the AV node

Conduction disturbances within the AV node may result from therapy with certain drugs, high vagal tone, and organic disease of the AV node and/or ventricular conduction system.

First degree AV block

First degree AV block occurs when AV conduction is prolonged, although all impulses are conducted.

Second degree AV block

Second degree AV block is characterised by intermittent AV conduction; some P waves are not followed by a QRS complex.

Third degree or complete AV block

Third degree or complete AV block is present when no sinus (or supraventricular) impulses are conducted into the ventricles; the P waves are not related to the QRS complexes which result from a ventricular escape rhythm (Fig. 11.14). Fortunately, most cats with complete AV block have an escape rhythm fast enough to sustain quiet daily activity; but evidence of any AV conduction disturbance in this species should prompt further diagnostic evaluation. Most cases have been associated with hypertrophic cardiomyopathy. Heart block is occasionally found in aged cats without detectable organic heart disease.

Abnormalities of serum electrolytes, especially potassium, can seriously affect the ECG.

Hyperkalaemia

Hyperkalaemia secondary to urethral obstruction in male cats is most common clinically (Fig. 11.14). Severe increases in serum potassium slow cardiac conduction velocity and shorten the refractory period. Progressive ECG changes occuring as serum potassium concentration rises include: peaked/tented T waves, flattening and eventual disappearance of the P waves (although the sinus node continues to function), slowing of the heart rate, progressive widening of the QRS complexes, and finally, ventricular asystole or fibrillation.

FURTHER READING

Bright, J.M., Golden, A.L., Gompf, R.E. et al. (1991) Evaluation of the calcium-blocking agents diltiazem and verapamil for treatment of feline hypertrophic cardiomyopathy. *J. Vet. Int. Med.* **5**: 272–282.

Dzimianski, M.T., McCall, J.W., McCall, C.A. (1986) Evaluation of heartworm immunodiagnostic test kits using well defined cat sera. *Proc. Heartworm Symp.* 159–161.

Pion, P.D., Kittleson, M.D., Rogers, Q.R. (1989) Cardiomyopathy in the cat and its relation to taurine deficiency. In: Kirk, R.W. (ed.) *Current Veterinary Therapy* **IX**: 251–262. W.B. Saunders Co., Philadelphia.

Pion, P.D., Kittleson, M.D. (1989) Therapy for feline aortic thromboembolism. In: Kirk R.W. (ed.) *Current Veterinary Therapy* **IX**: 295–301. W.B. Saunders Co., Philadelphia.

Rawlings, C.A. (1990) Pulmonary arteriography and hemodynamics during feline heartworm disease: effects of aspirin. *J. Am. Coll. Vet. Intern. Med.* **4**: 285–291.

Rush, J.E., Keene, B.W., Fox, P.R. (1990) Pericardial disease in the cat: a retrospective evaluation of 66 cases. *J. Am. Anim. Hosp. Assoc.* **26**: 39–46.

Turner, J.L., Lees, G.E., Brown, S.A. et al. (1989) Thiacetarsamide in normal cats: pharmacokinetic, clinical, laboratory and pathologic features. *Proceed. Heartworm Symp.*, pp. 135–141.

Zanotti, S., Kaplan, P. (1989) Feline dirofilariasis. *Compend. Cont. Educ.* **11**: 1005–1015.

12

Disorders of the Gastrointestinal System

W. GRANT GUILFORD

Gastrointestinal disease is common in small animal practice. It is often secondary to diseases of other organ systems. Gastrointestinal disorders can be acute or chronic. Animals with acute gastrointestinal disease can frequently be managed symptomatically (see later) but chronic, life-threatening or secondary diseases usually require an accurate diagnosis for appropriate therapy.

CLINICAL EXAMINATION

A complete history and physical examination are the keys to diagnosis. The history and physical examination define the client's complaint, determine patient profile, identify clinical signs of disease, indicate the severity of the disorder, suggest whether the condition is primary or secondary, and provide an initial list of differential diagnoses. In this latter regard, feline breed predispositions can assist the clinician (Fig. 12.1).

Clinical signs indicative of gastrointestinal disease are listed in Fig. 12.2. Those signs listed as specific problems are highly suggestive of gastrointestinal dysfunction. Those signs listed as non-specific problems are often associated with gastrointestinal disease but are also frequently seen with disorders of other body systems. It is important to note, however, that while the specific signs are strongly indicative of gastrointestinal dysfunction, few of these signs differentiate *primary* gastrointestinal disease from dysfunction *secondary* to other disorders (e.g. uraemic gastritis). The owner should

be questioned to determine which of these signs are present, the date of onset, which sign was noticed first, the frequency of occurrence and duration of a given sign, and the presence of exacerbating factors. Additional questions pertaining to the specific signs present should then be asked. For instance, the character of vomitus and bowel movements often provides useful information for differential diagnosis. The history is concluded by screening other systems of the body with appropriate questions to help detect systemic causes of gastrointestinal dysfunction.

Certain clinical presentations involving the above signs, alone or in combination, suggest serious disease (Fig. 12.3). Animals demonstrating such signs of serious disease should generally receive the benefit of diagnostic effort in addition to supportive therapy.

DIAGNOSTIC INVESTIGATIONS

While the history and physical examination are the most important parts of the diagnostic work-up, only on a few occasions (e.g. intestinal foreign body) will they reveal a specific cause. For complex or refractory gastrointestinal cases, a useful laboratory data base includes a complete blood count (CBC), serum chemistry profile with electrolyte levels, urinalysis, and faecal flotation and direct wet mount examination. The database is compiled in order to evaluate the patient for parasitism and systemic diseases, to identify any

SUSPECTED OR CONFIRMED BREED PREDISPOSITIONS	
Abyssinian	Megaoesophagus due to myasthenia gravis
Manx cat	Constipation, faecal incontinence
Siamese cat	Megaoesophagus, gastric retention, intestinal adenocarcinoma
Pedigree cats	Gingivitis/stomatitis

FIG. 12.1 Suspected or confirmed breed predispositions to gastrointestinal diseases.

CLINICAL SIGNS OF GASTROINTESTINAL DISEASE
Specific gastrointestinal problems
Dysphagia
Regurgitation
Vomiting
Bloat
Borborygmus
Flatulence
Diarrhoea
Dyschezia
Haematochezia
Tenesmus
Abdominal pain
Ascites
Icterus
Melaena
Faecal incontinence
Constipation
Non-specific gastrointestinal problems
Anorexia
Fever
Depression
Polydipsia
Shock
Dehydration
Weight loss
Polyphagia
Halitosis
Anaemia
Salivation

FIG. 12.2   Clinical signs of gastrointestinal disease.

additional incidental problems in another body system, and to facilitate management decisions such as choice of fluid therapy. If the database fails to provide a diagnosis, the choice of further diagnostic procedures is dictated by the nature of the primary problem (see below). The diagnostic work-up is concluded once safe and effective therapy or an accurate prognosis can be advised. It is important to reiterate that expensive diagnostic procedures are only applied to patients with chronic, intractable conditions, or to animals with warning signs of serious disease. For cats with acute manifestations of gastrointestinal disorders, unaccompanied by warning signs of serious disease, it is entirely appropriate to prescribe owner-administered symptomatic therapy.

GASTROINTESTINAL PROBLEMS

Vomiting

Vomiting is the forceful ejection of gastric content from the stomach. It occurs following stimulation of a brain-stem-based neural reflex. Vomiting is accomplished by pronounced contraction of the muscles of the diaphragm and abdomen. It is preceded by signs of nausea such as restlessness, hypersalivation, lip licking, frequent swallowing, and retching. Low pH or the presence of bile in the ejected material implies vomiting rather than regurgitation. Material of alkaline pH may be vomit (gastroduodenal reflux) or it may have been regurgitated. Great care must be taken to differentiate regurgitation from vomiting. The most reliable differentiating feature is the characteristic pronounced abdominal contractions of vomiting.

Vomiting is a very common problem in the cat and can be due to a multitude of causes (Fig. 12.4). The diagnostic procedures of value for the investigation of chronic vomiting are listed in Fig. 12.5 and described briefly below.

WARNING SIGNS OF SERIOUS GASTROINTESTINAL DISEASE
Chronic, frequent vomiting, regurgitation or diarrhoea
Evidence of shock (prolonged capillary refill time, weak pulse)
Marked depression or persistent anorexia
Marked weight loss, dehydration, or weakness
Yellow, pale or congested mucous membranes
Digested blood ('coffee grounds') in the vomitus
Large volume malodorous vomiting while food is withheld
Vomiting food more than 6 hours after ingestion (delayed gastric emptying)
Abdominal pain, distension, masses or effusions
Melaena

FIG. 12.3   Some warning signs of serious gastrointestinal disease.

CAUSES OF VOMITING
Acute vomiting
Food poisoning, intolerance or allergy Toxicities (household plants, insecticides, drugs) Gastrointestinal tract obstruction (linear foreign bodies, intussusception, hair balls) Toxaemias (pyometra, peritonitis) Viral gastroenteritis (panleukopenia, rotavirus, coronavirus) Bacterial gastroenteritis (*Salmonella, Campylobacter?*, others) Travel sickness
Chronic vomiting
Food intolerance/allergy Inflammatory bowel disease (chronic gastritis, lymphoplasmacytic enteritis, eosinophilic gastroenteritis etc.) Gastrointestinal tract obstruction (intussusception, pyloric stenosis, neoplasia) Gastrointestinal neoplasia Parasitism (*Ollulanus,* Ascarids, Physaloptera, *Giardia,* heartworm) Toxicities (lead) Constipation Chronic pancreatitis Endocrine diseases (diabetes mellitus, hyperthyroidism) Liver disease Uraemia Cardiomyopathy Neurologic diseases (dysautonomia, CNS diseases)

FIG. 12.4 Causes of vomiting.

History

Relevant history includes the likelihood of ingestion of linear foreign bodies (such as wool yarn or cotton) and the possibility of repeated access to rubbish, organophosphates, household cleaners or ornamental plants. Aggravation of vomiting by a certain diet raises the possibility of food intolerance or allergy. Almost any drug can cause vomiting as an idiosyncratic reaction. Concurrent polyuria/polydipsia suggests the presence of systemic disease such as diabetes mellitus, renal failure or hyperthyroidism, all of which can result in vomiting.

The frequency and chronicity of the vomiting, the volume and content of the vomitus, and the temporal relationship of the vomiting to the ingestion of food help determine the cause of the problem. Vomiting within minutes to a few hours after ingestion supports the presence of gastric inflammation or irritation. Vomiting of food more than 12 hours after ingestion is pathognomonic for delayed gastric emptying. Persistent vomiting of large volumes of liquid vomitus in spite of food restriction is highly suggestive of pyloric or upper intestinal obstruction. Occasional flecks of fresh blood in vomitus is not of concern but large amounts of digested blood ('coffee grounds') or melaena, suggest significant upper gastrointestinal haemorrhage. Yellow staining of vomitus is common no matter what the cause of vomiting: it is due to gastroduodenal reflux of bile and rules out complete pyloric obstruction.

Physical examination

A complete physical examination is essential. Particular attention is paid to attitude, hydration and cardiovascular status, all of which indicate the severity of the vomiting. Careful examination of the mouth and neck is important. Close attention should be paid to the base of the tongue where linear foreign bodies can catch. Examination of the base of the tongue is assisted by dorsally directed digital pressure between the mandibular rami. Careful palpation of the lymph nodes for lymphadenopathy and the neck for thyroid nodules should be performed (Fig. 16.4). Detection of tachycardia, arrhythmias, murmurs and weak

FIG. 12.5 Procedures for the diagnosis of chronic vomiting.

DIAGNOSIS OF CHRONIC VOMITING	
Procedure	**Usefulness**
Dietary trials	Food sensitivity
Complete blood count	Sepsis, toxaemia, eosinophilic gastritis, lead, hydration
Serum chemistry profile	Diabetes mellitus, uraemia hypoproteinaemia, liver disease, electrolyte levels
Urinalysis	Renal disease, liver disease, hydration, ketoacidosis
Blood gas	Acid-base status
Faecal flotation	Parasites
Faecal occult blood	Neoplasia, ulcers
Vomitus microscopic exam	*Ollulanus tricuspis*
Liver function test	Liver disease
Serum antibody/antigen tests	Heartworm, FeLV, FIV
T4 level	Hyperthyroidism
Survey radiographs	Obstructions, foreign bodies, liver and kidney size, masses, pancreatitis, peritonitis
Ultrasonography	Masses, metastatic neoplasia, mural thickenings
Contrast radiography	Gastric disorders, pyloric obstruction, gastric emptying, intestinal obstruction
Fluoroscopy	Gastrointestinal motility disorders
Endoscopy	Luminal and mucosal gastric, duodenal and large bowel disease
Cerebrospinal fluid (CSF) tap	Central nervous system diseases
Toxicology	Plasma cholinesterase, lead, serum osmolality (ethylene glycol)
Exploratory celiotomy	Full-thickness biopsy, gastrinoma, chronic pancreatitis

* Modified with permission from Strombeck D.R., Guilford W.G. (1990) *Small Animal Gastroenterology*, 2nd edn. Stonegate Publishing, Davis.

Fig. 12.5 Procedures for the diagnosis of chronic vomiting.

pulse suggests cardiomyopathy, a disorder that can result in vomiting. Both lymphosarcoma and hyperthyroidism are common causes of vomiting in cats. Methodical abdominal palpation is important. Distended gas-filled loops of bowel suggestive of obstruction may be apparent. Bowel infiltrated by inflammatory or neoplastic cells may feel thickened on palpation. Mesenteric lymphadenopathy or other abdominal masses may be detected but beware of confusing the easily palpable ileocolic valve region with an abdominal mass. The neurological examination should not be forgotten because persistent vomiting can result from CNS lesions.

Tabletop assessment

By the conclusion of the clinical examination, the clinician should be able to differentiate expectoration, gagging, retching (see below), regurgitation and vomiting, and should have assessed the severity of the condition and the fluid volume deficit (if any). The cause may be apparent or, more probably, the list of potential causes will have been narrowed.

Laboratory database

A laboratory database consisting of a CBC, serum chemistry panel, urinalysis and faecal flotation should be gathered. If available, a venous blood gas sample to determine acid-base status can be useful, as can a carefully interpreted faecal occult blood test if melaena is suspected. Look for evidence on the database of systemic diseases, such as kidney and liver insufficiency, toxaemias (e.g. pyometra, peritonitis), diabetes mellitus and lead toxicity. If the database points to any of these disorders, further diagnostic tests such as organ biopsy, liver function tests and lead levels may be required. Amylase and lipase have proved unreliable tests for chronic pancreatitis in cats. The database may detect significant or insignificant parasitism and aid the identification of eosinophilic gastritis. Perusal of the PCV, serum albumin, electrolyte panel and blood gas data helps tailor the fluid (crystalloid, plasma, blood) and electrolytes administered.

Survey abdominal radiographs

Gastrointestinal tract foreign bodies and intestinal obstruction can usually be diagnosed by survey radiographs. Radiographs also assess gastric size, position and content, detect gross abnormalities in liver and kidney size, and help detect abdominal fluid, abdominal masses, organ torsions, bowel perforation, peritonitis and pancreatitis. Radiographs showing tight clumping of the bowel gas pattern in mid-abdomen are characteristic of linear foreign bodies.

Controlled diets

If no diagnosis is apparent after performance of these initial diagnostic tests and there are no warning signs of serious disease, it is good practice to discharge the cat on a controlled diet for 2–3 weeks to determine if the vomiting is food responsive. The controlled diet should consist of a white meat (not fish) to which the cat has not had exposure in the last 6 months. An easily absorbable carbohydrate source, such as baby rice cereal into which the meat is diced, and vitamins and minerals should be added if the controlled diet is used for more than 2 weeks. If the diarrhoea does not respond to the controlled diet, the diagnosis should be pursued further with the following tests.

Contrast radiography

With the advent of endoscopy, the emphasis of gastrointestinal contrast radiography has moved towards procedures that assess gastrointestinal motility or detect intestinal obstructions or partial obstructions. Double contrast gastrograms allow

examination of the gastric mucosa and may be useful if an endoscope is unavailable. Liquid barium examinations may help detect gastric mural lesions missed by the endoscope and, if fluoroscopy is available, allow an appreciation of gastric motility. Administration of barium liquid will also detect gross obstructive disorders of the pylorus or intestine. Barium-coated food gives a crude estimate of gastric emptying time. Gastric emptying usually begins within 30 minutes of ingestion. Inadequate gastric motility is inferred by delayed gastric emptying without associated endoscopic or surgical evidence of an outflow obstruction.

Referral to a specialist facility

Most major cities now have a specialist facility. Such centres offer facilities such as abdominal ultrasound, endoscopy and fluoroscopy, all of which may provide sufficient information to avoid an unnecessary exploratory laparotomy.

Abdominal ultrasound and radiographs are complementary examinations. Ultrasound is more sensitive for the detection of abdominal masses including intraorgan miliary masses (e.g. metastatic neoplasia), mural thickenings, lymphadenopathy, pancreatitis and hepatic disorders.

Endoscopy is a sensitive technique for the diagnosis of such common disorders as chronic gastritis and inflammatory bowel disease without the attendant risks and morbidity of full-thickness surgical biopsy.

Fluoroscopy allows definitive diagnosis of gastric and intestinal motility disorders.

Exploratory laparotomy

Exploratory laparotomy may be required for the diagnosis of mural diseases of the gastrointestinal tract, mucosal lesions out of reach of the endoscope, gastrinomas, and low grade diseases of some organs such as chronic pancreatitis. Pyloric hypertrophy and large mass lesions of the gastric wall may be apparent on endoscopy, but definitive diagnosis may require full thickness biopsy. Full thickness biopsy of the intestine is disadvantaged by the increased likelihood of wound dehiscence. The biopsy sites of debilitated and hypoalbuminaemic animals are particularly likely to dehisce.

In these patients, full-thickness intestinal biopsy should be performed only after great circumspection and preferably in association with nutritional support.

Miscellaneous diagnostic evaluations

Various other tests may aid diagnosis in some cases of vomiting. Microscopic examination of the vomitus may reveal *Ollulanus tricuspis* larvae or, rarely, cytological evidence of neoplasia. Cerebrospinal fluid (CSF) taps or magnetic resonance imaging (MRI) may be required to detect CNS lesions causing vomiting.

Symptomatic therapy

Fluid therapy

Use lactated Ringer's with an additional 10–15 mEq/l of potassium chloride for all vomiting cats with the exception of those vomiting due to an upper duodenal or pyloric obstruction or those with blood gas evidence of alkalosis. Cats with these latter problems should be rehydrated with 0.9% sodium chloride with 15–20 mEq/l of potassium chloride. Avoid rehydration with potassium-free fluids. The volume of fluid required (mls) = deficit (% dehydration × bodyweight in grams) + maintenance (~ 50 ml/kg/day) + on-going losses in vomitus. Aim to replace the volume deficit over a 6–8 hour period. The intravenous route is preferred but the subcutaneous route is acceptable provided dehydration is not marked.

Diet

No food for 24–48 hours, followed by a bland diet, such as chicken, for 3–7 days is recommended. Feed three to four times per day in small amounts. If the diet is being used as a diagnostic tool, choose a protein source to which the animal has not had recent exposure (see above).

Antiemetics

These drugs are indicated only if vomiting is intractable. For a general purpose antiemetic, use prochlorperazine (0.1 mg/kg qid, SC) or chlorpromazine (0.5 mg/kg tid, SC). Metoclopramide has antiemetic action at the chemoreceptor trigger zone and in addition improves upper gastrointestinal motility. It is therefore most useful for vomiting due to drug reactions, toxaemias or motility abnormalities. Use metoclopramide at a dose of 0.2–0.4 mg/kg tid, SC. Cats appear peculiarly sensitive to the antidopaminergic actions of metoclopramide. The drug should be discontinued if disorientation, depression or hyperactivity are observed. Metoclopramide is also contraindicated if gastric obstruction is suspected. Anticholinergics, such as atropine, are contraindicated for routine use as antiemetics.

Inhibitors of gastric acid secretion

These drugs are indicated only if vomiting is associated with gastric erosions or ulcers (i.e. blood in the vomitus). They are not antiemetics, *per se*, but help reduce perpetuation of gastric mucosal lesions by gastric acid. Use cimetidine at a dose of 5–10 mg/kg tid PO or ranitidine at a dose of 3.5 mg/kg bid PO.

Locally acting protectants

Sucralphate binds to areas of denuded mucosa and is particularly useful for the treatment of gastric ulcers. Use at a dose of 30–50 mg/kg tid PO. Colloidal bismuth subcitrate (30 mg per cat q8–12h) has some local protective actions. Similarly, bismuth salicylate has protective and antisecretory activities of value in the non-specific treatment of gastroenteritis (0.5–1 ml/kg bid for 2–3 days).

Antibiotics

These drugs are primarily indicated if there is breach of the gastrointestinal mucosal barrier as indicated by fever or blood in the vomitus. Amoxicillin (10–20 mg/kg bid SC) is suitable.

Anti-inflammatory/immunosuppressive drugs

Because of the high incidence of inflammatory bowel disease in cats, symptomatic therapy of chronic vomiting with glucocorticoids is becoming widely practised. The use of these drugs without

CAUSES OF DIARRHOEA
Acute small bowel diarrhoea
Sudden change of diet Food poisoning, intolerance, or allergy Viral enteritis (panleukopenia, Coronavirus, Rotavirus, FeLV) Bacterial (*Campylobacter, Salmonella, Yersinia, Clostridium?, E. coli?*) Toxicosis (e.g. organophosphates) Toxaemias (pyometra, abscess, peritonitis)
Chronic small bowel diarrhoea
Bacterial overgrowth? (antibiotic misuse) Infectious enteritis (*Campylobacter*, FIV, FeLV) Parasites (*Giardia*, Helminths) Food intolerance or allergy Inflammatory bowel disease (eosinophilic, lymphocytic-plasmacytic, other) Infiltrative neoplasia (lymphosarcoma, mastocytosis) Partial obstruction (neoplasia, strictures, intussusception) Exocrine pancreatic insufficiency (rare) Liver failure Uraemia Hyperthyroidism
Acute large bowel diarrhoea
Acute idiopathic colitis Infectious colitis (*Salmonella, Campylobacter, Clostridium,* FeLV) Abrasive colitis (bones, hair, wrapping material) Toxaemias (pyometra, abscess, peritonitis) Toxicosis
Chronic large bowel diarrhoea
Chronic colitis (lymphocytic-plasmacytic, eosinophilic, histiocytic) Infectious colitis (FIP, FeLV, *Campylobacter,* histoplasmosis) Foreign material (hair?) Parasites (Cystisospora) Partial obstruction (neoplasia, strictures, ileocolic intussusception) Neoplasia (adenocarcinoma, lymphosarcoma) Uraemia

Fig. 12.6 Causes of diarrhoea.

a diagnosis is fraught with dangers and as a general rule their symptomatic use is discouraged.

Diarrhoea

Diarrhoea is an increase in the frequency, fluidity or volume of bowel movements. Diarrhoea can be due to primary disease of the gastrointestinal tract or may be secondary to a multitude of diseases of other organs (Fig. 12.6). The term 'small bowel diarrhoea' (malassimilation) refers to diarrhoea as a consequence of small intestinal dysfunction resulting from diseases of the intestine itself (malabsorption), or from diseases of digestive organs such as the pancreas and liver (maldigestion) that interfere with the ability of the small intestine to absorb food. The term 'large bowel diarrhoea' refers to diarrhoea resulting from diseases of the caecum, colon or rectum. In cats, chronic diarrhoea is less commonly reported by owners than chronic vomiting. In comparison with dogs, cats develop diarrhoea less commonly due to maldigestion or large bowel diseases.

History

The first goal of the history is to differentiate small bowel diarrhoea from large bowel diarrhoea (Fig. 12.7). This is important, because the diagnostic

FIG. 12.7 Differentiation of large and small bowel diarrhoea.

DIFFERENTIATION OF LARGE AND SMALL BOWEL DIARRHOEA

Clinical signs	Small bowel	Large bowel
Faecal volume	Large	Small
Faecal consistency	Loose	Loose to formed
Faecal mucus	Normal	Increased
Faecal fat	Increased	Normal
Faecal colour	Variable	Usually brown
Faecal blood	Usually none, occasionally melaena	Fresh blood frequent
Defecation frequency	Usually increased, 2-4 times/day	Always increased 4-10 times/day
Defecation urgency	Rare	Frequent
Tenesmus	None	Frequent
Weight loss	Common	Infrequent
Exacerbating factors	Diet changes High fat diets Poorly digestible diets	Stress and psychological factors may be important

and therapeutic approach differs with each category. Additional goals of the history are to identify potential causes of the diarrhoea, detect warning signs of serious disease, and identify any evidence of systemic disease (e.g. polydipsia/polyuria). With these aims in mind, questions to the client should include: (i) patient profile, parasite control programme and vaccination status; (ii) duration of the complaint; (iii) whether the diarrhoea ceases with fasting; (iv) historical associations (e.g. with a particular food, environment, stressful situations); (v) defaecation frequency; (vi) appearance of the faeces (mucus, presence of fresh blood, colour, volume, odour); (vii) presence of defaecation urgency, tenesmus or dyschezia.

Young animals are more prone to nutritional, microbial and parasitic causes of diarrhoea. Adverse reactions to food are a prominent cause of diarrhoea, and the history is a rapid way to identify responsible nutrients. For instance, chronic diarrhoea in young cats is frequently caused by an intolerance to milk. Osmotic diarrhoea, which usually results from malassimilation, is likely if the diarrhoea ceases when the animal is fasted. Secretory diarrhoea, which is usually due to infectious diseases, will often continue in the unfed animal. The frequency and appearance of bowel movements help differentiate large and small bowel diarrhoea (Fig. 12.7). Rapid transit time is associated with the yellow and green faeces due

to incompletely metabolised bilirubin. Melaena refers to black, tarry faeces resulting from upper gastrointestinal blood loss. Normal cats commonly have black faeces, however, and it is important not to assume black faeces are due to melaena. Increased quantities of faecal fat (steatorrhoea) impart a grey colour and rancid odour to the faeces. In the cat, steatorrhea is usually due to inflammatory bowel disease or hyperthyroidism, both very common causes of chronic diarrhoea.

Physical examination

Careful attention should be paid to the cat's attitude, hydration and cardiovascular status and to examination of the oral cavity, lymph nodes, thyroid glands and abdomen. Weight loss as a result of malassimilation may be apparent. Loops of bowel filled with fluid and gas may be palpated in animals with enteritis or obstruction. Detection of hepatomegaly raises the likelihood of hepatic disease. Palpation of the rectum may reveal faecal impaction or rectal masses. Examination of faeces adherent to the thermometer may detect melaena.

Tabletop assessment

By the conclusion of the clinical examination, the clinician should be able to differentiate small bowel from large bowel diarrhoea, and should have assessed the severity of the condition and the fluid volume deficit (if any). The cause of the diarrhoea is rarely apparent but the list of potential causes will have been narrowed.

Diagnostic evaluations

For complex or refractory cases of diarrhoea, the minimum laboratory database should include a CBC, a serum chemistry profile with electrolyte levels, a urinalysis, a faecal flotation for parasite ova, and a direct smear of saline-admixed fresh faeces for protozoa. Cats with diarrhoea in association with a peripheral eosinophilia usually have eosinophilic gastroenteritis but parasitism and mast cell neoplasia are also important possibilities. Panhypoproteinaemia (low serum albumin & globulin), which characterises protein-losing enteropathies, is uncommon in cats in comparison to dogs but is occasionally seen with severe inflammatory bowel disease or severe subacute enteropathy secondary to non-fatal panleukopenia. Serological tests for feline leukaemia (FeLV), feline immunodeficiency virus (FIV) and feline infectious peritonitis (FIP) may also be warranted. These diseases can be associated with chronic enteropathies. The FIP titre must be interpreted carefully. Serum thyroxine measurement is indicated in elderly cats with diarrhoea particularly if steatorrhea is observed. In cats with small bowel diarrhoea, a Sudan stain of fresh faeces for fat can be worthwhile. Large quantities of undigested fats raise the unlikely possibility of exocrine pancreatic insufficiency which can be confirmed by azocasein hydrolysis or radial enzyme diffusion tests but, as yet, not by serum trypsin-like immunoreactivity testing. If large bowel diarrhoea is suspected, a stained faecal smear or rectal scraping should be examined and may reveal inflammatory cells suggestive of colitis or fungi such as *Histoplasma*. Large amounts of neutrophils in a faecal smear or evidence of contagion are indications for faecal culture which is otherwise usually a low-yield procedure.

If no diagnosis is apparent after performance of these initial laboratory tests, and no warning signs of serious disease are apparent, it is customary to discharge the cat on a controlled diet for 2–3 weeks to determine if the diarrhoea is food responsive.

A similar controlled diet to that described for vomiting is appropriate.

If the diarrhoea fails to respond to the controlled diet, further tests are indicated. Because of the high incidence of inflammatory bowel disease, upper gastrointestinal biopsy is usually the next diagnostic procedure of choice. Where possible this should be performed by referral to an endoscopist to avoid the surgical morbidity of laparotomy. Full-thickness colon biopsies, in particular, should be avoided. Survey abdominal radiographs or contrast radiography rarely provide diagnostically useful information in cases of diarrhoea but, when they do, that information can be invaluable to patient well-being (e.g. partial obstruction). The advent of the endoscope has largely relegated absorption tests (such as xylose absorption) to obscurity. It should not be forgotten however, that endoscopic examination does not screen for the same spectra of diseases as do absorption tests (e.g. brush border abnormalities). Breath hydrogen analysis appears to be a useful absorption test in cats. The serum cobalamin/folate absorption test has not, as yet, been validated for use in cats. Miscellaneous other tests of occasional value are listed in Fig. 12.8.

Symptomatic therapy

Fluids and diet

The fluid and diet therapy of diarrhoea is similar to that described for vomiting. It has been suggested that cats with diarrhoea tolerate high fat diets better than high carbohydrate diets. This suggestion needs further investigation before widespread application.

Motility modifiers

Only indicated if diarrhoea is intractable. Use short courses of an opioid such as loperamide (0.08 mg/kg tid, PO). These drugs are contraindicated if the diarrhoea is due to invasive micro-organisms and must be used with care in cats. Metoclopramide (0.2–0.4 mg/kg qid, SC) is useful if diarrhoea is associated with ileus. Anticholinergics are contraindicated in diarrhoea.

FIG. 12.8 Procedures for the diagnosis of chronic diarrhoea.

DIAGNOSIS OF CHRONIC DIARRHOEA*	
Procedure	**Usefulness**
Complete blood count	Sepsis, toxaemia, eosinophilic gastroenteritis, hydration
Serum chemistry profile	Uraemia, protein-losing enteropathy, liver disease, electrolyte levels
Urinalysis	Renal disease, liver disease, hydration
Dietary trials	Food intolerance, food allergy
Blood gas	Acid-base status
Faecal flotation	Helminths, *Giardia*, cryptosporidia, Cystisospora
Faecal direct smear	Giardiasis, other protozoa, neutrophils
Baerman technique	*Strongyloides* larvae
Faecal Sudan stain	Steatorrhea
Faecal occult blood	Neoplasia, ulcers
Faecal digestion tests	Exocrine pancreatic insufficiency
Faecal culture	*Salmonella, Campylobacter*
Serum antibody/antigen tests	FeLV, FIV, FIP
Serum thyroxine level	Hyperthyroidism
Breath hydrogen test	Bacterial overgrowth?, carbohydrate malabsorption
Faecal total fat excretion	Fat malabsorption
Survey radiographs	Intussusception, foreign bodies, liver and kidney size, masses, pancreatic abscess, peritonitis
Ultrasonography	Masses, metastatic neoplasia, mural thickenings
Contrast radiography	Intestinal partial obstruction, neoplasia
Fluoroscopy	Gastrointestinal motility disorders
Endoscopy	Luminal and mucosal gastroduodenal and large bowel disease
Toxicology	Plasma cholinesterase, lead
ACTH stimulation test	Hypoadrenocorticism
Liver function test	Liver disease
Exploratory celiotomy	Full-thickness biopsy, chronic pancreatitis, phycomycosis, mycobacteria, focal neoplasia

* Modified with permission from Strombeck D.R., Guilford W.G. (1990) *Small Animal Gastroenterology*. 2nd edition. Stonegate Publishing, Davis.

Locally acting adsorbents and protectants

Activated charcoal (0.7–1.4 g/kg PO) is a useful adsorbent for the treatment of diarrhoea due to toxins. Kaolin and pectin are thought to have some adsorbent and perhaps protectant roles but there is little evidence to suggest that these are very effective medications. Bismuth subsalicylate is indicated for non-specific gastroenteritis (see above).

Antibiotics

Antibiotics have a number of adverse effects on the gastrointestinal tract and are likely to delay recovery if injudiciously used. They should only be used for the treatment of diarrhoea if the diarrhoea is haemorrhagic, a known pathogen has been cultured from the faeces, or there is evidence of bacterial overgrowth or sepsis. Fluoroquinolones are a good choice of antibiotic for the treatment of haemorrhagic diarrhoea because they are very effective against enteric pathogens. For severe haemorrhagic diarrhoea, ampicillin (10–20 mg/kg qid, IV) in combination with gentamicin (2.2 mg/kg tid, SC) provides effective broad spectrum coverage. However, because of potential nephrotoxicity, gentamicin cannot be used until after the animal has been rehydrated. Oral aminoglycosides should **not** be used for the treatment of diarrhoea. Metronidazole (10–20 mg/kg bid) for 5–7 days is useful if giardiasis or anaerobic bacterial overgrowth is suspected. In young cats with acute large bowel diarrhoea, an oral sulphonamide is sometimes useful because of the possibility of coccidiosis.

Anti-inflammatory/immunosuppressive drugs

As with chronic vomiting, symptomatic therapy of chronic diarrhoea with glucocorticoids is discouraged unless a diagnosis of inflammatory bowel disease has been made.

Gagging, retching and expectoration

Gagging is a reflexive contraction of the constrictor muscles of the pharynx resulting from stimulation of the pharyngeal mucosa. Retching is an involuntary and ineffectual attempt at vomiting. Retching is produced by contractions of the diaphragm and abdominal muscles, the same motor events that cause vomition. Expectoration is the ejection of airway and laryngopharyngeal mucus or discharges. Gagging and expectoration, alone or in combination, are common in cats. They are usually self-limiting and are commonly ascribed to accumulation of fur in the pharynx. Grass blades resting in the nasopharynx can produce similar signs. Diagnosis is usually made via history and oropharyngeal examination. Accumulation of fur can be minimized by regular combing.

CAUSES OF DIFFICULT OR PAINFUL PREHENSION AND MASTICATION*
Stomatitis/glossitis/gingivitis
Physical agents (electrical cord burns, trauma, insect bites) Caustic agents (petroleum products, alkalis, acids, thallium) Bacterial infections (*Bacteroides melaninogenicus*?) Viral infections (feline rhinotracheitis, calici, FeLV, FIV) Foreign bodies (imbedded plant material) Autoimmune diseases (pemphigus) Immune-mediated disorders (toxic epidermal necrolysis, idiopathic feline glossopharyngitis, eosinophilic granuloma) Immunodeficiencies Systemic disorders (uraemia, sepsis)
Oral/glossal neoplasia
Squamous cell carcinoma Fibrosarcoma Melanoma
Neurological disorders
Polyneuropathies Neuropathies of cranial nerves VII, IX, X, XII CNS lesions (cerebellar disorders, brain stem lesions, hydrocephalus)
Neuromuscular junction disorders
Myasthenia gravis
Musculoskeletal disorders
Temporomandibular joint disorders Nutritional secondary hyperparathyroidism Mandible fracture or subluxation
Miscellaneous disorders
Retrobulbar abscess Dental disorders (tooth root abscesses, fractured teeth)
* Modified with permission from Strombeck D.R., Guilford W.G. (1990) *Small Animal Gastroenterology*. 2nd edition. Stonegate Publishing, Davis.

FIG. 12.9 Causes of difficult or painful prehension and mastication.

FIG. 12.10 Causes of
oropharyngeal dysphagia
and regurgitation.

CAUSES OF OROPHARYNGEAL DYSPHAGIA AND REGURGITATION
Glossal disorders
Glossal neoplasia Neuropathies of cranial nerves VII, IX, XII Hydrocephalus, brain stem lesions
Pharyngeal disorders
Pharyngitis Neoplasia; nasopharyngeal polyps Foreign bodies Retropharyngeal lymphadenopathy Rabies Cricopharyngeal achalasia (rare)
Palate disorders
Congenital defects
Oesophageal disorders
Oesophagitis (persistent vomiting, gastro-oesophageal reflux, idiopathic papillomatous) Foreign bodies Hiatal disorders (herniation, gastro-oesophageal intussusception) Obstruction (stricture, neoplasia, vascular ring anomalies, perioesophageal masses) Megaoesophagus (dysautonomia, lead poisoning, myasthenia gravis, idiopathic) Motility abnormalities

Dysphagia and regurgitation

The term dysphagia refers to eating difficulty. Dysphagia should be differentiated from inappetence, a distinction that may escape the client. Dysphagia may result from disorders of the jaw, oral cavity, tongue, pharynx or oesophagus. Cats with disorders of the oral cavity, tongue or jaws have difficulty lapping liquids, grasping and chewing food. Inability to open the mouth is occasionally seen and is often a result of a retrobulbar abscess or, less commonly, abnormalities of the temporomandibular joints. The principal causes of prehension and mastication difficulty are listed in Fig. 12.9.

Animals with dysphagia due to pharyngeal or oesophageal disorders usually regurgitate. Regurgitation is the passive reflux of ingesta, usually from the oesophagus or pharynx. Unlike vomiting, it is not associated with signs of nausea or rhythmical abdominal contractions. Regurgitated food is usually undigested and may take on a tubular shape if originating in the oesophagus. It is rarely bile-stained. Regurgitation may occur immediately after eating or may be delayed for several hours. Patients affected by oropharyngeal dysphagia make exaggerated swallowing movements and usually food will drop from the mouth within seconds of prehension. In contrast, oesophageal dysphagia results in more delayed regurgitation and is usually not associated with exaggerated swallowing movements.

Regurgitation is an infrequent problem in the cat in comparison to the dog. It can occur as a result of any disease that obstructs the lumen of the oesophagus or damages the components of the swallowing reflex. Important causes of oropharyngeal dysphagia and regurgitation are listed in Fig. 12.10. Diagnostic procedures of value in the investigation of cats with these problems are listed in Fig. 12.11.

Halitosis

Halitosis is a relatively frequent complaint in dogs but is less frequent in cats. Common causes of halitosis are listed in Fig. 12.12. The most common of these include dental disease, high protein diets and inflammatory or necrotizing oral or pharyngeal lesions such as neoplasia or ulcerative stomatitis.

| DIAGNOSIS OF DYSPHAGIA AND REGURGITATION* ||
Procedure	Usefulness
Neurological examination	Cranial nerve disorders. CNS lesions, polyneuropathies
Oropharyngeal examination under general anaesthesia	Masses, foreign bodies
Serum chemistry profile	Uraemia
Blood lead	Lead toxicosis
Lymph node aspiration	Neoplasia
Survey radiographs	Dental & jaw disorders, megaoesophagus, perioesophageal masses, oesophageal or pharyngeal foreign bodies
Swallowing study	Megaoesophagus, motility disorders, stricture, oesophageal masses, vascular ring anomalies, hiatal disorders, perioesophageal masses
Ultrasound	Retropharyngeal disorders
Endoscopic examination of the nasopharynx	Masses, foreign bodies
Oesophagoscopy and biopsy	Oesophagitis, obstructive diseases
Exploratory surgery	Perioesophageal masses, hiatal disorders

* Modified with permission from Strombeck D.R., Guilford W.G. (1990) *Small Animal Gastroenterology.* 2nd edn. Stonegate Publishing, Davis.

FIG. 12.11 Procedures for the diagnosis of dysphagia and regurgitation.

Highly proteinaceous diets result in halitosis via excretion into the breath of odiferous products of protein fermentation such as ammonia, hydrogen sulphide, indoles and skatoles.

Most cases of halitosis can be diagnosed by history and a thorough physical examination of the oral cavity and pharynx. Occasionally, radiographs of the teeth, nasal cavity, pharynx or oesophagus are required. Examination of the pharynx with a dental mirror or endoscope and the nasal cavity with a rhinoscope is sometimes helpful. Management of halitosis depends on the primary cause but can include dietary manipulation and dental prophylaxis.

Drooling and xerostomia

Drooling can result because of excessive production of saliva (ptyalism) or because of failure to swallow saliva produced in normal quantities (pseudoptyalism). Prominent causes of drooling are listed in Fig. 12.13.

The diagnostic evaluation of drooling relies heavily on the history and physical examination (great care should be taken if rabies is suspected). Careful observation of the patient often differentiates drooling due to nausea or swallowing difficulty from the other causes of hypersalivation. Animals hypersalivating due to nausea will usually demonstrate other signs such as depression, lip-licking and retching. Animals drooling due to swallowing disorders will often show evidence of inability to swallow food.

Consequences of persistent drooling include cheilitis and acne. The treatment of hypersalivation is varied because of the wide disparity of causes.

Xerostomia, or dryness of the mouth, is uncommon. It is most often associated with feline dysautonomia.

Borborygmus and flatulence

Borborygmus is a rumbling noise caused by the propulsion of gas through the gastrointestinal tract. Gas is produced by aerophagia or bacterial degradation of unabsorbed nutrients. Excessive gas usually results from dietary indiscretions, but on occasion can herald more serious gastrointestinal disease such as malassimilation. Diets containing legumes are associated with gaseousness as they contain large quantities of indigestible

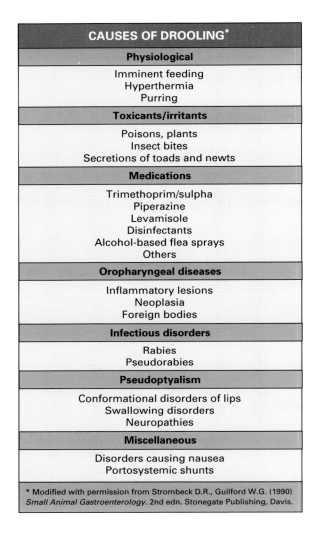

CAUSES OF HALITOSIS*
Dietary associated
Food remnants Highly proteinaceous diets Coprophagia
Diseases of the lips
Cheilitis
Oral cavity diseases
Inflammatory or necrotising oral lesions Foreign bodies
Pharyngeal diseases
Inflammatory or necrotising pharyngeal lesions Pharyngeal foreign bodies Tonsillar crypt foreign bodies
Nasal cavity and sinus disease
Inflammatory diseases Necrotising diseases
Dental disease
Periodontitis Gingivitis Tooth root abscesses Tartar
Oesophageal diseases
Megaoesophagus
Malassimilation
Systemic diseases
Uraemia
* Modified with permission from Strombeck D.R., Guilford W.G. (1990) *Small Animal Gastroenterology*. 2nd edn. Stonegate Publishing, Davis.

FIG. 12.12   Causes of halitosis.

CAUSES OF DROOLING*
Physiological
Imminent feeding Hyperthermia Purring
Toxicants/irritants
Poisons, plants Insect bites Secretions of toads and newts
Medications
Trimethoprim/sulpha Piperazine Levamisole Disinfectants Alcohol-based flea sprays Others
Oropharyngeal diseases
Inflammatory lesions Neoplasia Foreign bodies
Infectious disorders
Rabies Pseudorabies
Pseudoptyalism
Conformational disorders of lips Swallowing disorders Neuropathies
Miscellaneous
Disorders causing nausea Portosystemic shunts
* Modified with permission from Strombeck D.R., Guilford W.G. (1990) *Small Animal Gastroenterology*. 2nd edn. Stonegate Publishing, Davis.

FIG. 12.13   Causes of drooling: ptyalism and pseudo-ptyalism.

oligosaccharides. The management of these problems begins with a change to a highly digestible, low fibre diet with a moderate protein content. If dietary manipulation is not successful, consider investigation of the patient as described for the evaluation of small bowel diarrhoea.

Faecal incontinence

Faecal incontinence is the inability to retain faeces until defecation is appropriate. Clients sometimes fail to differentiate between the complaints of 'faecal incontinence' and 'diarrhoea'. The clinician should be careful to differentiate the two conditions, as they have some different causes and their work-ups and therapy are widely divergent.

Faecal incontinence can be due to large bowel disorders such as colitis that interfere with the reservoir capability of the rectum. It can also be due to failure of sphincteric mechanisms, usually through neurological dysfunction. Treatment is dependent on the primary cause. Symptomatic therapy includes the feeding of low residue diets and the use of diphenoxylate (0.05–0.1 mg/kg tid, PO) to increase sphincter tone.

Tenesmus

Tenesmus refers to persistent or prolonged straining that is usually ineffectual and often painful. Owners often incorrectly equate tenesmus with 'constipation'. Tenesmus is common in diseases of the lower gastrointestinal, urinary or reproductive tracts. The relevant organ system can usually be identified from the history and by physical examination. Whether the tenesmus is associated with micturition or defecation can also aid differentiation. Obstructive disorders of the large bowel are more commonly associated with tenesmus before evacuation (e.g. constipation), whereas irritative disorders (colitis) are often associated with persistent tenesmus after evacuation. In addition to examination of the large bowel, anus and perineum, the clinician should carefully palpate the bladder and closely examine the vagina or penis for evidence of pain, discharges, masses or calculi.

The diagnostic procedures are similar to those described for the evaluation of large bowel diarrhoea. In cats the most common cause of tenesmus is constipation.

Constipation

Diagnostic approach

Constipation is infrequent or absent defecation. Intractable constipation is called obstipation and has a guarded prognosis because irreversible degenerative changes in the colon may result. Constipation is a common presenting complaint and can result from many different causes (Fig. 12.14). In the cat the most common causes of constipation are ingestion of hair, tail-pulling neuropathies, pelvic fractures and idiopathic megacolon. Diagnosis is usually made by abdominal or rectal palpation. Neurological examination or pelvic radiography may reveal a cause.

Symptomatic therapy

The first considerations in the treatment of constipation are correction of any fluid and electrolyte derangements and attention to the

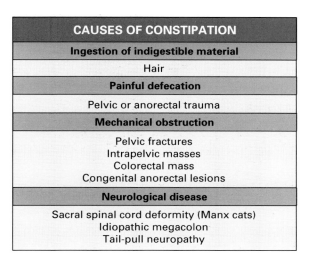

CAUSES OF CONSTIPATION
Ingestion of indigestible material
Hair
Painful defecation
Pelvic or anorectal trauma
Mechanical obstruction
Pelvic fractures Intrapelvic masses Colorectal mass Congenital anorectal lesions
Neurological disease
Sacral spinal cord deformity (Manx cats) Idiopathic megacolon Tail-pull neuropathy

FIG. 12.14   Causes of constipation.

primary cause if one can be identified. The initial approach to severely constipated patients should include anaesthesia, the administration of a warm-water lubricating enema, and manual fragmentation and removal of the hardened stool. Precautions include adequate preparation of the patient for anaesthesia (including rehydration) and the use of endotracheal intubation to prevent aspiration of regurgitated gastrointestinal content (which can be induced by the enema procedure). Phosphate enemas are contraindicated because of the likelihood of intoxication.

Animals with less severe constipation can be treated by regular warm-water lubricating enemas in association with softening agents such as dioctyl sodium sulphosuccinate (50 mg per cat q12–24h PO).

Prevention of subsequent constipation is best achieved by regular brushing of the cat's coat, use of bulk-forming laxatives such as psyllium fibre (1 tsp mixed with each meal) or bran (1–2 tblsp per 400 gm canned food), or the use of lubricant laxatives such as white petrolatum. Lactulose syrup (1–5 ml bid, PO) may be useful in some cats. Mineral oil should be avoided.

Abdominal pain

Clinical signs of abdominal pain include a hunched stance and stilted gait. Rapid evaluation

FIG. 12.15 Diagnostic procedures for the evaluation of abdominal pain.

EVALUATION OF ABDOMINAL PAIN*	
Procedure	**Usefulness**
Complete blood count	Sepsis, toxaemia, blood loss
Serum chemistry profile	Uraemia, liver disease, hyperlipidaemia
Blood gas	Acid-base status
Urinalysis	Kidney and liver disease
Faecal flotation	Parasitism
Survey radiographs	Masses, perforation, organomegaly, urinary calculi, foreign bodies, obstructions, peritonitis
Ultrasound	Masses, fluid, biliary and urinary calculi, kidney and liver disease, uterine disease, obstructions, torsions
Paracentesis	Fluid analysis
Diagnostic peritoneal lavage	Fluid analysis
Excretory urography	Renal and ureteral diseases
Contrast radiography	Obstruction, GI neoplasia
Gastrointestinal endoscopy	Gastric ulcers, foreign bodies, severe gastritis, inflammatory bowel disease, colitis, neoplasia
Exploratory celiotomy	Chronic pancreatitis, miscellaneous diagnosis and therapy

* Modified with permission from Strombeck D.R., Guilford W.G. (1990) *Small Animal Gastroenterology.* 2nd edn. Stonegate Publishing, Davis.

of the seriousness of the patient's condition is important. Diagnosis is usually made by localising the pain by palpation, identifying other signs (such as ascites or melaena) that incriminate a particular organ system, and the application of diagnostic tests (Fig. 12.15). Cranial abdominal pain is usually due to pancreatic or liver disease. Generalised abdominal pain is suggestive of peritonitis or severe enteritis. Abdominal pain developing several days after trauma raises the possibility of perforation of bowel, rupture of biliary or urinary tract, or necrosis of pieces of liver or spleen. Spasmodic pain is commonly due to contractions of a hollow viscus. Post-prandial pain can occur with gastrointestinal tract, pancreatic and biliary disorders.

Effective treatment of abdominal pain requires a diagnosis because many diseases associated with abdominal pain are life-threatening. Analgesic support during the painful episodes can be provided by meperidine at a dose of 4–5 mg/kg q4h SC or buprenorphine at a dose of 0.01 mg/kg q8–12h SC.

CLINICAL SYNOPSES OF COMMON GASTROENTERIC DISEASES

The following section presents brief reviews of the more prevalent primary gastrointestinal diseases of the cat.

Periodontal disease

Inflammation of the tissues surrounding the teeth is a very common complaint in cats. The most common cause is extension of gingivitis into the periodontal tissues. Treatment can include cleansing of the tooth crown and exposed root, gingivectomy to remove enlarged periodontal pockets, and extraction of loose teeth or teeth affected by external root resorption.

Gingivitis/stomatitis

Inflammation of the gums and oral mucosa can occur through a variety of systemic and local causes (Fig. 12.16). The most common cause of gingivitis is dental plaque or calculus. Herpes and calici viruses can cause ulcerative stomatitis. Cats affected by these viruses show sneezing, mucopurulent ocular and nasal discharge, depression and painful ulcers on the tongue and hard palate that prevent normal grooming. Chronic gingivitis in the absence of calculus is often associated with FIV infection. Successful treatment of gingivitis–stomatitis requires attention to the primary cause if identifiable. Dental scaling and 0.1% chlorhexidine mouth swabs are often necessary. Antibiotics such as amoxicillin (10–20 mg/kg bid, PO) and metronidazole (10–20 mg/kg bid, PO) may provide

CAUSES OF GINGIVITIS/STOMATITIS
Dental plaque/calculus
Physicochemical
Foreign bodies (plant material, fibreglass, bone fragments) Impacted food or hair Trauma; electrical burns Caustic or irritant chemicals; heavy metals
Micro-organisms
Bacteria? (*Bacteroides*) Viruses (calici, FIV, FeLV, herpes) Fungal agents (*Candida*)
Metabolic diseases
Diabetes mellitus Uraemia
Malnutrition
Protein-calorie malnutrition Hypervitaminosis A Niacin
Immune-mediated
Lymphocytic-plasmacytic stomatitis Pemphigoid diseases Drug reactions
Immunodeficiency
Neoplasia
Idiopathic

FIG. 12.16   Causes of gingivitis/stomatitis.

transitory benefit. Accumulation of calculus can be minimized by dry diets and use of a tooth brush.

Chronic lymphocytic–plasmacytic stomatitis is a serious disease of unknown cause. It has a variety of different names including chronic feline gingivitis–stomatitis and plasma cell gingivitis–pharyngitis. Cats of any age and breed can be affected but young pedigree cats may be predisposed. Signs include anorexia, dysphagia, drooling and halitosis. Intermittent exacerbations and relapses are common. Examination of the oral cavity shows proliferative or ulcerative stomatitis that can occur in a variety of localities including the gingiva, fauces, oropharynx and tongue. The mucosa about the premolars and molars is usually more severely afflicted than that about the incisor and canine teeth. Biopsies show heavy infiltration of plasma cells and lymphocytes. Lymphocytic–plasmacytic stomatitis requires aggressive therapy, which can

include teeth cleaning, debridement of necrotic tissue and extraction of any adjacent teeth. Extraction of all the premolar and molar teeth may be necessary and often results in remission of even lesions distant to the teeth. Administration of metronidazole (10–20 mg/kg bid PO) helps, at least on a temporary basis. A combination of metronidazole, aurothioglucose (1 mg/kg IM weekly until remission and then monthly for maintenance) and methylprednisolone acetate (20 mg SC every 3 weeks for 3 months) has given the author the best results in severe intractable cases. Care is needed with aurothioglucose as this gold salt is not licensed for use in cats and there is little information on efficacy and side effects in cats. In any case, no more than 12 consecutive weekly injections should be given. The first two injections should be test doses of 1 mg and then 2 mg. A CBC (including platelet count) should be checked for cytopenias every two weeks during induction and every month during remission. An occasional urinalysis should be performed to check for proteinuria. The prognosis for chronic lymphocytic–plasmacytic stomatitis is guarded.

Feline eosinophilic granuloma complex

The oral form of this disease complex usually commences as a shallow erosion on the upper lip, usually opposite the lower canine; it is often called 'rodent ulcer'. Lesions can also occur in the mouth, on the hard and soft palate and on the tongue. An important differential diagnosis is squamous cell carcinoma. Differentiation is made by cytology of a scraping from the lesion or by obtaining a biopsy. Biopsies of the affected area are infiltrated with eosinophils and mast cells. Treatment is either oral prednisone (1 mg/kg bid until remission, followed by decreasing dose over a 2–4 week period), intralesional triamcinolone (0.1–0.2 mg/kg), methylprednisolone acetate (20 mg SC) or surgical excision.

Oesophageal disorders

Signs of oesophageal disease include dysphagia, regurgitation and ptyalism. In the author's experience, the most frequent causes of oesophageal disease in the cat are foreign bodies; oesophagitis or strictures secondary to gastro–oesophageal reflux; and megaoesophagus secondary to dysautonomia or lead poisoning. Other causes of oesophageal disease are listed in Fig. 12.10. The most frequent foreign bodies are string, needles, fish hooks and bones. Diagnosis is usually made by radiography or endoscopy. Referral for endoscopic removal of the object is indicated.

Oesophagitis is uncommon in the cat because of its fastidious eating habits. Gastro-oesophageal reflux due to chronic vomiting, anaesthesia or hiatal disorders is the most common cause. The clinical signs are those of oesophageal disease but painful swallowing may be obvious. Diagnosis is usually made by history, clinical signs, endoscopy and occasionally barium swallows. Treatment can include metoclopramide (0.2–0.4 mg/kg tid PO), cimetidine (5 mg/kg bid PO) and sucralphate (30 mg/kg tid PO mixed with water and given as a slurry, preceding cimetidine by minimum of an hour). Hiatal disorders may require surgical correction. Oesophagitis can lead to oesophageal stricture. This is best treated by repeated balloon dilation.

Oesophageal motility abnormalities are uncommon. They may progress to oesophageal dilatation (megaoesophagus). Other clinical signs of dysautonomia may be apparent. The owners should be questioned about access of the cat to lead, that can result in megaoesophagus. Idiopathic megaoesophagus is particularly common in Siamese cats and is often associated with gastric emptying dysfunction. It may also result from oesophagitis. Diagnosis is reached by history, physical examination, radiography and fluoroscopy. Treatment is usually symptomatic and includes experimenting with diets of different consistency, use of elevated feeding bowls, or forced feeding via a gastrostomy tube.

Perioesophageal obstruction is seen occasionally in cats. Vascular anomalies are rare, the most common being persistent right aortic arch. Obstruction by mediastinal lymphoid tissue can also occur, usually as a result of mediastinal lymphosarcoma, thymoma or mediastinal lymphadenitis due to infections such as cryptococcosus. Diagnosis of perioesophageal obstruction is usually made by survey or contrast radiography.

Acute gastritis

Acute gastritis is common in cats. The history may reveal recent exposure to other cats raising the likelihood of viral infections. Recent ingestion of foreign material, spoiled food or carrion may also be reported. Damage to the mucosa results in episodic discomfort and vomiting. Occasionally lethargy, depression, haematemesis, fever, dehydration, polydipsia and anterior abdominal pain may be present. Diagnosis is made on the basis of history and physical examination. The clinical signs are self-limiting and treatment is supportive.

Chronic gastritis

Chronic gastritis is characterised by chronic persistent (occasionally sporadic) vomiting. Affected cats are usually otherwise bright and alert. Vomitus may contain bile, partly digested food, small amounts of blood or only clear liquid. There is no specific time relationship to eating. Specific types of chronic gastritis observed in cats include lymphocytic–plasmacytic gastritis (most common), eosinophilic gastritis and fibrosing gastritis. The latter disorder is probably an end-stage of the other forms of chronic gastritis and is also seen in association with *Ollulanus tricuspis*. The cause of chronic gastritis is usually not determined. Diagnosis is made on the basis of clinical signs, endoscopy and biopsy (via endoscopy). Contrast radiography is of little value. The gross appearance of the mucosa may be normal but histology reveals inflammatory cell infiltration in the lamina propria.

Treatment should be based on feeding a bland hypoallergenic diet because of the possibility of associated or causal dietary sensitivity. Eliminate any other potential causative factors such as drugs or toxic household plants. *Ollulanus tricuspis* can be treated with fenbendazole (50 mg/kg daily for 3 days) and perhaps pyrantel (20 mg/kg). Cats with a confirmed diagnosis of lymphocytic–plasmacytic or eosinophilic gastritis usually also require immunosuppressive therapy as described for inflammatory bowel disease (see below).

Acute gastroenteritis/enteritis/ enterocolitis

Acute gastrointestinal upsets are very common. They may affect just the stomach (gastritis), the stomach and small intestine (gastroenteritis) or the small and large intestine (enterocolitis). The clinical signs include a sudden onset of small bowel or a mixed small bowel/large bowel diarrhoea that is usually watery but sometimes bloody (dysentery). There is usually associated vomiting. Some animals show depression, fever, abdominal pain and de-hydration. Causes of acute diarrhoea are listed in Fig. 12.6. The clinical signs of these different causes of gastroenteritis are similar and diagnosis is most often based on history (e.g. likelihood of exposure to a toxin; change of diet; contact with other animals etc.). Panleukopenia stands out from the other causes because it usually affects young unvaccinated cats and because of the severity of the depression, deyhdration, diarrhoea (volum-inous and bloody) and leukopenia. Occasionally, FeLV or *Salmonella* spp infections will produce a similar picture to panleukopenia. Other viruses such as rotavirus and enteric coronavirus may be responsible for outbreaks of acute diarrhoea. A syndrome of transient third eyelid prolapse in association with self-limiting diarrhoea, probably of viral origin, has also been described. *Salmonella, Campylobacter* and Clostridial infections can pro-duce acute diarrhoea in cats as can *Yersinia pseudotuberculosis, Bacillus piliformis* and perhaps *Yersinia enterocolitica* and *E. coli*. These infec-tions often result in signs of enterocolitis rather than gastroenteritis. *Yersinia pseudotuberculosis* infections can be severe, resulting in pyogranulo-matous infiltration and enlargement of mesenteric nodes, liver and spleen. *Giardia* can produce acute to subacute or chronic diarrhoea (see below). The coccidia, *Cystisospora felis* and *Cystisospora rivolta*, are usually non-pathogenic but in some young cats appear to cause subacute large bowel diarr-hoea. Helminth parasites rarely cause significant diarrhoea in cats but two uncommon exceptions are *Strongyloides stercoralis* and *Strongyloides tumefaciens*.

Most causes of acute gastrointestinal upsets are self-limiting and cats will respond to supportive care regardless of the underlying cause. Because of this, few diagnostic procedures other than a faecal flotation and fresh smear for parasites such as Coccidia and Giardia are usually performed. A white blood cell count assists the diagnosis of panleukopenia. Serum electrolyte levels will aid the symptomatic treatment of the animal by assisting the choice of fluid therapy (particularly the amount of potassium to be added to the fluids). Blood urea nitrogen level (by dipstick) and urine specific gravity are sometimes determined to rule out acute renal failure as a cause of the diarrhoea. If history is supportive of an infectious cause and particularly if clinical evidence of enterocolitis is apparent, faecal cultures are warranted.

Symptomatic treatment of acute diarrhoea is discussed above. Panleukopenia requires broad spectrum antibiotic therapy in association with aggressive fluid and electrolyte therapy. Admini-stration of plasma may be helpful. Diarrhoea due to *Campylobacter* rapidly responds to erythromycin (10 mg/kg tid PO). Most other bacterial diarrhoeas will resolve with symptomatic therapy with or with-out fluoroquinolones, ampicillin or trimethoprim-sulpha. Unfortunately, *Yersinia pseudotuberculosis* and *Bacillus piliformis* infections are often fatal. Diarrhoea in association with Coccidian parasites is usually self-limiting if nutrition and hygiene are attended to but resolution appears to be hastened by the use of trimethoprim-sulphonamide prepara-tions (15–30 mg/kg q12–24h PO for 7 days). Most gastrointestinal helminths can be eliminated safely with pyrantel pamoate (10–20 mg/kg PO). Strongy-loides is treated with fenbendazole (50 mg/kg sid PO for 5 days).

Giardiasis

Giardia is a small bowel protozoan that can produce acute, chronic or episodic diarrhoea. The diarrhoea is usually suggestive of small bowel dysfunction, although excess mucus and, less com-monly, signs of mild colitis can be seen. Vomiting is uncommon. Diagnosis is usually made by detec-tion of cysts in faeces using zinc sulphate flotation. Motile trophozoites may also be observed in fresh faecal/saline smears. More than one faecal exam-ination may be necessary to detect the parasite. Treatment with metronidazole (20–25 mg/kg bid

PO) for 5–7 days is usually effective as is furazolidone (4 mg/kg bid PO) for 5 days.

Inflammatory bowel diseases

The idiopathic inflammatory bowel diseases (IBD) are a group of disorders characterised by persistent clinical signs of gastrointestinal disease associated with histological evidence of inflammation of undetermined cause in the lamina propria of the small or large intestine. IBDs are frequent causes of chronic vomiting and diarrhoea in cats. They are usually classified according to the type of inflammation present and the area of the gastrointestinal tract in which the inflammation predominates. The most frequent subclassifications recognised in cats are lymphocytic–plasmacytic enteritis and eosinophilic gastroenteritis. Other subclassifications of IBD seen less commonly in cats include lymphocytic–plasmacytic colitis, eosinophilic colitis and suppurative colitis. Rare cases of histiocytic and granulomatous IBD have been reported. The cause of IBD is unknown but appears to involve hypersensitivity to antigens (food, bacterial, mucus, epithelial) derived from the bowel lumen or mucosa.

Diagnosis of IBD is made by eliminating known causes of intestinal inflammation and then acquiring a biopsy of the mucosa. With the exception of suppurative colitis, the treatment of the different types of IBD is similar. A very important part of treatment is the use of a controlled diet such as chicken diced into baby rice cereal. The protein source is best chosen in relation to the animal's previous diet. Because acquired allergies may be an important reason for perpetuation of this disorder, it is best to avoid (if possible) any proteins the cat has been eating for the last 4–6 months. If colitis is present, the addition of fibre (psyllium; 1 tsp per meal) to the diet is useful.

In addition to the controlled diet, immunosuppressive therapy is required. For small intestinal disorders, use oral prednisone beginning at 2 mg/kg bid for 2 weeks followed by a decremental dose over 3 months. Intractable cats may require parenteral methylprednisolone injections (20 mg SC q 3–6 weeks). Refractory IBD may require metronidazole (15 mg/kg bid PO) or higher doses of prednisone (3 mg/kg PO bid) and the addition of azathioprine (0.3 mg/kg PO qod). The latter drugs are often required when eosinophilic infiltrates involve other abdominal organs in addition to the bowel (hypereosinophilic syndrome). Regular CBC (including platelet counts) should be performed during azathioprine therapy because of the risk of bone marrow suppression. Sulphasalazine, administered twice daily at 20–25 mg/kg for 1–2 weeks and then once daily for 2–5 weeks, can be safely and effectively used for lymphocytic–plasmacytic colitis.

Suppurative colitis in cats may have a different pathogenesis to the other types of IBD. Mild forms of suppurative colitis are often associated with fur-impacted faeces and it is possible that abrasion of the mucosa results in the suppurative response in some cats. Treatment includes lubricating laxatives such as white petrolatum, regular brushing of the coat and, if necessary, antibiotics such as ampicillin.

Gastrointestinal neoplasia

The majority of feline intestinal neoplasms are malignant. Lymphosarcoma and adenocarcinoma are the most common but visceral mast cell neoplasia is also observed with some frequency. The duodenum is more likely to be invaded by carcinomas from other organs such as the pancreas and liver than to develop primary neoplasia.

Prominent clinical signs of small intestinal neoplasia are chronic diarrhoea, vomiting, inappetence and weight loss. Large bowel neoplasia results in tenesmus and haematochezia. Signs due to intestinal neoplasia progressively worsen. Diagnosis is usually made by contrast radiography, ultrasound, or exploratory surgery and biopsy.

If the process is localised to one segment of the bowel, surgical resection is indicated. If metastasis has occurred, a systemic treatment such as chemotherapy must be selected. The prognosis for all non-resectable gastrointestinal cancers, including gastrointestinal lymphosarcoma, is guarded to poor.

Idiopathic megacolon

Idiopathic megacolon can affect cats of a variety of ages including kittens. The hallmarks of the disorder are a dilated colon with no evidence of physical or functional obstruction, and normal or near normal numbers of ganglion cells observed histologically in affected segments. Obstipation is the principal sign. Abdominal palpation and rectal examination are usually sufficient to identify an impacted colon and to rule out intestinal atresia and imperforate anus. Survey radiographs confirm megacolon and assess the pelvis. After evacuation, a barium or air enema will help establish if a narrowed rectal or colonic segment is present. If a narrowed segment is detected, proctoscopic evaluation with biopsy or surgical resection of the affected segment differentiates fibrous strictures, neoplastic proliferations and aganglionosis. Full-thickness (usually excisional) biopsy is required to detect aganglionosis. The treatment of choice for idiopathic megacolon is subtotal colectomy, which is very well tolerated by cats. Palliative medical therapies most often used are enemas, psyllium derivatives, and various other laxatives such as lactulose liquid (1–5 ml bid PO).

FURTHER READING

August, J.R. (ed.) (1991) *Consultations in Feline Internal Medicine.* W.B. Saunders Co., Philadelphia.

Sherding, R.G. (ed.) (1990) *The Cat. Diseases and Clinical Management.* Churchill Livingstone, New York.

Strombeck, D.R., Guilford, W.G. (1990) *Small Animal Gastroenterology*, 2nd edn. Stonegate Publishing, Davis.

13

Disorders of the Hepatobiliary System

SHARON A. CENTER

Clinical signs associated with mild or early hepatobiliary disease in the cat are usually vague. The underlying problem often remains ill defined until more serious organ impairment develops. It is unfortunate that liver disease in many cats is diagnosed only after jaundice is obvious and irreparable hepatic injury has developed. Cholestasis due to major bile duct occlusion is an exception because jaundice develops early and promotes definitive diagnosis at a time when aggressive surgical intervention can prevent permanent tissue injury. To achieve diagnosis of hepatobiliary disease at an early stage the clinician should aspire to use information provided by history, physical examination, clinicopathological tests, and abdominal radiography and ultrasonography. It is now possible to detect hepatic dysfunction before the development of jaundice by measurement of the serum bile acid concentrations following a 12-hour fast and 2 hours after ingestion of a meal. Early diagnosis of hepatobiliary disease before development of jaundice usually follows detection of increased liver enzyme activity over a course of several weeks or demonstration of increased serum bile acid concentrations that lead to ultrasonographic imaging of the liver or a liver biopsy. An algorithm presenting the diagnostic strategy for feline liver disease is shown in Fig. 13.1.

Liver disorders commonly encountered in cats can be grouped into general categories on the basis of histopathological findings (Fig. 13.2). The important physical and clinicopathological abnormalities and management of each of these disorders are detailed in the following discussion. The typical biochemical findings associated with each category are shown in Fig. 13.3.

EXTRAHEPATIC BILE DUCT OBSTRUCTION (EHBDO)

Clinical recognition may occur after a few days to a week of complete bile duct obstruction. Hyperbilirubinaemia develops within 36 hours and jaundice as early as 3 days. Urine urobilinogen values decrease to trace levels or are undetectable after 7 days. Acholic stools (pale grey faeces) can be noted as early as 4 days. Sudan III faecal stains will demonstrate the presence of steatorrhoea due to fat malabsorption as a result of an absence of bile salts in the alimentary canal. Non-painful gallbladder distention may be palpable as early as 12 days. Vitamin K_1-responsive bleeding tendencies can develop within 14 days. It is useful to realise that bleeding into the bowel may provide enough alimentary bilirubin to impart faecal colour and to produce urobilinogen.

Haematological abnormalities include development of anaemia that may be non-regenerative, as a result of chronic disease and malnutrition, or may be regenerative, reflecting major gastrointestinal blood loss usually associated with pyloric or duodenal ulcerations. A severe neutrophilic leukocytosis may also develop. Biochemical abnormalities (Fig. 13.3) include hyperbilirubinaemia that worsens with time (up to 50-fold normal bilirubin values) and remarkable increases in alkaline phosphatase (ALP), gamma glutamyl transferase (GGT), alanine aminotransferase (ALT, formerly SGPT) and aspartate aminotransferase (AST, formerly SGOT).[5,8] Serum bile acid concentrations may exceed 100-fold increases over normal values. Usually there is little difference between the fasting and postprandial serum bile acid concentrations.

On gross inspection, the EHBDO liver is enlarged and dark green/brown, and the common bile duct is dilated and tortuous proximal to the obstruction. Histologically, bile duct proliferation and luminal dilation is associated with a mixed cellular inflammatory infiltrate. Chronic EHBDO leads to periportal deposition of fibrous connective tissue which evolves into biliary cirrhosis. Recognition of a tensely dilated gallbladder and enlarged tortuous bile duct is accomplished easily using

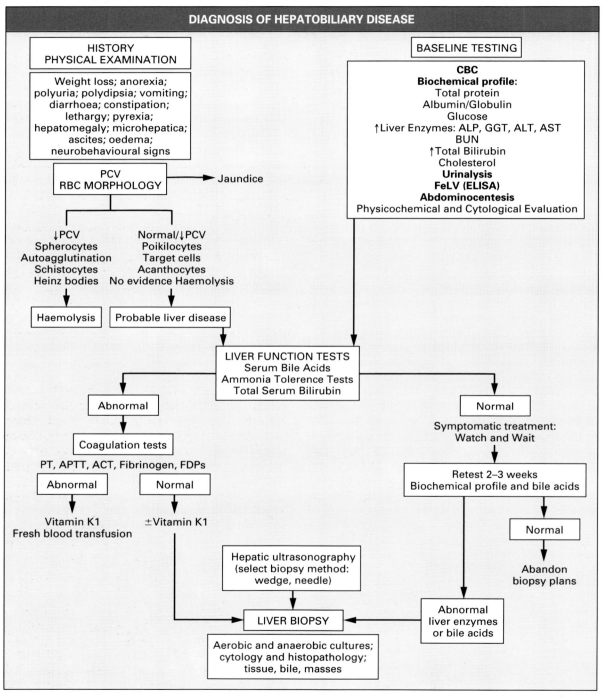

DIAGNOSIS OF HEPATOBILIARY DISEASE

HISTORY PHYSICAL EXAMINATION

Weight loss; anorexia; polyuria; polydipsia; vomiting; diarrhoea; constipation; lethargy; pyrexia; hepatomegaly; microhepatica; ascites; oedema; neurobehavioural signs

BASELINE TESTING

CBC
Biochemical profile:
Total protein
Albumin/Globulin
Glucose
↑Liver Enzymes: ALP, GGT, ALT, AST
BUN
↑Total Bilirubin
Cholesterol
Urinalysis
FeLV (ELISA)
Abdominocentesis
Physicochemical and Cytological Evaluation

PCV RBC MORPHOLOGY → Jaundice

↓PCV
Spherocytes
Autoagglutination
Schistocytes
Heinz bodies

Normal/↓PCV
Poikilocytes
Target cells
Acanthocytes
No evidence Haemolysis

Haemolysis

Probable liver disease

LIVER FUNCTION TESTS
Serum Bile Acids
Ammonia Tolerence Tests
Total Serum Bilirubin

Abnormal

Normal

Symptomatic treatment:
Watch and Wait

Coagulation tests

PT, APTT, ACT, Fibrinogen, FDPs

Abnormal

Normal

Retest 2–3 weeks
Biochemical profile and bile acids

Vitamin K1
Fresh blood transfusion

±Vitamin K1

Normal

Hepatic ultrasonography
(select biopsy method:
wedge, needle)

Abandon
biopsy plans

LIVER BIOPSY

Abnormal
liver enzymes
or bile acids

Aerobic and anaerobic cultures;
cytology and histopathology;
tissue, bile, masses

Continued

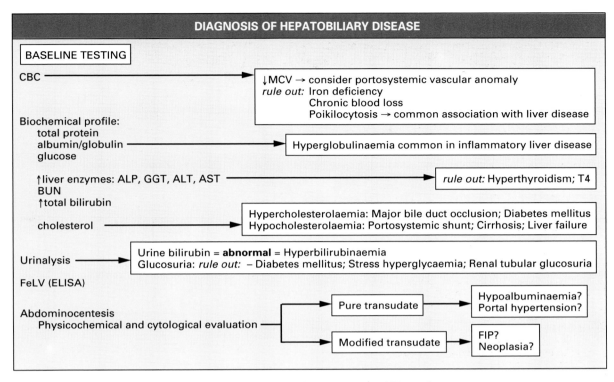

FIG. 13.1   Diagnostic algorithm for hepatobiliary disease.

ultrasonography. If these characteristics are obvious, the clinician should avoid percutaneous liver biopsy because of the potential for bile leakage from punctures in engorged intrahepatic bile ducts or inadvertent laceration of large bile ducts or gallbladder. Diagnosis of EHBDO should lead to laparotomy for surgical exploration of the biliary structures as soon as the cat's clinical status is stabilised.

A cholecystoduodenostomy or cholecystojejunostomy can be performed for biliary diversion if the common bile duct is occluded and inoperable. Although this can lead to chronic cholangitis associated with retrograde infection of the biliary tree with enteric organisms, good quality long-term survival is possible if antibiotics are used chronically to combat infection. If a resectable gallbladder lesion is identified, cholecystectomy can be performed. If a discrete, resectable bile duct stricture, mass or cholelith are detected, choledochotomy may be possible. Surgical resection of an obstructing neoplasm (most commonly

adenocarcinoma involving the common bile duct, pancreas or duodenum) is less rewarding because of the likelihood of metastasis or local recurrence.

Cholelithiasis (gall stones) is an uncommon cause of EHBDO and is difficult to diagnose with radiography because of the radiolucent composition of most choleliths. The most common type of cholelith in the cat is the pigment stone, a friable dark green composite. Ultrasonography detects their presence even before the biliary tree becomes obstructed. Predisposing factors in cholelith formation include the presence of impaired bile flow, epithelial biliary lesions, or infection. Surgical removal of choleliths provides at least temporary improvement but recurrence is possible if predisposing conditions remain unrecognised and uncorrected. If choleliths are surgically removed, the stone, bile, and liver tissue should be cultured and the liver should be biopsied. Post-operative treatments with an appropriate antibiotic and a hydrocholeretic are advised.

Gastrointestinal ulceration is common in cats

HEPATOBILIARY DISORDERS RECOGNISED IN THE CAT			
Extrahepatic bile duct obstruction	**Hepatic necrosis**		

Common bile duct stricture
Pancreatic inflammation/fibrosis
Duodenal inflammation
Neoplasia (bile duct adenocarcinoma)
Cholangitis
Common bile duct obstruction
Cholelithiasis
Sludged bile
Parasitic (liver flukes)
	Toxins
	Bacterial
	Fungal
	Drugs
	  (acetaminophen)
	Organophosphates
	Heavy metals
		Hypoxia
		Anaemia
		Shock
		Thromboembolism
		Congestive heart
		  failure
			Infectious disease
			Feline infectious
			  peritonitis
			Calicivirus
			Toxoplasmosis
			Septicaemia
			  (bacterial, fungal)
			Endotoxaemia

Cholangitis-cholangiohepatitis syndrome	**Hepatic lipidosis**		

Ascending inflammation up biliary tree
  Pancreatitis
  Duodenal inflammation
  Spontaneous reflux pancreatic enzymes, ingesta,
    micro-organisms
Cholelithiasis
Sludged bile (cause or effect?)
Parasitic (liver flukes)
Immune mediated
Copper accumulation (?)
	Idiopathic lipidosis
	Obesity
	Prolonged anorexia
		Secondary lipidosis
		Anaemia
		Chronic renal disease
		Gastrointestinal disease
		Neoplasia (hepatic or non-hepatic)
		Hyperthyroidism
		Diabetes mellitus
		Cardiomyopathy
		Energy restriction (diet foods)
		Hepatic diseases
		Protein malnutrition
		Chronic systemic inflammation/
		  infection	

Biliary cirrhosis	**Hepatic neoplasia**		
Chronic extrahepatic bile duct obstruction Chronic cholangitis-cholangiohepatitis syndrome	**Primary (rare)** Bile duct carcinoma/adenocarcinoma Hepatocellular carcinoma Haemangiosarcoma **Secondary/multisystemic** Lymphosarcoma Myeloproliferative disease Systemic mast cell neoplasia		
Portosystemic vascular anastomosis			
Congenital Left gastric vein (most common) Porto-azygous Portal-vena cava (single or multiple) Patent ductus venosus **Secondary (rare)**			

FIG. 13.2 Hepatobiliary disorders recognised in the cat.

with EHBDO. Treatment with cytoprotective agents, such as sucralphate (0.25 g PO tid), and H$_2$ blockers such as famotidine (1–2 mg PO sid, 1–2 mg IV bid) are recommended. The H$_2$ blockers which inhibit the cytochrome p450 oxidases (cimetidine and to a lesser extent ranitidine) should be avoided due to their potential to create drug interactions or intolerance.

INSPISSATED BILE

Sludged biliary secretions forming 'casts' with a rubbery consistency in intra- and extrahepatic bile ducts may develop in cats with cholestasis. It is thought that sluggish bile flow associated with cholestasis and resorption of water by the gall-bladder is aggravated by systemic dehydration and results in the formation of the tenacious bile concretions. This so-called 'inspissated bile' syndrome may also develop as a seemingly isolated event.[22,26] Surgical intervention is usually required for treatment. At surgery, cholecystotomy allows removal of the inspissated material. The gall-bladder and liver should be biopsied for cytological and histopathological examination and samples of bile and tissue should be cultured for aerobic and anaerobic bacteria. These procedures are carried out in an attempt to recognise an underlying cause. The major bile ducts should be flushed with sterile saline via a flexible catheter to eliminate inspissated bile. Care must be taken to avoid peritoneal contamination with bile. Fluid, electrolyte and antibiotic therapy (with or without the use of a hydrocholeretic agent such as dehydrocholic acid) and treatment of any underlying condition are important in post-surgical management.

CHOLANGITIS-CHOLANGIOHEPATITIS SYNDROME

In the absence of clinical evidence of hepatobiliary disease, histological evidence of mild cholangitis seems common in the cat. Clinically significant cholangitis (inflammation of the bile ducts) and cholangiohepatitis (inflammation of the bile ducts and surrounding hepatic tissue) usually present as an intrahepatic cholestasis syndrome: the cholangitis-cholangiohepatitis syndrome (CCHS). Clinical signs of CCHS are vague and recurrent in the early stages, when mild to moderate increases in the serum ALP, GGT, ALT and AST activities develop. Later, the cat becomes hyperbilirubinaemic and overtly jaundiced. In many cases jaundice develops before liver disease is considered seriously as a component of the cat's illness.

The CCHS usually develops in cats of more than 4 years of age. In one report of 21 cats with lymphocytic cholangitis, long-haired cats were over represented and 67% of the cats were less than 4 years of age.[19] However, review of CCHS cases in the author's hospital has not supported a breed or age predilection. Some cats with CCHS have inflammatory bowel disease that precedes development of the liver disease and this is similar to the situation in some humans where inflammatory bowel disease is associated with cholestatic liver injury.[24] Some cats develop CCHS subsequent to liver fluke infestation. Inflammation and fibrosis of the common bile duct and cholangitis may be associated with pancreatitis in cats and there seems to be a high frequency of interstitial pancreatitis and pancreatic fibrosis as an incidental finding in cats necropsied for a variety of reasons. This suggests that pancreatitis is a more common problem than is recognised clinically. Because the major pancreatic duct of the cat joins the common bile duct before it enters the duodenal wall, reflux of enzyme or bile rich fluids could initiate an inflammatory response concurrently in both systems. It is unknown whether spontaneous reflux of intestinal contents into the pancreatic duct occurs in the cat, though this phenomenon has been shown to occur experimentally in dogs during the postprandial interval. Such reflux could induce bile duct inflammation and fibrosis in the cat, considering that early major bile duct occlusion can cause histological changes in the biliary and periportal tissues similar to those of the CCHS syndrome.

Clinicopathological features of the CCHS include a mild non-regenerative anaemia and a neutrophilic leukocytosis with a left shift. Serum biochemical features include increased ALP, GGT and transaminase activities, hyperbilirubinaemia, hyperglobulinaemia and mild hypoalbuminaemia (Fig. 13.3). In anicteric cats, the fasting serum bile acid concentration may be normal or increased, but the 2-hour postprandial bile acid concentration is always increased when the syndrome is well developed.

Ultrasonographic examination may reveal a diffuse, multifocal, hyperechoic appearance to the liver. In some cases the biliary tree is prominent due to adjacent inflammation. Percutaneous needle biopsy can be used as successfully as a wedge biopsy taken at laparotomy for histological confirmation of the disease because of diffuse liver involvement. Grossly, the liver may appear swollen, pale in suppurative cholangiohepatitis, and soft or firm depending on the amount of inflammation, fluid retention and connective tissue proliferation. Surface contour may be smooth or irregular depending on the extent of regenerative hyperplasia and fibrosis. Thickened, dilated bile ducts with accentuation of the portal areas may be obvious on cut sections of liver.

Histologically, the CCHS can be categorised according to the predominant type of inflammatory cell in the portal triad and the degree of periductal hepatocyte involvement. The inflammatory cell component may be suppurative (neutrophils) or non-suppurative (lymphocytes, plasma cells), the latter form being most common.[15,22,26] Cytological imprints made from biopsy specimens may allow immediate recognition of the primary cell type involved (Fig. 13.4). If suppurative inflammation is recognised, liver tissue and bile should be cultured for aeroic and anaerobic

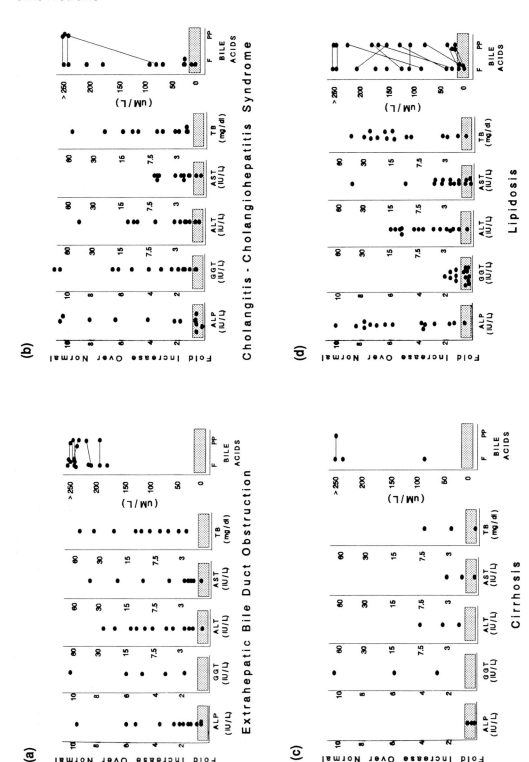

(a) Extrahepatic Bile Duct Obstruction

(b) Cholangitis - Cholangiohepatitis Syndrome

(c) Cirrhosis

(d) Lipidosis

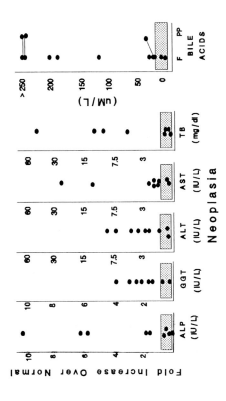

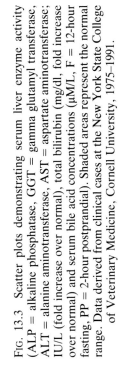

(f)

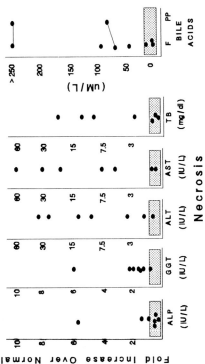

(e)

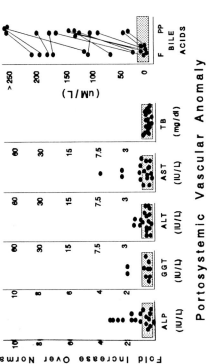

(g)

FIG. 13.3 Scatter plots demonstrating serum liver enzyme activity (ALP = alkaline phosphatase, GGT = gamma glutamyl transferase, ALT = alanine aminotransferase, AST = aspartate aminotransferase; IU/L (fold increase over normal), total bilirubin (mg/dl, fold increase over normal) and serum bile acid concentrations (μM/L, F = 12-hour fasting, PP = 2-hour postprandial). Shaded areas represent the normal range. Data derived from clinical cases at the New York State College of Veterinary Medicine, Cornell University, 1975–1991.

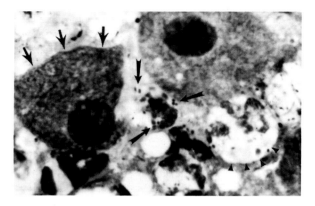

FIG. 13.4 Photomicrograph of impression smear made from a liver biopsy taken from a cat with suppurative cholangiohepatitis associated with cholelithiasis. A normal hepatocyte is indicated by the large arrows. Pleomorphic rod shaped bacterial organisms (medium sized black arrows) are identified both within neutrophils (black arrowheads) and extracellularly. *E. coli* was isolated from this specimen.

bacteria. Chronic CCHS usually involves a non-suppurative inflammatory process; it is possible that this develops subsequent to suppurative inflammation and is the result of immune-mediated self-perpetuating inflammation. It is probable that multiple pathogenic mechanisms are involved in the development of CCHS including cholelithiasis, pancreatitis, bacterial or parasitic infection, toxins and immune-mediated disorders.

Cats with the CCHS may present with clinical signs and laboratory features similar to those with EHBDO. Ultrasonographical examination can readily differentiate these disorders. If laparotomy is performed to explore the liver and collect biopsy specimens, the major bile ducts should be evaluated for patency, the gallbladder should be gently compressed to evaluate the potential for bile flow, and the biliary tree should be palpated carefully for mass lesions, choleliths or inspissated bile. The duodenum and pancreas should be inspected for evidence of inflammation or neoplasia. Bile and liver tissue should be collected for cytological and histological examination, and the specimens should be cultured for aerobic and anaerobic bacteria and antibiotic sensitivity testing. Antibiotics are indicated initially for all forms of CCHS: the suppurative form may require antibiotic treatment for 2 to 4 months or longer, and the non-suppurative form should be treated with an immunosuppressive regimen of corticosteroids. A dose of prednisolone of 2–4 mg/kg per day is prescribed initially and is reduced gradually over several weeks to a lower dose given on alternate days. It is speculated that chronic CCHS involves self-perpetuation of the injury by immune-mediated mechanisms. This can involve the release of antigens from injured liver and biliary tissues and stimulation of cytokine release which perpetuates the inflammation. Although the signs of CCHS may be controlled with glucocorticoids in many cats, cure should not be anticipated and intermittent therapy may be necessary as the disease activity waxes and wanes. Nevertheless, in one report, some cats with lymphocytic cholangitis had continued remission following glucocorticoid discontinuation.[19]

BILIARY CIRRHOSIS

Cirrhosis is an uncommon diagnosis in the cat and it is usually the sequel to chronic CCHS or EHBDO. In most cases, it is associated with hepatomegaly and a palpably firm liver texture; the development of ascites is rare. Biochemically, serum liver enzymes may be quiescent with the exception of GGT activity which may be increased markedly (Fig. 13.3). Fasting and 2-hour postprandial serum bile acids are increased and ammonia tolerance is abnormal.

Biliary cirrhosis is characterised by severe bridging portal fibrosis, bile duct proliferation and hyperplasia, and nodular regeneration. Non-suppurative inflammation is usually observed. Medical management is palliative and is tailored to the individual patient. It may include feeding a diet moderately restricted in protein; administration of an antibiotic that does not require hepatic biotransformation or elimination; provision of a doubled daily dose of water soluble vitamins; and intramuscular or subcutaneous administration of 5 mg of vitamin K_1 twice weekly. Glucocorticoids may be used if a prominent non-suppurative inflammatory infiltrate is identified. Care is warranted when glucocorticoids are administered because of the catabolic effects which may promote loss of body condition and development of encephalopathic signs.

HEPATIC NECROSIS

Acute hepatic necrosis results in markedly increased serum ALT and AST activities associated with smaller increases in the serum ALP and GGT activities (Fig. 13.3). Diffuse necrosis may cause hyperbilirubinaemia, hypoglycaemia, and co-agulation abnormalities that remain unresponsive to vitamin K_1. In some cases, diffuse necrosis leads to death prior to development of hyperbilirubinaemia.

Histological features are characterised by hepatocellular necrosis or degeneration that may develop in the absence of inflammation. Patterns described as zonal or focal may be labelled as toxin induced, but rarely is this proven.[26] The guardian position of the liver between the intestines and systemic circulation allows it to perform an important protective function. In health, the liver limits the systemic exposure to bacteria and toxins derived from the alimentary canal and transported via the portal circulation. The largest source of fixed macrophages, the reticuloendothelial Kupffer cells, are located in the liver. These cells provide essential macrophage activity which is important in the clearance of particulate material and organisms from the portal circulation. Because of its 'guardian' role, the liver may be preferentially injured by toxins or organisms of enteric origin. The metabolic functions of the liver (biotransformations, excretion of endogenous and exogenous substances) heighten its susceptibility to noxious and potentially necrotising insults. Acute gastroenteritis manifested clinically by vomiting and bloody diarrhoea may be associated with so-called toxic hepatopathy. Recognised causes of hepatic necrosis in cats include: feline infectious peritonitis; toxoplasmosis; calicivirus; *Bacillus piliformis*; endotoxaemia; septicaemia; toxicities from certain drugs (acetaminophen), chemicals, or plants; and hypoxaemia due to severe anaemia, circulatory failure, shock or thromboembolism.[17,23,26] Unfortunately, the initiating event or agent usually remains unidentified, necessitating symptomatic treatment.

Supportive care should be as complete as possible. Intravenous fluid therapy, with balanced polyionic fluids supplemented with glucose, water soluble vitamins and potassium, is essential. Parenteral antibiotics are recommended because of presumed injury to the hepatic 'guardian' function. Alimentation with foods that contain limited amounts of protein and ample carbohydrates should be accomplished through either a nasogastric or gastrostomy tube if the cat is uncooperative with oral feeding. If persistent vomiting is a problem, metoclopramide may be used as an antiemetic. Total parenteral nutrition is useful in severely debilitated patients. If it is suspected that toxic materials remain within the alimentary canal, a warm saline enema can be used to hasten their elimination. The use of super-activated charcoal (given by stomach tube or per rectum) or oral cholestyramine can also be beneficial in binding toxins.

HEPATIC LIPIDOSIS

Severe hepatic lipidosis is a common feline hepatobiliary disorder in North America. Affected cats are usually dehydrated, weak and jaundiced, and have been anorectic for at least a week.[9] Obesity followed by recent weight loss is common and many cats have a history of vomiting. Overt encephalopathic signs are uncommon. Physical examination usually reveals non-painful hepatomegaly. Severe hepatic lipidosis can be an idiopathic syndrome or develop secondary to another major organ system or hepatobiliary disorder (Fig. 13.5).[6]

Haematological features include a mild non-regenerative anaemia, poikilocytes (Fig. 13.6) and sometimes a mild neutrophilic leukocytosis. The serum enzyme activities demonstrate a unique pattern in lipidosis compared with other feline liver diseases (Fig. 13.3).[10] The serum ALP activity may be as high or higher than that associated with EHBDO while the GGT activity remains within the normal range or becomes only mildly increased. In all other feline liver diseases, the magnitude of the increase in GGT equals or exceeds that of ALP. The disproportionate increase in the magnitudes of the serum ALP and GGT activities may be used as a predictive indicator of lipidosis. This feature, coupled with ultrasonography revealing a diffusely hyperechoic liver,[25] increases the index of suspicion of lipidosis sufficiently to warrant liver aspirate or biopsy examination. Other

FIG. 13.5 Feline diseases associated with hepatic lipidosis. Retrospective study of cases at the New York State College of Veterinary Medicine, Cornell University, 1975–1986.

		DISEASES ASSOCIATED WITH HEPATIC LIPIDOSIS	
		Severity of cell vacuolation	
Cats	Primary disease	Severe	Mild to moderate
1	Anaemia	0	1
1	Portosystemic vascular anomaly	0	1
1	Hypereosinophilia	1	0
1	Gastrointestinal disease	1	0
1	Feline viral rhinotracheitis	1	0
2	Hyperthyroidism	1	1
2	Haemobartonellosis	1	1
3	Feline panleukopenia	1	2
3	Hernia (diaphragmatic)	3	0
4	Pancreatitis	3	1
5	Pneumonia	2	3
5	Chronic cystitis	2	3
5	Acute renal failure	2	3
6	Feline infectious peritonitis	3	3
6	Neurological disease	3	3
7	Chronic interstitial nephritis	1	6
8	Diabetes mellitus	1	7
15	Lymphosarcoma	8	7
15	Cardiomyopathy	7	8
17	Neoplasia (exclude LSA)	9	8
42	Idiopathic lipidosis	30	12
150		80	70

clinicopathological features of lipidosis include mild hyperglycaemia, hypokalaemia, marked hyperbilirubinaemia, and coagulation abnormalities.

Grossly, the liver appears enlarged with rounded margins and a yellow, greasy, friable texture with a prominent reticulated pattern. Definitive diagnosis requires examination of a liver aspirate or biopsy. Because there is diffuse liver involvement, needle procedures are successful. Tissue samples placed in formalin frequently float, due to their increased lipid composition. Cytological preparations stained with Wrights/Giemsa stains will demonstrate obvious hepatocellular cytosolic vacuolation (Fig. 13.7). Routine tissue processing for histopathology, that includes paraffin embedment of tissues for sectioning, results in loss of the vacuole lipid moieties. Frozen sections can be prepared for tissue staining with Oil red O or Sudan Black lipid stains to confirm the presence of fat within vacuoles. Two histological forms of hepatic vacuolation occur: macrovesicular and

microvesicular.[4,6,9,26] In some cats, macro- and microvesicular vacuolation coexist. It is speculated that small vacuoles represent a transition stage in lipid vacuole formation and that these coalesce to yield the macrovesicular appearance.[9]

Initial treatment should focus on establishing normal hydration, correcting electrolyte abnormalities, and providing sufficient nutritional support. Polyionic fluids that are judiciously supplemented with water soluble vitamins and with potassium chloride based on the serum or plasma electrolyte concentration and a commonly used sliding scale (Fig. 13.8) are administered intravenously. Parenteral (subcutaneous or intramuscular) vitamin K_1 is given at a dose of 5 mg sid or bid for 2 days and then once or twice weekly until full recovery. Vitamin K is given because of the dependency on derivation from gut microorganisms or ingested foods and because of the central role of the liver in rejuvenating vitamin K to its active form following activation of factors

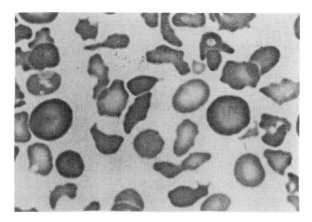

FIG. 13.6 Photomicrograph showing erythrocyte morphology typical of poikilocytosis in a cat. (Courtesy of Dr. T. French, Department of Pathology, New York State College of Veterinary Medicine, Cornell University).

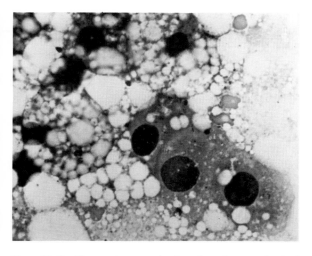

FIG. 13.7 Photomicrograph showing the cytological features of a hepatic aspirate taken from a cat with severe hepatic lipidosis showing diffuse severe cytoplasmic vacuolation of three hepatocytes. Three other hepatocytes are shown with only slight cytoplasmic vacuolation. Wrights-Giemsa stain.

POTASSIUM SUPPLEMENTATION FOR IV FLUIDS	
Serum potassium mEq/L	**Potassium chloride mEq added per 250 ml**
3.0–3.5	7
2.5–2.9	10
2.0–2.4	15
<2.0	20
Rate of KCl infusion should not exceed 0.5 mEq/kg/h	

FIG. 13.8   Potassium supplementation for IV fluids.

Nutritional support is initially provided by hand feeding, or by nasogastric intubation using a 3–5 French sized soft rubber feeding tube passed through the nose and positioned with the end just cranial to the gastric cardia. The tube is sutured and glued to the face and an Elizabethan collar is placed to prevent the cat from removing the tube. A liquefied diet can be given via oral and nasogastric tube routes.

When the critical condition of the cat is stabilised, a gastrostomy tube is inserted using either a percutaneous endoscopic placement (a method which has been well described elsewhere)[3,21] or via laparotomy. Mushroom-tipped catheters are preferable to balloon-tipped uretheral catheters for this purpose. A gastrostomy tube is the optimal mechanism of support for cats with hepatic lipidosis. These tubes seemingly are more comfortable to the patient than nasogastric tubes and can be easily managed in the home environment by most owners. Commercial feline maintenance diets can be mixed with water, passed through a food blender and processed with a fine gauge grinder or strained through cheese cloth to facilitate feeding through the gastrostomy tube, which should be flushed with a small quantity of warm water before and after feeding. Prior to feeding, the tube is aspirated to appraise the rate of gastric emptying. If food remains in the stomach 6 hours after feeding or if vomiting is a persistent problem, metoclopramide can be used (1–2 mg/kg IV infusion over 24 hours, 0.5–1.0 mg/kg via gastrostomy tube, 15–20 minutes prior to feeding). If the position of the tube is questionable, its exact location can be determined using radiography after an iodinated contrast medium (commonly used for urography) has been injected into the

II, VII, IX and X. Abnormal coagulation test results have been demonstrated in 50% of affected cats.[9] Administration of benzodiazepines as an appetite stimulant is contraindicated in this disorder as they are known to be involved in the genesis of hepatic encephalopathy, are dependent on hepatic metabolism for elimination, and do not ensure adequate energy intake.

feeding tube. If a tube becomes occluded, injection of a small amount of cola will usually dissolve the food obstruction within 10 minutes.

The unique nutritional requirements of cats affected with the lipidosis syndrome are poorly understood (Fig. 13.11). For most cases, we have successfully used routine maintenance diets and an energy intake equal to or exceeding 60 kcal/kg/day. In some cats, however, encephalopathic signs indicate the propriety of interventional treatment with oral lactulose, neomycin and the restriction of dietary protein. We also use l–carnitine (150–250 mg per cat/day) and taurine (250–500 mg/cat/day) as dietary supplements. Carnitine is selected on the basis of its physiological role in lipid oxidation: it acts as a transport factor in delivery of fat across the inner mitochondrial membranes. Determination of blood, liver tissue and urine carnitine moieties have been unable to demonstrate a carnitine deficiency in severely affected cats.[12,16] It still remains possible that l-carnitine supplementation ensures an optimal quantity of carnitine in the cellular areas where demands are greatest, and our clinical impression is that l-carnitine supplementation hastens recovery of cats but controlled studies have not been completed. Taurine supplementation is provided because of the severely reduced blood taurine concentrations in affected cats.[12] Their profoundly increased serum bile acids are largely conjugated with taurine, which may provide some protection against bile salt induced cholestatic injury.[12]

Although serum arginine concentrations are also reduced in affected cats, provision of a well balanced feline diet should replete any deficits. If a human enteral diet is used as a basis, additional arginine may be essential (1000 mg arginine/day). Diets that contain medium chain triglycerides should be avoided, because it appears that these promote lipidosis in the cat.[20] Because zinc deficiency develops in humans with severe liver disease[2] and because zinc deficiency leads to abnormalities in taste (dysgeusia), supplementation with zinc at 7–8 mg per day is recommended.[1] On a prophylactic basis, some clinicians provide antibiotics capable of modifying enteric flora. Because many cats with severe lipidosis are weak and lethargic, and often demonstrate neck ventroflexion, it is important to supplement water soluble vitamins (including thiamine) and to correct hypokalaemia. Thiamine supplementation is recommended at an initial dose of 100 mg IM or PO followed by 50 mg PO bid.

Currently, there is a recovery rate of 60% in cats with severe hepatic lipidosis that receive aggressive supportive care.[12] Cats with idiopathic disease seem to have a better survival rate than those with secondary lipidosis. It is prudent to consider the development of this disorder in any cat undergoing energy restriction for weight loss or in any obese cat that suddenly becomes anorectic or develops recurrent vomiting. Monitoring the serum biochemical profile for characteristic changes in the serum enzymes and maintaining a high level of suspicion allow for early therapeutic intervention and better recovery prospects.

HEPATIC NEOPLASIA

The most common hepatic neoplasia in the cat are metastatic or multisystemic, especially lymphosarcoma, myeloproliferative disorders and systemic mast cell disease. Primary hepatic neoplasia is uncommon, with the exception of the bile duct adenocarcinoma that usually develops in elderly animals. Clinical signs of hepatic neoplasia depend on the anatomic location of the tumour tissue. Common signs include chronic debilitation, non-regenerative anaemia, hepatomegaly, splenomegaly, palpable abdominal masses and jaundice. Increased serum enzyme activity and hyperbilirubinaemia are inconsistent (Fig. 13.3). Abdominal ultrasonography and sometimes abdominal radiography may reveal irregular liver margins, lobular involvement or discrete hepatic masses. Examination of a buffy coat blood smear may be diagnostic for lymphosarcoma, myeloproliferative disease or mastocytosis.

If abdominal palpation discloses diffuse hepatomegaly or discrete masses, or if ultrasonography is available to ascertain the diffuse or focal nature of the neoplasia, a needle aspirate of liver tissue may yield a rapid diagnosis. If a needle biopsy is collected, tissue imprints should be made for cytological evaluation to provide a chance for rapid definitive diagnosis. Consultation with veterinary personnel trained in cytopathology is suggested before a definitive cytological diagnosis is determined. In some cases, histopathology of the biopsied tissue is necessary to ascertain the diagnosis.

Once a diagnosis is made, treatment options may include focal tumour resection or debulking and chemotherapy. Despite the hepatotoxicity of some chemotherapeutic agents, and the reliance of some agents on hepatic biotransformation or elimination, reasonable protocols can be tailored for lymphosarcoma and mastocytosis. Empirical reduction of drug dosages are required for agents dependent on hepatobiliary elimination. Careful titration of cytotoxics and antimetabolites based on observed changes in white blood cell and platelet counts can be used to direct further dose reductions in subsequent treatments.

PORTOSYSTEMIC VASCULAR ANOMALIES

Most cats with portosystemic vascular anomalies (PSVA) demonstrate neurobehavioural signs at a young age. In addition to encephalopathic signs, anorexia, polyphagia, diarrhoea, vomiting, ptyalism and polydipsia may be apparent. Neurological signs reflect diffuse symmetrical central nervous system aberration and may include depression, aggression, head pressing, amaurosis, mydriasis and recurrent seizure activity. Signs may or may not be associated with protein-rich meals. Unexpectedly prolonged recovery from general anaesthesia or an exaggerated response to tranquillisers might increase suspicion of this disorder in some cats. There is no gender or breed predisposition.

Physical examination usually reveals a stunted body nature, prominent kidneys, and a unique copper coloured iris.[11] Systolic heart murmurs have been detected in some cats. Radiolucent urate renal or cystic calculi that have caused recurrent haematuria, stranguria or urinary tract obstruction are present in some cats. Renal, ureteral and cystic calculi are easily detected during abdominal ultrasonography for shunt identification.

Haematological features include poikilocytosis (Fig. 13.6) and microcytosis. Serum biochemical features include normal to mildly increased liver enzyme activities, especially ALP, presumably due to the young age of most cats at the time of initial diagnosis (Fig. 13.3).[11] Other features

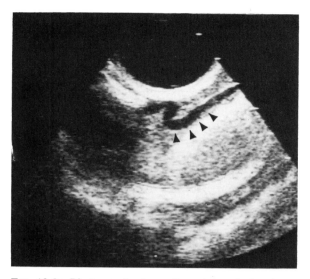

FIG. 13.9   Photograph of an ultrasonogram showing a left gastric vein shunt in a cat. The anomalous vessel is marked with black arrowheads. (Courtesy Dr. A. Yaeger, Section of Radiology, Department of Clinical Sciences, New York State College of Veterinary Medicine, Cornell University).

include a mild decrease in blood urea nitrogen (BUN), mild hypoglycaemia and mild hypocholesterolaemia. Ammonia biurate crystalluria develops inconsistently. Repeated urine sediment examination may sometimes disclose biurate crystals, especially after an encephalopathic episode. The most important test for recognition of PSVA is the demonstration of hepatic insufficiency (by use of a serum bile acid test) or ammonia intolerance.[7] If a PSVA is suspected, follow-up abdominal ultrasonography can sometimes document the presence of the shunting vascular anomaly; most cats in North America have a left gastric vein shunt that courses around the greater curvature of the stomach (Fig. 13.9). Radiographic portography is used to document the location of the shunting vessel; both lateral and ventrodorsal views are recorded to aid surgical correction (Fig. 13.10).

The preferred treatment of PSVA is by surgical occlusion of the anomalous vessel. Depending on the response of the portal circulation to anomalous vessel occlusion, there will be either complete or partial ligation, though before surgery it is impossible to predict which will be accomplished. Prior to and immediately after surgical correction, medical therapy is aimed at controlling or minimising episodes of hepatic encephalopathy. Medical management includes the feeding of a low protein diet with vitamin supplementation and the oral administration of lactulose and antibiotics capable of reducing intestinal ammonia production and absorption. Neomycin and lactulose are often used together orally because they are synergistic in action. Neomycin is not absorbed from the alimentary canal and can be administered chronically at a dose of 22 mg/kg PO bid to tid. Lactulose is administered initially at a dose of 0.055 ml/kg and

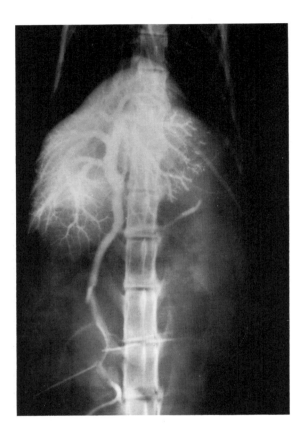

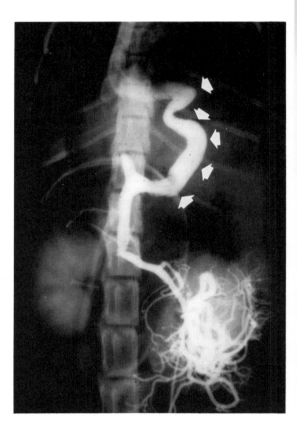

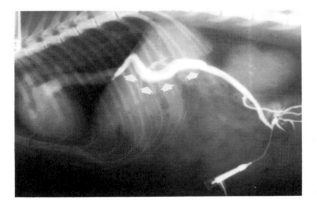

FIG. 13.10 Photographs of (above, left) ventrodorsal abdominal radiograph in a normal cat, (above, right) ventrodorsal and (left) lateral abdominal radiographs in a cat with a congenital portal vascular anomaly (same cat as illustrated in Fig. 13.9). Each radiograph was made immediately after injection of radiocontrast into a mesenteric vessel. The normal cat has abundant hepatic circulation as indicated by the contrast delineation of hepatic vasculature, whereas there is none in the cat with the portal vascular anomaly. The anomalous vessel is directly communicating with the vena cava and is marked with white arrows. Both radiographic views are required to differentiate this vessel from an intrahepatic ductus venosus. (Courtesy of Dr. A. Yaeger, Section of Radiology, Department of Clinical Sciences, New York State College of Veterinary Medicine, Cornell University).

MANAGEMENT OF FELINE HEPATOBILIARY DISORDERS

Therapeutic agent	Dose	Route	Frequency	Indications and comments
Antibiotics:				
Ampicillin	22 mg/kg	PO, SC, IV	tid	Broad-spectrum antibacterial; well concentrated in bile; renal excretion.
Amoxicillin	11-22 mg/kg	PO, IV	bid	Broad-spectrum antibacterial; well concentrated in bile; renal excretion.
Cefazolin	11-33 mg/kg	IM, IV	tid-qid	Broad-spectrum antibacterial; well concentrated in bile compared to other cephalosporins; renal excretion.
Enrofloxacin	2.5-5 mg/kg	PO	sid-bid	Broad spectrum antimicrobial; good absorption and tissue penetration. Avoid use in very young animals or those with epilepsy.
Chloramphen-icol	50 mg/cat	PO, IV	bid	Empiric dose reduction. Broad spectrum antibacterial; enterohepatic circulation; can cause anorexia and erythroid hypoplasia. Use in liver disease is controversial and restricted to situations where culture sensitivities direct its use. Relatively poor bile concentration.
Doxycycline	5 mg/kg 2.5 mg/kg	PO loading PO	dose once sid	Broad spectrum, good absorption and availability; good concentration in bile; faecal elimination. Sensitivity testing should direct its use because of the danger of inducing lipidosis with tetracyclines.
Metronidazole	7.5 mg/kg	PO, IV	bid-tid	Empiric dose reduction because clearance depends on hepatobiliary function. Good enteric absorption; useful against anaerobic organisms; used to modify flora responsible for encephalopathic toxins.
Neomycin	22 mg/kg	PO	bid-tid	Used to modify intestinal flora responsible for encephalopathic toxin production; inhibits ammonia-producers; synergistic with lactulose; is not systemically absorbed.

Antibiotics to avoid: tetracyclines, lincomycin, erythromycin, streptomycin, sulphonamides, trimethoprim-sulpha preparations. These drugs are either dependent on hepatobiliary processing for activation or elimination or are associated with idiosyncratic hepatobiliary reactions. Tetracyclines can induce hepatic lipidosis in other species warranting concern in the cat particularly susceptible to lipidosis.

Hydrocholeretic:				
Dehydrocholic acid	10-15 mg/kg	PO	tid	No documented proof of efficacy; is contraindicated in complete bile duct obstruction and in hepatic insufficiency. May be metabolised to lithocholic acid, a highly toxic bile acid capable of producing cholestasis.
Appetite stimulants:				
Diazepam	0.2 mg/kg	PO, IV	sid-bid	Contraindicated in severe hepatic dysfunction since
Oxazepam	0.2 mg/kg	PO	sid	benzodiazepines are involved in the genesis of hepatic encephalopathy. Short-lived response, side effects of ataxia and sedation; depends on liver for plasma clearance. Oxazepam is longer acting: effects seen in 1 hour may last 6-12 h.
Glucocorticoids:				
Prednisolone	2.2 mg/kg	PO, SC, IV	sid	Indicated for non-septic, active non-suppurative inflammation suspected to be immune-mediated, also
	taper dose to 0.5-1.5 mg/kg	PO	sid alternate day sid	used to curtail developing fibrosis. Catabolic; ↑protein deamination, ↑ammonia production; side effects: polyuria, polydipsia, immune suppression, appetite stimulation, disturbed sodium and water balance; may induce diabetes mellitus if high dose used chronically; contraindicated in hepatic lipidosis as it promotes lipolysis.
Treatment for gastro-duodenal ulceration				
H$_2$ blockers:				
Famotidine	1-2 mg/cat	PO IV	sid bid	Used to limit gastric acidity, new generation H$_2$ blocker; does not impede drug metabolising enzymes like cimetidine or ranitidine. The preferred H$_2$ blocker.
Cimetidine	5 mg/kg	PO, IV	bid-tid	Impedes hepatic p450 cytochrome oxidases leading to drug interactions.

continued

MANAGEMENT OF FELINE HEPATOBILIARY DISORDERS (continued)				
Therapeutic agent	**Dose**	**Route**	**Frequency**	**Indications and comments**
Ranitidine	0.5 mg/kg	PO, IV	bid	Impedes hepatic p450 cytochrome oxidases less so than cimetidine.
Gastric cytoprotection: Sucralphate	0.25 g/cat	PO	tid-qid	Locally stimulates prostaglandin production that assists with mucosal blood flow, mucin production, and ulcer healing. Not systemically absorbed.
Antiemetic: Metoclopramide	1-2 mg/kg 0.5-1 mg/kg	IV PO or in gastric tube 20 minutes before feeding	slow 24 h drip	Strong centrally acting antiemetic; also facilitates gastric emptying in cats with gastrostomy tubes in place.
Vitamins Vitamin K$_1$	5 mg/cat	IM, SC Never administer IV → anaphylaxis	sid	Bleeding tendencies due to vitamin K depletion (anorexia and antibiotic treatment derange vitamin K producing flora) and vitamin K malabsorption due to the absence of bile acids in intestines (complete bile duct occlusion; at 14 days). Corrects coagulation times by > 30% within 12 hours; begin therapy at least 12 hours before hepatic biopsy. Chronic use, 2 times weekly, recommended in acquired hepatic insufficiency.
Thiamine (B$_1$)	50 mg/cat	PO, IM	sid	Chronic anorexia in the cat is believed to lead to thiamine deficiency associated with neck ventroflexion and neurological signs (fixed dilated pupils, weakness, lethargy, tucked or curled posture). This is a safe prophylactic treatment.
Water soluble vitamins	doubled daily dose		sid	Abundant co-factors necessary for optimal intermediary metabolism. Water soluble vitamins are believed to be easily depleted in severe hepatobiliary disease especially those associated with anorexia.
Alteration of intestinal flora Ammonium ion trapping: Lactulose	0.25 ml/cat	PO	sid-tid	Used in hepatic encephalopathy to decrease intestinal ammonia production and absorption and to promote faecal elimination (cathartic effect). This is a non-digestible synthetic disaccharide broken down by gut flora to yield an acidic product. Too high a dose can produce severe diarrhoea, flatulence, cramping pains associated with gas production, dehydration, and a metabolic acidosis. Dose is titrated to stool consistency with 2-3 bowel movements per day of soft stool desirable.
Binding of toxins: Cholestyramine	0.25-0.5 g in 15 ml H$_2$O	PO	sid	Empiric dose approximated from human dose. A basic anion exchange resin capable of binding bile acids and endotoxins in the GI tract forming insoluble complexes that are excreted in faeces. Short term use only as chronic use leads to fat soluble vitamin depletion (malabsorption).
Activated charcoal	mix with water		sid	Binds toxins in GI tract. A formulation is available which is more miscible with water and has greater toxin binding capacity than generic activated charcoal.
Retention enemas: Lactulose	15-20 ml diluted 1:3; retain for 20-30 minutes. If faecal pH>6.0, repeat enema.		tid-qid	Enemas may be used to modify colonic contents acutely in encephalopathic patients. Warm saline cleansing enemas are initially used to flush the contents from the intestinal lumen mechanically. Retention enemas comprised of agents capable of altering bacterial flora responsible for toxin production or of impeding the absorption of ammonia, are given as retention enemas after the colon is cleansed.
Neomycin	15-20 ml 1% solution		tid-qid	

continued

MANAGEMENT OF FELINE HEPATOBILIARY DISORDERS (continued)				
Therapeutic agent	Dose	Route	Frequency	Indications and comments
Dietary supplements: (appropriate for cats with Hepatic Lipidosis, *unproved* efficacy)				
L-carnitine	150–250 mg/cat	PO	in food	Important cofactor promoting mitochondrial fatty acid oxidation. Use L-carnitine not D-L carnitine.
taurine	250–500 mg/cat	PO	in food	Important for bile acid conjugation. Assists in detoxification of bile acid effects.
arginine	1000 mg/cat	PO	in food	Necessary only if human enteral diets are fed.
zinc	7–8 mg/cat	PO	in food	Important intermediary metabolism co-factor deficiency can cause disordered taste perception in humans which may invoke anorexia. Consider if home formulated diet used.

FIG. 13.11   Therapeutic management of feline hepatobiliary disorders.

the dose is gradually titrated according to the stool consistency; several soft stools per day indicate an adequate dose. Amoxicillin at 10 mg/kg PO bid has been used to control encephalopathic signs in some cats. Metronidazole may be used to alter the gastrointestinal flora but at a smaller dose than normal; an empirical dose we have used with clinical success is 7.5 mg/kg PO sid to bid. Metronidazole relies on hepatic elimination and can produce ataxia and vestibular signs when toxic levels accumulate. If the encephalopathic signs are severe enough to preclude administration of oral medications, lactulose and neomycin retention enemas may be given (lactulose at 5–10 ml diluted 1:3 with water, and neomycin at 15–20 ml of a 1% solution, tid to qid).

Serum bile acid concentrations have been used to monitor the resolution of hepatic insufficiency. A gradual discontinuation of medical treatment and, eventually, a return to a normal feline diet, are advised if hepatic function tests are normal. In some cats, serum bile acid values have become normal within a month of surgery. In others, serum bile acids remain abnormal and chronic medical management is necessary. Some cats develop seizures before or after surgical ligation and require chronic management with low dose phenobarbital (initial dose 0.55 mg/kg PO sid to bid).

REFERENCES

1. Bauer J.E. (1989) Feline lipid metabolism and hepatic lipidosis. *12th Ann. Kal. Kan. Symposium* 75–78.
2. Bode J.C., Hanisch P., Henning H. et al. (1988) Hepatic zinc content in patients with various stages of alcoholic liver disease and in patients with chronic active and chronic persistent hepatitis. *Hepatology* **8**: 1605–1609.
3. Bright R.M., Burrows C.F. (1988) Percutaneous endoscopic tube gastrostomy in dogs. *Am. J. Vet. Res.* **49**: 629–633.
4. Burrows C.F., Chiapella A.M., Jezyk P. (1981) Idiopathic feline hepatic lipidosis: the syndrome and speculations on its pathogenesis. *Florida Vet. J.* (winter) 18–20.
5. Cantarow A., Stewart H.L. (1935) Alteration in serum bilirubin and bromosulphalein retention in relation to morphological changes in the liver and bile passages in cats with total biliary stasis. *Am. J. Pathol.* **11**: 561–581.
6. Center S.A. (1986) Hepatic lipidosis in the cat *Proc. 4th Annu. Vet. Med. Forum ACVIM, 2*: 13/71–13/76.
7. Center S.A., Baldwin B.H., de Lahunta A. et al. (1986) Evaluation of serum bile acid concentrations for the diagnosis of portosystemic venous anomalies in the dog and cat. *J. Am. Vet. Med. Assoc.* **186**: 1090–1094.
8. Center S.A., Baldwin B.H., King J.M. et al. (1983) Hematologic and biochemical abnormalities associated with induced extrahepatic bile duct obstruction in the cat. *Am. J. Vet. Res.* **44**: 1822–1828.
9. Center S.A., Crawford M.A., Guida L. et al.

A retrospective study of cats (n = 77) with severe hepatic lipidosis (1975–1990). (Submitted for publication).

10. Center S.A., Dillingham S., Baldwin B.H. et al. (1986) Serum gamma glutamyl transferase and alkaline phosphatase in cats with hepatobiliary disease. *J. Am. Vet. Med. Assoc.* **188**: 507–510.

11. Center S.A., Magne M.L. (1990) Historical, physical examination, and clinicopathologic features of portosystemic vascular anomalies in the dog and cat. *Sem. Vet. Med. Surg. (Sm. Anim.)* **5**: 83–93.

12. Center S.A., Thompson M., Wood P.A. et al. (1991) Hepatic ultrastructural and metabolic derangements in cats with severe hepatic lipidosis. *Proc. 9th Ann. Vet. Med. Forum ACVIM* 193–196.

13. Daniel G.B., Bright R., Ollis P. et al. (1991) Per rectal portal scintigraphy using ^{99m}technetium pertechnetate to diagnose portosystemic shunts in dog and cats. *J. Vet. Int. Med.* **5**: 23–27.

14. Edwards D.F., McCracken M.D., Richardson D.C. (1983) Sclerosing cholangitis in a cat. *JAVMA* **182**: 710–712.

15. Hirsch V.M., Doige C.E. (1983) Suppurative cholangitis in cats. *JAVMA* **138**: 1223–1226.

16. Jacobs G., Cornelius L., Keene B. et al. (1990) Comparison of plasma, liver and skeletal muscle carnitine concentrations in cats with idiopathic hepatic lipidosis and in healthy cats. *Am. J. Vet. Res.* **51**: 1349–1351.

17. Jones T.C., Hunt R.D. (1983) *Veterinary Pathology*, 5th edition, pp 1411–1442 Lea & Febiger, Philadelphia.

18. Jones E.A., Skolnick P., Gammal S.H. et al. (1989) NIH Conference. The γ-aminobutyric acid A (GABA A) receptor complex and hepatic encephalopathy. Some recent advances. *Ann. Int. Med.* **110**: 532–546.

19. Lucke V.M., Davies J.D. (1984) Progressive lymphocytic cholangitis in the cat. *J. Small Anim. Pract.* **25**: 249–260.

20. MacDonald M.L., Anderson B.C., Rogers, Q.R. et al. (1984) Essential fatty acid requirements of cats: pathology of essential fatty acid deficiency. *Am. J. Vet. Res.* **45**: 1310–1317.

21. Mathews K.A., Ginnington A.G. (1986) Percutaneous incisionless placement of a gastrostomy tube utilizing a gastroscope: preliminary observations. *J. Am. Anim. Hosp. Assoc.* **22**: 601–610.

22. Prasse K.W., Mahaffey E.A., DeNovo R. et al. (1982) Chronic lymphocytic cholangitis in three cats. *Vet. Pathol.* **19**: 99–108.

23. Sherding R.G. (1985) Acute Hepatic Failure. *Vet. Clin. N. Amer.* **15**: 119–132.

24. Vierling J.M. (1990) Hepatobiliary complications of ulcerative colitis and Crohn's disease. In: Zakim D. and Boyer T.D. (eds) *Hepatology: a textbook of liver disease* pp 1126–1158 W.B. Saunders, Philadelphia.

25. Yaeger A.E., Mohammed H.O. The accuracy of ultrasonography in the detection of severe hepatic lipidosis in cats. *Am. J. Vet. Res.* **00**: 000–000.

26. Zawie D.A., Garvey M.S. (1984) Feline hepatic disease. *Vet. Clin. N. Am.* **14**: 1201–1230.

14

Disorders of the Urinary System

DAVID F. SENIOR

INTRODUCTION

Diseases of the urinary system are among the most common problems leading to cats being presented for veterinary care. In young adult cats, lower urinary tract inflammation and urethral obstruction are the most common presenting complaints. In older cats, progressive loss of renal function leading to chronic renal failure predominates.

New knowledge of nutritional requirements for cats will probably change the incidence of lower urinary tract disease as commercial rations are reformulated.

The causes of chronic renal failure remain to be elucidated and the large proportion of idiopathic lower urinary tract disease makes management a challenge.

This chapter is arranged on a problem-oriented basis: azotaemia; proteinuria; renomegaly; lower urinary tract inflammation; disorders of micturition; and diagnostic techniques.

AZOTAEMIA

Azotaemia refers to the accumulation of protein metabolites in plasma when kidney function is reduced. Both serum creatinine and blood urea nitrogen (BUN) are used to determine the degree of azotaemia and kidney function can be estimated from these values. The aetiology of azotaemia can be prerenal, primary renal or postrenal and clinical differentiation of these three is the essential first goal of diagnosis in azotaemic cats.

Prerenal azotaemia occurs when dehydration or shock induce poor renal perfusion with subsequently reduced renal clearance of creatinine and urea or, rarely, when excessive amounts of urea are presented for excretion, for example in gastro-intestinal haemorrhage (Fig. 14.1).

Primary renal azotaemia is caused by conditions that directly damage or destroy functional kidney

CAUSES OF PRERENAL AZOTAEMIA
Reduced renal perfusion
Dehydration Shock: septic, hypovolaemic, haemorrhagic, hypoadrenocorticoidism
Excessive urea production
Gastrointestinal haemorrhage

FIG. 14.1   Causes of prerenal azotaemia.

tissue. It can have many causes but two broad syndromes are recognised: acute renal failure (ARF – a rapidly progressing form that may be reversible) and chronic renal failure (CRF – a slowly progressing form that is irreversible).

Postrenal azotaemia occurs when obstruction, rupture or perforation of the renal collection system, ureters or lower urinary tract prevents normal passage of urine from the body (Fig. 14.2). Both prerenal azotaemia and the obstructive form of postrenal azotaemia can induce intrinsic renal damage and ARF if the insult is sufficiently severe and prolonged.

Prerenal azotaemia can be differentiated from

CAUSES OF POSTRENAL AZOTAEMIA
Urethral obstruction
Muco-crystalline plugs Urolithiasis Granulomatous urethritis Neoplasia
Bilateral ureteral obstruction
Neoplasia
Urethra trauma
Gunshot Automobile accident

FIG. 14.2   Causes of postrenal azotaemia.

193

FIG. 14.3 Differentiation of prerenal and primary renal azotaemia.

DIFFERENTIATION OF PRERENAL AND PRIMARY RENAL AZOTAEMIA[a]		
	Prerenal	**Primary renal**
Dehydration	+	±[b]
Shock	+	±[b]
Urine specific gravity	>1.060	<1.035
Correction with fluid treatment	+	−

[a] Although other criteria including urine sodium concentration, urine/plasma creatinine ratio and fractional excretion of sodium (FE_{Na}^{+}) are used in human beings and dogs, values for these have not been established in the cat.
[b] Dehydration and shock can also be present in cats with intrinsic renal disease when both prerenal and primary renal components contribute to azotaemia.

primary renal azotaemia based on history, physical examination, urinalysis and response to treatment (Fig. 14.3). Recognition of postrenal azotaemia is based on the history and physical findings. Rupture of the lower urinary tract results in retroperitoneal accumulation of fluid in the sublumbar region, subcutaneous accumulation of fluid, or ascites, depending on the location and size of the defect. Uroperitoneum can be differentiated from ascites by measurement of creatinine in both serum and peritoneal fluid. Peritoneal fluid creatinine levels are higher than serum levels in uroperitoneum, whereas in ascites they are the same.[4] Rupture of a full bladder can be catastrophic in the cat because the extremely hyperosmotic urine induces rapid diffusion of extracellular water into the peritoneal cavity with subsequent hypovolaemic shock. Hyponatraemia is a common serum chemistry finding.

Differentiation of primary renal azotaemia into ARF and CRF facilitates accurate determination of aetiology, appropriate management and an accurate prognosis (Fig. 14.4).

Acute renal failure

In ARF there is a rapidly progressive loss of renal function due to an acute insult. Most patients develop oliguria initially; polyuria may occur in the recovery phase. Some causes of ARF induce polyuria initially rather than oliguria, for example gentamicin nephrosis. Affected patients develop

DIFFERENTIATION OF ACUTE AND CHRONIC RENAL FAILURE		
	ARF	**CRF**
Onset of signs	recent	prolonged[a]
General body condition	good	poor
Urine volume	low[b]	high
Red cell mass	normal	anaemic
Serum K^+	high (can be normal)	low (can be normal)[c]
Urine sediment	active	benign
Response to supportive Rx	recovery[d]	no recovery
Renal size	normal/large	small[e]
Renal biopsy	necrosis	fibrosis/atrophy

[a] Many cats with CRF maintain homeostasis with few (if any) signs until stress causes decompensation making the syndrome look acute.
[b] Some forms of ARF develop polyuria, not oliguria (e.g. gentamicin nephrosis).
[c] Recent addition of more potassium to commercial diets has reduced the tendency of cats with CRF to develop hypokalaemia.
[d] When the insult causing ARF is massive, recovery is not possible.
[e] The kidneys are enlarged in many forms of CRF (e.g. polycystic kidney disease) - see Fig. 14.8.

FIG. 14.4 Differentiation of acute renal failure and chronic renal failure.

AETIOLOGY OF ACUTE RENAL FAILURE		
Extension of prerenal insults	**Primary renal insults**	**Extension of postrenal insults**

Hypovolaemia
  dehydration
  haemorrhage
  hypoalbuminaemia
  hyponatraemia
  hypoadrenocorticoidism
 	
Cardiovascular failure
  CHF
  endotoxaemia
  prolonged anaesthesia
 	
Vascular failure
  thromboembolism
  NSAIDS
	Toxins
	  ethylene glycol
	  aminoglycosides
	  catecholamines
	  radiographic contrast
	    agent
	  haemoproteins
	  amphotericin B
	  cis-platinum
	  heavy metals
	  methoxyflurane
	    anaesthesia
	  Easter lily
	
	Other
	  hypercalcaemia
	  pyelonephritis
	  vasculitis/DIC
	  heat stroke
	  leptospirosis
		Urethral obstruction
		  mucocrystalline plugs
		  urolithiasis

FIG. 14.5 Aetiology of acute renal failure.

anorexia, vomition, lethargy and weakness. Physical examination may reveal 'uraemic' halitosis and palpation of the kidneys may be painful. The syndrome is characterised by rapidly rising serum creatinine and BUN in a non-anaemic cat with an active urine sediment. ARF can develop from severe prerenal or postrenal insults or from the direct effect of toxins or infectious agents on the kidney (Fig. 14.5).

Non-specific management of acute renal failure

A few aspects of management relate to combating specific causes of ARF but most management strategies are non-specific and are useful in all patients with ARF, regardless of aetiology. A primary goal should be to correct all prerenal and postrenal insults. Rehydration and normalisation of systemic and renal arterial blood pressure will facilitate return of normal renal perfusion.

Rehydration

Rehydration is best performed with lactated Ringer's solution or, if hyperkalaemia is present or suspected, normal (0.9%) saline. Lower urinary tract integrity and patency should be established by correcting rupture or obstruction.

If oliguria persists after rehydration, metabolic

MANAGEMENT OF METABOLIC ACIDOSIS AND HYPERKALAEMIA

Correction of Metabolic Acidosis
  Amount of HCO_3 required (mM) = 0.3 x BW kg x Base Deficit OR 0.5-1.0 mM/kg
 	
Correction of Hyperkalaemia (Temporary)
  Bicarbonate - as above
  Insulin/dextrose[a] Dextrose 50% 1.5 g/kg IV; 1 unit regular insulin/3 g dextrose
  Ca gluconate 10%[b] 0.5-1 ml/kg

[a] Administration of exogenous insulin may not be necessary because glucose may stimulate endogenous insulin release but the adequacy of the endogenous insulin release is not known in cats with ARF. [b] Counteracts the cardiotoxic effects of hyperkalaemia but does not reduce plasma K^+.

FIG. 14.6 Management of metabolic acidosis and hyperkalaemia.

acidosis and hyperkalaemia are frequently present. Correction of metabolic acidosis is only necessary with pH < 7.2 or serum HCO_3 < 14 mM/l. Hyperkalaemia may be managed temporarily with sodium bicarbonate, glucose/insulin, and calcium gluconate administration (Fig. 14.6).

Diuretics

Diuretics should be given to increase urine production in patients with oliguric ARF (Fig. 14.7). Diuretics given hours to days after the onset of ARF probably do not ameliorate the severity of renal damage but polyuric patients are easier to manage.

After rehydration and diuretic treatment, overhydration leading to pulmonary oedema can develop if rapid fluid administration is continued in the face of persistent oliguria. Intravenous fluid composition should be changed to 2.5% dextrose in 0.45% saline or 5% dextrose in water to prevent hypernatraemia. The rate of administration should be slowed to replace insensible losses (10–12 ml/kg bodyweight/day) + urine production + gastrointestinal losses (vomiting and diarrhoea).

Peritoneal dialysis

Persistent oliguria in ARF leads to life-threatening hyperkalaemia, extreme azotaemia and severe metabolic acidosis – all indications for peritoneal dialysis. Results of peritoneal dialysis are relatively poor because the severity of renal damage often prevents return of useful renal function and because of complications associated with dialysis, such as peritonitis.[21] In addition, expense may preclude or limit the use of dialysis in many patients. However, when performed prior to surgery to correct rupture of the urinary tract, dialysis to correct azotaemia is usually very successful.

After sterile placement of a dialysis catheter into the peritoneal cavity, dialysate (a specially formulated electrolyte fluid containing 1.5% dextrose) should be instilled into the abdomen and allowed to dwell for about 1 hour before being drained. After drainage, the next aliquot of dialysis fluid should be instilled and this procedure should be repeated until hyperkalaemia, metabolic acidosis and progressive azotaemia are controlled. Hypertonic dialysis solutions (containing up to 4.5% dextrose) can be used to correct overhydration because the drained volume will be greater than the volume of dialysate instilled. In rupture of the urinary tract, 3–5 exchanges are usually necessary to prepare the cat for anaesthesia. Lactated Ringer's solution with 2.5% dextrose added is an adequate dialysate in this instance if specially formulated dialysate is unavailable. In primary ARF, 12–15 exchanges per day may be necessary to stabilise the patient. Once stabilisation is achieved, 5–7 exchanges per day are usually sufficient for maintenance. Longer dwell times are used when exchanges are less frequent so that dialysate is constantly in the peritoneal cavity. If renal function does not improve to a level compatible with future dialysis-free life after 2–3 weeks of treatment, continued improvement is not likely.

Polyuria

Polyuria might be produced initially by some forms of ARF (e.g. nephrosis due to gentamicin and amphotericin B) but the development of

---

DIURETIC USE IN OLIGURIC ACUTE RENAL FAILURE

1. Mannitol[a] 0.5 g/kg bodyweight IV over 3-5 minutes, repeat if urine production does not increase.
2. Frusemide 2 mg/kg bodyweight IV, repeat at 4 mg/kg if no effect with the initial dose
3. Dopamine[b] 3-5 µg/kg bodyweight/min.

[a] Should not be given in extremely hypertonic patients or patients with congestive heart failure (e.g. ethylene glycol intoxication).
[b] Has been shown to be of some benefit in dogs when used in conjunction with frusemide but there are no data on efficacy in the cat. Must be given with an infusion pump to ensure accuracy.

FIG. 14.7 Diuretic use in oliguric acute renal failure.

polyuria after initial oliguria usually represents the commencement of a recovery phase. In addition, massive polyuria often follows relief of urethral outflow obstruction. During the polyuric phase, fluid therapy should prevent dehydration and diuresis associated hypokalaemia. Frequent assessment of bodyweight with appropriate changes in the administration rate of intravenous fluids are necessary to prevent dehydration, which could lead to further renal damage. Potassium supplementation is necessary to prevent hypokalaemia.

Control of vomition

Control of vomition can be difficult in ARF. The H$_2$-histamine receptor antagonist, cimetidine, given at 2.5 mg/kg bodyweight PO bid or ranitidine given at 2–4 mg/kg bodyweight PO bid, appears to reduce vomition in some cats – presumably by alleviating erosive gastritis. Metoclopramide given at 0.2 mg/kg bodyweight PO tid may also be of benefit. Cimetidine, ranitidine and metoclopramide are excreted by renal clearance, so doses should be reduced after the initial loading dose (see p 00). The centrally acting antiemetic chlorpromazine, given at 0.4–2 mg/kg bodyweight PO bid, may be more effective but can cause excessive drowsiness that can reduce appetite and the cat's level of activity. In addition, high doses of chlorpromazine may reduce blood pressure, so that dosing should be conservative, to effect.

Specific management of ARF

Ethylene glycol intoxication

Ethylene glycol intoxication is the most common cause of toxin induced ARF in cats[9] and the lethal dose is 6–8 ml/kg. In the first 12 hours after ingestion, intoxicated cats demonstrate ataxia, staggering and vomiting. Loss of plasma volume into the bowel due to the hypertonicity of ethylene glycol induces a rapid rise in PCV, and marked metabolic acidosis with a wide anion gap usually develops. By 12 hours, calcium oxalate monohydrate crystals (dumb-bell, hempseed and elongated four- or six-sided, occasionally with budding bullets) or dihydrate crystals (Maltese cross) may be observed in the urine sediment. Renal failure

with rapidly increasing serum creatinine usually develops after 2–3 days. Treatment with a specific antidote to inhibit alcohol dehydrogenase e.g. ethanol 95% given at 1 ml/kg bodyweight IV qid for 4 doses must be started within 8 hours after ethylene glycol ingestion to prevent ARF effectively. Intravenous crystalloid solutions to restore intravascular volume with added bicarbonate to control metabolic acidosis should be provided as necessary during the acute phase. Animals with severe renal failure (creatinine > 880 µM/l) seldom regain sufficient renal function to be maintained even if appropriate fluid treatment and dialysis are used to support the patient for several weeks.

Aminoglycoside intoxication

Cats appear to be relatively resistant to the nephrotoxic effects of aminoglycoside antibiotics although prolonged high doses can induce ARF. Affected patients develop polyuria and granular casts appear in the urine sediment. Gentamicin is the most commonly implicated drug. Several risk factors enhance the nephrotoxicity of gentamicin in other species (e.g. fever, dehydration, hypokalaemia) but it is not known if these are important in cats. Good supportive care can lead to return of significant renal function over a 2–3 week period.

Urethral obstruction

Postrenal azotaemia due to urethral obstruction is a common cause of ARF in cats. For a detailed description see p 207.

Chronic renal failure

The aetiology of chronic renal failure in cats is frequently obscure but many of the known causes are shown in Fig. 14.8. In CRF there is a slowly progressive loss of renal function. Affected patients develop mild polydipsia and polyuria, reduced appetite, vomiting and lethargy. Physical examination results are variable but may reveal 'uraemic' halitosis, pale mucous membranes, oral ulceration and abnormal kidney size and shape. The syndrome is characterised by slowly rising serum creatinine and BUN over months to years. Affected animals

AETIOLOGY OF CHRONIC RENAL FAILURE

Large Kidneys (> 3.2 x length of L 2)
Polycystic kidney disease (very large)
Lymphosarcoma[a]
Feline infectious peritonitis[a]
Hydronephrosis[a]
Amyloidosis[a]

Small Kidneys (< 2.3 x length of L 2)
Chronic generalised nephritis[a]: after irreversible ARF, idiopathic
Glomerular sclerosis
Pyelonephritis
Membranous glomerulonephritis
Nephrolithiasis[a]
Amyloidosis (particularly Abyssinian cats)[a]

[a] Kidneys can be normal size as well

FIG. 14.8 Aetiology of chronic renal failure.

are usually anaemic and the urine sediment is unremarkable.

Management of chronic renal failure

Although management of some specific forms of CRF vary with aetiology (e.g. chemotherapy in lymphosarcoma) most management strategies can be applied to the common problems encountered in almost all patients with CRF, i.e. polyuria and polydipsia, reduced appetite, vomiting, azotaemia, hyperphosphataemia, hyperparathyroidism, hypokalaemia, metabolic acidosis, anaemia and hypertension.

Diet changes

All dietary changes should be instituted gradually over several days. Adjustments to new metabolite excretion rates require more time in CRF so that extracellular fluid (ECF) volume and composition may not be properly maintained when dietary changes are too abrupt. Similarly, sudden environmental changes that alter the quantity or pattern of food and water intake should be avoided.

Water

Water should be available at all times. Some cats with CRF tend to become progressively dehydrated and develop a significant prerenal azotaemia that can lead to a crisis. Such patients may require periodic rehydration with parenteral fluids followed by 1–2 days of solute diuresis to reduce the degree of azotaemia. Owners can give subcutaneous fluids daily or every other day to prevent this tendency.

Reduced protein intake

Reduced protein intake decreases polydipsia and polyuria, improves the feeling of wellbeing, and lessens azotaemia and proteinuria. Cats with CRF should be fed approximately 20% of calories as protein. Protein intake should be 3.3–3.5 g/kg bodyweight/day with energy intake of 70–80 kcal/kg bodyweight/day.[16] The protein source should be of high biological value. Reducing the BUN to less than 13.2 mM/l (80 mg/dl), a level at which many cats can survive reasonably well, is a valid goal and dietary protein intake should be adjusted accordingly. However, this goal is often not achievable in cats with severely reduced glomerular filtration rate (GFR). The source of protein may be important. Metabolic acidosis was more severe in dogs fed low protein diets when the sole protein source was egg albumin.[18] It is not known if the same phenomenon occurs in cats.

Hyperparathyroidism, phosphate and calcitriol

Plasma parathyroid hormone (PTH) levels are increased in CRF due to both phosphate retention and reduced renal production of calcitriol. Phosphate retention tends to lower the serum ionized calcium level thus stimulating PTH production. Calcitriol normally inhibits PTH production by the parathyroid glands and PTH production increases when renal calcitriol production is diminished in CRF (Fig. 14.9).[12] Phosphate retention induces soft tissue mineralisation, including mineralisation of the kidneys, and hyperparathyroidism contributes to demineralisation of bone and shortened erythrocyte life-span (Figs 14.9 and 14.10). Phosphate retention and renal secondary hyperparathyroidism can be controlled by dietary restriction of phosphate, use of oral phosphate binders and administration of low dose calcitriol.

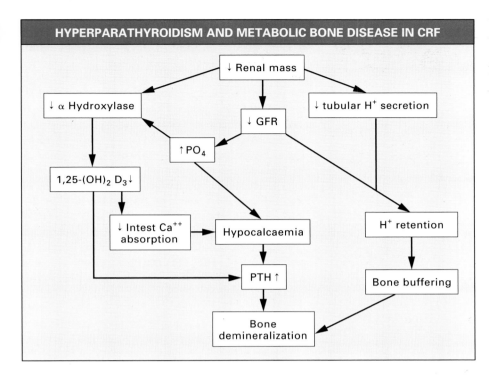

FIG. 14.9 Pathogenesis of hyperparathyroidism and metabolic bone disease in chronic renal failure.

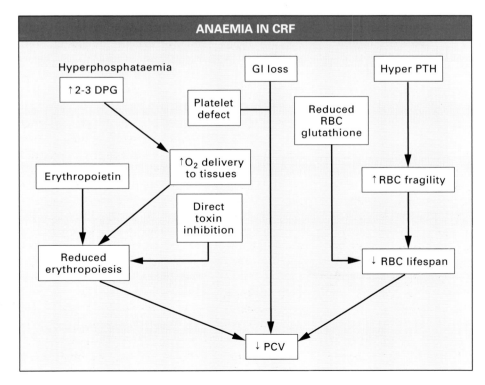

FIG. 14.10 Pathogenesis of anaemia in chronic renal failure.

Low protein diets tend to be low in phosphate. The currently recommended intake of phosphate for cats in CRF is 80–100 mg/100 kcal ME.[11] The calcium–phosphate ratio should be maintained at 1.2–1.5:1. The goal of phosphate restriction is to reduce serum phosphate levels to less than 1.78 mM/l (5.5 mg/dl). If dietary phosphate restriction alone fails to achieve a serum phosphate of 1.78 mM/l (5.5 mg/dl) or less, aluminium carbonate or aluminium hydroxide given at 10–30 mg/kg bodyweight PO tid or calcium acetate given at 30 mg/kg bodyweight PO tid are effective phosphate binders. Oral phosphate binders are ineffective in lowering serum phosphate levels in dogs fed normal non-phosphate restricted diets and the same is probably true in cats.[8] Cats tend to have an extreme aversion to oral administration of liquid forms of these supplements and so capsules or tablets should be given. Aluminium carbonate may be more effective than aluminium hydroxide. Calcium salts have been used in humans instead of aluminium salts because long-term use results in neuropathy secondary to aluminium accumulation in neural tissues. However, aluminium toxicity has not been reported in cats. Calcium acetate tends to cause hypercalcaemia before adequate control of hyperphosphataemia is achieved, and extreme care should be taken to monitor serum calcium levels when using a calcium salt to bind phosphate. Rapid soft tissue mineralisation can occur when hypercalcaemia develops with concurrent hyperphosphataemia.

Suppression of hyperparathyroidism

Calcitriol given at extremely low doses (1.5–3.5 nanograms per kg bodyweight sid) appears to inhibit PTH production directly and reduce serum PTH levels without a significant hypercalcaemic effect.[12] Low dose calcitriol treatment with correction of high parathyroid hormone levels tend to reduce hyperphosphataemia but all attempts should be made to normalise serum phosphate levels using low phosphate diets and phosphate binders before commencing treatment. Owners report that their pets 'feel better' with low dose calcitriol treatment.

Correction of hypokalaemia

Cats with CRF tend to develop hypokalaemia due to obligatory renal potassium loss. Acidified diets that are low in magnesium may contribute to the potassium loss. Hypokalaemia may induce more rapid progression of renal disease because of increased tubular ammoniagenesis. Serum potassium should be maintained at 4–5.5 mM/l. Concurrent metabolic acidosis also tends to increase renal tubular ammoniagenesis. Both hypokalaemia and metabolic acidosis can be treated using an alkaline potassium salt at 2–4 mM every 12 hours to effect or at 2.2 mM/100 kcal ME. Potassium gluconate and potassium citrate in slow release tablets are preferable to potassium chloride, which is more prone to cause gastrointestinal disturbances and does not correct metabolic acidosis.

Correction of anaemia

The pathogenesis of anaemia in CRF is shown in Fig. 14.10. Although many factors may contribute, lack of renal erythropoietin production appears to play a major role and supplementation with recombinant human erythropoietin, epoetin alpha, can correct the anaemia completely.[6] Although supplementation to produce a normal red cell mass in all patients would be optimal, about 25% of cats develop an immunological response to epoetin alpha which results in development of anaemia even more profound than initial pretreatment values. Fortunately, this immunological response dissipates once epoetin alpha treatment is discontinued and cats eventually return to pretreatment levels of anaemia. Thus, treatment with epoetin alpha is best restricted to patients with profound anaemia (PCV < 20%) where correction of the anaemia is likely to have a dramatic effect. Treated cats exhibit improved appetite and activity within 24–48 hours of first administration, long before the red cell mass shows any appreciable increase. The currently recommended dose of epoetin alpha in cats is 100 u/kg bodyweight SC twice weekly until a PCV of 25–28% is achieved, which usually takes 3–4 weeks. At this point, the dose should be reduced to 100 u/kg bodyweight weekly or 50 u/kg bodyweight twice weekly to maintain red cell mass. Excessive epoetin alpha administration can induce polycythaemia and increase the chance of immunogenicity.

Management of anorexia

Rejection of therapeutic diets is one of the most frustrating aspects of managing cats with CRF. Low protein diets can be less palatable, appetite is often reduced and cats with a rigid and restricted range of tastes tend to starve rather than eat diets that could improve their metabolic status.

Gradually increasing the ratio of new diet versus original diet in the ration often allows adjustment of protein and phosphate intake to some extent. Warming the food to increase aroma and adding highly flavoured (low sodium) gravy or chicken fat can make the diet more palatable. In some instances, handfeeding encourages sufficient food intake but this strategy is only successful when owners are very painstaking and patient. As oral treatment can be stressful and worsen anorexia in some cats, medications should be formulated according to individual preference for liquid, tablets or capsules. A home-cooked diet low in protein and low in phosphate is shown in Fig. 14.11. When cats stubbornly refuse to consume all therapeutic diets, consumption of a familiar regular diet is preferable to starvation.

Anaemic cats with CRF appear to have increased appetite when treated with epoetin alpha but this drug should not be used as an appetite stimulant in the absence of anaemia. Direct appetite stimu-lants – such as diazepam given at 0.05–0.2 mg/kg bodyweight IV bid, oxazepam given at 0.2–1 mg/kg bodyweight PO sid, or flurazepam hydro-chloride given at 0.2 mg/kg bodyweight PO sid – have all been shown to be effective in cats but chronic use beyond 2–5 days is not recommended. Also, the sedative effects of these drugs can be enhanced in CRF. Corticosteroids are not recom-mended as appetite stimulants in cats with CRF because of limited effect and potential side effects.

Vomition

Cats with CRF tend to vomit. The same principles used to control vomition in ARF can be applied to CRF.

Drug dose adjustment in renal failure

Renal clearance of many drugs and drug metab-olites is reduced in CRF. In addition, changes in protein binding and disruption of the blood–brain barrier causes the effect of some drugs to be enhanced. For example, normal doses of bar-biturates cause excessive sedation. In advanced CRF, administration of drugs cleared by the kidney should be reduced by decreasing the size of each dose or increasing the interval between doses.[19] This is very important if high plasma levels of the drug are associated with adverse side effects. If possible, potentially nephrotoxic drugs (such as aminoglycosides) should not be used. In drugs cleared entirely by the kidney, a normal initial loading dose can be given and subsequent admini-stration can be adjusted according to either of

---

HOME-COOKED LOW-PROTEIN/LOW-PHOSPHORUS DIET

115 g (1/4 lb) liver
2 large eggs (100 g) hard cooked
350 g (2 cups) cooked rice with no added salt
15 g (1 tablespoon) vegetable oil
5 g (1 teaspoon) calcium carbonate

Balanced vitamin and mineral supplement for cats

Dice and braise the liver, retaining fat.
Combine all ingredients and mix well.
Add water to improve the texture and palatability.
Yield 585 g (11/4 lb); 1397 kcal/kg as fed; 4700 kcal/kg on a dry matter basis

FIG. 14.11 A home-cooked low-protein/low-phosphorus diet for cats in chronic renal failure.[11]

the following (where Scr = serum creatinine in mg/dl):

Reduced dose, with the same interval between doses:

$$Adjusted\ dose = \frac{normal\ dose}{Scr}$$

Same dose, with an increased interval between doses:

$$Adjusted\ interval = normal\ interval \times Scr$$

PROTEINURIA

Renal excretion of protein is associated with loss of selectivity of the glomerular filtration barrier. If protein loss is sufficiently great, patients develop hypoalbuminaemia and oedema with hypercholesterolaemia, i.e. the nephrotic syndrome.

Aetiology of proteinuria

Most instances of glomerular proteinuria are associated with extrarenal inflammatory conditions leading to glomerular deposition of antigen–antibody complexes where the kidney is affected as an innocent bystander (Fig. 14.12). Fortunately, the proteinuria is usually not severe enough to cause the nephrotic syndrome; progressive loss of

CAUSES OF GLOMERULAR PROTEINURIA
Associated with nephrotic syndrome

Idiopathic
   membranous glomerulonephritis
   IgG, IgA, IgM, C'$_3$
   membranoproliferative glomerulonephritis

Not associated with nephrotic syndrome
FeLV FIV polyarthritis (infectious)   e.g. *Mycoplasma gatae*, L-form bacteria systemic lupus erythematosus tumours amyloidosis pancreatitis subacute bacterial endocarditis abscess

FIG. 14.12   Causes of glomerular proteinuria.

renal function to cause CRF does not occur and the proteinuria ceases once the underlying condition is resolved. In relatively few instances, idiopathic glomerular deposition of large amounts of immune complexes causes sufficiently severe proteinuria to induce the nephrotic syndrome (e.g. membranous glomerulonephritis). Affected cats can develop progressive loss of renal function with reduced GFR and ultimately CRF. While renal amyloidosis in dogs is associated with heavy proteinuria, marked proteinuria is not common in renal amyloidosis in cats.[5]

Diagnosis of proteinuria

A protein concentration on urine dipstick of 4+ ($\geq$ 200 mg/l) in any urine, and 3+ (30 mg/l) in dilute urine when the urine sediment is benign, suggests significant proteinuria. The gold standard diagnostic test is 24-hour protein excretion: the normal rate is < 30 mg/kg bodyweight/day and for glomerular proteinuria > 150 mg/kg bodyweight/day. As collection of 24-hour urine samples is impractical in clinical patients, urine protein to creatinine ratio ($U_{Pr/Cr}$) performed on a single urine sample can be used to estimate a 24-hour protein excretion (normal: $U_{Pr/Cr} \leq 1$; glomerular proteinuria: $U_{Pr/Cr} \geq 3$). Note that when using the Coumassie brilliant blue method of protein measurement, 24-hour protein excretion (mg/kg/day) $\approx 30 \times U_{Pr/Cr}$.[12] Urinary protein is best measured when urinary tract infection and urinary haemorrhage have been controlled because urinary protein loss associated with these conditions can confuse interpretation of the results.

Once significant proteinuria is identified, a routine work-up to screen for the major known causes of glomerular disease includes: FeLV and FIV tests, antinuclear antibody (ANA), lupus erythematosus (LE) cell preparation, joint tap (polyarthritis, LE), funduscopic examination (toxoplasmosis, granulomatous lesions), lipase and amylase (chronic pancreatitis), radiographs of both body cavities (abscess or tumour), abdominal ultrasound and echocardiography (endocarditis). Indicated tests may vary depending on the presenting clinical syndrome.

Prognosis may be predicted from the immunological type, location and severity of immune complex deposition based on immunofluorescence of histological biopsy specimens. Cats with IgG and C'3 deposits confined to the glomerular capillary wall tend to live longer than those with IgM and IgA deposition and those with deposition of any immune complexes in the subepithelial region.[2] The long-term prognosis for cats with severe glomerular proteinuria is not good because they tend to become progressively more azotaemic and advance inexorably into CRF despite all treatment.

Specific management of glomerular proteinuria

Predisposing causes should be treated and eliminated if possible (Fig. 14.12). Dimethyl sulphoxide (DMSO) has beneficial effects in amyloidosis of humans where serum amyloid A levels are reduced and amyloid deposition may decrease. Experience in dogs is limited, with variable results, and there are no reports of DMSO use in renal amyloidosis in cats. Prednisolone (given at 2–4 mg/kg bodyweight PO sid) has been reported to cause remission of nephrotic syndrome in cats with idiopathic glomerulonephritis but experience is limited.[13] Protein excretion should be monitored during treatment, which should be discontinued if proteinuria is enhanced.

Nonspecific management

Low protein diets tend to reduce the degree of proteinuria in cats with glomerular proteinuria but protein intake should not be reduced below 6 g protein/100 kcal ME (about 30% protein on a dry-matter basis in usual diets). This level of protein intake still allows maximal hepatic albumin production but further protein restriction may impair this and worsen hypoalbuminaemia. Low sodium diets can lessen oedema and ascites, particularly when fed in conjunction with the use of diuretics.

Diuretics (e.g. frusemide given at 1–4 mg/kg bodyweight/day PO) can lessen oedema and ascites but conservative doses and caution are advisable, particularly in azotaemic patients. Affected animals usually have reduced GFR and may have reduced plasma volume, so that cardiovascular collapse and severe prerenal azotaemia can develop rapidly.

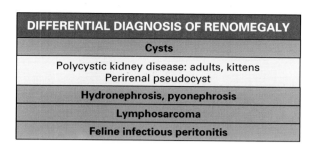

DIFFERENTIAL DIAGNOSIS OF RENOMEGALY
Cysts
Polycystic kidney disease: adults, kittens Perirenal pseudocyst
Hydronephrosis, pyonephrosis
Lymphosarcoma
Feline infectious peritonitis

FIG. 14.13   Differential diagnosis of renomegaly in the cat.

RENOMEGALY

The common causes of renomegaly in the cat are shown in Fig. 14.13.

Polycystic kidney disease

In polycystic kidney disease of adult cats, affected kidneys tend to be very large with an irregular surface. The cysts vary in size but are often large. The disease can be unilateral but is usually bilateral and affected cats develop CRF if both kidneys are affected. In unilateral disease, the affected kidney can be resected. In a congenital form reported in long-haired breeds, multiple small cysts were observed in the cortex and medulla and affected kittens died of renal failure in the first few months of life.[7]

Perirenal pseudocysts

Subcapsular or extracapsular fluid can accumulate around the kidneys, giving the impression of renomegaly. On palpation, the surface of the cyst cannot usually be distinguished from renal tissue. Intravenous pyelography and ultrasonography best demonstrate the outer cyst capsule with the smaller kidney inside. When the kidneys are very small, the combined kidney and cyst may not appear larger than a normal kidney or may even seem smaller. The disease is usually bilateral and the cause is unknown although the condition is often associated with CRF. The cyst fluid does not appear to be urine. Fluid accumulation can be prevented by surgical resection of the cyst capsule.

Hydronephrosis and pyonephrosis

Chronic obstruction to urine flow leads to hydronephrosis and, if the process is associated with infection, pyonephrosis. Affected kidneys can be very large if the disease is unilateral with normal function in the contralateral kidney. Ureteral malformation can cause congenital hydronephrosis; acquired hydronephrosis can develop from obstruction by uroliths and inadvertent placement of, or reaction to, a surgical ligature (e.g. during ovariohysterectomy). However, in many instances the aetiology is obscure. Bilateral hydronephrosis can be seen in CRF where the cause of obstruction is not identifiable.

Partial ureteral obstruction can induce polyuria because back pressure in the renal collecting ducts interferes with normal renal concentrating mechanisms. Both intravenous pyelography and ultrasonography reveal the thin outer rim of renal tissue surrounding the dilated renal pelvis. The best treatment is relief of obstruction, that can result in the return of significant renal function if instituted early enough. Unfortunately, early intervention is often not possible in unilateral hydronephrosis because affected cats remain free of clinical signs. If the cat is not azotaemic and the contralateral kidney appears to function normally on intravenous pyelography, surgical resection of the affected kidney is the best treatment for severe unilateral hydronephrosis and also for pyonephrosis.

Lymphosarcoma and feline infectious peritonitis (FIP)

Both lymphosarcoma and FIP cause bilateral enlargement of the kidneys but in most cases the degree of enlargement is not as great as that seen in polycystic kidney disease and unilateral hydronephrosis. The surfaces of affected kidneys are usually irregular because renal enlargement is not uniform. Affected animals may be azotaemic. Effective treatment of lymphosarcoma can lead to improvement in kidney function.

FELINE LOWER URINARY TRACT DISEASE

Both male and female cats frequently exhibit signs of lower urinary tract disease (LUTD) with

CAUSES OF LOWER URINARY TRACT DISEASE

Crystalluria[a]
Urolithiasis[a]
Excessive mucus production[a]
Urinary tract infection
Neoplasia
Idiopathic:
viral[b], glycosaminoglycan deficiency[b], allergic[b], immune-mediated[b]

[a] can cause obstruction
[b] relationship to LUTD currently not clear

FIG. 14.14 Causes of lower urinary tract disease in cats.

haematuria, pollakiuria, stranguria, and crying out during urination. Some cats, the vast majority of which are males, develop urethral outflow obstruction which leads to severe postrenal azotaemia and ARF if left untreated. The aetiology of LUTD in cats is shown in Fig. 14.14, and a routine diagnostic plan in Fig. 14.15.

Careful palpation of the bladder may reveal uroliths, thickened bladder wall and large masses. Urinalysis and urine culture are always best performed on specimens collected by cystocentesis (see p. 00). It is often necessary to use contrast radiography or ultrasonography to detect bladder uroliths as many have a flattened disc shape, which makes them difficult to palpate on physical examination and undetectable on plain radiographs.

The mineral composition of uroliths in cats is shown in Fig. 14.16[17] and must be determined accurately to ensure appropriate preventive measures. Crystallographic, x-ray diffraction and infra-red spectroscopy techniques are preferable to qualitative chemical analysis to determine the composition of uroliths and crystals. Most uroliths and crystals are composed of struvite,

DIAGNOSTIC TESTS FOR LUTD

Abdominal palpation
Urinalysis
Urine culture
Radiographs: plain, contrast
Tissue biopsy
Culture bladder wall
Crystal and urolith analysis

FIG. 14.15 Diagnostic tests for lower urinary tract disease in cats.

MINERAL COMPOSITION OF UROLITHS	
Mineral	%
Struvite (MgNH$_4$ PO$_4$. 6H$_2$O)	70.2
Calcium oxalate	10.6
Calcium phosphate	3.2
Uric acid and urates	5.6
Cystine	0.2
Mixed and compound	6.8
Matrix	3.3

FIG. 14.16 Mineral composition of uroliths in cats (n = 1200).

although heavy crystalluria with calcium oxalate and amorphous urates and phosphates is seen occasionally.

For management purposes, LUTD is best divided by aetiology into two broad areas: (i) caused by or associated with mineral precipitation; and (ii) not associated with mineral precipitation.

LUTD associated with mineral precipitation

Crystalluria and urolithiasis commonly induce or accompany LUTD. While a cause-and-effect relationship exists between urolithiasis and LUTD, the role of crystalluria is not so clear but large crystals may cause irritation as they pass through the urethra. Feeding a diet that prevents crystalluria will alleviate or eliminate clinical signs in a large proportion of affected cats.

Diets to prevent struvite crystalluria should be low in magnesium ($\leq$ 20 mg/100 kcal ME) and phosphorus ($\leq$ 150 mg/100 kcal ME). Urine pH should be maintained at $\leq$ 6.4 even during the postprandial alkaline tide. To achieve this, diets should be formulated with animal protein and mineral additives selected to promote formation of acidic urine. For example, MgCl$_2$ can be used instead of MgO as the magnesium source, and CaCl$_2$ instead of CaCO$_3$ as the calcium source.

Urolithiasis

Cystic uroliths commonly cause LUTD and formation of small uroliths may lead to urethral obstruction in male cats. On occasion, nephroliths may form but they do not induce LUTD.

Uroliths can be treated by medical dissolution or surgical resection. Before embarking on a dissolution protocol, the mineral composition of the urolith(s) should be identified because calcium oxalate uroliths cannot be dissolved by medical means and must be removed surgically. Supporting evidence of struvite urolithiasis includes moderate radiopacity and the presence of struvite crystals in the urine sediment. Calcium oxalate uroliths are more radio-opaque and are associated with calcium oxalate dihydrate or monohydrate crystals in urine.

Dissolution of struvite uroliths in cats can be induced by dietary management. Struvite urolithiasis in cats is not usually associated with urease-producing infection (e.g. *Staphylococcus intermedius*); however, urinalysis and, if necessary, urine culture and sensitivity should be performed to rule out concurrent infection. Concurrent antimicrobial treatment is not necessary to aid dissolution when UTI is not present but dietary inducement to dissolve struvite uroliths associated with urease-producing infections must be accompanied by continuous antimicrobial treatment. Dissolution of struvite cystic uroliths is usually achieved in 4–6 weeks and the dissolution diet should be fed for at least 30 days after uroliths are no longer visible radiographically.[15] (Nephroliths usually take longer to dissolve.) If uroliths fail to dissolve with appropriate dietary management and antimicrobial treatment, owner compliance may be poor or the uroliths may be composed of a mineral other than struvite. In such instances, surgical resection with appropriate quantitative analysis of the composition of the urolith may be the best approach.

Once uroliths have been dissolved or surgically resected, lifelong prevention strategies should be instituted based on known or suspected mineral composition. Dietary formulations (low in magnesium and phosphorus, with acidifier) to prevent struvite crystalluria have been outlined above. Prevention strategies for calcium oxalate urolithiasis and crystalluria are not established in the cat but extrapolation from data in humans and dogs suggests that a low protein diet alkalinised with potassium citrate to induce a urine pH of 7.0–7.5 is likely to be effective.

LUTD not associated with mineral precipitation

Urinary tract infection (UTI)

About 5–10% of cats with LUTD have UTI. Bacteriuria may accompany crystalluria and urolithiasis either as a cause of struvite precipitation, in the case of urease-producing bacteria, or as a secondary infection. Cats with perineal urethrostomy can be more prone to bacterial UTI when excessive blunt dissection around the penis is used to perform urethroplasty.[10] *Escherichia coli, Staphylococcus intermedius, Streptococcus* spp, and *Proteus mirabilis* are the most frequently isolated organisms. Although culture and sensitivity may be indicated in refractory infections, empirical treatment with sulpha-trimethoprim, enrofloxacin or amoxicillin with clavulanic acid is likely to be successful in more than 80% of previously untreated cats. In repeated infections, contrast radiography should be performed to identify primary underlying causes such as uroliths, neoplasia and diverticula.

Neoplasia

Bladder and urethral neoplasia is very rare in cats. Tumours have only been reported in cats older than 7 years and about 80% are malignant.[20]

The most common tumour types are shown in Fig. 14.17. Little information is available concerning treatment of urinary tract neoplasia in cats and the high percentage of malignancy suggests that the prognosis tends to be poor even if surgical resection is possible.

Idiopathic LUTD

A significant proportion of cats with LUTD continue to exhibit signs of lower urinary tract inflammation even though they are free of bacterial UTI, they are fed diets that prevent crystalluria, and radiographic studies indicate no identifiable anatomical defects or uroliths. Affected cats have haematuria, frequency and straining, and often urinate in inappropriate places. At the present time, the aetiology remains obscure. Current research investigating the role of viruses and immunologic response to endogenous Tamm-Horsfall protein is underway.

As the severity of idiopathic LUTD spontaneously waxes and wanes, many treatments have been thought to reduce clinical signs but no controlled studies have been performed to support these claims. Use of antibiotics, corticosteroids, progestagens, 50% DMSO administered intravesicularly, anticholinergic agents, diuretics, elimination diets, pentosan polysulphate (an exogenous glycosaminoglycan) and surgical placement of a copper

NEOPLASIA OF THE URINARY BLADDER			
	Number	%	Age range (years)
Epithelial			
Malignant			
transitional cell carcinoma	8	30	8-16
squamous cell carcinoma	4	15	6-15
adenocarcinoma	3	11	6-13
Nonepithelial			
Benign			
fibroma	1	(4)	8
leiomyoma	3	(11)	5-14
haemangioma	1	(4)	15
Malignant			
leiomyosarcoma	2	(7)	5-10
haemangiosarcoma	2	(7)	3
rhabdomyosarcoma (botryoid)	1	(4)	7
Lymphosarcoma			
lympho primary	1	(4)	8
lympho metastatic	1	(4)	3

Fig. 14.17 Neoplasia of the urinary bladder in 27 cats.[20]

ring into the bladder have all been tried. This wide range of treatments underscores the frustration experienced by veterinarians attempting to control a disease of unknown aetiology. Many of these treatments could be palliative and symptomatic, alleviating the clinical signs but are unlikely to address the primary cause.

Urachal diverticula

Diverticula are often observed at the position of the remnant urachus on cystograms of cats with LUTD. Development of diverticula usually reflects changes in intravesicular pressure associated with LUTD. They do not appear to cause a problem and they tend to disappear when LUTD is resolved.[14] Unless the bladder wall is thickened around the diverticulum and there is a history of recurrent UTI, resection of diverticula is not recommended.

Urethral obstruction

Urethral obstruction frequently occurs in male cats but is very rare in females. The obstructing material is usually mucus with loosely attached individual crystals but occasionally urethral obstruction is caused by mucus without crystals. The most common crystal type associated with the mucus is struvite although other minerals, such as calcium oxalate, can be involved. Formed uroliths can also cause obstruction. The common factor in the mucocrystalline plug form of urethral obstruction is mucus. Excessive mucus production or formation of abnormal mucus may play a role but the nature and cause of these changes remain unknown.

Prolonged urethral obstruction causes postrenal azotaemia with life-threatening metabolic changes. After complete obstruction for 2 days, dehydration, hyperkalaemia and metabolic acidosis become severe and the cardiotoxic effects of hyperkalaemia become life-threatening. Bradycardia, absence of a P wave, wide sine-wave QRS complexes and a 'tented' T wave are typical changes seen on ECG.

Affected cats must be handled very gently. An intravenous fluid line should be established and 2.5% dextrose in 0.45% saline should be given at a rate calculated to rehydrate the patient in 2–4 hours. Severe hyperkalaemia should be treated on an emergency basis (Fig. 14.6). Once cardiac stability has been achieved, urethral obstruction can be relieved.

Relief of obstruction

Tranquillisation is required so that the patient does not move during the procedure, e.g. with ketamine (2–10 mg IV). The lower dose is sufficient in semi-comatose cats while the high dose is necessary in metabolically normal patients. Gaseous anaesthesia is a safe alternative.

Obstructing mucocrystalline plugs are usually located in the narrow distal urethra. Larger uroliths may be located anywhere in the urethra. They tend to be more difficult to remove and may cause obstruction again after they are backflushed into the bladder.

Sometimes the obstruction can be removed by rolling the tip of the penis between the finger and thumb but this is rarely successful and urethral catheterisation is required. The penis should be retracted caudally by grasping the penile-preputial sheath while a small diameter open-ended catheter is advanced into the urethral lumen as saline is injected. The catheter should be nudged gently against the obstruction while saline is forced out of the catheter tip. Small pieces of mucocrystalline plug break off and flow out of the urethra around the catheter. Once the catheter has been advanced about 3 cm, the urethra can be clamped manually around the catheter to prevent antegrade flow of saline. Saline should then be instilled into the urethra under pressure. If the urethra is obstructed proximal to the tip of the catheter, the urethra dilates and the obstructing material is forced back into the bladder. Relatively easy retrograde passage of saline indicates that the urethra is clear. After relief of the obstruction, a well-lubricated 14 cm (5.5 inch) 3.5F catheter should be passed into the bladder. The bladder should be emptied by aspiration through the catheter then rinsed several times with 20–30 ml saline.

Catheters suitable for initial removal of obstructing material in the urethra include 2.5–2.8 cm (1–1.5 inch) 20 g over-needle catheter (with the needle removed) or 3.5F open-ended tom cat catheter. Ultrasonically vibrated needles adapted from dental scalers have also been developed. The constant fluid flow from these needles is often very effective but the contribution of the ultrasonic vibration is questionable. Extreme gentleness and care are required during initial reopening of the urethra because damage to the urethra leads to inflammation, with oedema of periurethral tissue and subsequent reobstruction. In addition, inappropriate force may cause urethral rupture. If catheterisation of the urethra is impossible, the bladder can be decompressed by cystocentesis with removal of 20–30 ml of urine using a 22 g needle. On occasion, an emergency perineal urethrostomy may be required to remove obstructing material.

When catheterisation has been achieved with minimal trauma, an indwelling urethral catheter should not be maintained because of the possibility of further urethral irritation and ascending infection. When trauma has been significant, a urethral catheter should be cross-taped and sutured in place for 24–48 hours. Suitable indwelling catheters include the 11.4 cm (4.5 inch) 3.5F tom cat catheter and the 11 cm (4.3 inch) 4F Jackson catheter. Medications to reduce urethral spasm and promote normal urination include: the α-adrenergic antagonist, phenoxybenzamine, given at 5 mg PO sid for 3–5 days to induce urethral smooth muscle relaxation; diazepam given at 2.5 mg PO bid for 3–5 days to reduce urethral striated muscle spasm, and prednisone given at 2.5 mg PO bid for 3–5 days to reduce urethral inflammation. Broad spectrum antimicrobial drugs should be administered and the indwelling catheter should remain in place for several days. Ideally, a closed urine collection system should be attached to the catheter to measure urine output and reduce the likelihood of ascending bacterial infection. Antimicrobial treatment may need to be changed when the catheter is removed because organisms resistant to the antimicrobial used during the period of catheterisation rapidly colonise the lower urinary tract. A culture and sensitivity test can aid the choice of antimicrobial drug.

Perineal urethrostomy may be necessary when excessive urethral trauma causes oedema and spasm with a cycle of recatheterisation and further urethral trauma. Perineal urethrostomy is only recommended when all attempts to establish normal urethral function have failed. A significant proportion of cats with perineal urethrostomy develop chronic LUTD due to UTI although this problem can be reduced if blunt dissection around the penis is minimised.[10]

Postobstructive diuresis

After prolonged urethral obstruction, some cats develop a postobstructive diuresis. The magnitude of diuresis may be small or massive (up to 30–50 ml/hr) and last up to 3 days. Postobstructive diuresis may be a normal response to overhydration from overzealous fluid replacement. In addition, back pressure during obstruction may cause renal collecting ducts to become unresponsive to vasopressin. During the polyuric phase, fluid therapy should prevent dehydration and diuresis associated hypokalaemia. The rate of intravenous fluid replacement should match urine production and body weight should be assessed frequently to prevent fluid overload or dehydration. Affected cats tend to become hypokalaemic during high volume diuresis and intravenous replacement fluid should be supplemented with potassium chloride to maintain a serum potassium level of greater than 3.5 mM/l (intravenous administration of potassium must not exceed 0.5 mM/kg bodyweight/hr). Once the cat is able to eat and drink, the rate of intravenous fluid administration should be reduced gradually over 12–24 hours to see if the cat becomes dehydrated. If normal hydration is maintained, intravenous fluid administration can be withdrawn.

DISORDERS OF MICTURITION

Aetiology

The lower urinary tract has two functional phases: storage and micturition. Disturbances of the storage and micturition phase lead to urination in inappropriate places and incontinence. A classification of disorders of micturition is shown in Fig. 14.18.

Considerable care should be taken to separate behavioural changes from organic disease. With behavioural changes the patient urinates in an inappropriate place but adopts a normal urination posture and urinates normally (see Chapter 7). Behavioural changes and urgency can be

DISORDERS OF MICTURITION
Storage Phase

Urgency
  inflammation of the bladder
  UTI, tumour, urolithiasis, idiopathic
Urethral sphincter incompetence
  spontaneous
    FeLV related, Manx cats
  induced
    trauma, perineal urethrostomy, bladder surgery
Atonic bladder
  overdistension due to obstruction
  sacral lesion (LMN disease)
  tail avulsion
Bypass of the bladder
  ectopic ureter
Upper motor neurone disease
  brain or spinal lesion above the sacrum

Emptying Phase

Urethral outflow obstruction
  mucocrystalline plugs
  sacral lesion, urolithiasis, stricture
  oedema, haemorrhage, inflammation (trauma)
Upper motor neurone disease (reflex dyssynergia)
  brain or spinal lesion above the sacrum

Behavioural

Threatening environment - spraying
  new house, new cat, new appliance, new child
  (pecking order change)
Unclean litter box
Senility

FIG. 14.18 Disorders of micturition – aetiological classification.

differentiated by urinalysis because urgency is usually associated with inflammation causing the appearance of erythrocytes or leukocytes in the urinary sediment. Bladder atony is usually consistent with a history of urethral outflow obstruction leading to overdistension. Abdominal palpation and radiographs reveal a large overdistended bladder.

Cerebral lesions and spinal lesions above the sacrum cause detrusor muscle contraction at reduced bladder volume and there may be little conscious control over urination. Complete neurological examination often reveals other localising signs of neurological disease. Neurological disease above the sacrum results in reflex dyssynergia where bladder contraction is not complete and flow of urine is punctuated by spasmodic contraction of the urethra.

Urethral sphincter incompetence can occur spontaneously in Manx cats. In other breeds, a large proportion of affected cats have concurrent FeLV infection but the relationship between FeLV infection and incontinence is not known.[3] Sphincter incompetence can be caused by pelvic and pudendal nerve damage due to pelvic fracture or surgical trauma such as perineal urethrostomy and cystotomy. Bladder and urethral tumours may be involved but they are rare. Sacral cord trauma secondary to tail avulsion may also result in functional urethral obstruction. Urethral outflow obstruction is most often caused by mucocrystalline plugs or uroliths. Urethral trauma leading to inflammation, haemorrhage and oedema due to passage of uroliths or traumatic catheterisation often causes temporary urethral obstruction. Rarely, urethral trauma can lead to permanent stricture formation. Ectopic ureter is uncommon in cats. Affected animals leak urine constantly or with changes in body position. If the disease is

WORK-UP FOR DISTURBANCES OF MICTURITION
Assessment of history
Age of onset Breed Previous trauma, urethral obstruction Threats in the environment Frequency of litter changes
Accurate description of the problem
Location of urination Frequency, straining, haematuria Conscious or unconscious urination
Physical examination
Bladder size, thickness, masses, uroliths, crepitus Neurological examination Clinical pathology Urinalysis, urine culture FeLV test
Radiology
Plain radiographs Cystography Retrograde urethrography IVP
Urodynamic tests
Cystometrogram Urethral pressure profile

FIG. 14.19 Comprehensive work-up for disturbances of micturition.

FIG. 14.20 Drugs used to normalise micturition.

DRUGS USED TO NORMALISE MICTURITION		
Problem	**Drug**	**Dose in Cats**
Bladder atony	bethanechol chloride	2.5-5 mg PO tid
	propranolol hydrochloride	0.2-1 mg/kg BW PO tid
Bladder spasm	atropine sulphate	0.02-0.04 mg/kg BW PO qid
	propantheline	7.5 mg PO sid-tid
Urethral incompetence	ephedrine hydrochloride	2-4 mg/kg BW PO bid-tid
	phenylpropanolamine	1.5 mg/kg BW PO tid
Urethral spasm	phenoxybenzamine	0.25-0.5 mg/kg BW PO tid-qid
		or 5 mg PO sid 3-5 days
	diazepam	2.5 mg PO bid
	dantrolene	0.5-2 mg/kg BW PO bid

unilateral, normal urination also occurs. Diagnosis is by intravenous pyelography. Thorough historical assessment is necessary to define the nature of the disturbance of micturition and clinical evaluation should be comprehensive and complete (Fig. 14.19).

Treatment

Behavioural stresses that cause inappropriate urination must be identified and eliminated. Relocation of food and litter, and separation of cats in multi-cat households will often alleviate stress and solve the problem. Clean litter is essential.

Upper motor neurone disease sufficiently severe to cause disorders of micturition usually carries a poor prognosis. Intervertebral disc disease is rare in cats, and other spinal and cerebral lesions (e.g. FIP, lymphosarcoma and other tumours of the CNS) can be difficult to diagnose antemortem. Spinal lymphosarcoma may respond to standard treatment protocols and allow improvement in disturbances of micturition.

Neurological lesions and detrusor atony can be addressed by treating the primary problem, which is rarely possible, and by giving appropriate medications to stimulate or suppress both bladder and urethral functions as necessary (Fig. 14.20). With acute functional urethral obstruction, regular catheterisation to empty the bladder until normal micturition is restored can prevent overdistension of the detrusor muscle. Overdistension with disruption of intercellular tight junctions causes permanent bladder atony.

Urethral outflow obstruction due to mucocry-

stalline plugs and uroliths is discussed above. Stricture formation presents special problems but early stricture formation in the urethra can be treated by dilation. The length of the stricture along the urethra determines prognosis: short strictures tend to respond better than long ones. Concentric catheters with a progressively wider outer diameter are suitable for dilation of mature strictures while angioplasty balloon catheters are easier to use and quite successful for treating recent strictures in which fibrous tissue is less organised.

Ectopic ureters can be treated by surgical implantation of the ureter into the bladder. Incontinence due to unilateral ectopic ureter can be treated by nephrectomy of the affected side if the kidney of the normal ureter has adequate function. Concurrent UTI should also be treated.

REFERENCES

1. Adams L.G., Polzin D.J., Osborne C.A., O'Brien T.D. (1992) Correlation of urine protein/creatinine ratio and twenty-four-hour urinary protein excretion in normal cats and cats with surgically induced chronic renal failure. *J. Vet. Int. Med.* **6**: 36–40.
2. Asther J.E., Lucke V.M., Newby T.J., Bourne F.J. (1986) The long-term prognosis of feline idiopathic membranous glomerulonephropathy. *J. Am. An. Hosp. Assoc.* **22**: 731–737.
3. Barsanti J.A., Downey R. (1984) Urinary incontinence in cats. *J. Am. Anim. Hosp. Assoc.* **20**: 979–982.
4. Burrows C.F., Bovee K.C. (1975) Metabolic changes due to experimental rupture of the canine urinary bladder. *Am. J. Vet. Res.* **35**: 1083–1088.

5. Chew D.J., DiBartola S.P., Boyce J.T., Gasper P.W. (1982) Renal amyloidosis in related Abyssinian cats. *J. Am. Vet. Med. Assoc.* **181**: 139–142.

6. Cowgill L.D., Feldman B., Levy J., James K. (1990) Efficacy of recombinant human erythropoietin (r-HuEPO) for anemia in dogs and cats with renal failure (abstr.) *Proc. 8th ACVIM Forum*, p 1128, Washington, DC.

7. Crowell W.A., Hubbell J.J., Riley J.C. (1979) Polycystic renal disease in related cats. *J. Am. Vet. Med. Assoc.* **175**: 286–288.

8. Finco D.R., Crowell W.A., Barsanti J.A. (1985) Effects of three diets on dogs with induced chronic renal failure. *Am. J. Vet. Res.* **46**: 646–653.

9. Grauer G.F., Thrall M.A. (1982) Ethylene glycol (antifreeze) poisoning in the dog and cat. *J. Am. Anim. Hosp. Assoc.* **18**: 492–497.

10. Griffin D.W., Gregory C.R. (1992) Prevalence of bacterial urinary tract infection after perineal urethrostomy in cats. *J. Am. Vet. Med. Assoc.* **200(5)**: 681–684.

11. Lewis L.D., Morris M.L. Jr, Hand M.S. (1987) *Small Animal Clinical Nutrition III*, Mark Morris Associates, Topeka, Kansas.

12. Nagode L.A., Chew D.J. (1991) The use of calcitriol in treatment of renal disease in the dog and cat. *Proc. Purina International Nutrition Symposium*, pp 39–49, Orlando, Florida.

13. Nash A.S., Wright, N.G., Spencer A.J., Thompson H., Fischer E.W. (1979) Membranous nephropathy in the cat: A clinical and pathological study. **Vet. Rec. 105**: 71–77.

14. Osborne C.A., Johnston G.R., Caywood D.C., O'Brien T.D., Kruger D.J., Lulich J.P. (1986) New insights into management of feline urinary tract disease. *Proc. 4th Annual Vet. Med. Forum*, pp 4/7–10, Washington, DC.

15. Osborne C.A., Lulich J.P., Kruger J.M., Polzin D.J., Johnston G.R., Kroll R.A. (1990) Medical dissolution of feline struvite urocystoliths. *J. Am. Vet. Med. Assoc.* **196**: 1053–1063.

16. Osborne C.A., Polzin D.J., Abdullahi S., Klausner J.S., Rogers Q.R. (1982) Role of diet in management of feline chronic polyuric renal failure: current status. *J. Am. Anim. Hosp. Assoc.* **18**: 11–20.

17. Osborne C.A., Sanna J.J., Unger L.K., Clinton C.W., Davenport M.P. (1989) Analysing the mineral composition of uroliths from dogs, cats, horses, cattle, sheep, goats, and pigs. *Vet. Med.* **8**: 750–764.

18. Polzin D.J. (1988) The influence of egg protein in reduced protein diets designed for dogs with renal failure. *J. Vet. Intern. Med.* **2**: 15–21.

19. Rivière J.E. (1984) Calculation of dosage regimens of antimicrobial drugs in animals with renal and hepatic dysfunction. *J. Am. Vet. Med. Assoc.* **185**: 1094–1097.

20. Schwarz P.D., Greene R.W., Patniak A.K. (1985) Urinary bladder tumors in the cat: A review of 27 cases. *J. Am. Anim. Hosp. Assoc.* **21**: 237–245.

21. Thornhill J.A., Riviere J.E. (1983) Peritonitis associated with peritoneal dialysis: Diagnosis and treatment. *J. Am. Vet. Med. Assoc.* **182**: 721–724.

FURTHER READING

Barsanti J.A., Finco D.R. (1986) Feline urinary incontinence. In: Kirk R.W. (ed.) *Current Veterinary Therapy IX*, pp 1159–1163, W.B. Saunders, Philadelphia.

Chew D.J., DiBartola S.D., Fenner W.R. (1986) Pharmacological manipulation of urination. In: Kirk R.W. (ed.) *Current Veterinary Therapy IX*, pp 1207–1212, W.B. Saunders, Philadelphia.

Fettman M.J. (1989) Feline kaliopenic polymyopathy/nephropathy syndrome. *Vet. Clin. North Am. [Small Anim. Pract.]* **19**(3): 415–432.

Moreau P. (1982) Neurogenic disorders of micturition in the dog and cat. *Compend. Contin. Educ. Pract. Vet.* **4**: 12–22.

Polzin D.J., Osborne C.A., Adams L.D., O'Brien T.D. (1989) Dietary management of canine and feline chronic renal failure. *Vet. Clin. North Am. [Small Anim. Prac.]* **19**(3): 539–560.

15

Disorders of the Reproductive System

TIMOTHY J. GRUFFYDD-JONES

In veterinary practice, the most common experience concerning the feline genital tract is in its removal. However, there is now greater interest in the breeding of pedigree cats and the problems that occasionally arise have led to more frequent requests to investigate reproductive failure. The last decade saw a considerable advance in our knowledge of the reproductive endocrinology of cats but causes of reproductive failure are still poorly understood. The husbandry systems applied to pedigree cats inevitably expose these animals to risk of infectious agents that are an important consideration in reproductive failure. Until recently, FeLV was undoubtedly the most important cause of feline infertility, but breeders have now largely eradicated FeLV from the pedigree population in many countries through self-imposed control measures. Other causes of reproductive failure have emerged to take the place of FeLV.

BASIC REPRODUCTIVE DATA

Basic normal reproductive patterns are outlined in Fig. 15.1. Pedigree cats show marked differences in many of the reproductive parameters compared with free-living mixed breed cats and, whilst exceptions exist, inter-breed variations are much more marked than intra-breed variations. These must be taken into account when considering whether the reproductive efficiency of an individual of a particular breed is satisfactory. For example, puberty at fifteen months would be late for a Siamese queen but not abnormal for a Persian. Similarly an average litter size of three would be within the breed variation for a Persian but significantly low for a Siamese or Burmese.

The evaluation of any reproductive problem should begin with a detailed reproductive history for not only the infertile cat but also all the other cats within the cattery. Comparisons of reproductive histories will enable assessment of whether a

---

BASIC REPRODUCTIVE PATTERNS

Type of reproductive cycle
  Seasonally polyoestrus; however, many pedigree cats show no period of anoestrus

Puberty
  Domestic mixed breed cats 5-8 months
  4-18 months in pedigrees
  Correlates with body weight
  Later in males than females
  Influenced by season of birth

Oestrous cycle duration
  Domestic mixed breed cats around 3 weeks
  Very variable in pedigree cats - orientals tend to show short, interoestrual periods
  Some other breeds, such as Persians, may show less frequent oestrus

Oestrus
  Domestic mixed breed cats - around 7 days
  Duration very variable in pedigree cats
  Tends to be longer in orientals - extended periods of oestrous behaviour are common

Ovulation
  Induced ovulator
  Responsiveness to coitus as a stimulation for ovulation is variable and influenced by day of oestrus and number of matings
  Ovulation around 36 hours after mating

Gestation
  Around 64 days but can vary from 59-70 days from time of mating

Litter size
  Domestic mixed breed cats - usually 4. Pedigree cats - more variable, frequently varying between 2 and 8.

FIG. 15.1 Basic reproductive patterns.

colony problem exists or the infertility is restricted to individuals. The initial history should include an assessment of any other disease problems and of the management – which is most satisfactorily investigated by visiting the cattery.

Breeders may be prepared to accept difficulty in breeding from one queen only and most requests to investigate reproductive failure originate from catteries experiencing difficulties with more than one cat. This does not necessarily point to an infectious or husbandry problem. Frequently cats in multicat pedigree households are related and therefore the possibility of an inherited reproductive problem should be considered. In addition, the reproductive management is likely to be consistent for all the queens in a cattery (for example, extensive use of progestagens) and this may be a predisposing factor in the development of reproductive problems.

REPRODUCTIVE FAILURE IN QUEENS

The first step in the investigation of reproductive failure in queens is to establish the stage in the reproductive process at which the problem arises.

The initial assessment is generally straightforward and is summarised in Fig. 15.2.

Failure of oestrus

The investigation of a queen failing to show oestrus is summarised in Fig. 15.3. The initial consideration for maiden queens is whether adequate time has been allowed for puberty, taking breed differences into account. The management of the cattery should be investigated with particular attention to lighting, as the seasonal nature of the reproductive cycle in free-living cats is dependent primarily on daylight length. Most pedigree cats are exposed to artificial lighting, that will abolish the period of anoestrus. A constant 14 hours of light will ensure reproductive activity.

The possibility of pseudopregnancy should be considered. Neutered toms, even if castrated before puberty, will frequently mount and mate with

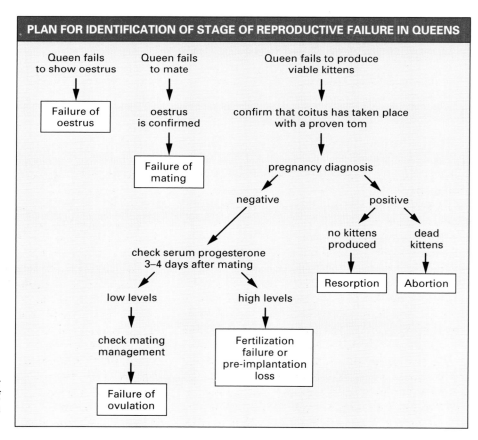

FIG. 15.2 Plan for identification of stage of reproductive failure in queens.

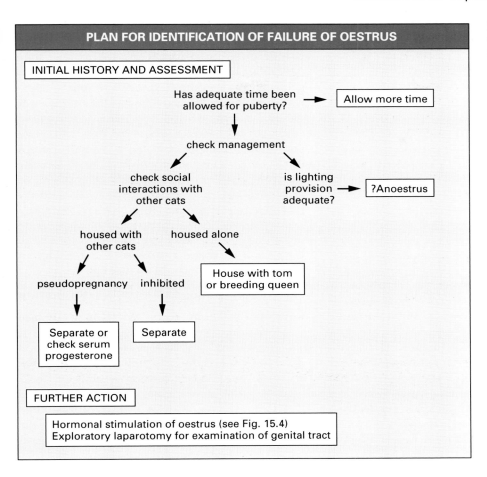

FIG. 15.3 Plan for investigation of failure of oestrus.

queens coming into oestrus. This may inhibit the normal display of oestrus and no oestrous behaviour is noted by the breeder. Mounting of queens by other queens in the same group may also lead to ovulation and pseudopregnancy.

Serum progesterone estimations will confirm whether or not pseudopregnancy is present. A progesterone concentration in excess of 10 nmol/l indicates active luteal tissue which, in the absence of pregnancy, indicates pseudopregnancy. If the progesterone concentration is low, the test should be repeated 3–4 weeks later in case the first sample had been collected just as a pseudopregnancy ended. If pseudopregnancy is confirmed, removal of toms from the group or isolating the affected queens should lead to a resumption of normal oestrous activity. (Adoption of this approach avoids the need to determine progesterone concentrations.)

Social interactions can play an important part in either stimulating or inhibiting the oestrual display. Even in the absence of oestrous behaviour, normal cycles of follicular activity are displayed by most queens and can be identified by vaginal cytological examination. Reluctant queens, particularly if housed in isolation, may show more interest in oestrus if housed with a stud tom, or at least within sight, smell and sound. An alternative strategy is to introduce the queen to a group of other active, breeding queens. In this situation synchrony of oestrus frequently develops and may stimulate oestrus in a previously reluctant queen. In contrast, oestrous behaviour may be suppressed in a timid, subordinate queen housed with a group

---

TREATMENT REGIMENS FOR INDUCTION OF OESTRUS

Pregnant Mare Serum Gonadotrophin (PMSG)
Days 1 and 2   100i.u.
Days 3 - 5   50i.u.

Follicle Stimulating Hormone (FSH)
2 mg daily for 5 days

FIG. 15.4   Treatment regimens for induction of oestrus.

of other cats. Such queens may show normal oestrous behaviour if housed individually.

If management problems have been ruled out, two major avenues of investigation remain. Hormonal induction of oestrus can be considered and regimes for this purpose are outlined in Fig. 15.4. They have proved reliable for use in mixed breed cats but the response in pedigree cats is more unpredictable. Generally queens of oriental breeds appear to be more responsive and may show superovulation, whereas Persians may be less responsive. The dosage may require adjustment accordingly. Underdosage is ineffective whereas overdosage carries the risk of superovulation and the possible development of ovarian cysts. An alternative strategy is to examine the genital tract at either laparotomy or laparoscopy. Congenital agenesis of part of the genital tract, including the ovaries, can occur but is not common.

Failure of mating

The stress induced by travelling and a change of environment may inhibit oestrous behaviour in queens transported to the stud tom for mating purposes as soon as oestrus is identified. Most queens will resume oestrous behaviour within a short period once adjusted to the new environment, although a small proportion fail to do so. This problem can be circumvented by rehousing the queen with or in close proximity to the selected stud tom in advance of anticipated oestrus to allow her time to settle. An alternative strategy is to transport the tom to the queen but many pedigree stud toms become conditioned to a particular environment and routine for mating, and are inhibited if moved to unfamiliar surroundings.

Oestrous behaviour is generally very characteristic. As it appears suddenly, with no distinctive preceding phase of pro-oestrus and minimal changes in the external appearance of the genitalia, there is little difficulty in identifying the optimal time for mating and acceptance of the tom. However, some queens may show extended periods of apparent oestrous behaviour that persist despite evidence of decline of follicular activity. In particular, some queens develop prolonged, more frequent oestrous periods if left unmated for several oestrous cycles. Vaginal cytology can be used to identify the true period of oestrus when mating should be accepted, but collection of vaginal smears may stimulate premature ovulation. Finally, mate preference is an explanation for failure to mate offered by some breeders and this possibility should not be discounted.

Failure to produce live kittens after mating

The investigation of queens failing to produce viable kittens after appearing to have mated is summarised in Fig. 15.5. A key to the investigation of such cases is to ascertain if ovulation has occurred. This can be determined readily by checking blood progesterone concentrations shortly (>3 days) after mating. A high level of progesterone (>10 nmol/1) demonstrates active luteal tissue whereas baseline progesterone concentrations (<3 nmol/1) indicate failure of ovulation.

Failure of ovulation

The most likely explanation for failure of ovulation is some deficiency of mating. Firstly, was the queen simply mounted by the tom with no coitus taking place? Close observation of mating is required to check for this possibility. The queen shows characteristic post-coital behaviour, often striking out at the tom as he dismounts and then violently rolling and squirming on her back before licking at her vulva. If this reaction is not observed, it is likely that coitus has not occurred. If in doubt, collect a vaginal smear shortly after mating to check for the presence of sperm.

If coitus can be confirmed, consider the mating management. Individual sensitivity of the ovulatory response varies. The number of matings may be an important factor and about a third of queens fail to ovulate after a single mating. Multiple matings

INVESTIGATION OF FAILURE TO PRODUCE LIVE KITTENS

Failure of ovulation

1. Check mating
   Is coitus occurring?
   Does the queen show a post-coital reaction?
   Vaginal smear for sperm
2. Check mating management
   Are multiple matings taking place within a short period?
3. Is the queen in 'true' oestrus?
   Check vaginal cytology
4. Consider hormonal treatment with eCG or LHRH

Fertilisation failure/pre-implantation loss

1. Has a proven tom been used?
2. Exploratory laparotomy 3-4 days after mating - collect and assess ova

Resorption and abortion

1. Check management, particularly diet
   Screen for taurine deficiency
2. Check for infectious diseases
   Screen for FeLV
   Is there any history of conjunctivitis?
   Screen for chlamydial infection
3. Check for endometritis

   Vaginal discharge   Vaginal discharge
          ↓   ↓
       Present   Absent
          ↓   ↓
   Trial therapy with prostaglandins   Uterine biopsy
4. Habitual resorption or abortion
   Monitor serum progesterone concentrations
   Check foetal numbers
   Progesterone implant

Fig. 15.5 Investigation of failure to produce live kittens.

may be required to ensure that such individuals ovulate successfully. The timing of the matings is also important and the receptivity of the queen may vary according to the day of oestrus. The time course of luteinising hormone (LH) release in response to a single mating is fairly short: maximal concentrations are achieved within 90 minutes and levels often fall to baseline by 8 hours. It may therefore also be important that the multiple matings take place within a short period. The practice adopted by some breeders of immediately removing the tom after a single, supervised mating may therefore lead to failure of ovulation and should be avoided. It is preferable to leave the queen and tom together throughout her period of oestrus to allow 'natural' multiple matings to take place.

If a queen fails to ovulate despite satisfactory mating management, hormonal supplementation to facilitate ovulation can be considered and 250 i.u. equine chorionic gonadotrophin (eCG) is administered. The treatment should be given close to a natural mating.

Fertilisation failure and pre-implantation loss

Pre-implantation loss may be associated with chronic endometritis (see later) but apart from this, neither of these two forms represents a significant cause of reproductive failure. The phenomenon of induced ovulation safeguards against asynchrony between deposition of sperm and ovulation. This is an important factor in contributing to the very high fertilisation rate in this species and fertilisation failure is rare. In any event, investigation generally necessitates specialised expertise and is beyond the scope of practice. It involves laparotomy for collection of eggs from the oviducts within the first 4 days of mating with a proven stud tom, or shortly afterwards from the uterus. The eggs can be checked for successful fertilisation and for morphological abnormalities. Diseases of the oviducts are rare in cats but laparotomy provides the opportunity for a gross examination of these structures, particularly to check for adhesions, which are found on rare occasions.

Pregnancy failure – resorption and abortion

Late pregnancy failures in the form of abortion, and particularly resorption, are the most common forms of reproductive failure in cats. Abortion may be self-evident but may pass unnoticed if the foetuses are eaten by the queen, or by other cats in the household. Resorption may be accompanied by a bloody vaginal discharge which may lead the breeder to the mistaken belief that abortion has occurred.

Resorption and abortion occur after implantation and therefore pregnancy diagnosis is the key to their identification. This procedure should be undertaken for all queens in catteries with reproductive problems. Pregnancy diagnosis is most often performed by abdominal palpation at around 4 weeks after mating. It is helpful to attempt to assess the number of foetuses; however, it may be difficult to do this accurately although it will usually be possible to make an assessment of whether a normal, low or high number is present. Pregnancy diagnosis can also be performed using ultrasound scanning. It may be possible to assess foetal viability by detecting foetal movements or heartbeats.

Infectious diseases

Several potential causes of resorption and abortion can be confirmed or eliminated at an early stage in investigation, particularly through screening for infectious diseases. If the breeder does not maintain an FeLV-free colony through regular screening, the cats should be tested. The prevalence of FeLV in pedigree cats has been greatly reduced by general implementation of the test and removal system by breeders and infection is now uncommon in this group. Nevertheless FeLV is a potentially important cause of pregnancy failure: it most often causes resorption at around 5–7 weeks of pregnancy with the sudden appearance of a pink or bloody vaginal discharge and reduction in abdominal size. Abdominal palpation will reveal small, irregular, soft 'doughy' conceptual swellings. Less commonly abortion occurs with passage of foetuses which have died at differing stages of gestation. If unrecognised and the queen is rebred again, the reproductive failure may occur earlier with each succeeding pregnancy and may eventually lead to preimplantation loss.

The role of viruses other than FeLV is less clear. Although clinically affected queens may abort, there is no convincing evidence to suggest that asymptomatic infections or carrier status cause reproductive failure. Abortion has been noted in some FIV-infected queens but it is not clear whether this was coincidental. In any event the prevalence of FIV is very low in pedigree cats.

Although *Chlamydia psittaci* has not been confirmed as a cause of reproductive failure, there is strong circumstantial evidence to implicate this organism in cases of abortion. This is based on frequent association between abortion and recent conjunctivitis or confirmed chlamydia infection in the queen, consistent isolation of chlamydia from the vagina of infected queens and occasional isolation from the aborted foetus (T.J. Gruffydd-Jones and D. Harbour, unpublished observations). Special attention should be paid to any affected queens or other cats in the household with a recent history of conjunctivitis which suggests the possibility of chlamydial infection. Infertile queens can be screened readily by determining serological chlamydia titres, high titres ($\geqslant 1.640$) indicating active or recent infection. Prolonged systemic treatment for around 4 to 6 weeks with oxytetracycline or doxycycline may eliminate *Chlamydia psittaci*. Treatment of all the cats in the household is advisable although the possibility of teeth discoloration as a side effect of systemic treatment of young kittens or pregnant queens must be considered.

Management

The second line of investigation that should be followed during the initial assessment of a resorption or abortion problem is to assess management in the cattery. In particular the diet should be investigated for the possibility of taurine deficiency. The importance of taurine deficiency as a cause of naturally occurring reproductive failure is not known but there is evidence from experimental studies that feeding a taurine deficient diet may lead to infertility. This may take the form of poor viability of kittens or birth of stillborn foetuses, abortion, resorption or earlier pregnancy failure. The taurine content of reputable commercial diets is monitored carefully but deficiencies may arise if a significant proportion of the diet is home-prepared (see Chapter 3).

Endometritis

The endometritis complex is now the most important diagnosed cause of reproductive failure in queens. It leads most often to resorption but may also cause birth of stillborn kittens, abortion or in severe cases pre-implantation loss. A history of a vaginal discharge unrelated to the immediate post-puerperal period should raise suspicion of endometritis, which should be investigated. Confirmation of diagnosis depends on histological assessment of uterine biopsies collected by full-thickness wedge biopsy at laparotomy. Vaginal swabs are of no value in diagnosis because the organisms involved are secondary opportunists that constitute part of the normal vaginal flora and it is impossible to interpret the significance of isolates. However, vaginal smears may be of value in confirming a neutrophilic preponderance in the discharge. In cases with a history of vaginal discharges, once the more readily diagnosable causes of pregnancy failure outlined above (particularly the infectious agents) have been discounted, trial therapy may be preferred by the breeder to confirmation of diagnosis by uterine biopsy.

In many cases of endometritis there is no reported vaginal discharge. Uterine biopsy is an important priority in such cases and is preferable to trial therapy in this situation. If the uterus shows severe gross enlargement, the prognosis for future successful breeding is guarded and ovariohysterectomy may be indicated. Histological examination of the uterus not only enables confirmation of endometritis but also allows some assessment of

the severity of the lesions and the likelihood of response to treatment.

It is not uncommon for multiple cases of endometritis to occur in the same household. This may lead to the misconception that the condition results from a primary bacterial infection and that a stud tom has played a role in its transmission. A more likely explanation is that the system of management predisposes the cats to developing endometritis. Repeated progestagenic dominance is the primary aetiological factor and either frequent use of progestagens or repeated pseudopregnancies increase the risk of endometritis developing. It is also possible that hereditary factors may influence susceptibility to endometritis and this may contribute to appearance of multiple cases in catteries where some of the individuals are related.

Prostaglandins are indicated for the treatment of endometritis. Various dosage regimes have been recommended. Treatment is usually given daily or every other day for up to 10 days. Initial treatment is PGF2α at a dosage of around 20–50 μg/kg SC increasing to 200–500 μg/kg. These drugs are generally well tolerated by cats although they are not licensed for use in this species in some countries. Their beneficial action is mediated through their ecbolic effect and prostaglandins do not appear to have a marked luteolytic action in cats. Broad spectrum antibiotics are generally given, although it is not clear if these have any beneficial effect. As the condition takes some time to resolve, prolonged antibiotic therapy is likely to be required if this is to be of any benefit.

The queen should be allowed at least one oestrus unmated before she is bred again, and it is important to ensure that ovulation and consequent progestational dominance are avoided by preventing mounting or mating of the queen by castrated toms or other cats maintained in the same group. It is also vital to avoid the use of progestagens in queens with a history of endometritis.

Some queens will breed again successfully following this management. The prospects for future breeding probably depend on the duration of the endometritis: the changes become irreversible in long-standing cases. In severe cases, particularly if untreated, the condition may progress to pyometra. In such cases the gross distension of the uterus with exudate is readily palpable and may lead to marked abdominal enlargement. Despite the severity of the condition, affected queens may be remarkably bright, still eating and free of any signs attributable to toxaemia. Medical treatment is unlikely to be effective in cases of advanced pyometra and ovariohysterectomy is indicated.

Hormone imbalances

There is little evidence to indicate that hormonal imbalances are a significant cause of reproductive failure in cats. Progesterone deficiency is blamed as a cause of habitual resorption or abortion but with little supportive evidence. Diagnosis of progesterone deficiency necessitates serial serum progesterone assay to document subnormal concentrations. Maximum luteal activity generally peaks between days 8–30 of pregnancy with progesterone concentrations of around 70–80 nmol/l that are maintained until just prior to parturition. Luteal regression occurs around days 45–50 of pregnancy, the foetoplacental units producing progesterone to maintain pregnancy during the latter stages. Progesterone deficiency is generally attributed to inadequate luteal function and therefore progesterone concentrations should be monitored from around 3–6 weeks. Inadequate progesterone deficiency at a later stage (after days 45–50) indicates inadequate foetoplacental production and may reflect the presence of only one or two foetuses. Unless prior pregnancy diagnosis has indicated a larger number of foetuses, this points to a low ovulatory rate. Although progesterone supplementation may allow such a pregnancy to be maintained, genetic factors are likely to dictate ovulatory rate and therefore the justification for treatment is questionable. Progesterone supplementation can be achieved in queens with luteal inadequacy by implanting a 10 mg progesterone implant within the first fortnight of pregnancy. This must be removed several days before the anticipated day of parturition.

REPRODUCTIVE FAILURE IN TOMS

The investigation of reproductive failure in toms is summarised in Fig. 15.6. The first step is to establish whether there is a failure to mate or an inability to produce kittens. In most cases the

---

INVESTIGATION OF REPRODUCTIVE FAILURE IN TOMS
Lack of libido
1. Check genitalia: penile hair ring persistent frenulum May show interest in females and mount but no coitus takes place 2. History/management Stress factors Change of environment 3. Unproven toms Onset of puberty Check serum testosterone concentrations Chromosomal karyotyping
Infertility
1. Check management: ? proven queens mated ? adequate matings 2. Check for general health 3. Semen collection 4. Chromosomal karyotyping

Fig. 15.6   Plan for investigation of reproductive failure in toms.

differentiation is clearly evident but close observation of mating may be necessary in some cases to determine whether coitus is taking place or the tom is only mounting the queen.

Failure to mate

The initial clinical examination should include a detailed inspection of the external genitalia. This will reveal any of the rare physical obstructions to mating, such as penile hair rings or persistence of the frenulum causing deviation of the penis. In such cases the tom may be observed to have normal libido and will mount the queen but show reluctance to proceed with coitus.

A lack of libido is a more likely reason for failure to mate and such toms show disinterest in oestrous queens. The most important cause of lack of libido in toms which have previously bred successfully is some psychological or stress factor. Toms can become strongly conditioned to mating in a particular pen. Libido can be readily inhibited if the tom is moved to an unfamiliar environment. Libido will usually be regained once the tom has had an opportunity to become accustomed to his new surroundings. Libido can also be inhibited in a young inexperienced tom after a 'difficult' mating with an aggressive queen showing an extreme 'rage reaction' as part of her post-coital behaviour. Such toms may be encouraged to mate again if care is taken to select docile, co-operative queens.

Allowance for adequate time for puberty must be made for toms who have never bred previously. Toms of some breeds, such as Persians, may not mature until nearly 2 years of age. Occasionally toms will show delayed puberty if maintained in isolation but this can be rectified readily by housing the tom with one or more breeding females. Failure of libido may also reflect some inherent endocrine disorder that may be identified by hormonal testing. Testosterone concentrations have not been well characterised in normal cats.

Chromosomal abnormalities may cause infertility. Although probably rare, they are readily recognisable in tortoiseshell male cats due to sex linkage of the orange gene (which is responsible for the tortoiseshell coat pattern). This is carried on the X chromosome and therefore heterozygosity for the gene is not possible in a normal male. Similar chromosomal abnormalities almost certainly occur in tom cats with other coat colour patterns. Cytogenetic analysis is not generally available but should be considered in the investigation of infertile toms, particularly if they fail to develop normal secondary male sex characteristics such as thickened jowls, penile barbs and a pungent odour to the urine.

Failure to produce kittens

Several points must be established before a tom should be investigated for infertility. It is important that he has been tried with a number of proven queens from separate households. The mating management must have been such as to ensure that the queens have had every opportunity to ovulate. Matings should have been observed and if there is any doubt as to whether coitus occurred the queens should be checked for ovulation a few days after mating by determining serum progesterone concentrations (see earlier).

Inadequate semen quality is the most probable explanation for failure to sire kittens. Techniques have been developed for semen collection involving electroejaculation[3,4] and the use of an artificial vagina[5,6] but require specialised expertise and are not generally available. Normal values for semen are shown in Fig. 15.7. The investigation of this form of infertility is aimed most practically at identifying subclinical disease that may be impairing spermatogenesis. There may be an impression of reduction in testicular size and abnormal testicular consistency, although this may be difficult to assess accurately on palpation. The prospects for successful breeding are much better for a tom showing infertility of this type who has bred successfully previously, and in such cases the loss of fertility may be only temporary. The outlook is much less favourable for an unproven tom.

MISCELLANEOUS REPRODUCTIVE CONDITIONS

Misalliance

Various hormonal treatments for prevention of pregnancy after mismating have been reported and these are summarised in Fig. 15.8, but most of them have not been evaluated adequately for either efficacy or safety. Serial injections of oestradiol have been demonstrated to prevent implantation by prolonging oviduct transport of the ova. If the queen is required for future breeding it may be preferable to allow her to carry her litter to term or, if not, to carry out ovariohysterectomy during early pregnancy.

SEMEN CHARACTERISTICS IN NORMAL TOMS		
Semen volume (ml)	Sperm count	Motility (%)
0.01–0.5	3–130×10^6	35–100

FIG. 15.7   Semen characteristics in normal toms.

TREATMENT REGIMENS FOR MISALLIANCE

Stilboestrol
    2 mg on days 2,3,7 and 10 after mating
Oestradiol benzoate
    0.5-1 mg 2-3 days after mating
Oestradiol cyprionate
    0.125-0.25 mg 2 days after mating
Megoestrol acetate
    2 mg within 2 days of mating

FIG. 15.8   Treatment regimens for misalliance.

Uterine torsion

Uterine torsion is a rare complication of pregnancy. It may cause an acute, life-threatening toxaemia but more commonly results in mummification of the incarcerated foetuses. After parturition the retained, mummified foetuses are still readily palpable.

Mammary hyperplasia

Fibrous hyperplasia of the mammary glands occurs occasionally either as a natural condition in pregnant queens or in cats of any sex following progestagen treatment. All the mammae are generally involved, becoming grossly enlarged and oedematous. In severe cases ulceration of the overlying skin occurs. The condition will resolve once the pregnancy ends (or is terminated prematurely) or following cessation of progestagen therapy. The main importance of the condition is in differentiation from mammary neoplasia.

Mastitis

Acute mastitis with abscessation and systemic signs is uncommon. It generally responds rapidly to antibiotic treatment and poulticing of the affected mammae.

REFERENCES

1. Davidson A.P., Feldman E.C., Nelson R.W. (1992) Treatment of pyometra in cats using PgF$_{2\alpha}$: 21 cases (1982–1990). *JAVMA* **200**; 825–828
2. Herron M.A., Sis R.F. (1974) Ovarian transport in the cat and the effect of estrogen administration. *Am. J. Vet. Res.* **35**: 1277
3. Pineda M.H., Dooley M.P., Martin P.A. (1984) Long-term study on the effects of electroejaculation on seminal characteristics of the domestic cat. *Am. J. Vet. Res.* **45**: 1038.
4. Platz C.C., Seager S.W.J. (1978) Semen collection by electroejaculation in the domestic cat. *JAVMA* **173**: 1353
5. Platz C.C., Wildt E.E., Seager S.W.J. (1978) Pregnancy in the domestic cat after artificial insemination with previously frozen spermatozoa. *J. Reprod. Fertil.* **5**: 279
6. Sojka N.J., Jennings L.L., Hamner, C.E. (1970) Artificial insemination in the cat (*Felis catus*). *Lab. Anim. Care* **20**: 198

16

Disorders of the Metabolic and Endocrine Systems

MARK E. PETERSON AND THOMAS K. GRAVES

Metabolic and endocrine diseases have become an important aspect of feline medicine. Disorders such as hyperthyroidism and, to a lesser extent, diabetes mellitus have been well characterised in the veterinary literature and appear quite commonly in feline practice. Less common disorders such as acromegaly, hyperadrenocorticism and hypoadrenocorticism have been recognised more recently. While these diseases may be quite rare, it is likely that they will be recognised more frequently as knowledge and expertise increase among the practitioners of feline medicine.

The historical, physical examination and biochemical findings in cats with endocrine disorders are wide-ranging and reflect the multitude of biological derangements caused by hormonal abnormalities. With that in mind, presentation of a cat with signs of multisystemic disease should raise an index of clinical suspicion of an underlying endocrinopathy. The clinical signs of endocrine disease are often quite vague and diagnosis can be a challenge. This chapter will discuss separately diseases of the pituitary, thyroid, parathyroid and adrenal glands and of the endocrine pancreas. It is important to appreciate, however, that clinical signs of these diseases often overlap.

DISORDERS OF THE PITUITARY GLAND

Primary disorders of the pituitary gland are rare in the cat. Those that are reported are primarily related to neoplasia (almost exclusively adenomas) of the pars distalis or pars intermedia. Pituitary dwarfism (growth hormone deficiency) has not been reported.

Acromegaly

Chronic hypersecretion of growth hormone (GH) results in acromegaly, characterised by overgrowth of connective tissue, bone and viscera. In the cat, as in man, acromegaly is most often caused by a GH-secreting tumour of the pituitary gland. In contrast to the dog, in which progestagen treatment or the increased circulating progesterone concentrations that occur during dioestrus can stimulate pituitary GH overproduction (without the development of a pituitary tumour), progestagens do not appear to stimulate GH secretion in the cat.

Clinical features

As in man, feline acromegaly appears to be associated with middle or old age. All reported cases of feline acromegaly have been mixed breed cats (domestic short- and long-hair) and the great majority have been males, which suggests a sex predilection.

From Fig. 16.1, which gives the frequency of clinical and laboratory findings in cats with acromegaly, it can be seen that the most commonly recognised clinical manifestation is insulin-resistant diabetes mellitus. Growth hormone displays powerful diabetogenic activity, mainly by inducing peripheral insulin resistance. Cats with acromegaly exhibit severe, persistent hyperglycaemia which is relatively refractory to insulin therapy and can only be controlled with extremely large doses of exogenous insulin (30–130 U/day of an intermediate or long-acting insulin). Therefore, acromegaly should be considered as an underlying cause of insulin resistance, especially in male cats. Despite the presence of such uncontrolled diabetes mellitus, the development of ketoacidosis is rare in cats with acromegaly.

The other three body systems that are commonly affected are the cardiac, renal and skeletal systems. Thus, development of cardiomyopathy,

CLINICAL AND LABORATORY FINDINGS IN ACROMEGALY	
	No. of cats (%)
Clinical Findings:	
Polyuria/polydipsia	14/14 (100)
Polyphagia	14/14 (100)
Hepatomegaly	14/14 (100)
Cardiomegaly	12/14 (86)
Renomegaly	11/14 (79)
Prognathia inferior	10/14 (71)
Heart murmur	9/14 (64)
Weight gain	8/14 (57)
Weight loss	8/14 (57)
Large head	8/14 (57)
Renal failure	7/14 (50)
Pot belly	7/14 (50)
Congestive heart failure	6/14 (43)
Spondylosis	6/14 (43)
Arthropathy	6/14 (43)
Large tongue	3/14 (21)
CNS signs	2/14 (14)
Laboratory Findings:	
Hyperglycaemia/glycosuria	14/14 (100)
Proteinuria	9/14 (64)
Hyperproteinaemia	8/14 (57)
Azotaemia	7/14 (50)
Hypercholesterolaemia	6/14 (43)
Hyperphosphataemia	6/14 (43)
Erythrocytosis	5/14 (36)
Raised alanine aminotransferase	4/14 (29)
Ketonuria	2/14 (14)
Raised alkaline phosphatase	1/14 (7)

From Peterson M.E., Taylor R.S., Greco D.S. et al (1990) Acromegaly in fourteen cats. *J Vet Intern Med* **4**:192-201

FIG. 16.1   Frequency of clinical and laboratory findings in cats with acromegaly.

nephropathy or arthropathy is common in long-standing feline acromegaly. The cardiomyopathy is often associated with systolic murmurs and signs of congestive heart failure, especially in the later stages of diseases. Although the kidneys may enlarge (see below), a protein-losing glomerulopathy leading to the development of chronic renal failure is often found. In some cats, arthropathy is also a prominent sign, evidenced by degenerative arthritis, spondylosis deformans and thickening of the bony calvarium.

As in man, cats with acromegaly experience GH-induced proliferation of connective tissue, which results in an increase in body size, most frequently manifested as marked weight gain and mild to moderate enlargement of the abdomen and face. Growth and hypertrophy of all organs in the body is also characteristic. Signs of neurological dysfunction occur in 25% of cats with acromegaly and most likely reflect the compressive effects of space-occupying pituitary tumours.

Serum biochemical features of feline acromegaly reflect the clinical findings of diabetes mellitus and renal failure. Urinalysis reveals glycosuria without ketonuria. Biochemical and haematological abnormalities are listed in Fig. 16.1.

Diagnosis

As already stated, acromegaly should be suspected in any cat with severe insulin-resistant diabetes mellitus (persistent hyperglycaemia despite daily insulin doses > 25 U/day), especially if other characteristic signs of acromegaly (particularly arthropathy or cardiomyopathy) are also present. The definitive diagnosis can be established by demonstrating markedly elevated circulating GH concentrations. Unfortunately, serum (plasma) GH determinations are not performed routinely by most commercial veterinary laboratories. It may be difficult for the practising veterinarian to obtain reliable results because of the unavailability of GH radioimmunoassays that have been validated for use in the cat and it should be noted that GH assays designed for humans will not give accurate measurements for feline GH.

Computerised tomography (CT) and magnetic resonance imaging (MRI), if available, are useful means to identify a mass in the region of the pituitary and hypothalamus, a finding that supports the diagnosis of acromegaly. In addition to documenting the presence of a pituitary tumour, determining the size and location of the tumour is helpful in establishing the mode of therapy (i.e. surgery, medical, radiotherapy) and to monitor the tumour's response to therapy.

Treatment

Obviously the veterinary profession has limited experience with the treatment of feline acromegaly, so that recommendations are highly subjective and are based on extrapolation of methods used in treatment of the human disease. Basically, three options can be considered: surgery, radiation therapy or medical management. The effects of surgery have not been evaluated in cats with GH-secreting pituitary tumours but surgical cure is most likely to result if the tumour is small and noninvasive. Pituitary radiation is probably a good alternative to neurosurgical therapy and has been used successfully in a limited number of cases. However although it may offer the best chance for control of feline acromegaly, the availability of radiation is limited. Medical treatment (e.g. dopaminergic agents or long-acting somatostatin analogues) works well in human patients with acromegaly but has been ineffective in cats.

Current medical management of acromegaly in cats entails symptomatic treatment of diabetes mellitus, chronic renal disease and heart failure. Severe insulin-resistant diabetes mellitus can generally be controlled using large doses of insulin in divided daily doses. Mild to moderate cardiac disease responds well to diuretic therapy. Despite the possibility that acromegaly may have been diagnosed late in the course of the disease, survival times have ranged from 8–30 months. However, all of the cats do die eventually or are euthanased because of the development of severe congestive heart failure, renal failure or an expanding pituitary tumour.

Cushing's disease

As in man and the dog, hyperfunctioning ACTH-secreting adenomas of the pituitary corticotrophs have been reported to cause hyperadrenocorticism (Cushing's disease) in cats. Feline hyperadrenocorticism, caused by a pituitary (or possibly hypothalamic) disorder, will be discussed in the section concerning the adrenal glands.

Diabetes insipidus

Diabetes insipidus is a rare disorder and most cats in which it has been diagnosed are young adults. The major clinical signs are marked polyuria and polydipsia (> 100 ml/kg/day; normal, 40–70 ml/kg/day), usually of several months' duration. The severity of clinical signs varies because diabetes insipidus may result from a partial to complete defect in either ADH secretion or action.

Diagnosis

Diabetes insipidus should be differentiated from the many other causes of polyuria and polydipsia including primary renal disease, diabetes mellitus, and hyperthyroidism (all much more common than diabetes insipidus). Primary (psychogenic) polydipsia, a rare disorder associated with compulsive water drinking, is a major differential for diabetes insipidus in the dog but has not been well documented in the cat.

In general, the results of routine haematological and serum biochemical testing in cats with diabetes insipidus are either normal or show mild dehydration (e.g. mild increases in PCV, total protein and sodium). In contrast, most of the other differential disorders for polyuria and polydipsia result in marked abnormalities in these screening tests (e.g. elevated serum BUN, creatinine, glucose). In diabetes insipidus, complete urinalysis is unremarkable except for persistently dilute urine (specific gravity less than 1.008–1.012) whereas the degree of dilution with other disorders associated with polyuria and polydipsia tends to be less severe (usually in the range of 1.012 to 1.025). The diagnosis of diabetes insipidus can be confirmed by performing an abrupt water deprivation test, together with an aqueous vasopressin stimulation test.

Treatment

There are many drugs that may be used to treat diabetes insipidus, including vasopressin tannate in oil (1–2 USP units every 1–3 days), desmopressin (1-desamino-8-D-arginine vasopressin; 1–2 μg SC and 1–2 drops intraconjunctivally), hydrochlorothiazide (2–4 mg/kg, bid, PO), and chlorpropamide (40 mg/day). Although vasopressin tannate in oil appears to be most effective in controlling polyuria in cats with diabetes insipidus, the drug is no longer available. Our preliminary studies indicate that desmopressin may not be as effective.

It should be noted that persistent polyuria and polydipsia do not pose a serious hazard for the cat as long as adequate water is available; therefore, treatment may not be necessary unless the polyuria is socially unacceptable to the owner. However, water should never be restricted because the inability to concentrate urine will lead to dehydration and possibly death.

DISORDERS OF THE THYROID GLAND

Hyperthyroidism

Hyperthyroidism (thyrotoxicosis) is a multisystemic disorder resulting from excessive circulating concentrations of the two thyroid hormones, thyroxine (T_4) and triiodothyronine (T_3). It is the most common endocrine disorder of middle-aged and old cats.

Causes

Functional thyroid adenomatous hyperplasia involving one or both thyroid lobes is the most common pathological abnormality associated with feline hyperthyroidism. Both thyroid lobes are enlarged in most cats (70%) with hyperthyroidism. Unilateral thyroid lobe involvement and ectopic thyroid gland adenomas are also seen. Functional thyroid adenocarcinomas causing hyperthyroidism are rare.

Clinical features

Hyperthyroidism occurs in cats with a reported range of 4–22 years (mean age, approximately 12–13 years). There is no breed or sex predilection. As the actions of the thyroid hormones are generally stimulatory, the clinical and historical signs of hyperthyroidism are usually manifested by evidence of increased thyroid hormone effects on one or more organ systems.

The most common signs associated with the disease are listed in Fig. 16.2. The clinical manifestations may be mild to severe and are modified by the duration of hyperthyroidism, presence of concomitant abnormalities in various organ systems, and the inability of a body system to meet the demands of excess thyroid hormone. Cardiac abnormalities occur commonly in feline hyperthyroidism and are listed in Fig. 16.3.

Cats with hyperthyroidism are usually restless; they can show a frantic, anxious expression and can be difficult to handle, becoming aggressive during restraint. They tend to have impaired

HYPERTHYROIDISM	
	% Cats
Weight loss	95-98
Hyperactivity/Difficult to examine	68-81
Polyphagia	65-75
Tachycardia	57-65
Polyuria/Polydipsia	45-55
Cardiac murmur	10-54
Vomiting	33-50
Diarrhoea	30-45
Increased faecal volume	13-28
Decreased appetite	19-28
Lethargy	15-25
Polypnoea (panting)	13-28
Muscle weakness	15-20
Muscle tremor	15-30
Congestive heart failure	10-15
Dyspnoea	10-15

FIG. 16.2   Frequency of historical and clinical signs in feline hyperthyroidism.

CARDIAC ABNORMALITIES IN HYPERTHYROIDISM	
	% Cats
Thoracic Radiography	
Cardiomegaly	50
Pulmonary oedema/Pleural effusion	10
Electrocardiography	
Sinus tachycardia	70
Increased R wave amplitude in Lead II	30
Intraventricular conduction defects	10
Atrial premature contractions/fibrillation	10
Ventricular premature contractions	2
Echocardiography	
Left ventricular hypertrophy	70
Hypertrophy of the interventricular septum	40
Left atrial dilation	70
Left ventricular dilation	45
Hyperdynamic wall motion (hypercontractility)	20

FIG. 16.3   Approximate frequency of cardiac abnormalities in feline hyperthyroidism detected with thoracic radiography, electrocardiography and echocardiography.

tolerance for stressful situations and for some the stress of a visit to the veterinary hospital may result in marked respiratory distress and weakness, with the development of cardiac arrhythmias (and even cardiac arrest) in a few cases. This decreased ability to cope with stress must be considered when planning diagnostic or therapeutic procedures.

Enlargement of one or both thyroid lobes can be detected in over 90% of cats with hyperthyroidism. The thyroid gland is not usually palpable in the normal cat. To palpate an enlarged thyroid gland, the cat's neck should be slightly extended with the head tilted backward (Fig. 16.4). Gently pass the thumb and index finger over both sides of the trachea, starting at the laryngeal area and moving caudally toward the thoracic inlet. As the thyroid lobes are loosely attached to the trachea, the enlarged lobe frequently descends caudally from its normal location adjacent to the larynx. In hyperthyroid cats in which thyroid gland enlargement is not palpable, the possibility that the affected lobes have descended into the thoracic cavity should be considered.

Apathetic or masked hyperthyroidism is a clinical form of thyrotoxicosis that develops in about 10% of cats with hyperthyroidism. In these cats, hyperexcitability or restlessness is replaced by depression and weakness as the dominant clinical features. Weight loss remains a common clinical

sign but is usually accompanied by anorexia rather than increased appetite. These cats frequently have cardiac abnormalities, including arrhythmias and congestive heart failure. Ventroflexion of the neck, which may reflect severe muscle weakness, may also be observed.

Screening laboratory tests

Screening laboratory tests (e.g. complete blood count, serum biochemical profile, urinalysis) should always be performed in a cat suspected of having hyperthyroidism. Results of these tests may show alterations that will aid in the diagnosis and may reveal the presence of a concurrent disorder not directly related to the hyperthyroid state, a situation that should not be surprising considering the old age of most cats with hyperthyroidism. Chest and abdominal radiographs, electrocardiogram, echocardiogram or other studies may also be warranted, especially if signs of congestive heart failure are present.

Thyroid function tests

Increased basal serum thyroid hormone concentrations are the biochemical hallmark of hyperthyroidism. Resting serum concentrations of both T_4 and T_3 are above the normal range in the vast majority of cases. Approximately 5–10% will maintain normal serum concentrations of T_3, however, despite clearly elevated T_4 concentrations. Therefore, a serum T_4 determination is usually of greater diagnostic value than determination of serum T_3.

We have demonstrated that serum concentrations of T_4 and T_3 can fluctuate in and out of the normal range over days in some cats with mild to moderate hyperthyroidism and it is therefore advisable to repeat the basal T_4 determination when a single normal or high-normal test result is found in a cat suspected of having hyperthyroidism. If the result is again in the normal to high-normal range, a T_3 suppression test is recommended.

The T_3 suppression test is performed by determining basal serum concentrations of T_4, administering exogenous T_3 at the dosage of 25 µg every 8 hours for 2 days and giving the last (seventh) dose on the morning of the third day. Approximately 4

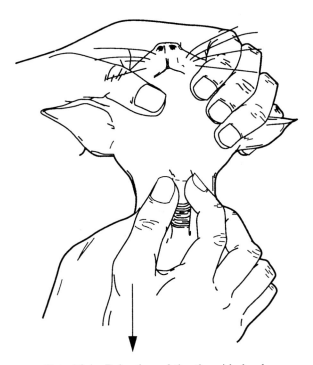

FIG. 16.4   Palpation of the thyroid glands.

TREATMENT FOR HYPERTHYROIDISM			
	Methimazole	**Surgery**	**Radioiodine**
Persistent hyperthyroidism	Low (dose-related)	Rare	Low (dose-related)
Complications:			
Hypoparathyroidism	Never	Common	Never
Permanent hypothyroidism	Never	Intermediate	Rare (dose-related)
Anorexia, vomiting	Common	Rare	Never
Haematological effects	Rare (thrombocytopenia, agranulocytosis, serum ANA)	Never	Rare (only with very high doses)
Neurological damage	Never	Rare (vocal cord paralysis, Horner's)	Never
Hospitalisation time required	None	1-3 days	1-4 weeks
Time until euthyroid	1-3 weeks	1-2 days	1-12 weeks
Relapse/recurrence	High	Intermediate	Low
Ease of treatment	Simple	Most difficult	Intermediate (not readily available)

FIG. 16.5 Advantages and disadvantages of treatment modalities for feline hyperthyroidism.

hours after the last dose of T_3 is administered, serum for determination of T_4 is collected again. In the normal cat, suppression of the serum T_4 concentration to approximately 50% or greater of the pretreatment value occurs after administration of T_3 at this dosage. In contrast, little to no decrease in serum T_4 concentration is found in cats with mild hyperthyroidism.

Treatment

Feline hyperthyroidism can be treated in three ways – surgical thyroidectomy, radioactive iodine (^{131}I), or chronic administration of an antithyroid drug. Antithyroid drug therapy is extremely useful as short-term treatment (3–6 weeks) in preparation for thyroidectomy. The advantages and disadvantages of each form of treatment are summarized in Fig. 16.5.

The treatment of choice for an individual cat depends on several factors, including age, presence of associated cardiovascular diseases or other major medical problems (e.g. renal disease), availability of a skilled surgeon or nuclear medicine department, and the owner's willingness to accept the form of treatment advised. Of the three, it must be emphasised that only surgery and radioactive iodine respectively, remove and destroy the adenomatous thyroid tissue and thereby 'cure' the hyperthyroid state. Use of an antithyroid drug will block thyroid hormone synthesis. However, because antithyroid drugs do not destory adenomatous thyroid tissue, relapse of hyperthyroidism invariably occurs within 24–72 hours after the medication is discontinued.

Antithyroid drugs

Methimazole and propylthiouracil (PTU) are the two antithyroid drugs available for use in the United States. Carbimazole, available in Europe, is predominantly converted to methimazole after administration, so the two drugs can be considered equivalent. They are actively concentrated by the thyroid gland, where they act to inhibit the synthesis of thyroid hormones.

Although all antithyroid drugs are effective in decreasing serum thryoid hormone concentrations, PTU produces a high incidence of mild to serious adverse effects which include anorexia, vomiting, lethargy, immune-mediated haemolytic anaemia and thrombocytopenia. Overall, studies show that methimazole and carbimazole are better tolerated and safer than PTU and can be considered the antithyroid drugs of choice for both the preoperative and long-term medical management of feline hyperthyroidism.

Initially, methimazole (or carbimazole) should be given at a dose of 10–15 mg/day, depending on the severity of the hyperthyroid state. This dosage ensures that serum T_4 concentrations will decrease to normal or low values within 2–3 weeks of treatment in most cats. During the first three months of therapy (a period when the most serious side-effects associated with medical therapy develop), the cats should be examined every 2–3 weeks in order to make necessary dose adjustments and to monitor for adverse effects. At each of these rechecks, serum T_4 concentrations and complete blood and platelet counts should be determined. If little or no decrease in serum T_4 concentration occurs during this initial treatment period, the daily dosage should be gradually increased (in 5 mg increments) after poor compliance by owners or difficulty in giving the medication has been excluded as the cause of persistent hyperthyroidism. Although a few cats appear to be 'resistant' to the effects of the drug, euthyroidism can be restored in virtually all cats if a high enough dosage of methimazole or carbimazole (25–30 mg/day in a few cases) is administered reliably on a daily basis.

In cats in which long-term antithyroid drug treatment is planned, the goal is to maintain serum T_4 values within the low-normal range with the lowest daily dosage, because some of the side-effects appear to develop less frequently with lower doses. Therefore, if serum T_4 concentrations fall to low or low-normal values during treatment, the daily drug dosage should be decreased by 2.5–5 mg increments and further testing continued at 2–3 week intervals until the lowest daily dose is found that will effectively maintain serum T_4 concentrations within the low-normal range. Although a few cases can be effectively controlled on a long-term basis with a daily dosage as low as 2.5–5 mg, the majority will require a dose of 7.5–10 mg/day. Other cats may continue to require dosages of 15–20 mg/day to maintain serum T_4 concentrations within normal range.

Mild clinical side-effects associated with methimazole or carbimazole treatment are relatively common (approximately 15% of cats) and are listed in Fig. 16.6. Some of these side effects are transient (e.g. anorexia, vomiting, lethargy) while others necessitate cessation of drug therapy. Clinical improvement, with resolution of anorexia, vomiting and lethargy, usually occurs within a few days after cessation of treatment. The most life-threatening side-effects (e.g. hepatopathy, thrombocytopenia, agranulocytosis) usually develop

SIDE-EFFECTS AND ABNORMALITIES ASSOCIATED WITH METHIMAZOLE	
	No. of cats (%)
Clinical signs:	
Anorexia	29/262 (11.1)
Vomiting	28/262 (10.7)
Lethargy	23/262 (8.8)
Excoriations	6/262 (2.3)
Bleeding	6/262 (2.3)
Laboratory findings:	
Eosinophilia	30/262 (11.3)
Lymphocytosis	19/262 (7.2)
Leukopenia	12/262 (4.7)
Thrombocytopenia	7/262 (2.7)
Agranulocytosis	4/262 (1.5)
Hepatopathy	4/262 (1.5)
Antinuclear antibodies	52/239 (21.8)
Positive Coombs' test	3/160 (1.9)

Modified from data in: Peterson M.E. et al (1988) Methimazole treatment of 262 cats with hyperthyroidism. *J Vet Intern Med* **2**:150-157

FIG. 16.6   Clinical side-effects and haematological and immunological abnormalities associated with methimazole treatment in cats with hyperthyroidism.

quickly after rechallenge with the drug, and alternative therapy with either surgery or radioiodine should be considered in these cases.

Although the most serious adverse effects of methimazole or carbimazole treatment usually develop during the first few weeks of drug administration, side-effects can occur at any time during treatment. After the first three months of therapy, serum T_4 concentrations should be measured at intervals of 3–6 months in order to monitor dosage requirements and response to treatment. Complete blood and platelet counts should be performed if agranulocytosis or thrombocytopenia are suspected.

Surgery

Thyroidectomy is a highly effective treatment for feline hyperthyroidism. All cases should be prepared for surgery by administration of an antithyroid drug to decrease the metabolic and cardiac complications associated with hyperthyroidism. If antithyroid drug treatment cannot be tolerated, a β-adrenergic blocker such as propranolol should be given at 2.5–5.0 mg tid as required, to decrease resting heart rate within the normal range and control hyperexcitability. In cats with congestive heart failure secondary to chronic thyroid hormone excess, propranolol should not be initiated until cardiac failure has been stabilised with diuretics (and digitalis when indicated). In these cases, propranolol should be used with caution, because the drug depresses myocardial function.

Anaesthetic management should include the judicious use of agents that have minimal cardiac arrhythmic effects. A variety of anaesthetic agents and techniques can be used and none has advantages that exclude use of all others, especially if the hyperthyroid state has been controlled with antithyroid drugs prior to surgery.

Techniques for unilateral and bilateral thyroidectomy have been described. Both intracapsular and extracapsular methods designed for removal of thyroid tissue while preserving parathyroid function have been used. However, with the intracapsular technique for thyroidectomy it can be difficult to remove the entire thyroid capsule (and therefore all abnormal thyroid tissue) while concurrently preserving parathyroid function. Small remnants of thyroid tissue which remain attached to the capsule may regenerate and produce recurrent hyperthyroidism. The main advantage of the extracapsular technique is that the incidence of relapse is less because the entire thyroid capsule is removed together with the thyroid lobe.

There are many potential complications associated with thyroidectomy, including hypoparathyroidism, Horner's syndrome and laryngeal paralysis (most commonly voice change). The most serious complication is hypocalcaemia, which develops after the parathyroid glands are injured, devascularised or inadvertently removed in the course of bilateral thyroidectomy. As one parathyroid gland is required for maintenance of normocalcaemia, hypoparathyroidism develops only in cats treated with bilateral thyroidectomy. After bilateral thyroidectomy, the serum calcium concentration should be monitored on a daily basis until it has stabilised within the normal range. In most cats with iatrogenic hypoparathyroidism, clinical signs associated with hypocalcaemia will develop within 1–3 days of surgery. Although mild hypocalcaemia is a common finding during this immediate postoperative period, laboratory evidence of hypocalcaemia alone does not indicate that treatment is required. However, if accompanying signs of muscle tremors, tetany or convulsions develop, therapy with vitamin D and calcium is indicated (see section on hypoparathyroidism). Although hypoparathyroidism may be permanent in some cats, spontaneous recovery of parathyroid function may occur weeks to months after surgery. In most cases, such transient hypocalcaemia probably results from reversible parathyroid damage and ischaemia incurred during surgery.

Serum thyroid hormone concentrations fall to subnormal levels for 2–3 months after hemithyroidectomy for unilateral thyroid lobe involvement but thyroxine supplementation is rarely required during this period. If bilateral thyroidectomy has been performed, thyroxine (0.1–0.2 mg/day) should be started 24–48 hours after surgery. Although thyroxine supplementation at this dosage can be safely continued indefinitely, the low serum concentrations of T_4 and T_3 that develop 24–48 hours after bilateral thyroidectomy may increase spontaneously to within the normal range some weeks or months later. Thyroxine administration can then be discontinued.

Because of the potential for recurrence of hyperthyroidism, all cats treated with surgical thyroidectomy should have serum thryoid hormone concentration monitored once or twice a year. In cases of recurrent thyrotoxicosis after bilateral thyroidectomy, treatment with either antithyroid drugs or radioiodine is favoured over further surgery because the incidence of surgical complications (especially permanent hypoparathyroidism) is considerably higher in subsequent operations.

Radioactive iodine

Radioactive iodine (radioiodine-131; ^{131}I) provides a simple, effective and safe treatment for cats with hyperthyroidism. Overall, use of radioiodine may be the optimum treatment for feline hyperthyroidism when nuclear medicine facilities are available. Radioactive iodine treatment involves a single, nonstressful procedure that is without associated morbidity or mortality, and no untoward systemic effects have been observed. Unlike surgery, anaesthesia is not required. A single ^{131}I treatment will restore euthyroidism in most cats with hyperthyroidism, whereas cats that remain persistently hyperthyroid can be successfully retreated with radioiodine and those that become hypothryoid can be supplemented readily with thyroxine. At present, the major disadvantage of radioiodine therapy is the unavailability of facilities that can handle ^{131}I safely and determine the ideal dose accurately.

Feline hypothyroidism

Naturally-occurring hypothyroidism is an extremely rare clinical disorder in the cat. The most common cause is iatrogenic destruction or removal of the thyroid gland (following radioiodine therapy or surgery) for treatment of hyperthyroidism. Although antithyroid drug overdosage could also produce hypothyroidism, this appears to be uncommon. The recommended treatment is daily administration of L-T_4, using an initial dose of 10–20 µg/kg/day.

DISORDERS OF THE PARATHYROID GLANDS

Primary hyperparathyroidism

Primary hyperparathyroidism is a disorder resulting from the excessive secretion of parathyroid

PRIMARY HYPERPARATHYROIDISM	
	No. of cats (%)
Clinical signs:	
Anorexia	4/7 (57)
Lethargy	4/7 (57)
Vomiting	2/7 (29)
Polyuria/polydipsia	2/7 (29)
Weakness	1/7 (14)
Weight loss	1/7 (14)
Mentally dull	1/7 (14)
Laboratory findings:	
Hypercalcaemia	7/7 (100)
Hypophosphataemia	2/7 (29)
Azotaemia	4/7 (57)
Isosthenuria	3/7 (43)
Increased alanine aminotransferase	2/7 (29)

Modified from data in: Richter K.P., Kallet A.J., Feldman E.C.: Primary hyperparathyroidism in the cat. In: Kirk R.W., Bonagura J.D. (eds): *Current Veterinary Therapy XI*. W.B. Saunders Co., Philadelphia. pp 380-382

FIG. 16.7   Clinical and laboratory findings in cats with primary hyperparathyroidism.

hormone (PTH) by one or more abnormal (usually neoplastic) parathyroid glands. In the cat, primary tumours of the parathyroid gland are very rare and may or may not be associated with hyperparathyroidism. Clinical signs include extreme listlessness, weakness, anorexia and vomiting (Fig. 16.7). Skeletal radiographs reveal loss of density of the scapulae and coarse bony trabeculation of the humeri. Treatment involves surgical removal of the parathyroid adenoma, which may result in normalisation of the serum calcium concentration and clinical recovery.

Hypoparathyroidism

Hypoparathyroidism is a metabolic disorder characterised by hypocalcaemia and hyperphosphataemia and either transient or permanent PTH insufficiency. In the cat, the most common cause of hypoparathyroidism is iatrogenic injury or removal of the parathyroid glands during thyroidectomy, and spontaneous (idiopathic) hypoparathyroidism is extremely rare. Hypocalcaemia causes the major clinical manifestations of hypoparathyroidism, by increasing the excitability of both the central and peripheral nervous systems. Peripheral neuromuscular signs include muscle tremors, twitches and tetany, while generalised convulsions are the predominant central nervous manifestations.

Diagnosis is based on history, clinical signs, laboratory evidence of hypocalcaemia and hyperphosphataemia, and exclusion of other causes of hypocalcaemia (e.g. hypoproteinaemia, malabsorption, pancreatitis, renal failure). After bilateral thyroidectomy, the potential development of hypoparathyroidism should be anticipated.

Treatment includes the use of calcium supplements and vitamin D. A complete description of treatment protocols for hypocalcaemia is available.[10]

DISORDERS OF THE ADRENAL GLANDS

Hyperadrenocorticism

Causes

Hyperadrenocorticism (Cushing's disease) results from excessive production of glucocorticoids by functional neoplasms of the adrenal cortex or bilateral adrenocortical hyperplasia. Adrenocortical hyperplasia results from overproduction of adrenocorticotrophin (ACTH) by neoplastic or, less commonly, hyperplastic pituitary corticotrophs (pituitary-dependent hyperadrenocorticism). While the syndrome is quite rare, both pituitary-dependent hyperadrenocorticism and functional adrenal tumours (adenoma and carcinoma) have been identified in the cat. Approximately 85% of cats with naturally-occurring hyperadrenocorticism have the pituitary-dependent form. Iatrogenic hyperadrenocorticism is a well recognised disorder in cats, although they tend to be more resistant to the effects of exogenous glucocorticoid excess than dogs.

Clinical features

Hyperadrenocorticism is a disease of middle-aged to older cats. As in human Cushing's disease, there is a strong female sex predilection. The clinical signs and abnormal laboratory findings are listed in Fig. 16.8. Affected cats are predisposed to develop insulin resistance, which is manifested by hyperglycaemia and overt diabetes. As in diabetic

HYPERADRENOCORTICISM	
	No. of cats (%)
Clinical findings:	
Polyuria/polydipsia	17/18 (94)
Pot-bellied appearance	17/18 (94)
Increased appetite	16/18 (89)
Hair loss	13/18 (72)
Muscle wasting	12/18 (67)
Obesity	11/18 (61)
Hepatomegaly	10/18 (56)
Infection	7/18 (39)
Thin skin	6/18 (33)
Weight loss	2/18 (11)
Diarrhoea	2/18 (11)
Laboratory findings:	
Hyperglycaemia	14/14 (100)
Hypercholesterolaemia	12/14 (86)
Glucosuria	14/17 (82)
Lymphopenia	8/12 (67)
Eosinopenia	7/12 (58)
Mature leukocytosis	5/12 (42)
High alkaline phosphatase	5/14 (36)

Fig. 16.8 Clinical signs and abnormal laboratory findings in cats with hyperadrenocorticism.

dogs with untreated hyperadrenocorticism and cortisol-induced insulin resistance, some cats will require high daily insulin doses to control severe hyperglycaemia and glucosuria. Unlike dogs, only about a third of the cats with hyperadrenocorticism have elevated serum alkaline phosphatase concentrations.

Pituitary-adrenal function tests

Basal serum cortisol determinations

Basal serum cortisol determinations are of little value in the diagnosis of feline hyperadrenocorticism. A large percentage of cats are likely to exhibit high-normal or high resting serum cortisol concentrations due to the effects of stress or non-adrenal disease. Conversely, a finding of normal serum cortisol concentrations should not be used to exclude the diagnosis.

ACTH stimulation tests

The ACTH stimulation test is a valuable screening test for hyperadrenocorticism and two regimens have been described. One method is to collect blood for determination of serum (or plasma) cortisol concentration before and at 60 and 120 minutes after IM administration of ACTH gel (2.2 U/kg). With this regimen, the maximal rise in cortisol concentrations occurs at 2 hours after gel administration in about half of the cats, whereas the remaining cats have peak values at 1 hour post-injection. Alternatively, the test may be performed by injecting synthetic ACTH (cosyntropin or tetracosactide) and measuring serum cortisol before and at 60–90 minutes after IV administration (0.125 mg). Regardless of the basal cortisol value obtained, diagnosis of hyperadrenocorticism depends upon demonstration of a post-ACTH cortisol concentration that is significantly higher than the normal range.

Recent studies have reported that a variety of chronic illnesses (not associated with hyperadrenocorticism) can influence ACTH-stimulated cortisol secretion in the cat. It is likely that the 'stress' associated with chronic illness results in some degree of bilateral adrenocortical hyperplasia in sick cats, which could account for an exaggerated cortisol response to ACTH. Therefore, the diagnosis of feline hyperadrenocorticism should be based primarily on the cat's history, clinical signs and routine laboratory findings, and not solely on the results of serum cortisol determinations.

Dexamethasone suppression tests

Low- and high-dose dexamethasone suppression tests are useful in the diagnosis of hyperadrenocorticism in the dog and in man, but the tests have not been well-standardised for the cat. A dosage of intravenous dexamethasone ranging from 0.010 to 0.015 mg/kg is sufficient for the consistent suppression of serum cortisol concentrations to low or undetectable values for at least 8 hours in normal healthy cats. However, further studies must be done before a low-dose dexamethasone suppression test can be considered a definitive diagnostic test for feline hyperadrenocorticism. As with the results of ACTH stimulation testing, a variety of illnesses other than hyperadrenocorticism may influence low-dose dexamethasone suppression test results. The high-dose test (0.1 mg/kg, IV) may be the preferred method of screening for hyperdrenocorticism, at least at this time.

Treatment

A number of different protocols have been attempted, with varying levels of success, in the treatment of spontaneous feline hyperadrenocorticism. Generally, no drugs have been found that can be used successfully to treat the disease in cats.

Surgical adrenalectomy is the most successful procedure and unilateral adrenalectomy is recommended for treatment of hyperfunctioning adrenocortical tumours. Bilateral adrenalectomy, followed by mineralocorticoid and glucocorticoid replacement therapy, may be the best treatment available for pituitary-dependent hyperadrenocorticism. Radiation therapy represents another possible treatment for pituitary adenoma.

Iatrogenic hyperadrenocorticism

Compared with dogs, cats are more resistant to the development of iatrogenic hyperadrenocorticism. Although clinical signs of the disease are rare, suppression of the feline pituitary-adrenal axis with exogenous glucocorticoids or with megestrol acetate can occur. Clinical signs of adrenocortical insufficiency (e.g. anorexia, lethargy, vomiting) are rarely observed following treatment with progestagens or glucocorticoids but the cat may develop clinical signs of iatrogenic hypoadrenocorticism if acutely stressed or if the drugs are given in high dosages and then stopped abruptly.

Hypoadrenocorticism

Causes

Adrenocortical insufficiency, or hypoadrenocorticism, results from deficient adrenal production of glucocorticoids or mineralocorticoids. In the cat, naturally occurring hypoadrenocorticism is caused by idiopathic atrophy of all three zones of the adrenal cortex (primary adrenocortical insufficiency). The resultant deficiency of both

PRIMARY HYPOADRENOCORTICISM	
	No. of cats (%)
Clinical signs:	
Lethargy	10/10 (100)
Anorexia	10/10 (100)
Weight loss	9/10 (90)
Dehydration	9/10 (90)
Weakness	9/10 (90)
Slow capillary refill time	5/10 (50)
Weak pulse	5/10 (50)
Microcardia	4/10 (40)
Vomiting	4/10 (40)
Polyuria/Polydipsia	3/10 (30)
Bradycardia	2/10 (20)
Laboratory findings:	
Azotaemia	10/10 (100)
Hyperphosphataemia	10/10 (100)
Hyponatraemia	10/10 (100)
Hyperkalaemia	9/10 (90)
Hypochloraemia	9/10 (90)
Hypercalcaemia	1/10 (10)
Anaemia	3/10 (30)
Lymphocytosis	2/10 (20)
Eosinophilia	1/10 (10)

Modified from data in Peterson M.E., Greco D.S., Orth D.S. (1989) Primary hypoadrenocorticism in ten cats. *J Vet Intern Med* **3**:55-58

FIG. 16.9   Clinical signs and laboratory findings in cats with primary hypoadrenocorticism.

glucocorticoids and mineralocorticoids causes the clinical signs.

Clinical features

Naturally occurring primary hypoadrenocorticism is a disease of young to middle-aged cats and there is no sex predilection. The clinical signs and laboratory findings are listed in Fig. 16.9. The extracellular fluid volume contraction associated with primary adrenocortical insufficiency often results in prerenal azotaemia and hyperphosphataemia. As in cases of canine primary hypoadrenocorticism, pretreatment urine specific gravities are variable but may be more dilute than would be expected in a cat with prerenal azotaemia.

Diagnosis

The most accurate screening test for hypoadrenocorticism is the ACTH stimulation test already described for hyperadrenocorticism. The finding of a low basal serum cortisol concentration with a subnormal or negligible response to ACTH is indicative of adrenocortical insufficiency.

Treatment

In cats with acute adrenal failure, initial therapy should be aimed at restoring the circulating blood volume, providing glucocorticoids, and correcting electrolyte disturbances. Initially, isotonic fluids (e.g. 0.9% saline) should be administered at the rate of 40 ml/kg/hour during the first 1–2 hours. Once fluid deficits are restored, the rate of fluid administration should be decreased to 60 ml/kg/day, given by continuous infusion or divided evenly over three treatments. Fluid administration is tapered when azotaemia resolves, electrolyte abnormalities are corrected, and the cat is eating and drinking on its own. Intravenous administration of glucocorticoids is extremely important in the initial management of severe adrenocortical insufficiency. In most cases, dexamethasone (0.5–1.0 mg/kg) is adequate and will not interfere with concurrent ACTH stimulation testing. Glucocorticoid replacement should be continued as prednisone (or prednisolone) at a dosage of 0.2 mg/kg/day, PO if possible.

Once stabilised, maintenance therapy for the cat with primary adrenocortical insufficiency consists of life-long mineralocorticoid and glucocorticoid supplementation. Either oral fludrocortisone acetate (0.1 mg/day) or intramuscular injections of repositol desoxycorticosterone pivalate (12.5 mg/month) can be given for mineralocorticoid therapy. Adjustment of the dosage of mineralocorticoid supplementation is based on serial serum electrolyte concentrations, determined every 1–2 weeks during the initial maintenance period. Glucocorticoid supplementation can be provided as prednisone or prednisolone (1.25 mg/day/PO) or IM methylprednisolone acetate (10 mg/month). With proper corticosteroid replacement therapy the long-term prognosis of feline adrenocortical insufficiency is excellent.

DISORDERS OF THE ENDOCRINE PANCREAS

Diabetes mellitus

Causes

In the cat, diabetes mellitus can be classified into three types – Type I (insulin-dependent), Type II (non-insulin-dependent), and Type III (secondary). Type I represents a cachectic, ketoacidotic cat in which life-long insulin therapy is absolutely crucial in order to prevent certain death. Type II diabetes mellitus describes an obese cat in which ketoacidosis does not develop, even when insulin therapy is withheld for prolonged periods. Although Type II diabetic cats may benefit from insulin therapy, they do not require insulin treatment to survive. Type III can result from a variety of factors such as primary pancreatic disease (e.g. pancreatitis), other endocrinopathies (hyperadrenocorticism and acromegaly) or drug therapy (glucocorticoids and progestagens).

Clinical features

Diabetes mellitus can develop in cats of any age, breed or sex. However, the disease is seen most often in middle-aged and older cats and appears to be more common in males. Diabetes mellitus without acidosis, stupor or coma can be referred to as uncomplicated diabetes. Polyuria, polydipsia, polyphagia and weight loss are classical signs but often go unnoticed by owners. Less commonly, diabetic cats may develop a plantigrade posture, probably due to peripheral neuropathy.

Ketoacidotic diabetes mellitus is characterised by persistent fasting hyperglycaemia, ketonuria and metabolic acidosis. In addition to a history consistent with previous uncomplicated diabetes mellitus, clinical signs in cats with ketoacidosis include polyuria, polydipsia, weight loss, anorexia, vomiting, diarrhoea, lethargy, weakness, dehydration and hypo- or hyperventilation.

Diagnosis

Diagnosis is dependent on a persistent hyperglycaemia and glycosuria, and must be correlated with at least three or four of the classical clinical signs (i.e. polyuria, polydipsia, polyphagia, weight loss). It should be kept in mind that hyperglycaemia in cats is often associated with stress, so that a diagnosis of diabetes mellitus should not be based on a single finding of hyperglycaemia.

Treatment

Treatment is based on the severity of the disorder and the presence or absence of ketoacidosis. Appropriate initial therapy is usually different in each of the three presenting types. Initial therapy of ketoacidosis requires a short-acting insulin whereas intermediate to long-acting insulins are used in the treatment of uncomplicated diabetes mellitus.

Ketoacidotic diabetes mellitus

The main objectives in the treatment of diabetic ketoacidosis are (1) to correct dehydration and electrolyte deficits using an isotonic fluid; (2) to provide adequate amounts of insulin to reduce hyperglycaemia gradually and stop ketogenesis; (3) to provide a carbohydrate substrate when required during insulin treatment; and (4) to identify precipitating factors (e.g. infection) in the disease process. The metabolic abnormalities associated with diabetic ketoacidosis should not be corrected too rapidly but over a period of 36–48 hours.

Short-acting insulin is used in the initial treatment of diabetic ketoacidosis, especially if depression, dehydration, anorexia and vomiting are present. On the other hand, a ketoacidotic cat with a good appetite and no signs of debilitation can be treated as an uncomplicated diabetic (see below).

Initially, the best way to control hyperglycaemia and ketoacidosis involves the use of low-dose intramuscular insulin therapy. With this treatment protocol, short-acting insulin is given IM at a loading dose of 0.2 U/kg, followed by hourly doses of 0.1 U/kg IM, until the blood glucose concentration falls below 250 mg/dl. Then short-acting insulin (initial dose, 0.5 U/kg) can be given subcutaneously every 6 hours. Subsequent doses should be adjusted by 0.5–1.0 units to maintain blood glucose concentrations between 100 and 250 mg/dl.

Frequent monitoring of the initial blood glucose response to insulin (at 1–2 hour intervals) is essential for successful management of diabetic ketoacidosis. Urine glucose determinations should not be used alone. When laboratory facilities are unavailable for blood glucose determinations, fairly accurate results can be obtained using reagent test strips.

When the blood glucose concentration reaches 250 mg/dl, the cat should be given a 2.5–5.0% dextrose drip (to prevent hypoglycaemia), and fluid therapy should be maintained until the cat is able to eat without vomiting. This dextrose provides a substrate for the exogenous insulin in the absence of intake of food. Once the cat is eating and does not vomit, treatment is continued with long-acting (ultralente or NPH) insulin using the protocol described below for an uncomplicated diabetic.

In cats with ketoacidosis, supplementation with potassium is important. As cats with hyperkalaemia upon presentation may rapidly become hypokalaemic as insulin and fluid therapy are initiated, frequent monitoring is important. Potassium supplementation for moderate to severe hypokalaemia is best provided by the addition of potassium chloride to the parenteral fluids (Fig. 16.10). The amount of potassium required varies according to renal function and dietary replacement.

Uncomplicated diabetes mellitus

The goals of treatment are to achieve an 'acceptable' level of blood glucose (100–250 mg/dl), to

SUPPLEMENTATION OF POTASSIUM FOR IV FLUID THERAPY IN DIABETES MELLITUS	
Serum potassium (mEq/l)	mEq of potassium to add to 250 ml fluids
>3.5	5
3.0-3.5	7
2.5-3.0	10
2.0-2.5	15
<2.0	20
Rate of potassium administration should not exceed 0.5-1.0 mEq/kg/h	

FIG. 16.10 Supplementation of potassium for intravenous fluid therapy in diabetes mellitus.

prevent ketosis, and to cause remission of clinical signs of the disease. Achieving strict euglycaemia is probably not of critical importance.

Therapy for uncomplicated diabetes should be initiated with either a long-acting insulin preparation given once a day or an intermediate-acting insulin administered twice a day. In most diabetic cats, hyperglycaemia can be controlled with once-daily administration of ultralente, but some will require twice-daily injections for adequate regulation. When compared with ultralente, NPH insulin has a more rapid onset and shorter duration of action. Therefore, it is unlikely that use of NPH would ever control hyperglycaemia satisfactorily when administered once a day. If an intermediate-acting insulin preparation is used, it is recommended that the cat initially receives insulin injections on a split dose (bid) schedule, with similar doses given at 12-hour intervals.

When initiating therapy with an intermediate- or long-acting insulin, it is best to start with a relatively low dose (0.25–0.5 U/kg/day) and slowly increase the dose as needed. The cat should be fed half of its energy allotment at the time of the morning insulin injection and the remainder approximately 12 hours later (at the time of the evening insulin injection when on a split dose regimen). Semi-moist food should not be fed to diabetic cats because of its high sugar content.

Low-dose syringes (e.g. $\frac{3}{10}$ cc U-100 syringes) or dilution of insulin may be helpful for accurate dosing, especially if U-100 insulin (100 U/ml) rather than U-40 insulin is used. Intermediate- or long-acting insulin preparations can be diluted in

sterile water or isotonic saline or prepared with a pH-adjusted diluent obtained from the manufacturer. Because sterile water and isotonic saline may affect the shelf-life of insulin, a new supply of freshly diluted insulin should be prepared at least every two months.

Initial regulation of the insulin dose is best done at home by the owner, because diet and exercise are two important variables that affect insulin requirements. During the first 1–2 weeks the owner should measure urinary glucose and ketone levels once or twice a day. Based on the urine glucose readings and clinical response (lessening of polyuria, polydipsia, and weight gain), the daily insulin dose should be adjusted by 0.5–1.0 unit increments every 3–4 days as directed by the veterinarian. After 7–14 days of treatment, the cat should be re-examined.

Initially, re-evaluation of the diabetic cat by monitoring serial blood glucose concentrations throughout the day is recommended at 1–2 week intervals until satisfactory glycaemic control is achieved. In the morning, the owner should inject insulin and feed the cat as usual. As soon as possible, the cat is brought to the hospital for the first blood glucose determination. Additional samples for blood glucose measurement should be collected at 1–2 hour intervals. Cats receiving twice-daily injections of insulin need to be monitored for 10–12 hours; after that time, they can be returned to their owners for the evening meal and insulin treatment. In cats treated with a single daily dose of insulin, monitoring of blood glucose levels at 1–3 hour intervals should, if possible, be continued for 24 hours to evaluate diabetic control adequately. In the latter circumstance, the cat's evening meal should consist of the same amount and type of food that it receives at home. Based on the results of these glucose determinations, adjustments in insulin dosage or type are made as necessary.

Once the diabetes is controlled, subsequent rechecks every few months are recommended. These should consist of a history, physical examination, review of the urine glucose measurements and determination of serial blood glucose concentrations (every 1–2 hours) for at least 10–12 hours. During long-term insulin treatment, owners should continue to monitor for recurrence of clinical signs, as well as measure urine glucose and ketone concentrations at least once or twice a week. If a cat is consistently glycosuric, or if ketonuria is detected on more than 2–3 consecutive days, the cat should be brought to the hospital for re-evaluation. If there is ever any doubt concerning the control of the diabetes, serial blood glucose determinations are recommended.

Hypoglycaemia

During both initial and long-term insulin treatment, owners should frequently be reminded to watch for signs of hypoglycaemia, including weakness, lethargy, shaking, ataxia, convulsions, coma and death. If mild signs of hypoglycaemia develop, the cat should be fed its normal food. If severe signs develop, a tablespoon of corn syrup, molasses or honey should be given orally. If no response to food or sugar water is observed within a few minutes, the cat should be taken to the veterinarian for the administration of intravenous dextrose. Whenever signs of hypoglycaemia occur, the insulin dose needs to be decreased until appropriate insulin dosage adjustments can be made based on serial blood glucose determinations.

FURTHER READING

1. Kraus K.H. (1987) The use of desmopressin in diagnosis and treatment of diabetes insipidus in cats. *Compend Cont Ed Prac Vet* **9**: 752–758.
2. Nelson R.W., Feldman E.C. (1988) Spontaneous hyperadrenocorticism in cats: 7 cases (1978–1987). *J Am Vet Med Assoc* **193**: 245–250.
3. Nelson R.W., Feldman E.C.: (1992) Treatment of feline diabetes mellitus. In: Kirk R.W., Bonagura J.D. (eds.) *Current Veterinary Therapy XI*. W.B. Saunders Co., Philadelphia pp 364–367.
4. Peterson M.E., Birchard S.J., Mehlhaff C.J. (1984) Anesthetic and surgical management of endocrine disorders. *Vet Clin North Am: Small Anim Pract* **14**: 911–925.
5. Peterson M.E., Kintzer P.P., Hurvitz A.I. (1988) Methimazole treatment of 262 cats with hyperthyroidism. *J Vet Intern Med* **2**: 150–157.
6. Peterson M.E., Greco D.S., Orth D.N. (1989) Primary hypoadrenocorticism in ten cats. *J Vet Intern Med* **3**: 55–58.
7. Peterson M.E., Randolph J.F. (1989) Endocrine diseases. In: Sherding R.G. (ed.) *The Cat: Diagnosis and Clinical Management*, pp 1095–1161 Churchill Livingstone, New York.
8. Peterson M.E., Ferguson D.C. (1989) Thyroid diseases. In: Ettinger S.J. (ed) *Textbook of Veterinary Internal Medicine: Diseases of the Dog and Cat*, 3rd edn. pp 1632–1675 W.B. Saunders Co., Philadelphia.
9. Peterson M.E., Taylor R.S., Greco D.S., Nelson D.S., Foodman M.S., Randolph J.F., Moroff S.D., Lothrop C.D. (1990) Acromegaly in fourteen cats. *J Vet Intern Med* **4**: 192–201.
10. Peterson M.E. (1992) Hypoparathyroidism and other causes of hypocalcaemia in cats. In: Kirk R.W., Bonagura J.D. (eds) *Current Veterinary Therapy XI*. W.B. Saunders Co., Philadelphia, pp 376–379.
11. Randolph J.F., Peterson M.E. (1992) Acromegaly (growth hormone excess) syndromes in dogs and cats. In: Kirk R.W., Bonagura J.D. (eds) *Current Veterinary Therapy XI*. W.B. Saunders Co., Philadelphia. pp 322–327.
12. Richter K.P., Kallet A.J., Feldman E.C. (1992) Primary hyperparathyroidism in the cat. In: Kirk R.W., Bonagura J.D. (eds) *Current Veterinary Therapy XI*. W.B. Saunders Co., Philadelphia, pp 380–382.
13. Thoday K.L., Mooney C.T. (1992) Medical management of feline hyperthyroidism. In: Kirk R.W., Bonagura J.D. (eds) *Current Veterinary Therapy XI*. W.B. Saunders Co., Philadelphia, pp 338–345.
14. Welches C.D., Scavelli T.D., Matthiesen D.T., Peterson M.E. (1989) Occurrence of problems after three techniques of bilateral thyroidectomy in cats. *Vet Surgery* **18**: 392–396.
15. Zerbe C.A., Refsal K.R., Peterson M.E. et al (1987) Effect of non-adrenal illness on adrenal function in the cat. *Am J Vet Res* **48**: 451–454.

17

Disorders of the Musculoskeletal System

DAVID BENNETT

Pathology of the musculoskeletal system is not particularly rare in the cat although disease may be present without obvious clinical signs. However, when lameness becomes evident it is often of great concern to the owner, since the cat is generally expected to show agility and grace in its movements.

Lameness may not show as an obvious limp but as a weakness or reduced exercise tolerance. The commonest cause is disease of the musculoskeletal system (Fig. 17.1) but other possible diagnoses must be considered, such as disease of the integument, nervous system, endocrine system and even the cardiovascular system. Traumatic disease, which is common in the cat, is not covered in this chapter.

ARTHRITIS

The classification of feline arthritis is shown in Fig. 17.2. There are two broad types: the degenerative and the inflammatory. Synovial fluid examination is a useful aid to the differential diagnosis of arthritis, particularly in distinguishing between these two broad groups. The degenerative fluids contain relatively few white cells, most of which are macrophages and lymphocytes; the inflammatory fluids contain many more white cells, most of which are polymorphonuclear cells.

Degenerative type

Traumatic arthritis

This type of arthritis follows a single acute injury to the joint such as may occur during a fall, road accident, or fights with other animals. There is usually pain and swelling of the joint and generally only one joint is involved. Many cases are not serious and will recover quickly with rest and confinement but all should be examined for more serious complications, e.g. ligament damage, which may need surgical treatment. Cases of traumatic arthritis can easily be confused with septic arthritis; if there is any doubt, synovial fluid examination should be performed.

Osteoarthritis

Osteoarthritis is a disease of moveable joints characterised by deterioration and abrasion of articular cartilage and by the formation of new bone at the articular margins. Osteoarthritis can be *primary*, where there is no obvious underlying cause, or *secondary*, where the arthritis is a result of some other joint disorder. For example, secondary osteoarthritis can occur in association with hip dysplasia, patellar luxation, congenital elbow subluxation, cranial cruciate rupture and repeated episodes of traumatic arthritis. The latter is sometimes induced by the natural and frequent activity of jumping, which could 'over-stress' certain joints.

Lameness is usually of a chronic nature and of insidious onset. As in other species, osteoarthritis may be asymptomatic. The problem is usually apparent in only a single joint, although many cases show bilateral pathology. The most typical radiographic feature is the presence of new bone deposits referred to as osteophytes, spurs, exostoses or as a 'lipping' of the joint margin (Fig. 17.3). Calcification of the articular soft tissues may be seen. Radiography is also helpful in identifying the cause of secondary osteoarthritis.

Most cases of osteoarthritis in the cat require no treatment but, where necessary, drugs shown in Fig. 17.4 can be used. They include, among others, non-steroidal anti-inflammatory drugs (which, however, are best avoided or used only

MUSCULOSKELETAL DISEASES	

Traumatic:
  Fractures
  Luxations/Subluxations
  Ligaments
Arthritis:
  Degenerative
  Inflammatory
Metabolic:
  Nutritional secondary hyperparathyroidism
  Osteogenesis imperfecta
  Renal secondary hyperparathyroidism
  Primary hyperparathyroidism
  Primary hypoparathyroidism
  Hypervitaminosis A
  Hypovitaminosis A
Neoplastic and neoplastic-like:
  Primary tumours –
    osteosarcoma
    juxtacortical osteosarcoma
    chondrosarcoma
    osteoma
    osteoid osteoma
    multilobular chondroma
    osteoclastoma
    undetermined sarcomas
    fibrosarcoma
    extraskeletal tumours of bone
    synovial sarcoma
    aneurysmal bone cyst
    fibrous dysplasia
    neoplasia of skeletal muscle
 	
  Metastatic neoplasms –
  true metastases
  direct extension of non-skeletal neoplasia –
    fibrosarcoma
    carcinoma
    others
	Neoplastic-like –
	    osteocartilaginous exostoses
	    synovial osteochondrometaplasia
	    synovial cyst
	Inherited, congenital and developmental:
	  Congenital deformities
	  Mucopolysaccharidosis
	  Patellar luxation
	  Hip dysplasia
	  Osteochondrosis
	Miscellaneous:
	  Myelofibrosis - osteosclerosis syndrome
	  Osteopetrosis
	  Hypertrophic pulmonary osteoarthropathy
	  Disuse osteopenia
	  Cranial cruciate ligament rupture
	  Osteomyelitis (suppurative)
	  Osteomyelitis (mycotic)
	  Temporomandibular ankylosis
	  Feline metaphyseal osteopathy
	Muscle disease:
	  Myositis
	  Localised myositis ossificans
	  Generalised myositis ossificans
	  Aortic thromboembolism
	  Myasthenia gravis
	  Hypokalaemic polymyopathy
	  Tetanus
	  Fibrotic myopathy
	  Dystrophy-like myopathies
	  Other myopathies
	  Gastrocnemius contracture
	  Gastrocnemius rupture
	  Neoplasia
	Diseases of vertebral column:
	  Intervertebral disc protrusions
	  Discospondylitis
	  Atlanto-axial subluxation
	  Feline hyperaesthesia syndrome

FIG. 17.1 Classification of feline musculoskeletal diseases.

as short courses when the lameness is particularly severe), low dose corticosteroids (again in short courses), and intra-articular sodium hyaluronate and polysulphated glycosaminoglycans.

Surgical treatment is seldom necessary. Correction of the underlying cause of the secondary arthritis is sometimes useful (e.g. ligament replacement, stabilisation of a luxating patella) and excision arthroplasty might be indicated with a painful arthritic joint (e.g. femoral head excision, condylectomy of the temporomandibular joint). Replace-ment arthroplasty is rare but arthrodesis can be used in a painful joint especially where instability is a feature.

Inflammatory type: infective arthritis

Infective arthritis is an inflammatory arthropathy caused by a microbial agent which can be cultured from the joint, i.e. viable organisms are present in the diseased joint and are contributing significantly to the pathology.

Bacterial arthritis (septic arthritis)

This is not uncommon in the cat and is usually associated with a bite wound penetrating the joint. However, bacteria can also localise to a joint via the blood stream or by extension from the periarticular tissue. Haematogenous localisation of infection can be associated with bacterial endocarditis, where several joints can be involved, and in young kittens it can be associated with an infected umbilicus, or with post-parturient uterine and mammary gland infection of the queen (see Chapter 5).

Various bacteria can be involved e.g., *Staphylococcus* spp., *Streptococcus* spp., *Pasteurella* spp., coliforms and anaerobes. Generally only a single joint is affected and the joint is usually swollen and painful on motion. Radiography may show extensive bony destruction (Fig. 17.5) although in early cases only soft tissue changes are present. Periosteal new bone and soft tissue calcification are other features seen in more chronic cases. Synovial fluid is usually increased in quantity, turbid and of reduced viscosity, and contains several thousand white cells, most of which are polymorphs. Synovial fluid should always be cultured, although the synovial membrane is more sensitive to culture.

Systemic antibiotics, preferably based on bacterial culture and sensitivity testing, are the treatment of choice. Useful antibiotics include ampicillin, amoxycillin and clavulanic acid, cephalosporins and clindamycin. Joint drainage and lavage are sometimes helpful and can be facilitated by the insertion of drains. The limbs should be bandaged to protect the drains, which should only be left in place for 3–4 days. Joints complicated by serious destruction may have to be treated by arthrodesis or excision arthroplasty, or even limb amputation.

Some cases of bacterial infective arthritis are complicated by persisting synovitis in the absence of viable organisms. It is assumed that the synovitis is associated with an immune response against bacterial antigens persisting within the joint cavity. Such cases will respond to corticosteroid therapy, although it is important to ensure that viable organisms are not present.

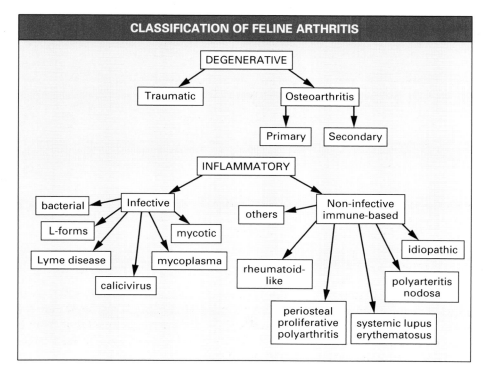

FIG. 17.2 Classification of feline arthritis.

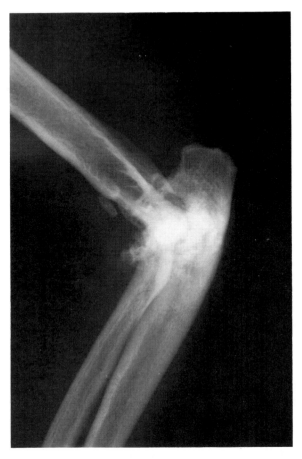

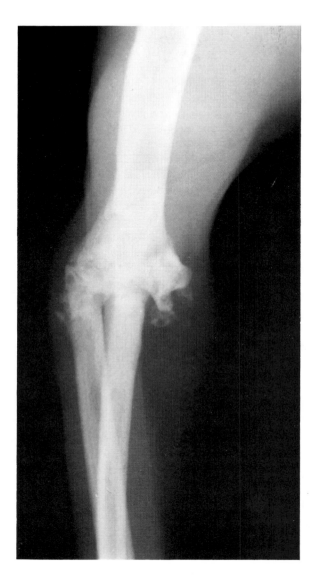

FIG. 17.3   (above) Lateral radiograph of the elbow joint of an 8-year-old DSH cat with advanced osteoarthritis. New bone deposition is evident. (right) Craniocaudal radiograph showing the osteoarthritis is secondary to a congenital subluxation of the humeroradial joint. In addition to the new bone, there is obvious bony remodelling.

Arthritis associated with bacterial L-forms

Bacterial L-forms (i.e. bacteria without a cell wall) can cause arthritis and subcutaneous abscessation. These are very difficult to grow in the laboratory even with specialised techniques and cultures are often negative. Such infections are resistant to many antibiotics, although most are susceptible to tetracyclines.

Feline Lyme disease

Lyme disease (or borreliosis) is caused by infection with the spirochaete *Borrelia burgdorferi*. The bacterium is transmitted by ticks (*Ixodes ricinus* in the UK, *Ixodes damini* and *Ixodes pacificus* in the USA). Cats can certainly be infected with the organism as shown by seroconversion but there is no clear account of clinical disease.[26] Clinical signs of Lyme disease reported in other species include lameness (single or multiple joints), fever, anorexia, lethargy, lymphadenopathy, muscle disease, meningitis, carditis, renal disease and neurological disease. The criteria for diagnosis of Lyme disease are given in Fig. 17.6.

Mycoplasmal arthritis

Mycoplasma gateae and *M. felis* are common local inhabitants of the oropharynx of healthy cats and are generally considered relatively non-pathogenic. However, both these organisms can produce polyarthritis and tenosynovitis, particularly in animals which are immunosuppressed in some way. The synovial fluid is watery and contains large numbers of white cells, most of which are polymorphs. The organism can be cultured on special media or sometimes visualised in a fluid smear using Wright-Leishmann and Giemsa stains. Treatment is with tetracyclines, tylosin, erythromycin, gentamycin or chloramphenicol.

Mycotic arthritis

Fungal infections of bone and joints are unlikely to be encountered in the UK, but can be seen in some areas of the United States. Disseminated systemic mycotic infections (e.g. *Cryptococcus,*

Histoplasma) may rarely invade joints haematogenously or by direct extension from an adjacent fungal osteomyelitis or dermatitis.

Calicivirus arthritis

A fleeting stiffness, soreness and lameness with high fever, probably caused by certain strains of calicivirus, has been reported in young kittens.[1,29] It is also known that a transient, sometimes protracted, arthropathy can occur as a complication to vaccination. Lameness occurs 5–7 days after vaccination and studies have shown calicivirus antigens within synovial macrophages. Arthritis associated with viable calicivirus within the joint has also been demonstrated. The arthritis is usually self-limiting and a complete recovery can be expected although the role of calicivirus in chronic inflammatory arthritis is not yet defined.

Inflammatory type: non-infective arthritis

The non-infective inflammatory arthropathies are defined as those where no micro-organisms can be cultured from the joint. Two types are identified – the crystal arthropathies (which are not reported in the cat) and the immune-based arthropathies. There are a number of different types of the latter and their classification is shown

DRUGS USED TO TREAT OSTEOARTHRITIS			
Therapeutic agent	Dose	Route	Frequency
Aspirin	10-15 mg/kg	PO	Every 48-72 h
Codeine	1-2 mg/kg	PO	bid
Phenylbutazone	13-16 mg/kg	PO	bid. Alternate weeks if continuous therapy required
Prednisolone	0.25-2.0 mg/kg	PO, SC, IV	bid. Reducing dose, alternate days
Prednisolone	0.25-0.5 tab.	PO	Once/twice a day
Chinchophen			
Hexamine[a]			
Dexamethasone	0.125-0.5 mg/kg	PO, IV, IM	sid
Flunixin[b]	1.0 mg/kg	PO	sid
Essential fatty acids[c]	1 cap./5 kg	PO	sid
Pentosan sulphate	0.1 ml	i-artic	4-5 injections at 5-7 day intervals
	3 mg/kg	SC	4-5 injections at 5-7 day intervals
Polysulphated glycosaminoglycans	0.1 ml	i-artic	Once a week for 4-5 weeks
Sodium hyaluronate	0.1 ml	i-artic	Single injection can be repeated

[a] Use with extreme caution since fatal gastrointestinal ulceration can occur.
[b] No clinical trials have been reported (Lees & Taylor 1991)
[c] Alternatively fish liver oil supplements can be given & fish diets encouraged

FIG. 17.4 Drugs used to treat osteoarthritis.

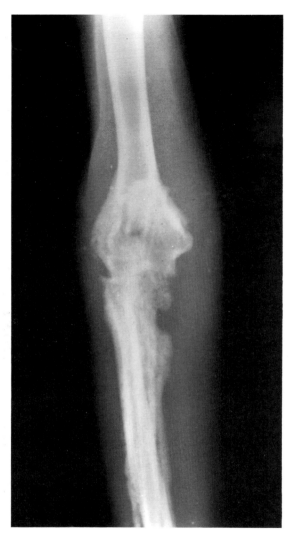

FIG. 17.5   Craniocaudal radiograph of the elbow joint of a 2-year-old DSH cat with a septic arthritis. Periosteal new bone is present and extends beyond the confine of the joint. The joint space is poorly defined, and small erosions are present.

in Fig. 17.2. The criteria for diagnosing the immune-based arthropathies are given in Fig. 17.7. Although they are classed as non-infective because no organism can be cultured from the joints, it is probable that infective agents or their antigens are involved in their pathogenesis.

Clinically, all the immune-based arthropathies can look similar. They are invariably polyarthritic or pauciarthritic (involving 2 to 4 joints) syndromes with a bilaterally symmetrical arthritis. The animal will present with a lameness characterised by a generalised stiffness or an obvious limp if an individual joint is severely affected. The lameness may shift from one limb to another and may be intermittent, particularly in the early stages. Systemic signs may be present (i.e. fever, anorexia, lethargy) and other body systems besides the joints may show disease. Joints may be swollen and painful on manipulation, although in many cases the clinical changes are subtle and difficult to appreciate. Synovial fluid is increased in quantity, of reduced viscosity and shows increased numbers of white cells, most of which are polymorphs. All cats with suspected immune-based arthritis should be tested for FeLV and FIV infection; although there is no definite aetiological association, the presence of these viruses can affect treatment and prognosis.

Rheumatoid-like arthritis (RA)

This is a rare chronic polyarthritis associated with bony destruction, visible on radiography. Severe joint derangement with luxation and sub-luxation can occur. Serum rheumatoid factor (an autoantibody against the patient's immunoglobulin) is often present.

Periosteal proliferative polyarthritis (PPP)

This can affect any joint but most often affects the carpus and hock, especially in the early stages. It is more common in male cats (Fig. 17.8). The most typical radiographical feature is the presence of extensive new bone which appears to be primarily periosteal in nature and which extends well beyond the confines of the joint (Fig. 17.9). Bony erosive changes within the joint are usually apparent. Enthesopathies also occur and show local erosion or proliferation of bone at tendon and ligament attachments. The possibility that there is an aetiological association with feline syncitium-forming virus has not been proven.

Systemic lupus erythematosus (SLE)

This is a rare multisystemic disease of the cat in which a variety of clinical signs can occur depending on which body systems are involved. The polyarthritis is bilaterally symmetrical and is non-erosive in nature. Hence radiographic examination of the joints usually reveals only soft tissue changes (Fig. 17.10) e.g. increased periarticular soft tissue density, loss of the intra-articular fat pads of the stifle joints, distension of joint capsules. Besides lameness, other clinical signs include those related to glomerulonephritis, haemolytic anaemia, thrombocytopenia, meningitis, dermatitis etc. (Fig. 17.11). The presence of circulating antinuclear antibody is an important diagnostic criterion. Certain other autoantibodies can be demonstrated in individual cases.

Idiopathic polyarthritis (IP)

Idiopathic polyarthritis is a term used to classify types of immune-based arthritis which do not satisfy the criteria for RA, PPP and SLE. It is divided into four types according to whether or not certain associations are present. Type I is uncomplicated polyarthritis; in Type II the arthritis is associated with infections elsewhere in the body (e.g. conjunctivitis, urinary tract infection, uterine infection, respiratory tract infection, skin infection); in Type III gastrointestinal disease is associated with the arthritis; and in Type IV neoplastic disease is present elsewhere in the body. Most cases show multiple joint involvement, although single joint disease is also possible.

In Type II cases, it is useful to confirm the focus of infection by culture techniques, where this is feasible. The author has seen cases of chlamydial conjunctivitis associated with arthritis and lameness; culture of the conjunctiva, the demonstration of chlamydial antigens on a conjunctival smear or the presence of increased levels of

DIAGNOSIS OF LYME DISEASE	
Criterion	**Remarks**
1. History of exposure to ticks	Ticks found on animal or animal lives in tick infested area. Ticks can infest dogs and cats and not be noticed by their owners.
2. Seasonal incidence	The incubation period can be very variable and thus disease signs can occur at any time.
3. Presence of clinical features	Signs include fever, lethargy, inappetence, lameness (limp in 1 or more limbs, stiffness), swollen joint or joints, neck pain, carditis (heart block), glomerulonephritis, neurological signs (aggression, seizures, behavioural changes). Clinical features are very non-specific.
4. Laboratory aids to diagnosis	Confirmation of inflammatory (poly) synovitis by synovial fluid analysis (increased WBC, mainly PMNs) or synovial membrane biopsy for histology. Confirmation of meningitis by CSF analysis (increased WBC, protein content, creatine phosphokinase level). ECG abnormalities with cardiac disease. Confirmation of glomerulonephritis by renal biopsy.
5. Positive serological test (IFT or ELISA) for anti-*Borrelia* antibodies	Animals can seroconvert without ever showing disease.
6. Prompt response to antibiotic therapy	In some chronic cases the pathology may be more associated with an immune response against *Borrelia* antigens.
7. Culture of spirochaetes from blood, urine, synovia, CSF and tissues	Culture of *B. burgdorferi* is very difficult.
8. Identification of *Borrelia* organisms or antigens in blood, urine, synovial fluid and tissue biopsies such as skin and synovium	Not fully evaluated. Organisms may be isolated from individuals without clinical signs of disease.
9. Exclusion of other possible causes of the clinical signs by careful clinical evaluation and laboratory testing.	Depends on available resources.

Before Lyme disease can be diagnosed, criteria 1, 3 and 4 (relevant to clinical manifestations), 5 and 9 should be satisfied as a minimal requirement. Ideally criterion 6 should be satisfied in most cases.

FIG. 17.6   Criteria for the diagnosis of Lyme disease in the cat.

DIAGNOSIS OF IMMUNE-BASED POLYARTHROPATHIES

Rheumatoid-like arthritis (RA):
1. Stiffness after rest.
2. Pain or tenderness on motion of at least one joint.
3. Swelling of at least one joint.
4. Swelling of one other joint within three months.
5. Symmetrical joint swelling.
6. Subcutaneous nodules.
7. Erosive changes on joint radiographs.
8. Serological test positive for rheumatoid factor.
9. Abnormal synovial fluid.
10. Histopathology of synovium.
11. Histopathology of subcutaneous nodules.

Seven criteria must be fulfilled, including two of criteria 7, 8 and 10. Criteria 1, 2, 3, 4 and 5 should be present for at least six weeks.

Periosteal proliferative polyarthritis (PPP):
1. At least four joints affected.
2. Periosteal articular new bone on radiographs.
3. Erosive changes on joint radiographs.
4. Enthesopathies on radiographs.

Criteria 1, 2 and 3 must be satisfied.

Systemic lupus erythematosus (SLE):
1. Multisystem disease. Most common manifestations include polyarthritis, skin disease, anaemia, glomerulonephritis.
2. Antinuclear antibody present in blood.
3. Immunopathological features consistent with clinical involvement should be present.

Criteria 1 and 2 must always be satisfied.

Polyarteritis nodosa (PN):
1. Symmetrical polyarthritis.
2. Necrosis and inflammation of blood vessels seen on biopsy of synovium, and other tissues.

Idiopathic:
Includes all cases of polyarthritis which do not satisfy criteria for RA, PPP, SLE or PN.
Type I - No associations.
Type II - Arthritis associated with infection elsewhere in body.
Type III - Arthritis associated with gastrointestinal disease.
Type IV - Arthritis associated with neoplastic disease.

FIG. 17.7   Criteria for diagnosing the immune-based polyarthropathies.

circulating chlamydial antibodies can help in diagnosis. Calicivirus infection can also initiate arthritis, although it is uncertain whether this should be classed as an immune-based disease or primarily an infective arthritis.

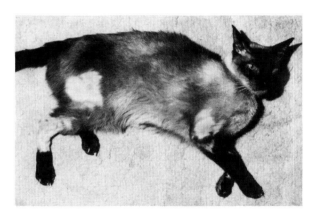

FIG. 17.8   A 7-year-old male castrate Siamese with periosteal proliferative polyarthritis. This cat presented with generalised stiffness, inability to jump and a reluctance to exercise. All the limb joints were thickened, and showed pain on manipulation. The cat showed periods of pyrexia and inappetence.

Cases of Type II arthritis should be treated by clearing the infective process, and anti-inflammatory treatment may also be required. Diagnosis of the gastrointestinal problem in Type III cases is desirable and, again, specific treatment is necessary. The most common neoplastic process in Type IV cases is some form of myeloproliferative disease; diagnosis involves a bone marrow biopsy and the prognosis is dictated by the nature of the neoplasm.

Others

Polyarteritis nodosa has been described in the cat and can cause a polyarthritis. It is characterised by widespread necrosis and inflammation of small and medium-sized arteries in many tissues and organs, including the joints. Drug-induced arthritis has not been reported convincingly in the cat as it has in the dog.

Treatment of immune-based arthritis

Treatment depends to some extent on the type of arthritis which is diagnosed and reference has already been made to the treatment of the idiopathic Types II, III and IV where the underlying association is more relevant than the joint disease itself.

Glucocorticoids (e.g. prednisolone) are most often used to treat immune-based arthritis. In acute onset cases, high doses of prednisolone can be used, e.g. 2–4 mg/kg bodyweight for 2 weeks, after which the dose is gradually reduced over 6–8 weeks, provided that clinical remission persists. It is hoped that the drug can be stopped eventually, although in some cases a maintenance dose is necessary, ideally on an alternate day basis. In the more chronic cases, such as the rheumatoid-like disease and periosteal proliferative polyarthritis, there is no advantage in giving high dose therapy.

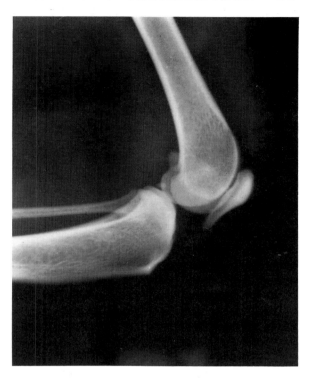

FIG. 17.10   Lateral radiograph of the stifle joint of a 4-year-old DSH spayed cat with a non-erosive polyarthritis. There is loss of the fat pad shadow, consistent with a synovial effusion. It is usual with non-erosive polyarthritis to see only soft tissue changes on the joint radiographs. This cat was positive for circulating antinuclear antibody, and also had a protein-losing nephropathy, and was diagnosed as a case of SLE.

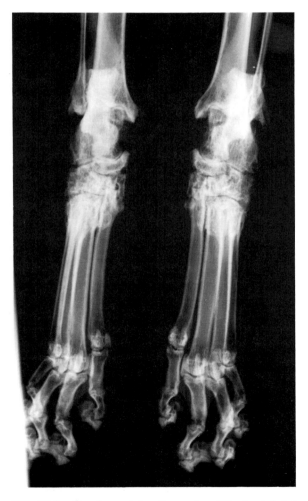

FIG. 17.9   Craniocaudal radiographs of the hock joints of a 4-year-old DSH cat with periosteal proliferative polyarthritis. Note the new bone formation affecting the hock joint. Synovial fluid samples from several joints of this cat had high polymorph counts.

Such cases are managed better with low dose corticosteroids when there is a clinical problem. Alternatively, chronic cases can be treated with a combination of prednisolone and cytotoxic drugs. Cyclophosphamide is often used at a dose of 2.0 mg/kg bodyweight once a day for four consecutive days of each week. Corticosteroids are given each day at a dose of 0.5–2.0 mg/kg.

If cytotoxic drugs are used, complete blood cell counts should be carried out every 10 days or so. If the white cell count falls below 6000/μl the drug dose should be reduced by 25%; if it falls below 4000/μl the drug is stopped for one week and then reinstituted at half the original dose. Cytotoxic drugs are stopped one month after complete remission is achieved although the prednisolone may be continued for longer. Cyclophosphamide

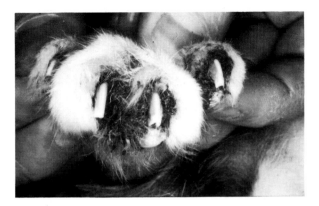

FIG. 17.11   Photograph of one of the paws of a 2-year-old DSH cat with systemic lupus erythematosus. This cat had an exudative paronychia in addition to a polyarthritis.

should not be used for longer than 4 months because of potential bladder complications. Cats should be protected from possible pathogens when undergoing immunosuppressive treatment, which is potentially a problem in the case of FeLV or FIV infected cats.

Chrysotherapy can be used in the rheumatoid-like disease and periosteal proliferative polyarthritis although gold is a very toxic drug. It can be given by injection (sodium aurothiomalate 2.5 mg IM once a week for 6 weeks). A less toxic oral preparation is now available (auranofin) which has been used in the dog but the author has no experience of its use in the cat.

METABOLIC BONE DISEASES

Nutritional secondary hyperparathyroidism (nutritional osteopenia, juvenile osteopenia)

This condition is caused by the feeding of a diet low in calcium and high in phosphorus – classically a meat-only diet (see Chapter 3). Resorption of bone to release calcium is an important homeostatic mechanism but the skeleton becomes weakened after prolonged release of parathyroid hormone, resulting in bone pain and deformities. Affected kittens often show a generalised stiffness or limp and become miserable and lethargic. Pathological

fractures occur and these can involve the vertebrae and produce neurological disturbances.

Radiography reveals poor bone mineralisation (Figs 17.12 and 17.13) and will show pathological fractures. Such fractures are usually minimally displaced and are best treated conservatively,

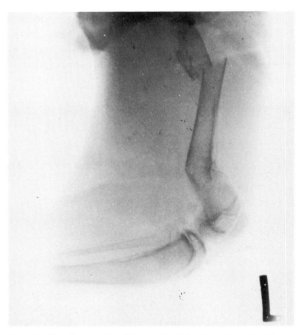

FIG. 17.12   Lateral radiograph of the hindleg of a kitten with nutritional secondary hyperparathyroidism. The mineralisation is poor, and there is a double pathological fracture of the femur.

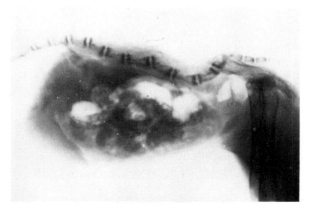

FIG. 17.13   Lateral radiograph of the lumbar spine of a kitten with nutritional secondary hyperparathyroidism. Note the marked deformity of the vertebral column.

although pathological fractures of the spine may necessitate euthanasia. Pelvic and thoracic deformities may cause defaecatory or reproductive, and respiratory problems respectively.

Rickets (osteomalacia) is virtually unknown in the cat. It is clinically similar to nutritional secondary hyperparathyroidism and the two diseases are distinguished by the radiographic appearance of the growth plates: in rickets the physes are increased in thickness, whereas in nutritional secondary hyperparathyroidism they are of normal thickness.

Osteogenesis imperfecta

This is an inherited bone disease characterised by poor mineralisation and excessive bone fragility. Clinically the disease mimics nutritional secondary hyperparathyroidism, and the term was often used incorrectly in the older literature to describe the nutritional disease. However, the disease does occur in kittens and should be suspected in young kittens presenting with osteopenia but being fed a normal diet.

There are two types – osteogenesis imperfecta congenita and osteogenesis imperfecta tarda (Fig. 17.14). Osteogenesis imperfecta has a poor prognosis; treatment, by supplementation with calcium and phosphorus, is unrewarding and euthanasia is usually necessary, since the generalised skeletal pain is difficult to control. Juvenile idiopathic osteopenia is a similar disorder but it has a better prognosis and has not been recognised in the cat.

Renal secondary hyperparathyroidism

Renal disease (e.g. glomerulonephropathy, chronic nephritis, amyloidosis, congenital renal disease) can lead to phosphorus retention with a compensatory fall in blood calcium. The latter initiates the release of parathyroid hormone, which causes calcium release from the skeleton. The renal pathology could also interfere with the production of 1,25 dehydroxycholecalciferol, the active metabolite of vitamin D, which is involved in the normal calcification of bone matrix, and osteomalacia can result.

It is generally the older cat which is affected, and there may be clinical signs related to the renal disease. The bony demineralisation may cause

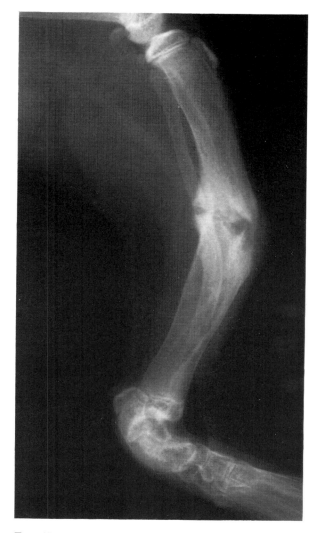

FIG. 17.14 Lateral radiograph of the lower hindlimb of a 5-month-old kitten with osteogenesis imperfecta. There is poor skeletal mineralisation, with a midshaft tibial fracture showing angulation. There is obvious curvature of the fibula and deformity of the fibular tarsal bone. This cat was receiving a balanced proprietary diet. The animal was euthanased because of generalised skeletal pain and deformity.

bone pain, soft bones (e.g. those of the jaw), loose teeth and pathological fractures. Radiography will show the poor bony mineralisation (Fig. 17.15) and resorption of alveolar socket bone, and loss of the lamina dura dentes. If feasible, treatment should be to halt the renal disease and is usually directed towards reducing the excretory load of the kidneys and providing substances that the kidney is failing to conserve. Calcium, as the gluconate or lactate, should be given with care, and additional vitamin D may be advisable.

Primary hyperparathyroidism

This rare condition is caused by a primary hyperplasia or a neoplasia of the parathyroid glands. Bone demineralisation occurs, which may show as polyostotic lesions on radiography. Pain, lethargy and reluctance to move are clinical features.

Primary hypoparathyroidism

This condition is the result of a lymphocytic parathyroiditis. There is very little clinical effect on the skeleton; anorexia, muscle spasms, lethargy and tetany are described. Treatment necessitates

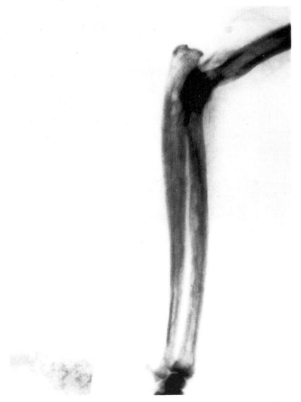

FIG. 17.15 Lateral radiograph of the left foreleg of an old cat with renal secondary hyperparathyroidism. Note the uneven mineralisation of the radius and ulna, particularly of the cortices.

initial intravenous and subcutaneous calcium, followed by oral calcium lactate and vitamin D. Iatrogenic primary hypoparathyroidism can also develop as a sequel to injury or removal of the parathyroid glands at the time of thyroid surgery, most often after bilateral thyroidectomy of hyperthyroid cats.

Hypervitaminosis A

The feeding of excessive amounts of liver to cats results in hypervitaminosis A (see Chapter 3).[32] It is most often seen in adult cats which have been on a liver-rich diet for several years, and is characterised by bony proliferation within the cranial and thoracic spine (Figs 17.16–17.18) and within the limb joints. Vitamin A is important in the regulation of osteoblasts and osteoclasts, and skeletal disease will occur if there is an excess or a deficiency of the vitamin. Excess liver given to young kittens will cause not only a secondary hyperparathyroidism, but also interference of bone growth.[3] Lipid infiltration of parenchymatous organs is also a feature of the toxicity.

The clinical signs in the older cat include stiffness, pain and an obvious limp. The spine is often ankylosed, and the neck shows reduced movement. Grooming becomes difficult and the animal's coat becomes unkempt. Affected limb joints may be enlarged, painful and with reduced motion. Sometimes a foreleg lameness can be associated with a neurological deficit, due to spinal exostoses compressing the peripheral nerve roots to the forelimbs.

Hypovitaminosis A

The prevalence of this disease is difficult to assess. It is seen in young kittens where the maternal supply of vitamin A is deficient. It causes bulky cranial and vertebral bones, resulting in a reduced size of the vertebral canal, cranial vault and neurovascular foraminae. Pressure on the brain, spinal cord and peripheral/cranial nerves results in a variety of neurological signs. The bony changes occur during about the fifth week after birth. Radiography of the skull will show an increased thickness of bones, especially those surrounding the posterior fossa of the brain. Although treatment by dietary supplementation

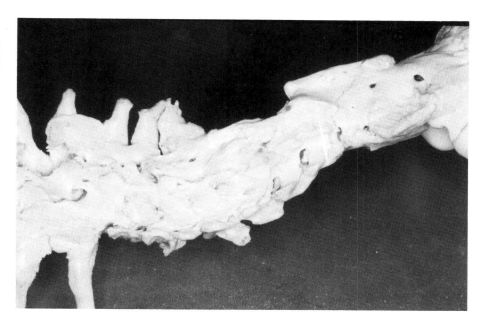

FIG. 17.16 Photograph of a post-mortem specimen of the cervical spine of a cat with hypervitaminosis A. There is a marked proliferation of new bone causing complete ankylosis.

with vitamin A is possible, euthanasia is often advisable if neurological signs are severe.

NEOPLASTIC & NEOPLASTIC-LIKE LESIONS

Primary tumours

Osteosarcoma is the most common primary bone neoplasm of the cat. It tends to occur in aged, female domestic short-haired cats – the average age is 11 years, with a range of 2–20 years. The humerus, femur and tibia are commonly affected, and the tumour may localise in any part of the bone. Most limb bones can be affected, as well as the sacrum, coccyx, pelvis, ribs and skull. Osteosarcoma associated with a previous fracture has been reported.

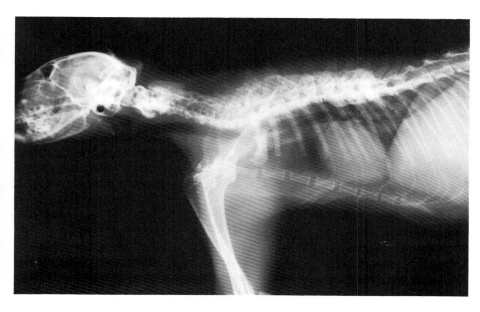

FIG. 17.17 Lateral radiograph of the cervical and thoracic spine of a cat with hypervitaminosis A. New bone deposits are obvious, particularly within the thoracic spine.

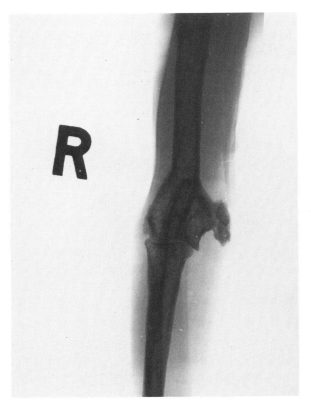

FIG. 17.18   Craniocaudal radiograph of the right elbow joint of a cat with hypervitaminosis A. There is new bone on the medial side of the distal humerus.

Pain and swelling over the neoplasm are the usual clinical features, and the onset of lameness can be sudden. Reduced movement of associated joints is usual.

The radiographic appearance is very variable. There may be predominant osteolysis characterised by radiolucency within the bone, thinning and loss of the cortices: this is more likely to be seen with tumours of the appendicular skeleton (Fig 17.19). 'Sunbursting' and periosteal new bone may also be seen, and are more likely with axial tumours. In other cases the tumours appear very radiodense, and the radiodensity may extend into the soft tissues and have an irregular outline. Pathological fractures are not uncommon. Osteosarcoma can sometimes be difficult to distinguish from osteomyelitis or a traumatic bone fracture; a biopsy may be necessary.

In general, osteosarcomas metastasise slowly in cats, although there have been reports of spreading to the lungs, regional lymph nodes and kidneys. Treatment by surgical excision of the mass or by amputation of the affected limb is often successful. The other primary tumours are summarised in Fig. 17.20.

Secondary neoplasms

Secondary spread of primary soft tissue neoplasms to the skeletal system appears to be rare. They include mammary gland carcinoma and bronchial carcinoma (see Fig. 17.21).[28] Tumours can also affect bone by local pressure and invasion (see Fig. 17.21).

Metastasis of pulmonary carcinoma to the digits is an interesting syndrome. Spread is generally to

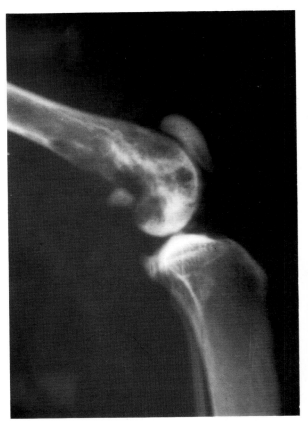

FIG. 17.19   Lateral radiograph of the stifle joint of a 13-year-old spayed DSH cat. There are obvious areas of radiolucency within the distal femur. Histological examination confirmed a diagnosis of osteolytic osteosarcoma.

PRIMARY MUSCULOSKELETAL TUMOURS			
Tumour	**Clinical features**	**Radiographic features**	**Treatment**
Osteosarcoma	Mainly older cats. No particular predilection sites	Osteolysis or osteosclerosis (see Fig. 17.19)	Slow to metastasise. Amputation possible
Juxtacortical osteosarcoma (parosteal osteosarcoma)	Arises from outer surface of cortex	Irregular, poorly-defined mass of variable mineral density	Unlikely to metastasise. Surgical excision or debulking
Chondrosarcoma	Incidence low	Bone destruction, mineralisation. Poorly defined margins. 'Snowflake' appearance	Radical local excision or limb amputation. Pulmonary metastases reported
Osteoma	Benign, mainly affects skull	Well circumscribed radiodense mass	Surgical excision
Osteoid osteoma	Small core of calcified osteoid tissue surrounded by mantle of sclerotic bone	Dense radiopaque bone, surrounded by zone of even denser radiopacity	–
Multilobular chondroma (chondroma rodens)	Usuallly arises from flat bones of skull. Locally invasive	Bony destruction	Local excision. Malignant transformation can occur
Osteoclastoma (giant cell tumour)	Affects limb bones	Expansile destructive lesion. Cortices thinned, trabeculae within lesion ('soap-bubble' appearance) (see Fig. 17.22)	Slow-growing and slow to metastasise. Local excision or limb amputation (see Fig. 17.23)
Fibrosarcoma	Long bones	Osteolysis	Limb amputation
Synovial sarcoma	Reported within joints	Bony destruction within joint. Soft tissue density. Irregular periosteal response	Rapidly metastasise
Synovioma	Mainly affects tendon sheaths within the limbs. Presents as swelling within limbs, with or without lameness	Soft tissue density	Local resection, although recurrence common. Limb amputation
Aneurysmal bone cyst	Benign blood-filled spaces and solid areas of spindle cell stroma containing osteoid and giant cells. Mainly appendicular skeleton	Discrete radiolucent area with thin cortex	Local resection can be attempted
Fibrous dysplasia	Developmental abnormality. Can affect whole skeleton or individual bones. Immature osseous trabeculae within fibrous matrix	Can be of bizarre appearance. Areas of radiodensity. Periosteal new bone	Local excision or limb amputation when affects individual bone. Euthanasia if generalised
Other bone sarcomas	There are many tumours reported in the cat which have not been accurately classified		
Tumours of skeletal muscle (e.g. rhadomyosarcoma)	Difficult to diagnose in early stages. Progressive lameness. Severe muscle atrophy and pain. Joint contractures occur		Poor prognosis usually. Euthanasia. Amputation if low malignancy

FIG. 17.20   Summary of the main features of primary musculoskeletal tumours in the cat.

multiple digits and the pulmonary lesion may be very small and difficult to identify, even at post-mortem examination.[28] These cats present with lameness and there is swelling of one or more digits. The lesions are painful and there is often permanent exsheathment of the claw (Fig. 17.24). Radiography shows bone loss of the 3rd (and sometimes 2nd) phalanx with irregular new bone proliferation and obvious soft tissue opacity (Fig.

17.25). These pulmonary carcinomas can metastasise to other sites, e.g. muscle, kidney, heart, skin; metastasis to the muscle will also produce a painful lameness. Radiography of the thorax rarely shows the pulmonary tumour. Diagnosis can usually be confirmed by digital amputation and histological evaluation. The prognosis is very poor and euthanasia is recommended.

SECONDARY MUSCULOSKELETAL TUMOURS			
Tumour	Clinical features	Radiographic features	Treatment
True metastases Bronchial carcinoma	Spread to the digits very common. Respiratory signs are rare	Bone loss of 3rd phalanx. Irregular calcification. Soft tissue density. Primary lung lesion rarely visible.	Euthanasia
Other carcinomas	Rare. Primary may be evident, e.g. mammary carcinomas	Bony destruction.	Euthanasia
Lymphosarcoma	Reported affecting joints of cats		Poor prognosis
Direct extension of neoplasm into bone Fibrosarcoma of soft tissue	Regularly reported	Bone lysis	Local resection may be possible
Multicentric subcutaneous fibrosarcoma	Fast growing. Cats less than 5 years of age. Associated with C-type oncornavirus (feline sarcoma virus)		Metastases to muscle and lungs as well as local invasion of bone. Feline sarcoma virus is a rare recombinant form of FeLV. Most cats FeLV antigen positive. Very poor prognosis
Squamous cell carcinoma	Mainly oral cavity. Bones of skull and mandible	Bone loss. Soft tissue swelling and density. Occasional periosteal new bone	Prognosis very poor
Others (Lymphosarcoma, lymphoma, rhabdomyo-sarcoma, melanoma, haemangiosarcoma, reticulum cell carcinoma, meningio-sarcoma, mandibular epidermoid carcinoma, fibro-meloblastoma, neurofibro-sarcoma, fibromatous epulis of malignant fibrous histocytoma)	Local bone pathology	Bony destruction and/or proliferation	Treatment depends on histopathology of initial biopsy

FIG. 17.21   Summary of the main features of secondary musculoskeletal tumours in the cat.

Neoplastic-like lesions

Osteocartilaginous exostoses

Solitary form

These are benign, slow-growing tumours of cartilage origin and are characterised by a cartilagenous cap that gives rise to cancellous bone by endochondral ossification. These lesions are most often diagnosed in mature cats, 2–4 years of age. Lameness of insidious onset is the presenting sign. The lesion develops at the physeal regions of the long bones, and is difficult to see on radiography in the early stages. The exostoses have a broad base and with time take on a dense, smoothly irregular appearance with a defined border. The underlying bone is generally not affected, although local bony erosion may occur. Treatment is by local surgical resection and the prognosis is good, although regrowth does occur. When malignant transformation (e.g. to osteosarcoma or chondro-sarcoma) is diagnosed, amputation is advisable.

Multiple form

Multiple osteocartilaginous exostoses or feline osteochondromatosis has been reported occasionally.[30] The multiple lesions are characterised by enlarging masses most frequently affecting the axial skeleton, e.g. ribs, scapulae, vertebrae, skull and pelvis (in decreasing order of frequency). Limb bone involvement is rare. The radiographic features of the individual tumours are similar to those seen with solitary osteocartilaginous exostosis. The lesions usually develop in young mature cats and the prognosis is very poor, no cat surviving beyond one year after onset of clinical signs. Histologically the lesion in the early stages is similar to a solitary osteochondroma but in time, the appearance is more consistent with a sarcoma. It has been suggested that a retrovirus infection may be involved in the aetiology, because C-type particles have been found in the tumours and several cats were FeLV positive.[30]

Synovial osteochondrometaplasia

This condition (also called synovial osteochondromatosis) is characterised by osseous and cartilaginous masses formed by hyperplastic metaplasia

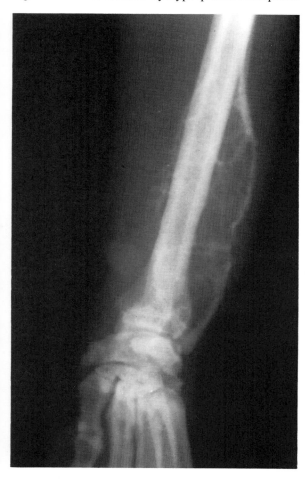

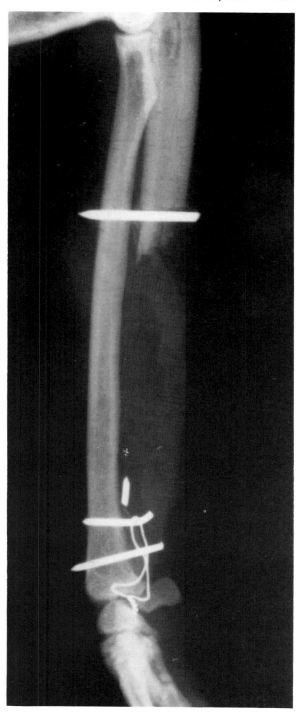

FIG. 17.22 Craniocaudal radiograph of the lower forelimb of a 12-year-old DSH cat, showing the 'soap bubble' appearance characteristic of an osteoclastoma affecting the ulna.

FIG. 17.23 Lateral radiograph of the lower forelimb after resection of the diseased ulna shown in Fig. 17.22. A bone graft was inserted to replace the styloid process of the ulna.

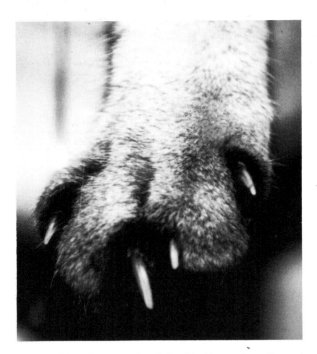

FIG. 17.24 Photograph of the hindfoot of an 8-year-old cat with metastatic spread of bronchial carcinoma to the 3rd phalanx of digit 3. The cat presented with lameness, painful swelling of the digit and permanent exsheathment of the claw.

of synovial cells. The cartilaginous masses often undergo calcification. The bony and cartilaginous lesions are found embedded within the synovial layer, although on X-ray films they may appear as free joint bodies. The disease is often confined to a single joint and can cause lameness, particularly in the later stages. It has been reported in the metacarpal joints and in the stifle and elbow.[30] Because of their position within the synovial lining, these lesions cannot be removed easily: surgical stripping of the synovium is possible, but surgical access will always be limited.

Synovial cyst

Synovial cysts are benign lesions which originate from the synovium of joints, bursae or tendon sheaths. They appear as a subcutaneous mass which may occasionally produce cutaneous ulceration.[31] They are difficult to distinguish from cutaneous and subcutaneous neoplasms. Local

excision is usually successful in treating these lesions.

INHERITED CONGENITAL AND DEVELOPMENTAL DISORDERS

Congenital deformities

Congenital deformities are rare in the cat, but several have been reported. The main deformities are summarised in Fig. 17.26.

Mucopolysaccharidosis

The mucopolysaccharidoses are a group of diseases due to inborn errors of glycosaminoglycan

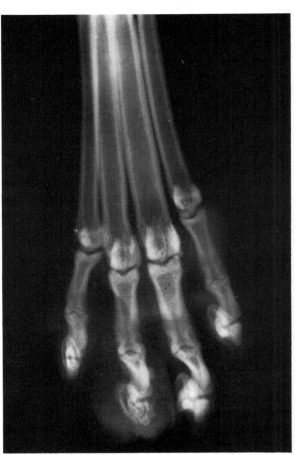

FIG. 17.25 Craniocaudal radiograph of the hindfoot of the cat in Fig. 17.24. There is soft tissue swelling, destruction of P3 and calcification affecting digit 3. Digital metastasis of bronchial carcinoma is well documented in the cat.

SUMMARY OF SOME CONGENITAL ABNORMALITIES

Abnormality	Clinical features	Other features	Comments
Absence of tail	No tail vertebrae - the 'rumpy'. Small no. tail vertebrae - the 'rumpyriser'. Several tail vertebrae, but deformed - the 'stumpy'. Several tail vertebrae, normal appearance - the 'longie'.	Spina bifida may be present leading to incontinence, defecation problems. Pelvic and rear limb deformities, microperforate anus.	Inherited dominant trait with incomplete penetrance, semi-lethal. Manx cats.
Kinked tail	Angular deformity between coccygeal vertebrae.		Recessive trait.
Polydactyly	Extra digits, especially forefeet.		Inherited. Common. Rarely requires any special treatment other than trimming of claws.
Syndactyly	Fusion of digits		Rare
Ectrodactyly	Absence of all or part of a digit.		Inherited. Rare. Affects forefeet.
Amelia and hemimelia	Absence of a limb (amelia) or the whole or part of distal limb (hemimelia).		Rare. Hemimelia of radius and ulna most common.
Peromelus ascelus	Absence of hindlimb		Rare.
Arrested development of long bones of forelimb	Failure of forelimb bones to grow their natural length (Kangaroo cats).		Rare. Inherited, possibly sex-linked, affects females.
Congenital duplication	Various types have been described.		Rare.
Mandibular ramus aplasia	Abnormal ossification of the mandible resulting in micrognathia.		Rare.
Arthrogryposis	Inability to flex and extend joints/ persistent flexion		Rare.
Achondroplasia	Dwarfism. Muscle weakness, particularly of hindlimbs. Death at 1-4 months of age.	Ascites, enlarged liver, spleen and lymph nodes. Hepatic storage disease.	Autosomal-recessive.
Scottish ear-fold chondrodysplasia	If homozygous, coccygeal vertebrae deformed (short tail), shortened metacarpal, metatarsal and phalangeal bones. Fusion of bones, tarsal exostosis.	Folded pinnae.	Deformities can be avoided, but folded pinnae retained if mate fold-ear to normal prick-ear.
Congenital hypothyroidism	Disproportionate dwarfism, lethargy, juvenile hair coat. Delayed closure of fontanelles, delayed appearance of epiphyses, irregular fragmented epiphyses, cortical thickening of the long bones.	Mental retardation, hydrocephalus.	Rare.
Maxillofacial compression (Peke, face, dished face)	Shortening of the maxilla and mandible - brachycephalic appearance.	Predisposed to respiratory, pharyngeal and ocular disease.	Persian, Angora and Himalayan breeds.
Craniofacial malformation in Burmese	Enlarged cranial cavity, duplicated or missing cerebral hemispheres. Eyes missing or small. Nostrils/nasal cavities may be missing. Upper jaw and palate may be partially duplicated.		
Thorax abnormalities	Additional thoracic vertebrae sternebrae, pairs of ribs.	Caudal displacement of heart.	Rare.
Fusion of cervical spine (Klippel-Feil anomaly)	Neurological deficits.		Rare.
Spina bifida	Closure defect of vertebral arches.	Meningocoele, meningomyelocoele, syringomyelia, sacrococcygeal agenesis, rachischisis.	Inherited, associated with gene for taillessness in Manx cats. Rare in other breeds.
Pectus e cavatum	Complete or partial depression of sternum with associated flattening.	May be associated with chronic respiratory disease.	Can be treated by surgical resection of the deformed sternum.

Fig. 17.26   Summary of some of the congenital abnormalities recognised in cats.

(mucopolysaccharide) metabolism. They are lysosomal storage diseases typified by a deficiency of a specific enzyme involved in the degradation of glycosaminoglycans. Although several different types have been described in man, only types I and VI have been reported in the cat.[4,18,23]

Feline mucopolysaccharidosis VI is an inherited autosomal recessive disease that occurs in Siamese and Siamese-cross cats. Affected cats excrete excess dermatan sulphate in the urine: there is a decreased activity of arylsulphatase B. Clinical features include broadening of the maxilla, corneal clouding, pectus excavatum and diffuse neurological abnormalities. The animals often have a crouching gait with abduction of the stifles, and pain and crepitus in several joints. The epiphyseal and metaphyseal areas of the long bones are enlarged and irregularly shaped. Neck manipulation is painful, and there is increased muscle tone in the limbs. Most cats have a chronic mucoid ocular discharge and chronic upper respiratory tract infection. Chronic diarrhoea occurs in some cases. Clinical signs begin at an early age, although affected animals may not be presented until adult. The radiographic features include bilateral hip luxation/subluxation, coxa valga, fusion of the cervical vertebrae, flaring of the ribs at the costochondral junctions and irregular osseous proliferation of the ends of the long bones. Diagnosis is confirmed by the demonstration of urinary glycosaminoglycans, identification of excessive amounts of dermatan sulphate and confirmation of decreased arylsulphatase B activity. Urinary glycosaminoglycans can be demonstrated with a urine spot test using toluidine blue stain or a commercial reagent. Examination of a blood smear, stained with Wright-Giemsa stain, will demonstrate coarse granular material in over 90% of neutrophils. The granules stain metachromatically blue with toluidine blue. There is no treatment and the prognosis is poor, although some cats can cope for several years.

Feline mucopolysaccharidosis 1 is thought to be an autosomal recessive disease, and has been described in white domestic short-haired cats. Affected cats excrete increased amounts of dermatan and heparin sulphate in the urine associated with a deficiency of α-L iduronidase. The clinical and radiographic features are similar to the type VI disease, except that long bone epiphyseal dysplasia is not a feature. The laboratory features include the presence of glycosaminoglycans in the urine, although metachromatic granules are not present in the circulating neutrophils. Again there is no treatment, but affected cats can survive comfortably for several years.

Patellar luxation

Medial congenital patellar instability has been reported in the cat.[10] Devon Rex may show a susceptibility, although it can occur in other breeds including the domestic short-hair. The clinical features include intermittent 'locking' of the stifle, followed by extension of the joint to release the patella, abnormal gait and carriage of the limb. Some cases show medial rotation of the tibial tuberosity and a shallow trochlear groove; angular and torsional deformities of the femur and tibia are not usually present. Diagnosis is made by clinical examination, although radiography can help.

Some mild cases do not require surgical treatment. The techniques used to correct medial patellar luxation in the cat are similar to those used in the dog, and are basically designed to realign the extensor mechanism of the stifle.

Congenital lateral patellar luxation is rare in the cat. Traumatic patellar luxation is also seen, usually as a result of direct trauma to the stifle joint. It is usually a medial luxation and is corrected by a tightening of the lateral joint capsule. Medial patellar luxation can occur secondary to hip luxation and correction of the hip abnormality will generally correct the patellar instability.

Hip dysplasia

Hip dysplasia occurs in the cat but seldom produces clinical signs. It is said to be more common in the Siamese. The radiographical features are similar to those of the dog. When they occur, clinical signs include a crouching hindleg gait, intermittent limp, inability to jump or climb, reluctance to defaecate, and howling in pain. Crepitus and pain may be detected on manipulation of the hip joints. Treatment may include pectineal myotomy and femoral head resection, although mild cases can be managed conservatively.[14]

MISCELLANEOUS BONE & JOINT DISEASES

Myelofibrosis – osteosclerosis syndrome

Myelofibrosis is characterised by fibroblastic proliferation and varying degrees of collagen deposition in the marrow cavity. Primary (idiopathic) myelofibrosis is defined as a chronic myeloproliferative disease, associated with myeloid metaplasia of the liver, spleen and lymph nodes and abnormal growth of haematopoietic cells in the bone marrow. Secondary myelofibrosis occurs as a non-specific reactive change following prolonged bone marrow damage. Osteosclerosis (increased bone density) may occur in some cases of myelofibrosis, although it may not be apparent radiographically; it may also be associated with feline leukaemia virus infection[9] and has been reported as a terminal development in cats with naturally occurring erythroleukaemia.

Osteopetrosis

Osteopetrosis refers to a generalised skeletal sclerosis or a generalised increase in skeletal mass, and can occur in the cat as an acquired or congenital problem. The difference between the terms osteopetrosis and osteosclerosis is not precisely defined: however, osteopetrosis is usually considered a generalised disease, and the increase in skeletal mass is obvious on radiography. The radiographic changes include a generalised increase in bone density of the vertebrae, cortical thickening of the long bones with loss of normal trabecular structure and additional irregular osseous structures within the medullary cavity. There are a number of different aetiopathogenetic mechanisms incriminated in acquired osteopetrosis, although many cases go unexplained.[22]

Hypertrophic pulmonary osteoarthropathy

This is very rare in the cat. It is characterised by periosteal proliferation of new bone along the shafts of the limb bones, and most cases are associated with an intrathoracic mass. In two cases reported in the cat, the forelimbs were more affected than the hindlimbs, and the phalanges were unaffected. The bony reaction was more extensive and less regular than seen in other species.

Disuse osteopenia

This is a bony loss in an individual bone or limb or in the entire skeleton caused by a lack of weight-bearing and normal body stress. It is most often seen in a limb not being used because of fracture healing. The osteopenia may be evident on the radiographs, and is reversible once normal stresses are reapplied to the bone.

Cranial cruciate ligament rupture

Rupture of the cranial cruciate ligament is a rare disease and is most often associated with major trauma. In such cases there may be other ligament damage, and luxation/subluxation of the femorotibial joint is not unusual. However, recently there have been reports of cruciate failure in the cat not associated with major trauma.[17] It is also suggested that these cases may be associated with cardiomyopathy, and hence with an increased anaesthetic risk.

Osteomyelitis (suppurative)

Osteomyelitis is most often caused by a bacterial infection of bone. Bone may be infected by penetrating wounds (e.g. bites), by extension from the soft tissues or by haematogenous seeding (very rare). Many cases of osteomyelitis can be related to previous orthopaedic surgery. Nail bed infections can occur and must be differentiated from carcinoma affecting the third digit. Cats with chronic periodontal disease will often have a dense osteoproductive lesion (osteomyelitis) surrounding the affected alveoli with bony lysis at the apices of the affected tooth roots.

Acute osteomyelitis refers to the early stages of infection. Chronic osteomyelitis occurs when the infection continues for an extended period, and may result in disseminated infection within the bone. Aerobic and anaerobic (or mixed) infections can occur. *Staphylococcus* and *Streptococcus* infections are most often seen but many other organisms can be involved, such as coliforms, *Pasteurella* or *Pseudomonas*. Lameness is usually obvious, associated with localised bone pain. Soft tissue swelling is often apparent. Other signs may be related to bone fractures (e.g. non-union), penetrating wound or infected soft tissue. Discharging sinuses may be evident, and fever and systemic illness may or may not be apparent. Radiography is useful to help establish the diagnosis (Fig. 17.27). Bone lysis or sclerosis may be seen. Periosteal new bone, which may extend a considerable distance along the length of the affected bone, may be present, as may sequestra, soft tissue swelling, loss of fascial planes and increased soft tissue density. Collection of bone

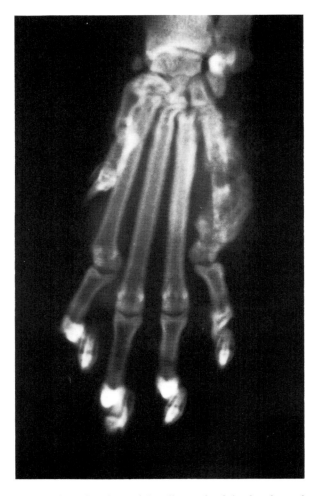

FIG. 17.27   Craniocaudal radiograph of the forefoot of a 2-year-old-male DSH. There is a bacterial osteomyelitis of metacarpal bone 5 following a bite wound. There is sequestrum formation within the shaft of the bone.

for culture is important for confirmation of diagnosis and providing antimicrobial drug sensitivities.

Treatment of bacterial osteomyelitis often involves surgical drainage and antibiotics. In acute osteomyelitis, drainage may be necessary to release exudate. Surgical drains can be inserted and in some cases multiple drill holes are made through the bone cortex to allow medullary drainage. Local drains also allow irrigation with saline and antibiotic solutions. The animal should be hospitalised to enforce strict rest whilst the drains are in place (normally 4–7 days) and should then be confined within the owner's house for another 2 weeks. The antibiotic should always be given systemically, preferably orally, and selected according to antibiotic sensitivity testing. The systemic antibiotics are continued for 4–6 weeks. Most organisms are sensitive to ampicillin and cephaloridine; some gram negative organisms only respond to gentamycin or kanamycin, and anaerobic infections usually respond to lincomycin, clindamycin, metronidazole, cephaloridine and amoxycillin/clavulanic acid. Gentamicin can be given locally by implanting polymethylacrylate beads, impregnated with the antibiotic, into the tissues adjacent to the infected bone: the beads are removed after 3–4 weeks. The gentamicin acts locally, and there is less chance of toxicity (e.g. renal damage).

The treatment of chronic osteomyelitis is similar to that of acute osteomyelitis. In addition, areas of diseased bone or sequestra must be removed surgically, and some surgical implants may also have to be removed. Surgical drains and prolonged systemic administration of antibiotics are advisable. Chronic osteomyelitis may resolve completely with treatment, although some cases may fail to respond and others resolve only to relapse. Limb amputation or local resection of the diseased bone and the use of a replacement bone graft can be used in those cases which do not respond to drainage and antibiotics.

Fungal (non-suppurative) osteomyelitis

Mycotic infection of bone in cats is rare in the UK. Coccidioidomycosis, cryptococcosis, blastomycosis, histoplasmosis, aspergillosis and streptomycosis have all been described.

Temporomandibular ankylosis

This has been reported in cats which are presented with difficulty in opening their mouths.[33] There is obvious mechanical impediment and any attempts to force open the jaw cause pain. The cats are unable to groom or eat properly, and may lose weight. Radiography may show loss of the temporomandibular joint space and proliferation of bone around the joint, which is often most evident in the zygomatic space on the ventrodorsal view (Fig. 17.28). Although there may be no history of trauma, it is thought that this is the most likely explanation of this clinical syndrome. The trauma may occur several months before the onset of clinical signs. Treatment involves the surgical resection of part of the zygoma, mandibular condyle and vertical ramus to free the ankylosis.

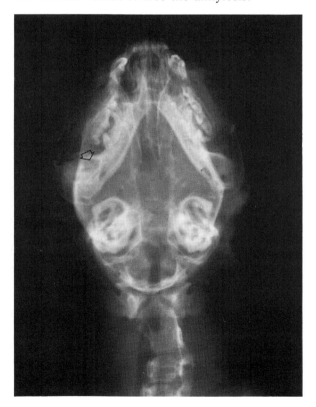

FIG. 17.28 Ventrodorsal radiograph of the skull of a DSH cat with inability to open the mouth. There is new bone deposition within the caudal left zygomatic space (arrowed) which obliterates detail of the temporomandibular joint space and vertical ramus of the mandible. The cat had a history of facial trauma several months previously.

Feline metaphyseal osteopathy

This syndrome is characterised by bony resorption from the metaphyses, generally resulting in pathological fractures. It most often affects the proximal femoral metaphyses but can affect others, and there may be multiple lesions. Both immature and adult cats can be affected. The aetiology of this disease is unknown, although metaphyseal necrosis has been produced, especially in kittens, by intravenous inoculation of herpesvirus.[15]

MUSCLE DISEASE

Myositis

Bacterial myositis often occurs in association with penetrating (particularly bite) wounds. Treatment includes drainage, local antisepsis and systemic antibiotics. Occasionally foreign bodies, such as teeth, claws, plant materials or airgun pellets, may be lodged in the tissue and require surgical removal. Foreign bodies may be associated with non-healing sinuses, and radiography may be helpful. Other causes of myositis, such as parasitic and immune-based, are not well documented in the cat. Cases of *Spirocerca lupi* infection of the oesophagus are reported in cats in Africa and southern USA. Such lesions are nodular, and cause vomiting and regurgitation; treatment is by surgical excision.

Localised myositis ossificans

This is characterised by heterotopic non-neoplastic bone formation in a single muscle, group of muscles or other soft tissue (Fig. 17.29). The lesion can be associated with lameness, and sometimes surgical resection will produce clinical improvement.

Generalised myositis ossificans

In this rare disorder, widespread muscle degeneration results from excessive fibrous tissue development with dystrophic calcification and ossification. The affected animal is stiff, with reduced movement of many joints. Many limb muscles contain firm nodules. Only skeletal muscle is affected, and shows fibrosis and ossification; the latter is seen on radiography.

Aortic thrombo-embolism

Iliac thrombosis is a well known syndrome in the cat. The animal presents with an inability to stand on its hindlegs, and there is an absence of femoral pulses. The resultant ischaemia affects peripheral nerves and muscles (see Chapter 11).[13]

Myasthenia gravis

Myasthenia gravis results from a failure of normal neuromuscular transmission, and may be congenital or acquired. The latter type is thought to be an autoimmune disease where antibodies against acetylcholine receptors can be demon-strated. Both types have been described in the cat. Clinical signs include generalised muscle weakness, dyspnoea, muscle tremor, ataxia and collapse when the animal is exercised.[5] A change in voice and difficulty in prehension and swallowing of food are also reported. Diagnosis is confirmed by response to anticholinesterase drugs, e.g. edrophonium (2.5–5.0 mg I/V). Electrophysiological testing can also help. Treatment is with oral pyridostigmine bromide or neostigmine; the maintenance dose will vary from case to case. Prednisolone therapy and possible surgical thymectomy should be considered if autoimmunity is thought to be involved.

Hypokalaemic polymyopathy

This condition has been widely reported in the USA but is rare in the UK.[16] The clinical signs

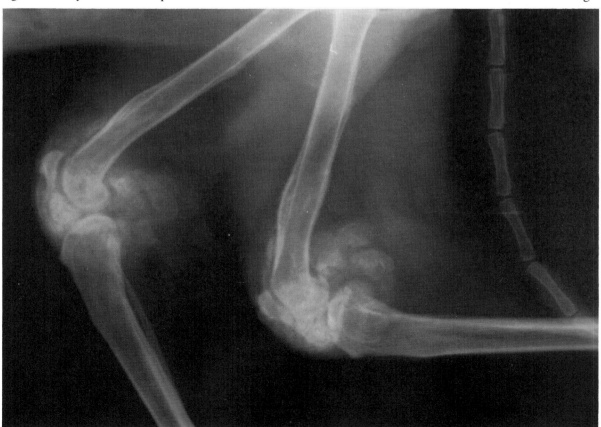

FIG. 17.29   Lateral radiograph of both hindlegs of a DSH, showing calcification and ossification of the soft tissue adjacent to the stifle joints. This is an example of myositis ossificans. Periosteal new bone, affecting both femora and tibiae, is also present.

include acute onset of muscle weakness, ventral flexion of the neck, reluctance to walk, stiff gait, easy fatigability and apparent muscle pain.[7,8] There is a severe hypokalaemia, thought to be caused by prolonged excessive urinary loss of potassium; this appears to be the result of renal dysfunction, which can be detected by routine blood testing. The potassium loss is worsened by a dietary insufficiency. The feeding of an acidifying agent may also increase potassium loss, and certain drugs (e.g. diuretics, corticosteroids) may accelerate renal potassium losses.[7] The hypokalaemia, once present, will cause further renal disease. Hypokalaemic polymyopathy is believed to occur in the Burmese cat as a breed problem, when it is referred to as Burmese sporadic myopathy. This was first reported by Mason[27], the age of onset varying from 4 to 10 months. Affected cats developed ventroflexion of the neck, with chin pressing on the anterior sternum, which could occur during rest or when walking. During locomotion the head would nod up and down rhythmically as though co-ordinated with limb movement. The forelimbs were stiff, straight and hypermetric; the hindlimbs would flex normally but were widespread and ataxic. Pupil dilation and claw protrusion occurred during handling, stress or fright. Affected animals could only walk a short distance and convulsions were also reported. The animals would improve spontaneously and show complete normality before relapsing days or weeks later. The condition was originally thought to be a thiamine deficiency but was later associated with hypokalaemia.[2,19] Muscle weakness and hypokalaemia have also been seen secondary to renal tubular acidosis and in a cat with primary hyperaldosteronism.

Treatment of cats with hypokalaemic polymyopathy is by oral potassium, preferably as potassium gluconate, at a dose of 5–10 M Eq./day, given in two divided doses. Palatable flavoured oral powders may also be available. Once clinical improvement has occurred and potassium levels are back to normal, the oral potassium supplement can be reduced; maintenance supplements of 2–6 M Eq of potassium/day may be necessary, or a diet which contains potassium at 0.7–0.9% of dry matter. Intravenous potassium therapy is best avoided unless the hypokalaemia is very severe, in which case the potassium should be administered at a rate of 0.5–1.0 M Eq/kg/hr. The potassium chloride should be diluted in a balanced electrolyte solution, such as lactated Ringer's solution, and administered via an infusion pump because highly concentrated potassium-containing solutions must be infused carefully to avoid phlebitis and potential fatal hyperkalaemia. During such infusions, serum potassium must be monitored together with ECG recordings. Fluids that do not contain the concentrations of potassium capable of replacing the deficit rapidly should not be used, because they may actually worsen the hypokalaemia by a dilution effect. An alternative treatment is to infuse dopamine (0.5 ug/kg/min), which causes translocation of potassium from the intracellular to the extracellular fluid.

Tetanus

The cat is resistant to tetanus, but the disease has been reported in this species. The muscle rigidity may initially be localised to the area of the wound site. This may progress to generalised muscle stiffness and rigidity. Severely affected animals lie on their sides, with rigidly outstretched limbs and tails turned dorsally. Opisthotonus is common. Ears are drawn closely together, with wrinkling of the skin of the forehead. Spasms of the extraocular muscles cause intermittent enophthalmus and protrusion of the third eyelids. Spasm of facial and masticatory muscles result in narrowed palpebral fissures, curling of the lips and inability to open the mouth. Treatment is with tetanus antitoxin, antibiotics and supportive care. The muscle spasms may be controlled with phenothiazines, barbiturates and diazepam. Recovery can occur.

Fibrotic myopathy

Fibrous replacement of the semitendinosus muscle has been described.[25] The lameness was characterised by marked flexion of the hip, stifle and hock, and the leg was advanced with an abruptly shortened anterior stride. The muscle was felt as a taut band. The cause of the fibrotic myopathy was undetermined. The author has seen fibrous replacement of muscles associated with neoplastic change (e.g. rhabdomyosarcoma); the muscle feels taut and painful.

Dystrophy-like myopathies

Two cases have been described characterised by varying muscle fibre diameter, internal nuclei, moderate degeneration and necrosis of solitary muscle fibres, and slight to moderate endomysial and perimysial fibrosis. Very few regenerating muscle fibres were present. Only one of the cats showed lameness, characterised by an inability to jump and a 'kangaroo-like' gait; chronic vomiting was also a feature. Two young littermate Siamese cats were reported with weakness, ultimately resulting in an inability to support body-weight. Muscle histology included irregular atrophy and hypertrophy of muscle fibres, individual muscle fibres showing degeneration and fragmentation with aggregation of histiocyte cells and lack of muscle fibre regeneration.

Other myopathies

There have been reports of a degenerate myopathy in cats fed vitamin-E deficient diets not containing unsaturated fatty acids[12] and a clinical case of vitamin-E deficiency.[6] The cat in the latter case was presented with swollen muscles in fore- and hind-limbs associated with difficult and painful movement. Histology included pale, swollen muscle fibres, loss of cross-striations, hyaline degeneration and necrosis with flocculation granules and myophagia by macrophages. Some swollen myofibrils showed proliferation of sarcolemmal nuclei and occasional centralisation of the nuclei. Chronic inflammatory cells were also present. Other myopathies of unknown aetiology have been reported.[11,20]

Contracture of the gastrocnemius muscle/tendon

A bilateral case of gastrocnemius contracture with hyperextension of both tarsal joints was treated successfully by surgical lengthening of the gastrocnemius tendons. The author treated a congenital case in a 3 month-old kitten by holding the hock joint in flexion with two transarticular pins, which were later removed.

Rupture of the gastrocnemius tendon

Rupture of any tendon can occur in association with a penetrating wound and sometimes with blunt trauma applied to the tendon and overlying skin. However, stretching and tearing of the gastrocnemius tendon can occur as an entity, mainly in overweight, middle-aged cats. There appears to be a failure of the tendon over time, with gradual development of a plantigrade posture (due to an inability to extend the hock). The tendon of the superficial digital flexor is usually intact, and therefore the digits flex when the hock 'collapses'. If the whole Achilles (or calcanean) tendon is ruptured, the digits remain in a normal or extended position when the deformity is accentuated. The damaged tendon needs to be sutured, and the sutures protected by holding the hock in extension by the use of a transfixation screw between the tuber calcis and distal tibia or an external fixator. A plantigrade stance may also be seen in cases of intertarsal and tarsometatarsal luxation/subluxation, in cats with sciatic nerve injury, spinal cord injury or diabetes mellitus. The relevant clinical, radiographic and laboratory features will help the differential diagnoses.

DISEASES OF THE VERTEBRAL COLUMN

Intervertebral disc protrusions

Dorsal disc protrusions are common in cats over 15 years old and are often multiple, although rarely associated with clinical signs.[21] Clinical cases have been reported but are rare. Plain radiography is seldom of diagnostic help, because calcification of intervertebral discs is rare in the cat, and narrowing of disc spaces often occurs without any disc protrusion. Myelography will help to localise the lesions. Treatment may be medical (corticosteroids) or surgical (decompression laminectomy and disc removal). Disc explosions also occur and are associated with major trauma; cord damage is caused by an impact injury and the prognosis depends on the severity of clinical disease. Treatment is with corticosteroids.

Bacterial discospondylitis

Infection localising to the disc spaces is rare in the cat. It is assumed to be blood-borne and the urinary tract may be the site of origin. The clinical signs are stiffness and a painful neck or back;

DIFFERENTIAL DIAGNOSES OF THE FELINE HYPERAESTHESIA SYNDROME

Trauma (especially fracture pelvis, fracture/separation tail)
Bite wounds (especially around base of tail)
Inflammation (myositis, osteomyelitis)
Dermatitis (including 'miliary eczema')
Pansteatitis (yellow fat disease)
Intervertebral disc disease
Bacterial discospondylitis
Polyarthritis
Myeloproliferative disease
Abdominal pain
Hypervitaminosis A
Aortic thromboembolism
Spondylosis deformans and ankylosing hyperostosis
Hip dysplasia
Osteopetrosis
Hyperparathyroidism
Idiopathic

FIG. 17.30   Differential diagnoses of the 'feline hyperaesthesia syndrome'.

neurological deficits may also be present. Radiography may help to confirm the diagnosis; the radiographic features include narrowing of the disc space, sclerosis of bone at the vertebral end plates and destruction of bone within the end plates, giving the disc space an irregular or widened appearance. Treatment is with long-term antibiotics, possibly in conjunction with surgical curettage of the lesions. If neurological deficits are present, decompression techniques may be applicable.

Penetrating bite wounds at the tail base have been associated with an infective spondylitis of the coccygeal vertebrae.

Feline hyperaesthesia syndrome

This describes cats which present with apparent pain and hyperaesthesia on handling, especially over the lumbar spine. A number of possible diagnoses must be considered (Fig. 17.30) but there are many idiopathic cases where no diagnosis is established. Such cases may respond to corticosteroid, phenobarbital or megestrol acetate therapy, although some necessitate euthanasia.

REFERENCES

1. Bennett D., Gaskell R.M., Mills A., Knowles J., Carter S.D., McArdle F. (1989). Detection of feline calicivirus antigens in the joints of infected cats. *Vet. Rec.* **124**: 329–332.
2. Blaxter A.C., Lieverley P., Gruffydd-Jones T., Wotton P. (1986). Periodic weakness in Burmese kittens. *Vet. Rec.* **118**: 619–620.
3. Clark L., Seawright A.A. (1968). Skeletal abnormalities in the hindlimbs of young cats as a result of hypervitaminosis A. *Nature* **217**: 1174–1176.
4. Cowell K.R., Jezyk P.F., Haskins M.E., Patterson D.F. (1976). Mucopolysaccharidosis in a cat. *J. Am. Vet. Med. Ass.* **169**: 334–339.
5. Dawson J.R.B. (1970). Myasthenia gravis in a cat. *Vet. Rec.* **86**: 562-563.
6. Dennis J.M., Alexander R.W. (1982). Nutritional myopathy in a cat. *Vet. Rec.* **111**: 195–196.
7. Dow S.W., Fettman M.J., Le Couteur R.A., Hamar D.W. (1987). Potassium depletion in cats: renal and dietary influences. *J. Am. Vet. Med. Ass.* **191**: 1569–1575.
8. Dow S.W., Le Couteur R.A., Fettman M.J., Spurgeon T.L. (1987). Potassium depletion in cats: hypokalaemia polymyopathy. *J. Am. Vet. Med. Ass.* **191**: 1563–1568.
9. Flecknell P.A., Gibbs C., Kelly D.F. (1978). Myelosclerosis in a cat. *J. Comp. Path.* **88**: 627–631.
10. Flecknell P.A., Gruffydd-Jones T.J. (1979). Congenital luxation of the patellae in the cat. *Feline Pract.* **9**(3): 18–20.
11. Gardner D.G. (1967). Skeletal myonecrosis in a cat. *New Z. Vet. J.* **15**: 211–213.
12. Gershoff S.N., Norkin S.A. (1962). Vitamin E deficiency in cats. *J. Nutr.* **77**: 303–308.
13. Griffiths I.R., Duncan I.D. (1979). Ischaemic neuromyopathy in cats. *Vet. Rec.* **104**: 518–522.
14. Holt P.E. (1978) Hip dysplasia in a cat. *J. small Anim. Pract.* **19**: 273–276.
15. Hoover E.A., Griesemer R.A. (1971). Bone lesions produced by feline herpesvirus. *Laboratory Investigation* **25**: 457–464.
16. Hopkins A.L. (1989). Sporadic feline hypokalaemic polymyopathy. *Vet. Rec.* **125**: 17.
17. Janssens L.A.A., Janssens G.O., Janssens D.L. (1991). Anterior cruciate ligament rupture associated with cardiomyopathy in three cats. *Vet. Comp. Orthop. Traumat.* **4**: 35–37.
18. Jezyk P.F., Haskins M.E., Patterson D.F., Mellman W.J., Greenstein M. (1977) Mucopolysaccharidosis in a cat with arylsulfatase B deficiency. A model of Maroteaux-Lamy syndrome. *Science* **198**: 834–836.
19. Jones B.R., Alley M.R. (1988). Hypokalaemic myopathy in Burmese kittens. *New Z. Vet. J.* **36**: 150–151.
20. Joshua J.O. (1965). *The Clinical Aspects of Some Diseases of Cats.* William Heinemann Medical books, London.
21. King A.S., Smith R.N. (1960). Disc protrusion in the cat: distribution of dorsal protrusions along the vertebral column. *Vet. Rec.* **72**: 333–337.

22. Kramer P., Fluckiger M.A., Rahn B.A. & Cordey J. (1988). Osteoporosis in cats. *J. small Anim. Pract.* **29**: 153–164.

23. Langweiler M., Haskins M.E. & Jezyk P.F. (1978). Mucopolysaccharidosis in a litter of cats. *J. Am. Anim. Hosp. Ass.* **14**: 748–751.

24. Lees P., Taylor P.M. (1991). Pharmacodynamics and pharmacokinetics of flunixin in the cat. *B. Vet. J.* **147**: 298.

25. Lewis, D.D. (1988). Fibrotic myopathy of the semitendinosus muscle in a cat. *J. Am. Vet. Med. Ass.* **193**: 240–241.

26. Magnarelli L.A., Anderson J.D., Levine H.R. & Levy S.A. (1990). Tick parasitism and antibodies to *Borellia burgdorferi* in cats. *J. Am. Vet. Med. Ass.* **197**: 63–66.

27. Mason K.V. (1988). A hereditary disease in Burmese cats manifested as an episodic weakness, with head nodding and neck ventroflexion. *J. small Anim. Pract.* **24**: 147–151.

28. May C. & Newsholme S.J. (1989). Metastasis of feline pulmonary carcinoma presenting as multiple digital swelling. *J. small Anim. Pract.* **30**: 302–310.

29. Pedersen N.C., Laliberte L. & Ekman S. (1983). A transient febrile limping syndrome of kittens caused by two different strains of feline calici virus. *Feline Pract.* **13**(1): 26–35.

30. Pool R.R. (1981). Osteochondromatosis. In: Bojrab M.J. (ed.) *Pathology in Small Animal Surgery*, pp 641–649. Lea & Febiger, Philadelphia.

31. Prymak C. & Goldschmidt M.H. (1991). Synovial cysts in five dogs and one cat. *J. Am. Anim. Hosp. Assoc.* **27**: 151–154.

32. Seawright A.A., English P.B. & Gartner R.J.W. (1967). Hypervitaminosis A and deforming cervical spondylosis of the cat. *J. Comp. Path.* **77**: 29–39.

33. Sullivan M. (1989). Temporomandibular ankylosis in the cat. *J. small Anim. Pract.* **30**: 401–405.

FURTHER READING

Bennett D. (1976). Nutrition and bone disease in the dog and cat. *Vet. Rec.* **98**: 313–320.

Bennett D. (1985). The musculoskeletal system. In: Chandler E.A. et al. (ed.). *Feline Medicine & Therapeutics*. Blackwell Scientific Publications, Oxford.

Bennett D., May C., Carter S.D. (1992). Lyme disease. In: Raw M-E., Parkinson T.J. (eds.). *Veterinary Annual* **32**: Butterworth Scientific, Surrey.

Bennett D., Nash A.S. (1985). Feline immune-based arthritis: a study of 33 cases. *J. small Anim. Pract.* **29**: 501–523.

Biletto W.C., Patnaik A.K., Schrader S.C., Mooney S.C. (1987). Osteosarcoma in cats: 22 cases (1974–1984). *J. Am. Vet. Med. Ass.* **190**: 91–93.

Liu S-K., Dorfman H.D., Patnaik A.K. (1974). Primary and secondary bone tumours in the cat. *J. small Anim. Pract.* **15**: 141–156.

Pedersen N.C., Pool R.R., Morgan J.P. (1983). Joint diseases of dogs and cats. In: Ettinger S.J. (ed.), *Textbook of Veterinary Internal Medicine. Diseases of the Dog and Cat*, 2nd Edn., Chapter 84. W.B. Saunders, Philadelphia.

Schrader S.C., Sherding R.G. (1989). Disorders of the skeletal system. In: Sherding R.G. (ed.), *The Cat: Diseases and Clinical Management*. Churchill Livingstone, New York.

18

Disorders of the Nervous System

SIMON J. WHEELER

The neurological examination provides information regarding the function of the components of the nervous system. The clinical signs seen with lesions of various parts of the nervous system form well-defined syndromes. This chapter describes these syndromes and the diseases that cause them.

NEUROLOGICAL EXAMINATION

Many accounts of the neurological examination are available – see Further Reading. Cats are not always co-operative and so detached observation of the patient is an important part in the process. It is appropriate to concentrate on the presenting problem, but not to neglect other parts of the cat, particularly in view of the high incidence of multifocal neurological disease and multisystemic involvement seen in cats.

LOCALISATION OF LESIONS

Brain

Diseases of the brain usually produce neurological deficits that fit into one of four categories: forebrain, brainstem, cerebellum and vestibular. The signs seen are summarised in Fig. 18.1. Multifocal neurological signs are common in cats but often they present with features that fit predominantly into one of these four categories.

Forebrain lesions

Forebrain lesions typically cause seizures, behavioural change and alteration in mental status. Many cats will circle compulsively in wide arcs towards the side of the lesion. Lateralising signs

CLINICAL SIGNS IN BRAIN LESIONS	
Forebrain	
General signs	Lateralising signs - Contralateral to lesion
Seizures	Conscious proprioception deficits
Behaviour change	Menace deficits
Circling	Visual deficits
Altered mental status	Diminished facial sensation
Depression	Mild facial weakness
Brainstem	
General signs	Lateralising signs - Ipsilateral to lesion
Depression	Hemiparesis or asymmetrical tetraparesis
Marked gait abnormalities	Conscious proprioceptive deficits
Tetraparesis	Cranial nerve palsies
Cerebellum	**Vestibular**
Tremor	Head tilt
Ataxia	Ataxia
Dysmetria	Nystagmus
Hypermetria	
Menace deficits	

FIG. 18.1 Summary of clinical signs seen in brain lesions.

occur contralateral to the lesion and include conscious proprioceptive (CP) deficits, mild weakness of the facial muscles and diminished facial sensation.

Brainstem

Brainstem lesions cause severe gait abnormalities, with hemiparesis or tetraparesis. Interference with the ascending reticular-activating system causes depressed mental status. Cranial nerve palsies are present, usually causing some or all of the following: facial paralysis, loss of facial sensation, temporal muscle atrophy, loss of blink, swallowing difficulties and head tilt (see Vestibular disease, below). All deficits are present on the same side as the lesion.

Cerebellar lesions

Cerebellar lesions produce dysmetria, hypermetria, ataxia and tremor. With uncomplicated cerebellar disease there are no CP deficits. Menace deficits with normal vision may be seen, but young kittens do not have a normal menace response.

Vestibular diseases

Vestibular diseases cause head tilt and ataxia. Nystagmus is usually present but may not be apparent in chronic cases. It is important to differentiate between central and peripheral vestibular disease – see Fig. 18.2. The most reliable feature of central vestibular disease is the presence

of CP deficits ipsilateral to the lesion. If nystagmus is present, the slow phase is towards the side of the lesion. In central vestibular disease, the character or direction of the nystagmus may change when the head position is altered. The head tilt is usually toward the side of the lesion. However, in some cases of central vestibular disease, the head tilt is away from the side of the lesion. This is the paradoxical head tilt seen in lesions involving the cerebellar input to the vestibular system.

Spine

Lesions of the spinal cord can be localised to one of four regions; the pattern of deficits seen is shown in Fig. 18.3. Lesions of the C1–C5 cord segments cause upper motor neurone-type deficits in forelimbs and hindlimbs. Predominantly unilateral signs may be seen with asymmetrical lesions. Lesions in the C6-T2 segments cause lower motor neurone-type deficits in one or both forelimbs and upper motor neurone signs in the hindlimbs. Lesions in segments T3-L3 cause upper motor neurone signs in the hindlimbs. Lesions in segments L4-S2 do not affect the forelimbs but cause lower motor neurone-type deficits in the hindlimbs.

Spinal cord lesions can interfere with bladder function. Lesions of the sacral segments cause lower motor neurone deficits in bladder function, with urinary incontinence and a flaccid bladder that is expressed easily. Lesions cranial to the sacral segments cause an upper motor neurone deficit in bladder function which results in urinary retention and overflow, with a bladder that is difficult to express.

The caudal spinal cord segments do not correspond anatomically with the vertebrae of the same notation. The lumbosacral segments are more cranially positioned than the corresponding vertebrae; the sacral segments lie in the caudal lumbar vertebrae, and the spinal cord ends in the sacrum. Thus, lesions of segments L4-S2 could involve the vertebral column as far forward as the L3 vertebra.

The neurological examination also gives information about the severity of the lesion. Mild lesions cause ataxia and CP deficits, moderate lesions cause paresis and severe lesions cause paralysis. The presence or absence of deep pain

VESTIBULAR DISEASE		
	Peripheral	**Central**
Head tilt	Yes	Yes
Ataxia	Yes	Yes
Proprioceptive deficits	No	Ipsilateral
Paresis	No	Ipsilateral
Nystagmus	Yes	Yes
Variable nystagmus[a]	No	Yes
Other cranial nerves	VII	Multiple
Horner's syndrome	Possible	Very rare
[a]Direction or character of nystagmus changes when head position is altered		

FIG. 18.2 Differential features of peripheral and central vestibular disease.

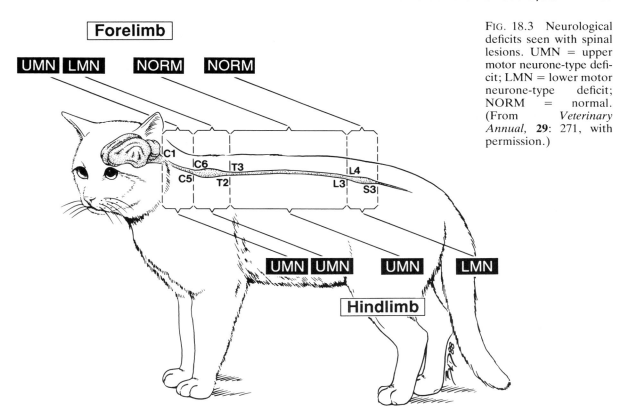

Forelimb

| UMN | LMN | | NORM | | NORM |

C1
C6 T3
C5 T2 L3 L4
S3

UMN UMN UMN LMN

Hindlimb

FIG. 18.3 Neurological deficits seen with spinal lesions. UMN = upper motor neurone-type deficit; LMN = lower motor neurone-type deficit; NORM = normal. (From *Veterinary Annual*, **29**: 271, with permission.)

sensation is an important prognostic sign. Deep pain is assessed by observing the cat's behavioural response to a firm pinch of the toes. Flexion of the limb alone is not an indicator of intact deep pain; this is merely a local reflex. If deep pain sensation is absent, the prognosis is poor.

Peripheral nerve, neuromuscular junction and muscle

Diseases of these structures produce a range of signs of varying severity. Peripheral polyneuropathies may cause ataxia, tetraparesis, depressed reflexes or tetraplegia. In mild cases, a plantigrade stance may be the only abnormality. Peripheral neuropathies generally cause lower motor neurone-type deficits; thus, diminished reflexes and neurogenic muscle atrophy are seen. Neuromuscular junction disorders may present in a similar fashion or as exercise intolerance or episodic weakness,

for example, in myasthenia gravis. Myopathies may present as weakness or stiffness.

DIAGNOSTIC TESTING

Once the lesion has been localised, a provisional differential diagnosis can be reached. Further identification requires use of certain ancillary tests.

Routine laboratory evaluations

A complete blood count, serum biochemistry analysis and urinalysis are valuable in assessing the general health of the cat. The feline leukaemia virus (FeLV) and feline immunodeficiency virus (FIV) status of the cat should be established. Specific biochemical tests of liver function are indicated if hepatic disease is suspected. Clinical pharmacology is necessary in monitoring anticonvulsant therapy.

Cerebrospinal fluid (CSF) analysis

Cerebrospinal fluid analysis is a useful indicator of nervous system disease. Abnormal CSF correlates well with neurological disease but normal CSF findings cannot be relied on to indicate absence of disease. However, with the high prevalence of inflammatory and neoplastic central nervous system (CNS) diseases in cats, CSF analysis is valuable. Methods of collection and analysis are covered elsewhere (see Further Reading).

Radiology

Radiology is a useful ancillary aid in the evaluation of many neurological cases. Radiographs of the skull are useful in trauma and otitis media. In some cranial meningiomas, there is radiographically-apparent bony thickening of the calvarium over the tumour. However, most intracranial lesions require computed tomography (CT) to reveal them. Spinal radiographs are valuable in some instances (for example, trauma) but myelography is required to demonstrate most spinal tumours.

DISEASES OF THE BRAIN

Forebrain

Seizures

Seizures are the most frequent manifestation of forebrain disease in cats. Seizures can be classified in various ways but a grouping based on the underlying pathogenesis is useful, as follows:

Intracranial causes – idiopathic epilepsy
 – structural lesions
Extracranial causes – metabolic
 – toxic.

Causes of seizures are given in Fig. 18.4.

Idiopathic epilepsy

Idiopathic epilepsy is less common in cats than in dogs. A diagnosis of idiopathic epilepsy can only be reached once all other possible causes have been eliminated. Careful clinical evaluation of epileptic cats reveals a surprisingly high incidence

CAUSES OF SEIZURES
Intracranial

Idiopathic epilepsy
Organic brain diseases:
  Neoplasia
  Inflammation and infectious disease
  Ischaemic encephalopathy
  Storage diseases
  Thiamine deficiency
  Hydrocephalus

Extracranial

Metabolic:
  Hepatic
  Hypoglycaemia
  Azotaemia
  Hypocalcaemia
Toxicity:
  Organophosphorus
  Organochlorine
  Strychnine
  Lead
  Medications
  Ethylene glycol

FIG. 18.4   Causes of seizures.

of structural brain diseases. Following a seizure, the neurological examination may be abnormal for a day or more.

Anticonvulsant therapy for idiopathic epilepsy is appropriate but suitable drugs are limited in availability. Phenobarbitone and diazepam are the most suitable; other anticonvulsants do not possess suitable pharmacokinetic properties in cats. Phenobarbitone is usually given at 2–3 mg/kg bid; diazepam at 2–5 mg orally tid. If phenobarbitone is prescribed, it is important that serum concentrations are checked periodically, at least twice yearly and 2 weeks after any change in dosage. The therapeutic range is 15–45 µg/dl, and the serum sample should be collected prior to the administration of the dose of medication. Serum biochemistry should be monitored regularly, at least every 6 months. Idiopathic epilepsy can be managed successfully in cats, provided that medication is given regularly and carefully monitored.

Status epilepticus

Status epilepticus occurs in cats with various conditions, including trauma, toxicity and uncontrolled idiopathic epilepsy. The priority in managing this situation is to control the seizures rather than to find the cause. Intravenous medication is used initially with diazepam (0.25–1.0 mg/kg) or, if the cat fails to respond, intravenous phenobarbitone (2–4 mg/kg). A patent airway must be maintained and oxygen given. Intravenous fluids should be administered and dextrose given if the serum glucose concentration is low. Once seizures have been controlled, the origin of the problem can be investigated.

Intracranial diseases

If the neurological examination reveals persistent deficits, the likelihood of a structural intracranial lesion is high. The following discussion describes the diseases that are most likely to be encountered (Fig. 18.5).

CAUSES OF FOREBRAIN SIGNS
Ischaemic encephalopathy
Trauma
Inflammation and infectious disease
Neoplasia
Storage disease
Hydrocephalus
Hepatic encephalopathy
Spongiform encephalopathy
Toxicity

FIG. 18.5   Causes of forebrain signs.

Ischaemic encephalopathy

Ischaemic encephalopathy causes an acute onset of neurological signs indicating asymmetrical forebrain dysfunction. Behavioural change, seizures, altered personality and circling are typical. There is ischaemia of the cerebral cortex, generally in the distribution of the middle cerebral artery, although other parts of the brain can be involved. The aetiology is unknown. The differential diagnosis includes trauma and toxicity. Trauma can usually be ruled out by historical information; toxicities will not be so markedly asymmetrical. Some cases of inflammatory disease present acutely but they tend to be multifocal.

The diagnosis is based on the acute, nonprogressive nature of the condition and the elimination of other causes. The CSF is noninflammatory, with only a mild increase in cell count and increased protein.

Treatment with corticosteroids (dexamethasone 2 mg/kg IV) is indicated in the acute phase. Anticonvulsants are indicated if seizures occur. The prognosis is good but residual deficits may remain.

Cranial trauma

Cranial trauma presents as various neurological disorders; seizures, forebrain or brainstem signs are most frequent. The diagnosis is usually apparent from historical or physical findings. However, cats in status epilepticus can suffer significant self-inflicted injuries that give the appearance of previous trauma.

With cerebral trauma, there is a tendency for increased intracranial pressure and subsequent caudal brain herniation. Affected cats show deteriorating clinical signs, with progressive tetraparesis, reduced consciousness, sluggish pupillary reflexes and respiratory depression. This is in contrast to brainstem trauma, where there is acute nonprogressive tetraplegia and coma. Differentiation is important as the former is potentially reversible but the latter is usually not.

Management of the cat with cranial trauma must consider all body systems in addition to the nervous involvement. Seizures should be controlled as discussed above, and a patent airway must be maintained. If increased intracranial pressure is suspected, this can be managed by hyperventilation with oxygen to reduce pCO_2, corticosteroids or osmotic diuresis. Mannitol (0.25 g/kg) may be used for this purpose, but should be restricted to situations where other therapy has failed. Frusemide (0.7 mg/kg IV), given 15 minutes after mannitol, enhances the therapeutic effect. Depressed skull fractures should be surgically elevated and antibiotics given to cats with open fractures. General nursing care is vital, with particular attention to the bladder, nutrition and fluid balance. The prognosis for forebrain injuries is relatively good, even when marked deficits are present.

Inflammatory disease

Inflammatory disease of the CNS is a significant cause of neurological dysfunction in cats.

Forebrain features can predominate; or inflammatory diseases can cause cerebellar signs, or may present with central vestibular signs. In general, however, the signs tend to be multifocal and are therefore discussed in detail in the section Multifocal Inflammatory Diseases. Feline infectious peritonitis (FIP) is one of the most common causes.

Storage diseases

Storage diseases are also multifocal. They can cause predominantly forebrain signs or may present signs of central vestibular dysfunction, but they are discussed in detail in the Cerebellum section (Lysosomal Storage Disease).

Neoplasms

Cerebral tumours are relatively frequent. Meningiomas are the most common; typically, they involve the convexity of the cerebral cortex, and they may be multiple. Diagnosis is based on the clinical signs and the progressive nature of the disease. Radiographs may reveal an area of thickened bone in the calvarium over the neoplasm, but the best method of diagnosis is by CT scanning. Treatment by surgical resection is effective in selected patients.

Hydrocephalus

Hydrocephalus is usually secondary to CNS diseases obstructing CSF flow. Cases should be investigated to determine whether there is an underlying cause, such as inflammatory disease or neoplasia. In some cats, no origin is determined; these cases are probably congenital. Identification of hydrocephalus is best achieved by CT scanning; other radiological contrast methods are less suitable.

Metabolic encephalopathy

Hepatic encephalopathy causes various clinical signs in cats, but forebrain signs predominate. Behavioural changes, visual deficits, pupillary abnormalities and ptyalism are all common. Hepatic dysfunction leads to increased concentrations of neurotoxic substances in the circulation. The underlying hepatic disease is usually a congenital portosystemic shunt. The blood urea nitrogen may be low, and the blood ammonia and serum bile acid concentrations elevated. The liver may appear small on radiographs. Treatment with a protein-restricted diet and oral neomycin or lactulose is useful, to stabilise the cat's clinical condition. Surgical ligation of shunts is required for successful long term management.

Some cats with underlying hepatic disease become comatose, particularly following an additional stress (for example, anaesthesia). Oral protein intake should be stopped, neomycin and lactulose given by enema, and attention paid to fluid and electrolyte balance.

Other causes of forebrain signs are given in Fig. 18.5 and are covered elsewhere in this chapter.

Brainstem

Brainstem presentations are relatively unusual in cats. **Inflammatory disease** and **neoplasia** occur in this location.

Trauma of the brainstem

Trauma of the brainstem can occur following road accidents. There is paralysis and loss of consciousness at the time of the accident. This is in contrast to brain herniation where the signs are progressive. Generally, the pupils are mid-sized, in contrast to the dilated, unresponsive pupils seen in herniation. The prognosis is poor in brainstem injury following trauma.

Thiamine deficiency

Thiamine deficiency is associated with a variable clinical picture, but brainstem signs are often seen. Ataxia, cranial nerve deficits and ventroflexion of the neck are characteristic; seizures may be seen late in the disease. The condition is seen in cats fed diets high in raw fish, that contain the enzyme thiaminase, or cooked meat. Mild cases respond to thiamine supplementation, but those which are advanced have a poor prognosis.

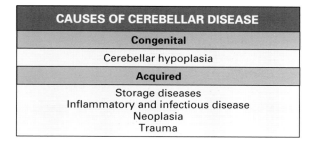

FIG. 18.6   Causes of cerebellar disease.

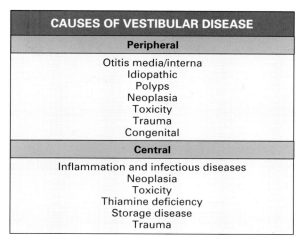

FIG. 18.7   Causes of vestibular disease.

Cerebellum

Causes of congenital and acquired cerebellar disease are shown in Fig. 18.6.

Cerebellar hypoplasia

Infection of pregnant queens, or kittens less than 3 weeks of age with panleukopenia virus causes cerebellar hypoplasia in affected kittens. Characteristic cerebellar signs of ataxia, tremor and hypermetria are seen. The condition is seen at a few weeks of age, but is not progressive – an important feature in differential diagnosis. Treatment is not possible but affected cats can lead a relatively contented life.

Lysosomal storage diseases

Lysosomal storage diseases are multisystemic disorders of young cats, with abnormal accumulations of metabolites within cells caused by deficiencies of specific degrading enzymes. The accumulations cause loss of function, primarily in the CNS. The enzyme deficiency is a result of specific genetic deletions or mutations. Most are inherited as autosomal recessive or X-linked traits.

Progressive cerebellar signs are common although careful evaluation usually reveals multifocal deficits. The main condition to be considered in differential diagnosis is cerebellar hypoplasia (see above). Cats with storage diseases can be differentiated by the progressive nature of the disease and the multifocal signs. Inflammatory conditions should also be considered and can usually be eliminated by CSF evaluation. Confirming the diagnosis is by a combination of studying familial patterns and evaluation of serum, white blood cells or various biopsies. There is no specific treatment and the prognosis is poor.

Vestibular

Vestibular disease can be peripheral or central in origin (Fig. 18.7).

Peripheral vestibular disease

Otitis media/interna

Otitis media/interna is a common cause of peripheral vestibular disease in cats. In addition to the vestibular signs, paralysis of the facial nerve and ipsilateral Horner's syndrome may be seen because of the proximity of the respective innervation to the structures of the middle ear. External evidence of otitis may be seen and radiography can demonstrate involvement of the tympanic bullae.

Many medications and topical agents used in ear cleaning and treatment can damage the vestibular and cochlear components, particularly if the tympanic membrane is not intact. For this reason, saline is the best fluid for ear irrigation; antiseptics and detergents should be avoided. Irrigation should be performed gently, as vigorous flushing or massage can cause ear drum perforation.

Idiopathic vestibular syndrome

Signs of peripheral vestibular disease are seen in cats where no underlying disease process can be detected. Signs are usually acute in onset and nonprogressive. Specific causes must be eliminated before a diagnosis of idiopathic vestibular syndrome is reached. Otoscopic examination (with the cat under anaesthesia) and bulla radio-graphs are the minimum requirements. The prognosis is good; some of the features resolve in time but the head tilt may persist.

Polyps

Polyps arising from the auditory canal are found in the nasopharynx and the middle ear, the latter causing vestibular signs. Otitis may occur secondary

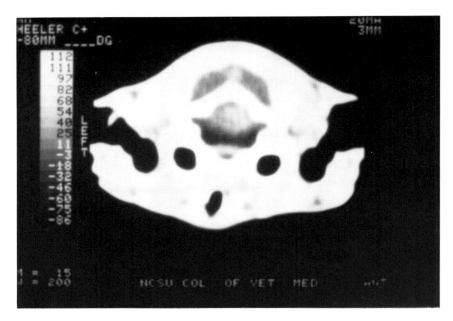

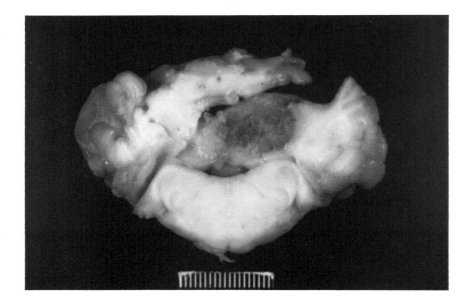

Fig. 18.8 Top: CT image of cat with central vestibular disease. There is a hyperdense region in the caudal fossa, ventral to the osseous tentorium. Bottom: Brain section from same cat. There is an area of discoloration in the cerebellum, caused by *Cladosporum* spp.

to the presence of the polyp. Physical, otoscopic and radiographic examinations will confirm the diagnosis. Treatment is by surgical resection.

Neoplasia

Squamous cell carcinoma may arise within the middle or inner ear. These tumours are usually aggressive, destroying bone in the bulla and skull. External evidence of otorrhoea may be seen. Radiography is useful, and collection of tissue by external means or bulla osteotomy provides the definitive diagnosis. The prognosis is poor.

Ototoxicity

Systemic medications, particularly the aminoglycoside antibiotics, may be toxic to the auditory and vestibular systems. As mentioned above, direct application of antiseptic solutions into the middle ear can be toxic.

Trauma

Trauma can occasionally cause peripheral vestibular disease in cats.

Congenital disease

Rare cases of congenital vestibular disease are seen in some purebred cats; the signs may resolve but residual deficits may remain.

Central vestibular disease

The conditions that cause central vestibular disease generally have a progressive nature and carry a poor prognosis. Thus, the differentiation between central and peripheral disease is important. Furthering the diagnosis can be difficult. Analysis of CSF and CT scanning are useful (Fig. 18.8).

Inflammatory diseases

Inflammatory diseases may present with central vestibular signs. Feline infectious peritonitis is one of the most common causes.

Neoplasia

Neoplasia of the brainstem and vestibular nuclei occur in cats but are less frequent than forebrain tumours.

Toxicities

Toxicities may present with central vestibular signs, particularly lead and mercury.

Thiamine deficiency

Thiamine deficiency causes vestibular signs but other manifestations are also seen, including seizures, depression, ataxia, ventroflexion of the neck and pupillary abnormalities (see brainstem signs above).

Storage diseases

Storage diseases may present with signs of central vestibular dysfunction.

Multifocal diseases

The high prevalence of inflammatory CNS disease in cats dictates that multifocal presentations will be encountered frequently. Cervical pain is particularly common and other body systems may be involved. Where CNS inflammatory disease is suspected, the diagnosis should be pursued by CSF collection and possibly CT scanning. Serological testing may be useful in identifying the aetiology.

Degenerative conditions also cause multifocal neurological signs. Of particular importance are storage diseases and spongiform encephalopathy.

Infectious diseases

Virus infections

Feline infectious peritonitis virus

Feline infectious peritonitis virus is a relatively common pathogen, with CNS involvement most often seen in the dry form of the disease. Seizures, vestibular signs, cerebellar signs and paraparesis are common, and the progression is insidious. The CSF is usually abnormal with increased protein and a mixed, predominantly neutrophilic pleocytosis. There is no definitive treatment and the prognosis is poor.

Feline leukaemia virus and feline immunodeficiency virus

Feline leukaemia virus and feline immunodeficiency virus may cause nonspecific neurological syndromes related to brain, spinal cord and nerve. Serological testing for these viruses is appropriate in any cat with neurological disease of obscure aetiology.

Rabies virus

Rabies virus infection occurs in cats. Behavioural changes are seen early in the disease, usually followed by the furious form and later paralysis. Rabies must be considered in the differential diagnosis if environmental circumstances are compatible with the disease. The course of action to be taken is described in Chapter 23.

Pseudorabies (Aujesky's disease)

Pseudorabies can produce neurological signs in cats, usually causing pruritus and self mutilation. The disease progresses rapidly and the prognosis is poor.

Bacterial infections

Bacterial CNS infections are rare but should be considered, particularly following skull trauma. Diagnosis is by CSF evaluation and culture. Treatment with appropriate antibiotics (usually ampicillin or high doses of chloramphenicol) may be beneficial.

Mycotic infections

Several fungal diseases have a predilection for the feline CNS. *Cryptococcus neoformans* is the most common, usually following upper respiratory infection. Other organisms may be involved, depending on the geographical location. Forebrain signs or more obvious multifocal manifestations are seen. Evaluation of CSF is useful and will show mild pleocytosis, possibly with eosinophilia. Serological tests are available for some organisms. The possibility of immunosuppression related to FeLV or FIV should be considered. Treatment with systemic antifungal drugs (for example, flucytosine, amphotericin B and ketoconazole) may be useful but the prognosis is generally poor.

Protozoal infections

Toxoplasma gondii is an unusual cause of CNS inflammatory disease in cats. Infections may be related to virus-induced immunosuppression. Serological testing may be useful in reaching a diagnosis. Treatment with clindamycin may be useful but the prognosis is guarded.

Parasitic infections

Rare cases of parasitic migration cause CNS signs in cats.

Degenerative diseases

Spongiform encephalopathy

A multifocal neurological syndrome has recently been reported in cats. Gait abnormalities, behavioural change and hypermetria predominate in the multifocal presentation. The disease is progressive and the prognosis is poor. The underlying pathological change is grey matter vacuolation, particularly involving the cerebral cortex and brainstem nuclei, and is similar to scrapie and bovine spongiform encephalopathy. The aetiology is unknown.

DISEASES OF THE SPINE

Tetraparesis and tetraplegia

A cat with neurological deficits in all four limbs may have a lesion at any of the following locations: intracranial, cervical spine (C1-C5), cervicothoracic spine (C6-T2), generalised neuromuscular, or multiple lesions. Differentiation is based on the findings of the neurological examination described above.

NEUROLOGICAL DEFICITS IN ALL LIMBS
Intracranial disease
Cervical spinal cord diseases
Trauma Neoplasia Inflammation and infectious diseases Hypervitaminosis A Multiple cartilaginous exostoses Congenital defects Disc disease
Peripheral neuropathy, neuromuscular junction and muscle diseases
Potassium depletion myopathy Polyneuropathy Myasthenia gravis Organophosphorus and carbamate toxicity Fenthion toxicity Myositis

FIG. 18.9   Neurological deficits in all limbs.

Trauma, neoplasia, inflammatory conditions and occasional congenital abnormalities are causes of cervical spinal cord disease (Fig. 18.9).

Trauma

Traumatic injury to the cervical spine is relatively unusual. Cervical fractures can be serious and lead to respiratory failure. Many spinal fractures can be managed conservatively if the neurological examination suggests a favourable prognosis (see below).

Neoplasms

Neoplasms occur in the cervical and cranial thoracic segments but are less common than in the thoracolumbar spine. Of particular importance are tumours of the nerve roots in the brachial plexus outflow segments (C6-T2). These tumours cause lower motor neurone signs, usually in one forelimb, but progress to cause upper motor neurone signs in the hindlimbs and possibly the contralateral forelimb.

Inflammatory disease

Inflammatory disease (described above) can cause cervical spinal dysfunction and should be considered in differential diagnosis.

Congenital abnormalities

Atlantoaxial subluxation occurs in cats, causing tetraparesis and cervical pain. Surgical treatment may be indicated and the prognosis is good.

Hypervitaminosis A

Hypervitaminosis A causes deposition of a massive amount of supplementary bone at various sites in the skeleton, including the cervical spine. This causes pain and neurological deficits, particularly in the forelimbs. The condition arises from an excessive intake of vitamin A, usually because of excessive amounts of liver in the diet (see Chapters 3 and 17). Similarly, multiple cartilaginous exostoses can affect the cervical spine.

Other causes of cervical spinal disease (disc extrusion, vertebral diseases, discospondylitis) are rare.

Paraparesis and paraplegia

There are several conditions that must be considered in the acutely paralysed cat. Trauma, ischaemic neuromyopathy (aortic embolism) and neoplasia are the most important. In more chronic cases, neoplasia and disc-related conditions are more likely.

Trauma

Trauma usually results from road accidents. Most cases are readily recognised by historical or physical information, but accurate client information regarding trauma is relatively less common in cats than in dogs. Radiography will confirm the diagnosis. Many cats respond well to conservative treatment by cage rest or application of a body cast. Surgical intervention may be appropriate if there is myelographic evidence of cord compression, the fracture is unstable or the cat is in severe pain. Acute spinal injuries may benefit from one treatment with high dose corticosteroids (dexamethasone 2 mg/kg IV; methylprednisolone sodium succinate 30 mg/kg IV) but long-term use is not indicated.

FIG. 18.10 Lateral radiograph of spine of paralysed cat. Neurological signs indicated T3-L3 lesion. Note area of increased opacity in dorsal thorax, ventral to vertebral column. Diagnosis – lymphosarcoma.

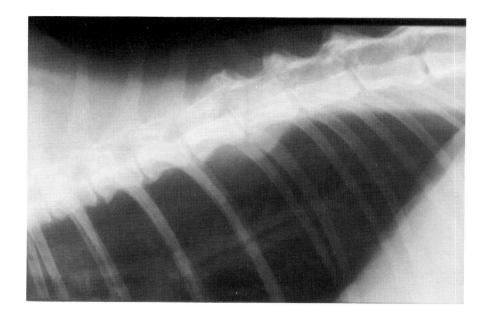

Ischaemic neuromyopathy (aortic thromboembolism)

Ischaemic neuromyopathy is a common cause of acute paraplegia (see Chapter 11).

Neoplasms

Neoplasms of the spinal cord and associated structures are common. Lymphosarcoma is the most prevalent; vertebral tumours are rare. Most cases of spinal lymphosarcoma occur in cats less than 3 years old, and the progression of the clinical signs is relatively acute. Thus, neoplasia must be considered in all cats, regardless of age or acuteness of signs. Thoracic and lumbar tumours are most common, causing neurological signs in the hindlimbs.

Diagnosis of spinal tumours depends largely on myelography. Plain radiographic abnormalities are unusual. Occasionally tumours involve the vertebrae. In some cases of lymphosarcoma, a soft tissue mass is visible in the thorax, ventral to the area of the spine involved (Fig. 18.10). Cerebrospinal fluid may be abnormal but is unlikely to provide definitive information. In spinal lymphosarcoma, systemic signs are usually not apparent but the majority of these cats are FeLV-positive.

The diagnosis is based on a compatible clinical course, positive FeLV test and myelographic evidence of an extradural mass. Biopsy and mass removal may be performed if definitive pathological confirmation is required.

Surgical removal alone is not adequate and must be accompanied by other treatment strategies. Combination chemotherapy and radiation therapy are beneficial. The neurological status will improve with treatment, but most cats succumb to the systemic effects of the disease in time.

Disc disease and discospondylitis

Disc protrusions occur frequently in cats but clinical signs related to spinal cord compression are rare. Cats with myelographic evidence of spinal cord compression should have decompressive surgery. Discospondylitis is also rare and is generally seen with other manifestations of infection (for example, subcutaneous abscesses).

Congenital spinal deformities

Spina bifida is seen occasionally, particularly in the Manx breed.

Ischaemic myelopathy

Ischaemic myelopathy causing peracute, asymmetrical neurological deficits is rare. The diagnosis is based on the absence of a compressive lesion on myelography. Conservative treatment is indicated.

DISEASES OF THE PERIPHERAL NERVE, NEUROMUSCULAR JUNCTION AND MUSCLE

Peripheral polyneuropathy

Diabetic neuropathy

Diabetic neuropathy occurs in some cats with diabetes mellitus. Affected cats are paraparetic with a plantigrade stance. Definitive diagnosis of polyneuropathy requires electrophysiological evaluation.

Inherited hyperchylomicronaemia

Inherited hyperchylomicronaemia causes peripheral neuropathy. Single limb paralysis is usually seen first but evaluation of the patient reveals more widespread peripheral nerve involvement, including cranial nerves. Peripheral nerves are compressed by the lipid granulomas that develop. The condition may improve if the hyperchylomicronaemia is reduced.

Ischaemic neuromyopathy

Ischaemic neuromyopathy is the most common peripheral neuropathy in cats but the clinical signs of acute paraplegia are initially more suggestive of spinal disease (see above).

Neuromuscular junction disorders

Myasthenia gravis

Myasthenia gravis may cause typical episodic weakness (Fig. 18.11) related to exercise, regurgitation, muscle tremors, dysphonia and neck flexion. Aspiration pneumonia may develop with megaoesophagus. Both congenital and acquired forms of the disease are seen, and Abyssinian and related breeds may have a relatively high incidence. The diagnosis is based on the clinical signs and may be confirmed by the intravenous administration of edrophonium hydrochloride (0.25–0.5 mg IV) – the 'edrophonium response test'. Here, cats with acquired myasthenia gravis rapidly become normal for a period of several minutes. The disease is immune-mediated, with antibodies directed against the acetylcholine receptor. Treatment with pyridostigmine hydrochloride (0.5–3.0 mg/kg/per day orally) and corticosteroids is indicated.

EPISODIC AND EXERCISE-INDUCED WEAKNESS
Myasthenia gravis
Polymyositis
Potassium depletion myopathy
Hepatic encephalopathy
Hypoglycaemia

FIG. 18.11   Episodic and exercise-induced weakness.

The congenital form of the disease is rare and is caused by a defect in the postsynaptic acetylcholine receptors at the neuromuscular junction.

Organophosphorus, carbamate and fenthion toxicity

Organophosphorus, carbamate and fenthion are widely used as insecticides in small animals and can be toxic to cats. The compounds interfere with neuromuscular transmission by inactivating acetylcholinesterase, the enzyme that degrades acetylcholine in synapses. There is autonomic overstimulation and neuromuscular dysfunction. With organophosphorus and carbamate toxicity, there is muscular stiffness and a rigid gait with tremors and fasciculations. In fenthion toxicity, weakness predominates (Fig. 18.12). Plasma cholinesterase concentrations may be depressed. Treatment is by reducing further absorption in acute cases, by bathing or gastric lavage as appropriate. Atropine is used to counteract the parasympathetic signs. Pralidoxime hydrochloride (20 mg/kg by IM or slow IV injection) is indicated in organophosphorus toxicity, but it should not be used in carbamate toxicity. Diphenhydramine (4 mg/kg IV or 2 mg/kg orally) can relieve muscle weakness and tremors in fenthion toxicity. Here, absorption of the toxin is rapid, so

FIG. 18.12 Cat with fenthion toxicity, caused by application of excess insecticide. Courtesy Dr. R.S. Bagley.

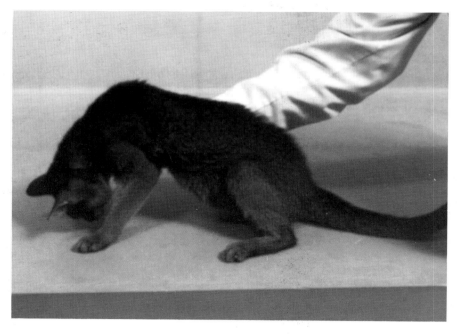

attempts to remove it by bathing are unlikely to be useful.

Myopathy

Potassium-depletion myopathy

Potassium-depletion myopathy is the most commonly recognised muscle disease reported in cats during recent years. Affected cats show acute muscle weakness with a typical posture of neck flexion and the head carried low. The gait is stilted and the cats are reluctant to walk. Muscles may be painful on palpation and exercise induces collapse.

Differential diagnosis includes myasthenia gravis, polymyositis and generalized polyneuropathy. The diagnosis is confirmed by demonstrating a low serum potassium (less than 3.0 mEq/1) in a clinically affected cat. Other causes of hypokalaemia (for example, alkalosis, hyperinsulinaemia or recent fluid therapy) must be eliminated. Creatine kinase concentrations are usually elevated. For further details, see Chapter 17.

Polymyositis

Polymyositis is rare. Typical clinical signs of stiffness, weakness and painful muscles may be seen in toxoplasmosis or in cats with idiopathic polymyositis.

Paralysis of one forelimb

Lesions of the spinal cord, nerve roots, brachial plexus and peripheral nerves can cause paralysis of one forelimb (Fig. 18.13). Spinal cord conditions will usually show upper motor neurone signs in the ipsilateral hindlimb.

Traumatic avulsion of the brachial plexus nerve roots

Traumatic avulsion of the brachial plexus nerve roots is the most likely diagnosis in acute cases.

NEUROLOGICAL DEFICITS IN ONE LIMB
Forelimb
Brachial plexus root avulsion Brachial plexus neoplasia C6-T2 spinal lesions: neoplasia, inflammation Brachial plexus neuropathy
Hindlimb
Pelvic fracture Iatrogenic injury - fracture repair, injection Neoplasia - spinal

FIG. 18.13   Neurological deficits in one limb.

This usually occurs without limb fractures but can occasionally complicate such cases. In addition to the limb deficits, an ipsilateral Horner's syndrome or loss of the panniculus reflex may be seen. The prognosis is poor.

Radial nerve paralysis

Radial nerve paralysis is extremely rare; iatrogenic injury during humeral fracture repair is the most likely cause.

Idiopathic paralysis

Some cats are seen with an acute onset of brachial plexus dysfunction and no history or signs of trauma. The unusual feature of this condition is that the cats recover spontaneously. The aetiology is unclear.

Neoplasia

Neoplasia is the most likely diagnosis in chronic cases of forelimb paralysis. Most tumours occur in the nerve roots and may invade the spinal cord substance. Diagnosis can be difficult, but there may be myelographic abnormalities if the tumour infiltrates the dura mater. Lymphosarcoma is the most common cause and treatment is as described above.

Paralysis of one hindlimb

Pelvic fractures

Traumatic pelvic fractures are the most common cause of hindlimb neurological dysfunction (Fig. 18.14). Sacroiliac luxations, sacral wing fractures and iliac shaft fractures are highly likely to have damaged the lumbosacral trunk. The fracture is likely to heal but neurological deficits may remain. Reflex testing can be difficult in patients with fractures. The absence of hock flexion on testing the withdrawal reflex and decreased sensation in the foot are good indicators of neurological damage. Care must be taken in repairing pelvic fractures as iatrogenic damage can occur, particularly in iliac repair.

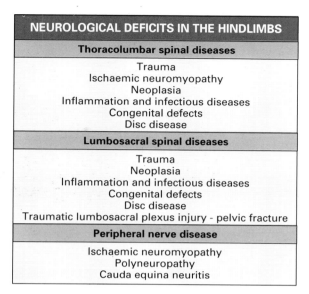

NEUROLOGICAL DEFICITS IN THE HINDLIMBS
Thoracolumbar spinal diseases
Trauma Ischaemic neuromyopathy Neoplasia Inflammation and infectious diseases Congenital defects Disc disease
Lumbosacral spinal diseases
Trauma Neoplasia Inflammation and infectious diseases Congenital defects Disc disease Traumatic lumbosacral plexus injury - pelvic fracture
Peripheral nerve disease
Ischaemic neuromyopathy Polyneuropathy Cauda equina neuritis

FIG. 18.14   Neurological deficits in the hindlimbs.

Sciatic neuropathy

Sciatic neuropathy occurs in two particular situations. During intramedullary pin fixation of a fractured femur, retrograde placement of the pin in the proximal fragment can damage the sciatic nerve. This can be avoided by keeping the limb adducted during pin placement. Pins can migrate proximally after placement, usually causing marked pain and neurological deficits. If sciatic damage occurs, the offending pin must be removed and an alternative method of fixation used. The sciatic nerve can be explored and débrided; if it is transected, anastomosis or grafting may be required. The prognosis for traumatic sciatic neuropathy is guarded.

The second situation where iatrogenic sciatic neuropathy occurs is following intramuscular injections in the caudal thigh. This site should not be used for injections; alternatives are available. Affected cats usually show signs at the time of injection. The prognosis depends on the material injected and whether the injection was near to or into the nerve. The prognosis is guarded or poor.

Neoplasia and spinal cord diseases are rare causes of hindlimb monoparesis.

BLADDER DYSFUNCTION

Neurogenic urinary dysfunction occurs in association with various disease conditions. Spinal diseases are common causes of urinary incontinence. The important clinical feature to determine is the nature of the incontinence (Fig. 18.15). Other considerations apply in evaluating bladder dysfunction – see Chapter 14 for discussion of other causes of urinary incontinence.

VISCERAL AND BLADDER DYSFUNCTION
Spinal lesions
Sacrocaudal fracture
Dysautonomia
FeLV-related

FIG. 18.15   Visceral and bladder dysfunction.

Sacrocaudal fractures cause tail paralysis, but are often complicated by urinary and faecal incontinence and even hindlimb paresis. The site of the fracture cannot account for these neurological signs; in fact, there is avulsion of the nerve roots from the caudal aspect of the spinal cord. This complication should be considered in any tail fracture. The prognosis can be good with appropriate management. It is important to empty the bladder regularly, preferably by manual expression or alternatively by intermittent aseptic catheterisation.

FURTHER READING

Blaxter A.C., Holt P.E., Pearson G.R., Gibbs C., Gruffydd-Jones T.J. (1988) Congenital portosystemic shunts in the cat: a report of nine cases. *J. small Anim. Pract.* **29**: 631.

Burke E.E., Miose N.S., DeLahunta A., Erb H.N. (1985) Review of idiopathic feline vestibular syndrome in 75 cats. *J. Am. Vet. Med. Ass.* **187**: 941.

Chandler E.A., Gaskell C.J., Hilbery A.D.R. (eds) (1985) *Feline Medicine and Therapeutics.* Blackwell Scientific Publications, Oxford.

Cuddon, P.A. (1989) Acquired immune mediated myasthenia gravis in a cat. *J. small Anim. Pract.* **30**: 511.

DeLahunta A. (1983) *Veterinary Neuroanatomy and Clinical Neurology* 2nd edn W.B. Saunders Co., Philadelphia.

Evans, R.J. (1989) Lysosomal storage diseases in dogs and cats. *J. small Anim. Pract.* **30**: 144.

Fenner, W.R. (1991) Inflammations of the nervous system. In: August J.R. (ed.) *Consultations in Feline Internal Medicine*, p. 507. W.B. Saunders Co., Philadelphia.

Griffiths I.R. (1987) Central nervous system trauma. In: Oliver J.E., Hoerlein B.F., Mayhew I.G. (eds) *Veterinary Neurology* W.B. Saunders Co., Philadelphia.

Griffiths I.R., Duncan I.D. (1979) Ischaemic neuromyopathy in cats. *Vet. Rec.* **104**: 518.

Jaggy A., Oliver J.E. (1990) Chlorpyrifos toxicosis in two cats. *J. Vet. Int. Med.* **4**: 135.

Kornegay J.N. (1989) Congenital cerebellar diseases of dogs and cats. In: Kirk R.W. (ed.) *Current Veterinary Therapy X* p. 838. W.B. Saunders Co., Philadelphia.

Kornegay J.N. (1978) Feline infectious peritonitis; the central nervous form. *J. Am. Anim. Hosp. Ass.* **14**: 580.

Kornegay J.N. (1981) Feline Neurology. *Compendium on Continuing Education* **3**: 203.

Mansfield P.D. (1990) Ototoxicity in dogs and cats. *Compendium on Continuing Education* **12**: 321.

Moise N.S. Flanders J.A. (1983) Micturition disorders in cats with sacrocaudal vertebral lesions. In: Kirk R.W. (ed.) *Current Veterinary Therapy VIII*, p. 722. W.B. Saunders Co., Philadelphia.

Nafe L.A. (1984) Topics in feline neurology. *Vet. Clin. N. Am. small Anim. Pract.* **14**(6): 1289.

Rochlitz I. (1984) Feline Dysautonomia (Key-Gaskell Syndrome): a preliminary review. *J. small Anim. Pract.* **25**: 587.

Wheeler S.J., Clayton Jones D.G., Wright J.A. (1985) Myelography in the cat. *J. small Anim. Pract.* **26**: 143.

Wheeler S.J., (ed.) (1989) *Manual of Small Animal Neurology.* BSAVA Publications, Cheltenham

Wheeler S.J. (1989) Spinal tumours in cats. *Vet. Ann.* **29**: 270.

19

Blood Disorders: Interpreting the Feline Haemogram

AL H. REBAR

Quantitative and qualitative evaluation of the peripheral blood, i.e. determination of the complete blood count (CBC), is an essential part of the laboratory evaluation of any ill cat. The CBC includes white cell, red cell, and platelet measurements, as well as morphologic evaluation of the various cell types in the peripheral blood film. The CBC provides general information regarding health status and also specific information about primary diagnosis in certain haematopoietic diseases.

WHITE CELL RESPONSES

White cell data are evaluated first, primarily because abnormalities in the white cell compartment often predict abnormalities in the other compartments as well. White cell measurements include the total white cell count and the white cell differential. Although differentials are nearly always reported as percentages, they should only be interpreted as absolute values. Absolute differential counts are obtained by multiplying differential percentages by total leukocyte counts. Reference ranges for absolute differentials in the cat are presented in Fig. 19.1.

In general, white cell counts can be used to differentiate inflammatory conditions from non-inflammatory ones as well as to recognise evidence of stress (high levels of circulating glucocorticoids) and systemic allergy. They cannot be used to identify specific causes of inflammatory disease such as bacterial and viral infections.

Inflammatory responses

Typical features of inflammatory leukograms in the cat are summarised in Fig. 19.2. Leukogram findings in inflammation are somewhat dependent upon the duration of the inflammatory process.

REFERENCE RANGES FOR ADULT LEUKOCYTE COUNTS	
Total white cell count	7000-17,000/µl
Neutrophils	6000-12,000/µl
Band cells	0-300/µl
Lymphocyte	1000-5000/µl
Eosinophil	0-750/µl
Basophils	0-200/µl
Monocytes	0-850/µl

FIG. 19.1   Reference ranges for adult feline leukocyte counts.

The typical leukogram in cats with acute to subacute inflammatory disease is leukocytosis characterised by neutrophilia and increased numbers of immature neutrophils (band cells) in circulation. Such a response is also termed a regenerative left shift and usually merits a favourable prognosis. The leukocytosis indicates that bone marrow production and release of granulocytes is keeping pace with and exceeding the utilisation of leukocytes by the inflammatory focus (foci) in the tissues. The left shift implies that marrow stores of mature neutrophils are being reduced and immature forms are being called into action. Other features of the typical acute inflammatory leukogram include monocytosis (indicative of tissue necrosis) and lymphopenia (discussed below).

Less commonly, acute inflammation is characterised by leukopenia with a left shift (degenerative left shift). As before, monocytosis and lymphopenia are often present. In these cases, leukopenia implies that tissue demand is overwhelming the capacity of the marrow to respond. These cats are often clinically depressed and the prognosis is accordingly guarded.

Chronic inflammatory leukograms are usually harder to recognise than those of acute inflammation. In chronic inflammation, increased marrow production of granulocytes is balanced by increased tissue utilisation in inflammatory foci so that total white cell count is only slightly elevated or normal. There is usually no or minimal left shift. Lymphocyte counts are also usually normal so that often the only abnormality noted is monocytosis, once again indicating tissue necrosis and a demand for phagocytosis. It is emphasised that the presence of monocytosis alone is sufficient to indicate an inflammatory process.

Leukograms with persistent eosinophilia constitute a special class of inflammation and are worthy of special comment. Eosinophilic inflammation is reflective of system allergic phenomena. In the cat, diseases associated with eosinophilic inflammation include systemic mastocytosis, pulmonary infiltrates with eosinophilia (PIE), heartworm disease, and the plaque form of the eosinophilic granuloma complex. Ectoparasitic diseases associated with lymphadenopathy may also manifest persistent eosinophilia. Most cases of intestinal parasitism in adult animals are not a cause of eosinophilia because a systemic reaction to the parasites does not occur.

Systemic toxaemia

Neutrophil morphology on the peripheral blood film can be used to assess the presence or absence of systemic toxaemia in inflammation. Systemic toxaemia interferes with the differentiation of neutrophil precursors at the level of the bone marrow, resulting in arrest of cytoplasmic or nuclear maturation. The most common cause of systemic toxaemia is bacterial infection, but other causes include tissue necrosis or various toxins.

Cat neutrophils are particularly sensitive to toxaemia, and netrophils containing Doehle bodies, a mild form of toxicity, are occasionally found even in the blood of clinically normal cats. Doehle bodies are aggregates of precipitated cytoplasmic RNA which are seen as rod-shaped to irregular blue cytoplasmic inclusions (Fig. 19.3). More severe signs of toxaemia include generalised foamy cytoplasmic basophilia, cellular giantism and irregular nuclear lobation. Cytoplasmic basophilia reflects general retention of cytoplasmic RNA with failure of formation of normal neutrophil granules. Both giantism and abnormal nuclear configuration indicate nuclear maturation arrest (Fig. 19.4).

Stress leukogram

From a haematological perspective, stress refers to the presence of high circulating levels of endogenous or exogenous glucocorticoids. Glucocorticoids cause reduced margination and longer circulating half lives of neutrophils and increased peripheral sequestration of lymphocytes and eosinophils. The net effects of these influences is mild leukocytosis with mature neutrophilia, lymphopenia, and eosinopenia. The most reproducible and reliable of these changes is lymphopenia; feline lymphocyte counts of less than 1000 to 1500/μl are usually the result of stress.

Stress leukograms take time to develop. Following a single pharmacological dose of prednisone, a stress leukogram develops in approximately 4

FEATURES OF INFLAMMATORY LEUKOGRAMS				
	Acute inflammation	Overwhelming inflammation	Chronic inflammation	Allergic inflammation
TWBC	↑	↓	normal to slight ↑	normal to ↑
Neutrophils	↑	↓	normal to slight ↑	normal to ↑
Bands	↑	↑	normal to slight ↑	normal to ↑
Lymphocytes	↓	↓	normal	variable
Monocytes	↑ or normal	↑ or normal	↑	normal to slight ↑
Eosinophils	normal	normal	normal	↑

↑ increased absolute numbers
↓ decreased absolute numbers

FIG. 19.2 Typical features of inflammatory leukograms.

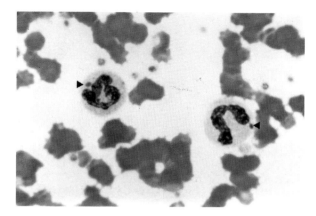

FIG. 19.3   Toxic feline neutrophils. Arrows indicate Doehle bodies.

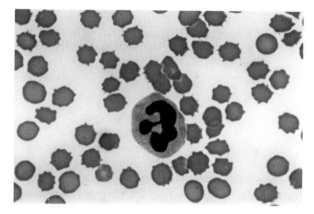

FIG. 19.4   Toxic neutrophil. Features of toxicity include the extremely large cell size and atypical nuclear shape.

hours. The response will persist for approximately 24 hours, assuming no more steroid is given. In cases of prolonged steroid therapy, 72 hours may be required before the stress leukogram resolves.

Elevated levels of endogenous glucocorticoids are a feature of almost all inflammatory processes; hence the lymphopenia seen in association with acute inflammation. Animals with chronic inflammatory processes are also stressed; however, chronic inflammation is usually accompanied by antigenic stimulation, an event which tends to elevate lymphocyte counts. The net effect of these counterbalancing influences is that lymphocyte counts in chronic inflammation are usually in the reference range.

Physiological leukocytosis

Totally distinct from the leukocytosis of stress or inflammation is the leukocytosis seen with excitement. Excitement causes increased blood flow (epinephrine effect); increased blood flow washes cells normally marginating on vessel walls back into the bloodstream. Normally, for every freely circulating leukocyte another is marginated; thus, excitement can effectively double the total white cell count. The cat is unique in that the leukocytosis is primarily the result of lymphocytosis rather than neutrophilia. The author has seen instances where lymphocyte counts in cats have reached 20,000/µl as a result of excitement. Lymphocyte morphology in these instances is normal.

Physiological leukocytosis is a transient phenomenon. It occurs immediately when blood flow increases and can disappear just as suddenly when blood flow returns to normal. In this way, physiological leukocytosis is quite distinct from either stress or inflammatory responses.

Non-inflammatory leukopenia

Non-inflammatory, non-neoplastic leukopenia is relatively common in the cat. Non-inflammatory leukopenia is distinguished by the lack of a left shift. It can be accompanied by marked non-regenerative anaemia and/or thrombocytopenia, or it may occur as an isolated haematological event. Regardless of the presentation, profound non-inflammatory leukopenia in the cat is an unfavourable finding which is usually associated with feline leukaemia virus (FeLV) related disease, feline immunodeficiency virus (FIV) infection, or feline panleukopenia infection. In all cases, bone marrow suppression is the underlying lesion. All cases warrant bone marrow evaluation and FeLV and FIV testing. Even if test results are positive, conservative support therapy should be considered, as a number of these patients do recover.

Leukaemia

Leukaemia (haematologic neoplasia) is a fairly frequent disorder in cats because of the high incidence of FeLV disease. Leukaemia in cats may involve white cells, red cells or platelets, either alone or in combination. In fact, the morphology of leukaemia may change from sampling to sampling in the same patient. Additionally, feline leukaemias may present as pancytopenia without malignant cells in circulation (aleukaemic leukaemia – marrow involvement only), leukopenia with rare malignant cells in circulation (subleukaemic leukaemia), or leukocytosis with large numbers of malignant cells in circulation (leukaemic leukaemia). In fact, the most common laboratory finding is profound non-regenerative anaemia!

Due to the large numbers of forms feline leukaemia can take (Fig. 19.5), the disease syndrome is best referred to as myeloproliferative disease. Whenever myeloproliferative disease is suspected, FeLV testing is indicated. Infection with FIV, while associated with severe leukopenia or anaemia, is not generally associated with leukaemia.

MYELOPROLIFERATIVE DISORDERS

1. Myelogenous (granulocytic) leukaemia -
   neutrophilic
   eosinophilic
   basophilic
2. Myelomonocytic leukaemia
3. Erythroleukaemia – neoplasia of both red cells and white cells
4. Erythaemic myelosis – red cell leukaemia
5. Lymphocytic leukaemia
6. Megakaryocytic myelosis – platelet leukaemia, blast cell form
7. Primary thrombocythaemia – platelet leukaemia
8. Non-neoplastic myeloproliferative disorders - myelofibrosis
   polcythaemia vera

FIG. 19.5   Classification scheme for myeloproliferative disorders of the cat.

RED CELL RESPONSES

Measures of red cell mass in the CBC include total red cell count, haemoglobin, and haematocrit. Red cell indices – mean corpuscular haemoglobin (MCHC), mean corpuscular volume (MCV) and mean corpuscular haemoglobin concentration (MCH) – describe the average characteristics of the red cells in a patient. They are also generally included as a part of the CBC and can be useful in the classification of various red cell disorders.

Polycythaemia

From a clinical perspective, increased red cell mass is polycythaemia. The flow chart in Fig. 19.6 summarises the clinical approach to the diagnosis of polycythaemia. Polycythaemia may be either relative or absolute. Relative polycythaemia is the result of haemoconcentration (dehydration) and is by far the most common form of polycythaemia seen in cats. In most cases, it is easily recognised because elevated measures of red cell mass are accompanied by elevated total protein. Absolute polycythaemia can be either secondary or primary. Secondary absolute polycythaemia can result from inappropriate increased production of erythropoietin as happens in rare cases of renal disease or renal neoplasia. Alternatively, it can occur in conditions where there is reduced oxygenation to the tissues (e.g. pneumonia) and an appropriate compensatory increase in erythropoietin production. Primary absolute polycythaemia, (polycythaemia vera) is an extremely rare myeloproliferative disorder.

Anaemia

Decreased circulating red cell mass is anaemia, by far the most common haematological syndrome seen in cats. Anaemia can be caused by or associated with a wide variety of diseases; whenever anaemia is recognised, every effort must be made to elucidate its origin.

The approach to differentiating anaemias is summarised in Fig. 19.7. From a pathophysiological perspective, all anaemias are either regenerative or non-regenerative. Regenerative anaemias are those in which the bone marrow responds appropriately by producing and releasing increased numbers of normal immature red cells into the circulation. Non-regenerative anaemias are those in which the marrow does not respond appropriately and young red cells are not released in adequate or significantly increased numbers.

The initial step in classifying an anaemia as regenerative or non-regenerative is the evaluation of blood films. In routine Romanowsky-stained blood films, immature RBCs are larger than normal and stain bluish because of their higher than normal content of RNA and their lower than normal complement of haemoglobin. These large

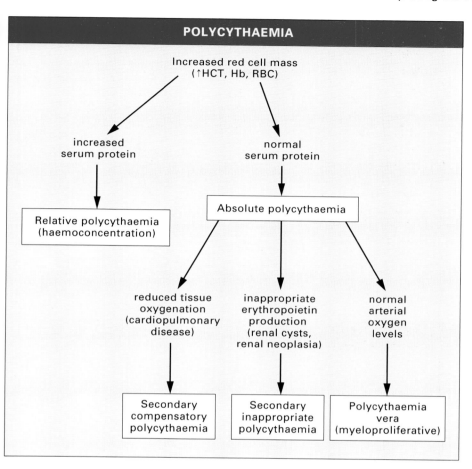

FIG. 19.6 General approach to the differentiation of polycythaemia.

bluish red cells are called polychromatophils and blood films which contain many of them are said to exhibit polychromasia and anisocytosis (variable red cell size). These observations on the peripheral blood film are often supported by the red cell indices; blood samples with large numbers of polychromatophils have a high normal or elevated MCV and a low normal or reduced MCHC.

Whenever anaemia is present and there is a suggestion of polychromasia, a reticulocyte count is indicated to establish whether the anaemia is regenerative. Reticulocyte counts are made on new methylene blue stained blood films. A small amount of EDTA-anticoagulated blood is mixed with an equal volume of new methylene blue. The combination is incubated for 30 minutes at room temperature and then air-dried smears are made.

Reticulocytes are easily identified because the new methylene blue precipitates the RNA they contain as a deep blue reticulum. The cat has three types of reticulocytes: aggregate, punctate, and intermediate (Fig. 19.8). Aggregate reticulocytes have an abundant network of precipitated reticulum; the punctate type contain only scattered focal precipitates; and intermediates contain an intermediate amount of precipitate. Only aggregate reticulocytes are counted. The count is determined by enumerating the number of aggregate reticulocytes/1000 RBCs and dividing by 10 to obtain a percentage. As a general rule, the aggregate reticulocytes correlate with the polychromatophils of the Romanowsky-stained smear but counts based on the new methylene blue stain are regarded as more accurate because they are more easily seen.

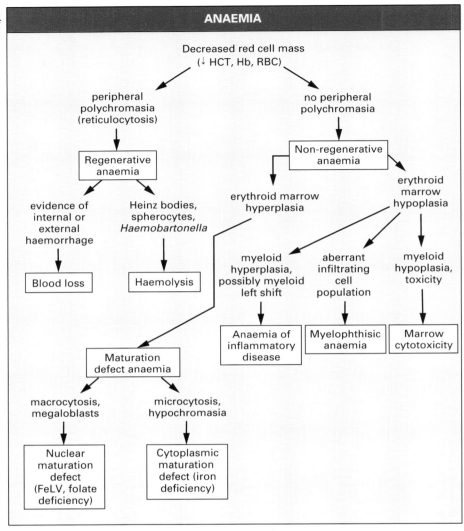

Normal cats have reticulocyte counts of up to 2%. By definition, anaemic cats with elevated counts have regenerative anaemias while anaemic cats without reticulocytosis have non-regenerative anaemias.

Regenerative anaemias

Regenerative anaemias include those caused by haemorrhage and haemolysis. In haemorrhagic anaemias, red cells are lost from the body but circulating red cell lifespan is normal; in contrast, the essential factor of haemolytic anaemia is shortened red cell lifespan. Blood loss anaemia can result from many non-specific causes. The causes of haemolysis are fewer and in many cases can be identified on the peripheral blood film. The principal haemolytic anaemias of cats are immune mediated haemolytic anaemia, Heinz body haemolytic anaemia, and haemobartonellosis.

Immune-mediated haemolytic anaemia

Immune-mediated haemolytic anaemia results from the occurrence of an antigen/antibody reaction

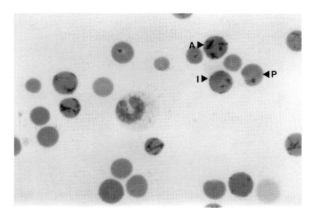

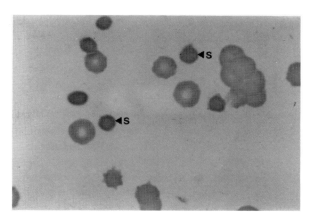

FIG. 19.8   Reticulocyte smear (new methylene blue) in the cat. Aggregate (A), punctate (P), and intermediate (I) forms of reticulocytes are seen in the upper right field.

FIG. 19.9   Acute immune-mediated haemolytic anaemia. Spherocytes are seen as small intensely stained red cells that lack central pallor. An aggregate of agglutinated red cells in seen in the upper right field.

on the red cell surface. The antibodies may be directed against the red cell itself or against antigens, such as drugs or infectious agents, which adhere to the red cell membrane. The presence of antigen/antibody complex on the red cell activates the complement cascade, leading to either intravascular lysis or extravascular red cell destruction by splenic and hepatic macrophages.

Immune-mediated haemolytic anaemia is generally a severe anaemia of rapid onset with profound polychromasia and anisocytosis. The most consistent relatively specific morphological finding is spherocytosis (Fig. 19.9). Spherocytes are small round red cells that stain intensely and lack central pallor. They are often present in large numbers in cases of immune mediated haemolysis but may also occur in low numbers in other diseases. They may be difficult to recognise in feline blood films because cat red cells are already small and somewhat lacking in central pallor.

Auto-agglutination (three-dimensional clumping of RBCs) may also be present (Fig. 19.9). If so, it confirms the diagnosis without need of additional tests. Unfortunately, because of the normally expected heavy rouleaux in cat blood, auto-agglutination is difficult to establish. If agglutination is suspected from peripheral blood films, it should be investigated by placing a drop of well mixed EDTA blood on a slide, adding an equal volume of isotonic saline, and adding a coverslip. If clumping is still present, it is likely

to be the result of agglutination rather than rouleaux.

Whenever clinical signs and peripheral blood data suggest a possible immune-mediated haemolytic anaemia and auto-agglutination is not seen, a direct antiglobulin test (DAT, or Coombs' test) is indicated for confirmation. The DAT is performed by mixing washed red cells with seven serial dilutions of commercially available species specific anti-IgG and anti-complement antibody. Agglutination of the red cells in the bottom of any of the tubes (as determined by microscopic evaluation of a wet preparation) establishes the diagnosis of immune mediated haemolysis.

The causes of immune-mediated haemolytic anaemia are diverse. Most are probably secondary rather than resulting from antibodies directed against the cat's own red cells (a true auto-immune phenomenon). For example, immune haemolysis may accompany haemobartonellosis, FeLV infection, and lymphosarcoma. In many cases an underlying cause is never determined; these cases are best described as idiopathic immune mediated anaemias. Regardless of cause, the vast majority respond dramatically to immunosuppressive doses of glucocorticoids.

Heinz body haemolytic anaemia

Heinz bodies are masses of precipitated haemoglobin that result from the oxidation of the protein (or globin) portion of haemoglobin. Heinz bodies are rigid and interfere with red cell flexibility. Flexibility is essential to normal red cell lifespan; cells measuring 5.5µ in diameter must routinely squeeze through splenic sinusoidal openings of 2–3µ. When cells containing Heinz bodies squeeze through such openings, that portion of the cell containing the Heinz body may be trapped behind, resulting in cell lysis (intravascular haemolysis). In some cases, the Heinz bodies may be so large that the entire cell may be unable to traverse the sinusoidal opening. When this occurs the cell will eventually be phagocytised by sinusoidal macrophages (extravascular haemolysis). The net effect in both instances is shortened red cell lifespan.

Red cells have internal biochemical systems which protect globin against oxidant action under normal circumstances; consequently, Heinz body haemolysis is only seen when these protective mechanisms are overwhelmed. The cat red cell is particularly sensitive to oxidant damage, primarily because its globin contains a high proportion of sulphur-containing amino-acids which are readily oxidised. Normal cats may have Heinz bodies in up to 10% of their red cells without any clinical evidence of haemolysis. Furthermore, we have seen sick cats (particularly those with metabolic disorders such as liver disease, hyperthyroidism and diabetes mellitus, where elevated levels of circulating oxidants might be expected) with Heinz bodies in over 80% of their red cells and no evidence of haemolysis!

Clearly, diagnosis of Heinz body haemolytic anaemia in the cat requires both the presence of a highly regenerative anaemia and identification of Heinz bodies. On Romanowsky stained smears, Heinz bodies appear as nipple-like projections from the red cell surface (Fig. 19.10). They stain like haemoglobin and may be difficult to recognise. Confirmation of the presence of Heinz bodies can be obtained with new methylene blue stains. With new methylene blue, Heinz bodies stain a sky blue which is quite distinctive from the deeper blue of the precipitated reticulum of reticulocytes.

Once the diagnosis is established, efforts should be made to identify the underlying cause. A number of oxidant drugs have been historically implicated as causes of Heinz body haemolytic

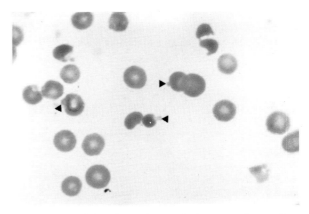

FIG. 19.10   Heinz body haemolytic anaemia. Heinz bodies are indicated by arrows. Two red cell fragments are seen in the upper right field.

anaemia in the cat, including aspirin, acetaminophen, and urine acidifiers such as D-L methionine.

Haemobartonellosis

Feline infectious anaemia, caused by *Haemobartonella felis*, is the principal infectious haemolytic anaemia of the cat. The disease may be either a primary infection or occur secondarily to immunosuppresive disorders such as feline infectious peritonitis (FIP) or FeLV infection.

The primary disease is a typical haemolytic anaemia characterised by anisocytosis and polychromasia. Agglutination may be present, suggesting an immune component to the disease. *Haemobartonella felis* organisms, (basophilic spherical bodies measuring approximately 1µ in diameter) are generally found in chains on the surface of affected red cells. Parasitaemia is both cyclic and transient; blood films may need to be examined on 4–5 consecutive days to ensure that the organisms are observed. At times of peak parasitaemia, the degree of anaemia, polychromasia and reticulocytosis are generally at their lowest level and vice versa. This inverse relationship is a reflection of the way in which the infection is handled by the host. Organisms build up in the blood until parasitised RBCs are removed in large numbers by splenic macrophages. This reduces the degree of parasitaemia while increasing the degree of anaemia and marrow responsiveness. Not surprisingly, splenomegaly is a frequent accompaniment of this disease. In its primary form haemobartonellosis responds quickly to tetracycline therapy and the prognosis for recovery is fair to good.

Secondary haemobartonellosis is far more common than the primary form and the outlook is much worse. *Haemobartonella felis* is an opportunistic organism which often manifests as a feature of severe immunosuppressive states. In this circumstance the anaemia is generally non-regenerative, primarily because of the incapacity of the marrow to respond. Large numbers of organisms are often found in peripheral blood films. These can be removed by tetracycline therapy but this does nothing to alleviate the severely anaemic state. Because of the close association of haemobartonellosis and immunosuppressive conditions, animals should be tested for conditions such as FeLV, FIV and FIP whenever the diagnosis of haemobartonellosis is made.

Non-regenerative maturation defect anaemias

Like the regenerative anaemias, non-regenerative anaemias can be grouped into two categories: maturation defect anaemias and hypoproliferative anaemias. While peripheral blood findings may be useful in some non-regenerative anaemias, in most cases marrow evaluation is needed to establish a definitive diagnosis.

Maturation defect anaemias are the result of acquired marrow abnormalities characterised by nuclear/cytoplasmic asynchrony affecting either red cell precursors only or all marrow precursors generally. Maturation defect anaemias are of two types: nuclear and cytoplasmic.

Nuclear maturation defects

Nuclear maturation defect anaemias are relatively common in cats. Clinically, they are mild to severe non-regenerative anaemias, usually accompanied by some degree of leukopenia and thrombocytopenia because all marrow elements are affected. Red cell morphology may be suggestive of the underlying nature of the anaemia. There may be anisocytosis with occasional large red cells (macrocytes). If the problem is marked, MCV may even be elevated while MCHC remains normal.

Additionally, rare to occasional abnormal nucleated red cells may be seen. These cells are abnormally large with fully haemoglobinised cytoplasm, and large round immature nuclei with abnormally clumped chromatin. These abnormal red cells, with young nuclei and mature cytoplasm, reflect arrested nuclear development in the marrow and are known as megaloblasts.

While peripheral blood findings are often suggestive of the problem, marrow evaluation is generally required for definitive diagnosis. The marrow is hypercellular even in the face of peripheral pancytopenia; this is a case of increased but ineffective production of blood cells by the marrow. All cell lines have evidence of arrested nuclear development with increased proportions of immature precursors. Numerous red cell precursors are megaloblastic. In the white cell series, most nuclei do not develop past the myelocyte stage even though granulocyte cytoplasm differentiates fully. The few band, metamyelocyte, and segmented nuclei present generally are deficient in their chromatin content (chromatin density), and nucleoli (which are never seen normally in these stages) are readily apparent. Megakaryocytes (platelet precursors) are perhaps the most bizarre of all. Normal megakaryocytes are large cells with 8–16 nuclei linked into a single nuclear mass. Megaloblastic megakaryocytes are smaller and often contain only one large nucleus or two at most.

The overall features of megaloblastic bone marrow are best described as marrow dysplasia. Caution must be taken in differentiating these changes from true leukaemia. In marrow dysplasia all cell lines are affected, while in most leukaemias abnormal precursors of a single cell line replace all other marrow elements. Megaloblastic marrow dysplasia may be a preneoplastic change, but it may also be reversible.

The cause of the nuclear maturation defect anaemias is generally a functional folic acid or vitamin B12 deficiency. These vitamins are required for DNA synthesis and therefore cell division. In animals generally, impaired folate metabolism is the usual cause. In the cat the most common cause is FeLV infection. The virus appears to interfere with nuclear development directly, although the possibility of megaloblastosis developing as a result of competition for nutrients between marrow precursors and a rapidly developing tumour has also been suggested.

Cytoplasmic maturation defects

Cytoplasmic maturation defect anaemias result when there is normal nuclear development but arrested cytoplasmic maturation. In most cases this means interference with the formation of haemoglobin. By far the most common of these is iron deficiency (severe blood loss) which only affects the red cell series. It causes distinctive microcytic hypochromic anaemia; blood films are characterised not only by the small size of the RBCs but also by marked poikilocytosis (variable in red cell shape) and red cell fragmentation. There is usually an accompanying thrombocytosis.

Marrow findings include a marked erythroid hyperplasia with a maturation arrest at the late rubricyte/metarubricyte stage. Arrested cells are smaller than normal, primarily because red cell precursors continue to divide until they have nearly a full complement of haemoglobin; furthermore, they accumulate in the marrow because the degree of haemoglobinisation also regulates release of red cells into the circulation.

Non-regenerative hypoproliferative anaemias

Hypoproliferative anaemias are the most common of all the anaemias in animals. Peripheral blood morphology is almost always unremarkable; as in the maturation defect anaemias, diagnosis often depends upon marrow evaluation. Hypoproliferative anaemias fall into three general categories 1) anaemia of inflammatory disease; 2) myelophthisic anaemias; and 3) anaemias due to marrow cytotoxicity.

Anaemia of inflammatory disease

The anaemia of inflammatory/chronic disease is perhaps the most common anaemic syndrome seen in any of the domestic species. It is mildly to moderately severe (in the cat, haematocrits range from 25 to 35 per cent) and is normocytic normochromic. Pathogenesis of this syndrome is somewhat controversial but involves interference with

mobilisation of iron to red cell precursors. Changes include decreases in serum iron levels, reductions in serum transferrin, and accumulation of iron in marrow macrophages. Morphologically, the marrow is usually characterised by granulocytic hyperplasia, increases in marrow macrophage and plasma cell numbers, and mild erythroid hypoplasia. Whenever inflammatory leukograms are present in conjunction with anaemia, this syndrome should be suspected. Confirmation depends upon demonstration of the changes described above.

Non-regenerative hypoproliferative anaemias are commonly associated with renal and hepatic disease and often represent a special case of the anaemia of inflammation. The pathogenesis of these conditions is varied; consequently, peripheral blood morphology is also varied.

Myelophthisic anaemia

Myelophthisic anaemias result from replacement of normal marrow by an abnormal cellular infiltrate which may be either non-neoplastic or neoplastic.

The principal non-neoplastic syndrome is myelofibrosis, which is the replacement of marrow by normal connective tissue. In the cat, myelofibrosis may be a primary FeLV-related myeloproliferative disorder or secondary to a variety of causes. Secondary myelofibrosis represents the logical endpoint of severe marrow stromal damage, or bone marrow scarring. Possible causes include exposure of bone marrow to ionising radiation, toxic drugs and chemicals, and prolonged high levels of oestrogen. In cases where the cause is not identified, myelofribrosis is referred to as idiopathic.

The primary causes of neoplastic myelophthisis are the lymphoid and haemopoietic neoplasms, which routinely involve the marrow. Less commonly, other disseminated neoplasms can fill the marrow causing a myelophthisic syndrome.

Regardless of cause, myelophthisic syndromes cause profound non-regenerative anaemias, usually associated with profound leukopenias. Platelet response is less predictable, as both thrombocytopenia and thrombocytosis occur with about equal frequency. Marked red cell poikilocytosis is reported in dogs but less well documented in cats.

Diagnosis is confirmed via bone marrow biopsy.

When myelophthisis is suspected, aspirates for cytology and core biopsies for histopathology should be collected. Generally aspirates from neoplastic myelophthisis will be highly cellular, and the diagnosis is made easily. The marrow will rarely be so tightly packed with cells that aspirates cannot collect them; in these cases examination of marrow cores are required for diagnosis. Similarly, aspirates in cases of myelofibrosis are usually hypocellular and core biopsy is required for diagnosis.

Anaemia due to marrow cytotoxicity

Acute marrow cytotoxicity may be caused by various infectious and non-infectious aetiologies. Infectious causes are largely viral – primarily feline panleukopenia virus and FeLV. Non-infectious causes are diverse and include ionising radiation, chemotherapy for cancer, and oestrogen toxicity.

Marrow cytotoxicity causes progressive pancytopenia. Consequently patients may present with bleeding problems (thrombocytopenia), overwhelming infections (granulocytopenia) or extreme lethargy with pale mucous membranes (anaemia). As with myelophthisic syndromes, diagnosis depends on examination of the marrow. Both aspirates and core histopathology biopsies may be required.

Toxicity in marrow precursors is more easily recognised. Changes include cytoplasmic basophilia and vacuolation, nuclear vacuolation, bizarre nuclear shapes, and cytonuclear dissociation.

If the process is more advanced, hypocellular aspirates are the rule. Core biopsy is required to prove that the marrow contains markedly reduced numbers of precursors (aplastic anaemia). When the diagnosis of aplastic anaemia is confirmed, a specific cause can be sought from the history. In most cases, regardless of cause, prognosis is guarded; few aplastic anaemias are reversible.

PLATELET RESPONSES

Platelet measurement in the CBC include platelet count and platelet morphology. The principal abnormalities noted are thrombocytopenia and thrombocytosis.

Thrombocytopenia falls into three categories: consumptive, hypoproliferative and sequestration.

Consumptive thrombocytopenias are conditions where production in the marrow is normal but peripheral utilisation is increased. The most frequent causes of consumptive thrombocytopenia are disseminated intravascular coagulopathy and immune-mediated thrombocytopenia. Hypoproliferative thrombocytopenia can occur in any of the hypoproliferative pancytopenias described above. Sequestration thrombocytopenia results from pooling of platelets in the spleen in cases of hypersplenism; this condition is extremely rare in cats. Differentiation of consumptive from hypoproliferative thrombocytopenias depends on marrow examination; consumptive processes have normal to increased numbers of megakaryocytes while hypoproliferative syndromes have decreased numbers.

Peripheral thrombocytosis is less often of clinical significance than thrombocytopenia. Very high counts can be present in cases of FeLV-related platelet leukaemias. In these instances, morphologically-abnormal platelets are usually observed.

FURTHER READING

1. Alsaker R.D., Laber J., Stevens J., and Perman V. (1977) A comparison of polychromasia and reticulocyte counts in assessing erythrocytic regenerative response in the cat. *J. Am. Vet. Med. Assoc.* **170**: 39.
2. Boyce J.T., et al. (1986) Feline leukemia virus-induced thrombocytopenia and macrothrombosis in cats. *Vet. Pathol.* **23**: 16.
3. Cain G.R., Suzuki Y. (1985) Presumptive neonatal isoerythrolysis in cats. *J. Am. Vet. Assoc.* **187**(1): 46–48.
4. Center, S.A., Randolph, J.F., Erb, H.N. (1990) Eosinophilia in the cat – a retrospective study of 312 cases: 1975–1986. *J. Am. Anim. Hosp. Assoc.* **26**: 349–358.
5. Cotter, S.M. (1977) Anemia associated with feline leukemia virus infection. *J. Am. Vet. Med. Assoc.* **175**: 191.
6. Cotter, S.M. and Holzworth, J. (1987) Disorders of the hematopoietic system. In Holzworth, J. (ed) *Diseases of the Cat: Medicine and Surgery.* W.B. Saunders Co., Philadelphia, p. 755.
7. Degen, M.A. and Breitschwerdt, E.B. (1986) Canine and feline immunodeficiency. *Comp. Cont. Ed.* **8**: 313, 379.
8. Fan, L.C., Dorner, J.L., and Hoffmann, W.E. (1978). Reticulocyte response and maturation in experimental acute blood loss anemia in the cat. *J. Am. Anim. Hosp. Ass.* **14**: 219.

9. Gorman, N.T. and Werner, L.L. (1986) Immune-mediated diseases of the dog and cat. *Br. Vet. J.* **142**: 395, 403, 491, 498.

10. Grindem, C.B. (1985) Morphological classification and clinical and pathological characteristics of spontaneous leukemia in ten cats. *J. Am. Anim. Hosp. Ass.* **21**: 227.

11. Harvey, J.W. (1980) Feline hemobartonellosis. In Kirk, R.W. (ed.) *Current Veterinary Therapy VII.* W.B. Saunders Co., Philadelphia, PA.

12. Harvey, J.W., Shields, R.P. and Gaskin, J.M. (1978) Feline myeloproliferative disease: Changing manifestations in peripheral blood. *Vet. Pathol.* **15**: 437.

13. Hirsch, V., and Dunn, J. (1983) Megaloblastic anemia in the cat. *J. Am. Anim. Hosp. Ass.* **19**: 873–880.

14. Hjelle, J.J. and Grauer, G.F. (1986) Acetaminophen-induced toxicosis in dogs and cats. *J. Am. Vet. Med. Assoc.* **188**: 742.

15. Hoover, E.A., Kociba, G.J., Hardy, W.D., Jr., and Yohn, D.S. (1974) Erythroid hypoplasia in cats inoculated with feline leukemia virus. *J. Natl. Cancer Inst.* **53**: 1271.

16. Kociba, G.J. (1983) Serum erythropoietin changes in cats with feline leukemia virus-induced erythryoid aplasia. *Vet. Pathol.* **20**: 548.

17. Lewis, H.B., and Rebar, A.H. (1979) *Bone Marrow Evaluation in Veterinary Practice.* Ralston Purina Co., St. Louis.

18. Madewell, B.R. (1983) Ferrokinetic and erythrocyte survival studies in healthy and anemic cats. *Am. J. Vet. Res.* **44**: 424.

19. Maede, Y. (1987) Methionine toxicosis in cats. *Am. J. Vet. Res.* **48**: 289.

20. Marsh, J.C., Boggs, D.R., Cartwright, G.E. and Wintrobe, M.M. (1967) Neutrophil kinetics in acute infection. *J. Clin. Invest.* **46**: 1943.

21. Meyers-Wallen, V.N. (1984) Hematologic values in healthy neonatal, weanling, and juvenile kittens. *Am. J. Vet. Res.* **45**: 1322.

22. Pederson, N.C. (1987) Isolation of a T-lymphotropic virus from domestic cats with an immunodeficiency-like syndrome. *Science* **235**: 790.

23. Perman, V. (1988) Peculiarities of the anemic cat. *Proceedings of the 55th Annual Meeting American Animal Hospital Association*, pp. 78–82.

24. Perman, V. and Schall, W.D. (1983) Diseases of the Red Blood Cells. In Ettinger, S.A. (ed.) *Textbook of Veterinary Internal Medicine.* W.B. Saunders Co., Philadelphia, PA.

25. Prasse, K.W., Kaeberle, M.L. and Ramsey, F.K. (1973) Blood neutrophilic granulocyte kinetics in cats. *Am. J. Vet. Res.* **34**: 1021.

26. Prasse, K.W. and Mahaffey, E.A. (1987) Hematology of normal cats and characteristic responses to disease. In Holzworth, J. (ed.) *Diseases of the Cat: Medicine and Surgery.* W.B. Saunders Co., Philadelphia, p. 739.

27. Prasse, K.W., Seagrave, R.C., Kaeberle, M.L. and Ramsey, F.K. (1973) A model of granulopoiesis in cats. *Lab. Invest.* **28**: 292.

28. Schechter, R.D., Schalm, O.W., and Kaneko, J.J. (1973) Heinz body hemolytic anemia associated with the use of urinary antiseptics containing methylene blue in the cat. *J. Am. Vet. Med. Assoc.* **162**: 37.

29. Searcy, G.P. (1980) Bone marrow failure in the dog and cat. In Kirk, R.W. (ed.) *Current Therapy VII.* W.B. Saunders Co., Philadelphia, PA.

30. Weiser, M.G. and Kociba, G.J. (1982) Persistent macrocytosis assessed by erythrocyte subpopulation analysis following erythrocyte regeneration in cats. *Blood* **60**: 295.

31. Weiser, M.G. and Kociba, G.J. (1983) Sequential changes in erythrocyte volume distribution and microcytosis associated with iron deficiency in kittens. *Vet. Pathol.* **20**: 1.

32. Weiser, M.G. and Kociba, G.J. (1983) Erythrocyte macrocytosis in feline leukemia virus associated anemia. *Vet. Pathol.* **20**: 548.

20

Disorders of the Eyes

SIMON M. PETERSEN-JONES AND JOHN R.B. MOULD

The majority of feline ocular diseases result from trauma or infection or are related to systemic disorders. Fortunately, the orbital and periocular conformation of the cat has been altered less by selective breeding than that of the dog. Consequently cats suffer comparatively rarely from ocular disease resulting from poor conformation. Inherited ocular disorders are also not as commonly recognised in cats as in dogs.

OPHTHALMIC EXAMINATION

Ophthalmic examination of cats can be performed using routine equipment. It should be carried out carefully, methodically and with a good knowledge of the normal appearance. Full details of ophthalmic examination techniques can be found in standard textbooks and are not repeated here. A systematic examination of the eye will become routine with experience and need not be time consuming. The following equipment will be required:

Pen torch
Simple magnification
Direct ophthalmoscope
Condensing lens for indirect ophthalmoscopy (optional)
Kimura spatula for taking conjunctival smears (any blunt blade-like instrument can be used)
Microscope slides
Bacteriology swabs
Fluorescein drops or impregnated strips
Local anaesthetic drops (proparacaine/ proxymetacaine)
Schirmer tear test papers

Disorders are dealt with in this chapter on an anatomical basis. It is wise, however, to take a 'whole eye' approach as a localised ocular lesion may well be accompanied by changes elsewhere in the eye. General physical examination is also important, as ocular disease may be secondary to a systemic disorder.

GLOBE AND ORBIT

Congenital disorders

Microphthalmia

Microphthalmia is a congenitally small eye. It may be bilateral or unilateral. The severity varies: some microphthalmic eyes are slightly smaller than usual, whereas others are very small and cystic. Accompanying intraocular abnormalities may include cataract, persistent pupillary membranes and retinal dysplasia.

Strabismus (squint)

Convergent strabismus (cross eyed) is inherited in the Siamese. Acquired strabismus may result from trauma, or denervation of extraocular muscles.

Acquired disorders

Prolapse

Prolapse of the globe is complete displacement anterior to the plane of the lids. The feline globe is well protected by the bony orbit and will only prolapse after severe trauma. Intraocular damage may accompany prolapse and should be assessed. A widely dilated non-responsive pupil indicates avulsion of the optic nerve. Fractures of the skull (e.g. the zygomatic arch and mandible) may also be present. The condition requires rapid treatment and the cornea should be kept moist until the globe can be surgically repositioned. This is facilitated by a lateral canthotomy to enlarge the palpebral fissure. Following repositioning, the eyelids are sutured closed until the swelling subsides.

Even with prompt correct management, the high possibility of damage to blood vessels, nerves and extraocular muscles means that the prognosis for a functional eye is guarded.

Exophthalmos

Exophthalmos is abnormal anterior displacement of the globe and may be due to retrobulbar space-occupying lesions such as abscesses, tumours or haemorrhage. In addition to anterior displacement, the globe may be deviated in another plane, and the third eyelid protruded. It is important to distinguish exophthalmos from buphthalmos (an enlarged eye due to glaucoma) as both cause a 'prominent eye'. The chronically glaucomatous eye has obvious intraocular changes, whereas an exophthalmic eye is essentially normal, but may develop exposure keratitis. If the patient is viewed from above, the exophthalmic eye is obviously displaced anteriorly whereas the globe with buphthalmos appears only slightly more prominent.

Haematology, radiography and ultrasonography, in addition to the clinical examination, can help in reaching a diagnosis.

Orbital abscesses may result from the penetration of foreign bodies from the oropharynx or from root infections of the upper molars. Abscessation results typically in a rapid onset of exophthalmia associated with pain (especially on opening the mouth), pyrexia and a neutrophilia with a left shift. Retrobulbar abscesses may be drained under general anaesthesia via the mouth. The oral mucosa behind the last upper molar tooth is incised and a blunt dissection made dorsally to reach the retrobulbar area.

Orbital tumours tend to manifest exophthalmos in a more insidious fashion and are not initially associated with pain. They may be primary (arising from the many tissues of the orbit), or they may enter the orbit by extension from periorbital structures (e.g. frontal sinuses, ethmoidal region of the nasal chambers) or result from metastasis from distant sites. Lymphoma may also occur in the orbit. The prognosis for orbital tumours is guarded as most are malignant.

Enophthalmos

The globe may retract into the orbit as a result of dehydration, loss of retrobulbar fat, or muscle atrophy. Protrusion of the third eyelid also occurs. Enophthalmos may also be a feature of Horner's syndrome.

Buphthalmos

Enlargement of the globe due to glaucoma will be considered later.

Panophthalmitis

Inflammation of the entire globe may result from penetrating wounds, or develop from an anterior or posterior uveitis. Penetrating wounds should always be treated aggressively with topical and systemic antibiotics (and surgical management when appropriate), as established bacterial endophthalmitis carries a very guarded prognosis.

Phthisis bulbi

Phthisis bulbi is a shrunken globe resulting from severe intraocular disease such as chronic uveitis or end stage chronic glaucoma. Enucleation should be considered, as these eyes may be at risk of developing sarcomas.

THE EYELIDS

Congenital and neonatal disorders

Coloboma

Coloboma is a congenital discontinuity of the ocular tissue. Occasionally agenesis of the lateral portion of the upper eyelid occurs. The affected eyelids may be unable to cover the cornea completely when closed and facial hair may contact the cornea, resulting in keratitis. Reconstructive surgery is indicated and referral to a specialist recommended.

Ankyloblepharon

Ankyloblepharon is fusion of the eyelids and is normal in kittens until 10–14 days of age. Occasionally ankyloblepharon persists into adult life and treatment is simply to incise along the presumptive opening of the eyelids.

If an infective conjunctivitis occurs before the lids separate (ophthalmia neonatorum), the eyelids become distended due to the accumulation of purulent material. There may be some discharge of pus at the medial canthus. If left untreated, ulcerative keratitis or even corneal perforation can develop. The eyelids should be opened and the conjunctival sac irrigated. Culture and sensitivity testing should be performed and a broad-spectrum antibiotic applied topically four times daily while awaiting results.

Distichiasis and ectopic cilia

Distichia are cilia emerging from the eyelid margin; ectopic cilia are cilia emerging through the conjunctival lining of the eyelid. They occur rarely in cats, first emerging in the young adult. If irritation results, the offending cilia should be permanently removed. Electrolysis is used to destroy distichia; local excision of the offending hair root is performed to remove ectopic cilia.

Acquired conditions

Abnormalities of lid position

Entropion, an inward turning of the eyelids, is encountered occasionally. It is usually secondary to chronic blepharospasm due to painful ocular lesions. The underlying lesion should be investigated and the eyelid everted surgically if necessary. Ectropion, an outward turning of the eyelid, is usually the result of cicatrix formation and is also uncommon.

Blepharitis

The outer surface of the eyelids consists of normal skin and therefore may be involved in any generalised dermatitis. There may also be an accompanying conjunctivitis. The causes of blepharitis include mycoses, bacterial infections (such as from bite wounds) and, less commonly, mite infestations. Pemphigus lesions may affect the lids, particularly the medial canthus.

Eyelid lacerations

Lacerations of the eyelids are common. They should be repaired surgically to allow healing by first intention. When the eyelid margin is involved, the first suture should be placed close to the margin to reform it accurately (ensuring the suture ends cannot abrade the cornea).

Eyelid tumours

These are rare in cats with the exception of squamous cell carcinomas which appear as slow growing ulcerative lesions. White cats are most commonly affected. Histopathological confirmation by biopsy is indicated. Metastasis to the regional lymph nodes occurs commonly and should be considered when giving a prognosis. Small squamous cell carcinomas can be excised. Larger lesions may be treated by radiation or cryotherapy. Fine needle aspirate or biopsy of the local lymph node to check for metastasis should be considered.

THE THIRD EYELID

The third eyelid plays an important role in protecting the cornea and contributing to and spreading the tear film, thereby maintaining a healthy ocular surface. It should never be removed unless infiltrated extensively by a tumour. Smooth muscle under sympathetic control usually keeps the third eyelid retracted. It will protrude passively if the globe is retracted into the orbit. Foreign bodies can lodge between the third eyelid and the cornea.

Prominence of the third eyelid

Prolapse or protrusion of the third eyelid is common in cats (Fig. 20.1).

Lacerations of the third eyelid

Large lacerations should be repaired with 6–0 cat gut or synthetic absorbable sutures, ensuring that the sutures do not abrade the cornea.

Prolapse of the gland of the third eyelid

This is uncommon in cats. The prolapsed gland appears as a pink medial canthal swelling. It is best to try to conserve the gland by suturing it to the periosteum of the medio-ventral orbit rim.

FIG. 20.1 Differential diagnosis of increased prominence of the third eyelid.

DIFFERENTIAL DIAGNOSIS OF INCREASED PROMINENCE OF THE THIRD EYELID	
Cause	**Accompanying signs**
Increased orbital volume displacing third eyelid (e.g. abscess, cellulitis, tumour)	Exophthalmos, difficulty repelling the globe into the orbit, pain (abscess), difficulty or pain on opening the mouth
Decreased orbital volume (e.g. dehydration, cachexia, phthisis bulbi)	Enophthalmos
Viral diarrhoea and other gastrointestinal upsets	Gastrointestinal
Horner's syndrome (sympathetic denervation)	Ptosis, miosis, enophthalmos
Ocular irritation or pain (e.g. foreign body)	Depends on aetiology, may have conjunctival, corneal or intraocular abnormalities
Symblepharon (e.g. following feline herpesvirus infection)	Conjunctival bands or partial obliteration of the fornices, corneal lesions may be present, may have tear overflow

Neoplasia

Tumours affecting the third eyelid are encountered occasionally. Haemangiomas, haemangiosarcomas, lymphoma and fibrosarcoma have been reported, as have adenocarcinomas of the gland of the third eyelid.

THE TEAR FILM AND NASOLACRIMAL DUCT SYSTEM

Tears are produced from the lacrimal gland, the gland of the third eyelid, mucus secreting glands of the conjunctiva (goblet cells) and lipid-producing glands within the eyelid (meibomian glands). For a normal tear film, the combined secretions must be distributed effectively by the lids and third eyelid. The presence of a normal tear film is paramount for a healthy ocular surface. Tears drain into the nasolacrimal duct system via the upper and lower puncta on the inner conjunctival surface of the eyelids near the medial canthus.

Epiphora

In this condition, tears overflow and run onto the face. Tear overflow may result from increased tear production or from obstruction of drainage. Increased lacrimation results from ocular irritation or pain (e.g. corneal ulceration). Epiphora in the absence of increased lacrimation can be investigated by instilling fluorescein dye into the conjunctival sac and observing its appearance at the ipsilateral naris. This test is intended to assess the overall drainage process but the value is limited by the fact that in many normal cats fluorescein will not appear at the nose. Cannulation and flushing of the upper or lower punctum will test actual patency of the nasolacrimal duct system. Sedation in addition to the application of a local anaesthetic is usually necessary. The puncta are small and a fine nasolacrimal cannula (e.g. 26 gauge) is required.

Some breeds of cats with short noses, such as Persians, often have epiphora despite the presence of a patent nasolacrimal duct system. In these cats, the prominent eyes and flattened face result in a shallow lacrimal lake at the medial canthus. Tears are therefore squeezed onto the face when the cat blinks, rather than being forced into the drainage system, and epiphora results.

Congenital absence of part of the drainage system is an occasional cause of epiphora in the cat. Acquired obstruction can result from conjunctival adhesions (e.g. following feline herpesvirus infection) and it is often impossible to re-establish patency of the nasolacrimal duct system in such cases.

Keratoconjunctivitis sicca ('dry eye')

This is uncommon in the cat. The Schirmer tear test, in which a strip of filter paper is positioned so that one end is between the cornea and lower lid, is used to measure tear production. The result for a normal cat is approximately 17 (+/− 5) mm of wetting in one minute. A result below 5 mm/min is diagnostic of dry eye. The condition results in irritation and the affected cornea lacks lustre and may develop a mild keratitis. It is an occasional sequela to feline herpesvirus infection. Another possible cause is denervation of the tear producing glands. In these cases the denervated glands are hypersensitive to parasympathomimetics, and one or two drops of a 1% pilocarpine solution twice daily in food can be a useful adjunct to the standard treatment of frequent administration of topical tear substitutes. Parotid duct transposition is reserved for patients in which medical therapy does not control the condition.

CONDITIONS OF OCULAR SURFACE

The ocular surface consists of the conjunctiva and cornea. The conjunctiva lines the eyelids and is reflected at the fornix to overlie the globe as far as the limbus, where the epithelium is then continuous with the corneal epithelium. The cornea is large and clear and is coated by the precorneal tear film.

Congenital disease

Dermoids

A dermoid is a piece of skin-like tissue (often bearing hairs) which during embryological development became associated with the cornea and/or conjunctiva, usually at the lateral canthus. They are familial in the Birman. Removal is by superficial keratectomy, conjunctival resection or both.

Acquired disease

Conjunctivitis

Conjunctivitides of various aetiologies are common in cats, and their general features are summarised in Fig. 20.2. The clinical signs are conjunctival hyperaemia, oedema (chemosis) and serous or purulent ocular discharge. Chemosis in the cat may be so severe that the swollen conjunctiva balloons out from beneath the lids. There

FELINE CONJUNCTITUS			
Aetiology	**Signs**	**Diagnosis**	**Treatment**
Herpesvirus	Severe inflammation Corneal involvement Respiratory signs	Signs Swabs – viral culture	Trifluridine* Idoxuridine Covering antibiotics
Calicivirus	Conjunctivitus Cornea unaffected Respiratory signs	Signs Swabs – viral culture	Idoxuridine Covering antibiotics
Chlamydia psittaci	Chronic conjunctivitus	Signs Scrapes – fluorescent antibody staining Serology	Topical and systematic tetracycline for 4 weeks
Mycoplasma	Pale or hyperaemic conjunctivae Pseudo-diptheritic membrane	Swabs Scrapes	Tetracycline Chloramphenicol Gentamicin
Trauma (e.g. foreign body)	May result in severe chemosis	Signs	Remove foreign body Covering antibiotics
Bacterial (unusual in cat)	Mucopurulent discharge	Swabs for bacteriology	Broad spectrum antibiotic
Follicular (usually a non-specific response)	Multiple small round pale nodules on conjunctiva	Signs Swabs Scrapes Serology	Treat the cause
*trifluridine is not yet available as an opthalmic preparation in the UK			

FIG. 20.2 Feline conjunctivitis.

may be accompanying corneal changes and upper respiratory signs depending on the aetiology. Standard texts describe typical clinical signs, clinical course and diagnostic tests for each agent. However, many infections are mixed so that the clinical appearance may not match the textbook description and it may not be easy to make a definitive aetiological diagnosis initially. Definitive diagnosis of herpesvirus infection is not always easy and interpretation of conjunctival smears for chlamydial or mycoplasmal infection requires expertise. It is best to establish with a diagnostic laboratory what tests are offered, what samples are required and how these should be handled to optimise the chances of a definitive diagnosis. A general approach is to take conjunctival swabs (before local anaesthetics are administered) and place them in the recommended transport media. A local anaesthetic is then applied, the lower lid is everted and a sterile spatula is drawn across the conjunctival surface. A small bead of translucent material is collected and gently smeared on two clean glass microscope slides. The material is fixed and one slide stained with a Giemsa type stain for cytology and the other sent to the laboratory for appropriate special staining, e.g. fluorescent antibody staining.

In the absence of a specific diagnosis, the most useful therapeutic agent is probably tetracycline, administered topically and orally, and continued for at least one week after clinical signs have resolved.

Symblepharon

Symblepharon refers to adhesions of the conjunctival or corneal surfaces and usually follows severe conjunctivitis (e.g. feline herpesvirus infection) in young animals. It is a very variable condition and may involve conjunctival adhesions partly obliterating the fornix, adhesions of the third eyelid to the lids (Fig. 20.3), occlusion of the nasolacrimal puncta or the presence of an opaque conjunctiva-like membrane on the corneal surface. There may be a marked difference in the degree to which the two eyes are affected. Each case must be assessed on its merits. The only treatment is surgical but specialist procedures may be required and the prognosis is guarded.

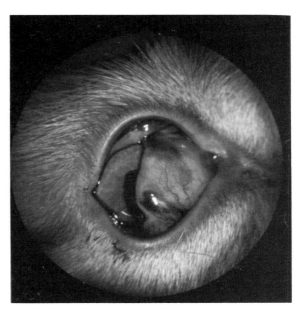

FIG. 20.3   Symblepharon resulting in permanent protrusion of the third eyelid. There are prominent adhesions running from the third eyelid to upper and lower lids.

Fortunately many cases require no attention, although there may be a cosmetic difference between the two eyes.

Corneal injuries

Treatment depends on the depth and extent of the wound. Covering antibiotics should be given and if necessary a third eyelid flap can be used to support the cornea while it heals. Immediate surgical repair is essential if the wound is full thickness resulting in an iris prolapse. After flushing debris from the prolapsed iris and removing adherent fibrin, the iris is replaced into the anterior chamber and the cornea repaired with 8–0 polyglactin 910 suture. Balanced salt solution should be used to reform the anterior chamber. Postoperatively, topical atropine and antibiotics are given.

Corneal ulceration

Corneal ulceration is a full thickness defect in the corneal epithelium. Its presence may be demonstrated by the use of topical fluorescein and the depth assessed by examination with the aid of magnification. Corneal ulcers cause pain and, if progressive, lead to corneal perforation.

Ulcers may result from mechanical trauma, chemicals, infections or exposure (e.g. following ketamine anaesthesia without application of a protective ointment to the cornea). Secondary bacterial infection can lead to a deepening of the ulcer. Herpesvirus infection in young cats can cause deep ulceration, whereas in adult cats it causes a superficial branching type known as a dendritic ulcer (most readily demonstrated by Rose Bengal staining). Herpesvirus associated ulcers are treated with antiviral drugs. Most corneal ulcers and abrasions heal rapidly, but in some cases third eyelid flaps or even conjunctival flaps may be required.

Eosinophilic keratoconjunctivitis

This is characterised by a proliferative lesion, often bilateral, affecting the superficial cornea and adjacent conjunctiva. The lesions are pink, vascularised and typically have an adherent white exudate, often described as like cottage cheese in appearance (Fig. 20.4). Eosinophils or eosinophilic material is seen within scrapings from the lesions.

The condition responds extremely well to mego-estrol acetate therapy. To avoid the possible side effects of this drug, however, topical corticosteroids should be the first line therapy, although they are usually less effective.

Corneal sequestrum or cornea nigrum

Corneal sequestrum or cornea nigrum is a unique feline condition of unknown aetiology in which there is necrosis of the corneal stroma, which takes on a black or brown appearance (melanin is not involved). In the UK, colour point cats are most commonly affected. The lesion starts as a painless brown discoloration of the central corneal stroma. This progresses to a dense black superficial plaque which often induces corneal vascularisation and can cause pain (Fig. 20.5). The epithelium may or may not remain intact. After several months the sequestrum often sloughs spontaneously. If the lesion is painful, superficial keratectomy should be performed to remove it, but this is a specialist procedure. When the lesion sloughs or is excised, a deep defect can result and the support of a third eyelid flap may be required.

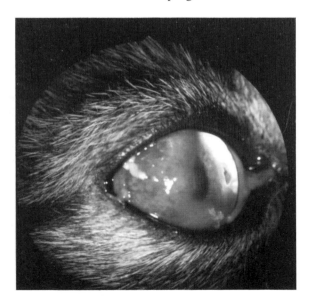

FIG. 20.4 Eosinophilic keratoconjunctivitis. Dense inflammatory tissue is invading the cornea and there is a whitish exudate on the surface.

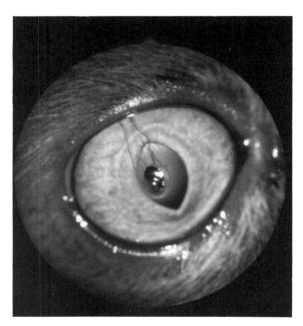

FIG. 20.5 Cornea nigrum. A black necrotic plaque is present in the superficial cornea and there are prominent new blood vessels approaching from the 12 o'clock area.

THE ANTERIOR CHAMBER AND ANTERIOR UVEA

The anterior portion of the uveal tract consists of the iris and ciliary body.

Congenital conditions

Persistent pupillary membranes (PPMs)

These are remnants of uveal vascular tissue present within the anterior chamber during embryological development, which normally regress completely within the first three weeks of life. PPMs originate from the anterior surface of the iris in the region of the minor arterial circle and may attach to another portion of the iris or the anterior lens capsule (associated with a focal cataract) or the posterior surface of the cornea (associated with corneal opacity). Treatment is not usually necessary.

Iris cysts

These hollow, roughly spherical structures are often darkly pigmented. They originate from the posterior surface of the iris and appear around the pupil or occasionally break away to float freely in the anterior chamber. Their spherical shape and the fact that they can be transilluminated helps distinguish them from neoplasms.

Acquired conditions

Anterior uveitis

Anterior uveitis is inflammation of the iris and ciliary body and is one of the most important conditions in feline ophthalmology, firstly because it is relatively common and secondly because it may be a sign (and sometimes the most obvious or only sign) of systemic disease.

Clinical signs

The clinical appearance of anterior uveitis is very variable. The condition may be mild or severe, acute or chronic, active or quiescent, and this variability determines the individual manifestation. There may also be accompanying posterior uveitis, manifest as focal or generalised chorioretinitis, retinal detachment or haemorrhage. These posterior signs may be obscured by opacity in the anterior segment or they may predominate with relatively mild anterior signs.

Pain The degree of discomfort varies.
Aqueous flare The inflammation results in leakage of protein and cells into the aqueous (aqueous flare). This may be detected by shining a sharply focused beam of light across the anterior chamber.
Keratic precipitates are accumulations of inflammatory cells and exudate on the posterior cornea. Usually they are situated ventrally and may be obscured from view by the lower and third eyelids. They vary from punctate opacities to larger yellow fatty-looking deposits ('mutton fat' precipitates) or even a generalised film covering a large area of the ventral posterior cornea. Focal precipitates may be very persistent and will darken with time.
Hypopyon is the accumulation of inflammatory cells in the anterior chamber, usually ventrally. The appearance may be modified by the presence of fibrin, leading to the formation of an irregular clot, or erythrocytes giving a brown or reddish appearance (Fig. 20.6). Haemorrhage may occur.

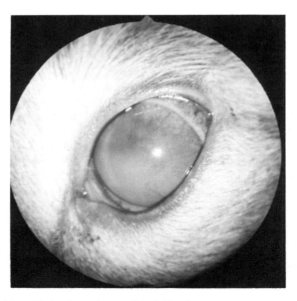

FIG. 20.6 Anterior uveitis following trauma. Most of the anterior chamber is filled with a fibrino-purulent exudate. The visible iris is inflamed and there is redness of the conjunctiva.

Miosis Inflammatory mediators cause contraction of the iris sphincter muscle resulting in a constricted pupil.

Synechiae are adhesions of the iris. Iris-lens adhesions are posterior synechiae and iris-cornea adhesions are anterior synechiae. Miosis increases iris-lens contact, favouring the formation of posterior synechiae. Where the adhesions are focal, they give rise to an irregular pupil which may be more obvious after mydriatic administration.

Iris rests are deposits of posterior iris pigment on the anterior lens following rupture of synechiae. They are permanent and remain as indicators of past uveitis.

Rubeosis iridis is the abnormal presence of prominent blood vessels on the anterior iris. These may be genuine new vessels or congested existing vessels.

Iris nodules are focal accumulations of inflammatory cells in the iris stroma appearing as dull, grey, slightly raised, circular areas.

Chronic changes may include: iris atrophy, which is recognisable as a darker, thinner translucent iris; cataracts (focal or extensive); glaucoma, due to the accumulation of inflammatory material and cells within the aqueous drainage pathways or extensive posterior synechiae, preventing the passage of aqueous through the pupil and resulting in an anterior bulging of the iris (iris bombé).

Aetiology

The following are recognised causes of uveitis. More complete details of general clinical signs, diagnosis and treatment are found in Chapter 23.

Feline Leukaemia Virus (FeLV) may cause anterior or posterior uveitis or the growth of solid masses in the anterior uvea. Retinal haemorrhage and degeneration may also occur if the FeLV infection causes a severe anaemia. Ocular lesions may be the most obvious presenting sign of FeLV in some cases although there will usually be other signs such as lymphomegaly. A recent study suggested that FeLV was not a major cause of ocular disease, other than via the secondary effects of severe anaemia.[2]

Feline Infectious Peritonitis (FIP) manifests variable ocular lesions. There may be a typical anterior uveitis, sometimes with a prominent reddish fibrinous clot in the anterior chamber, or posterior lesions with retinal vasculitis, haemorrhages or detachment and optic neuritis. When retinal detachment is extensive, the appearance may resemble that seen in hypertension.

Feline Immunodeficiency Virus (FIV) manifests most commonly as anterior uveitis, but inflammation of the pars plana and posterior changes have also been seen.

Toxoplasmosis typically causes chorioretinitis with localised inflammation and possibly detachment, but it can also cause anterior uveitis.

Systemic fungal infections usually cause posterior uveitis with areas of swollen discoloured retina, possibly with detachment and haemorrhage. Cryptococcus is the most common agent in endemic areas. These infections are very rare in the UK.

Idiopathic and other causes of uveitis include septicaemia/bacteraemia, ocular trauma, and deep corneal ulcers. A recent survey found that the aetiology remained obscure in 70% of cases despite full investigation.[4] Several immunopathological mechanisms have been incriminated but these are difficult to demonstrate in the individual case.

Diagnosis

All cats with anterior uveitis should receive, in addition to an ocular examination, a full clinical examination. Where there is no obvious cause of the uveitis, tests for FeLV, FIP, FIV and toxoplasmosis should be carried out as well as haematology and biochemistry. Confirmation of cryptococcosis is by demonstrating the organism in aspirates or tissues.

Management

Non-specific therapy for anterior uveitis consists of anti-inflammatory medication, topically and often systemically, and mydriatics. Topical corticosteroids should be used at a frequency of 4–6 times daily initially, reducing gradually over a period of weeks or according to response. Corticosteroids which are reasonably potent and have good corneal penetration should be chosen (e.g. prednisolone acetate, dexamethasone phosphate). Mydriatics relieve the pain of ciliary muscle spasm and dilate the pupil, thereby decreasing the area of iris-lens contact and reducing the risk of synechiae formation. Atropine 1% is used to produce a reasonably dilated but not maximal pupil. Initially it is applied 2–4 times daily. Topical atropine can have a systemic effect in small patients. Cats dislike the bitter taste of atropine, and ointment is better tolerated than drops.

Other acquired conditions

Neoplasia

Lymphosarcoma has been mentioned previously. Other anterior uveal tumours include melanomas (pigmented or non-pigmented, diffuse or nodular) (Fig. 20.7); adenomas and adenocarcinomas of the ciliary body; and secondary tumours. Most of the primary tumours of the uveal tract are malignant; therefore early enucleation should be considered and the prognosis is guarded. Enucleation with curative intent is not indicated for secondary tumours or where metastatic spread has already occurred.

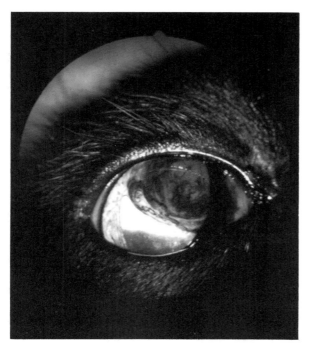

FIG. 20.7 Amelanotic melanoma in the dorso-medial iris of the right eye.

Hyphaema

Blood in the anterior chamber may result from trauma, uveitis, coagulopathies, or intraocular tumours. It may be associated with systemic disorders such as hypertension (e.g. due to cardiomyopathy, hyperthyroidism or chronic renal failure). The underlying cause should be identified and treated.

Glaucoma

Glaucoma is an elevation in intraocular pressure which is detrimental to the eye. In the cat, it most commonly occurs secondary to anterior uveitis or anterior uveal neoplasia. Primary glaucoma is not recognised. Anterior lens luxation occurs occasionally but the presence of the lens in the anterior chamber does not invariably cause a secondary glaucoma. Glaucoma often appears to cause remarkably little pain and affected individuals are often only presented once buphthalmos (and often marked vision loss) has developed. Occasionally congenital glaucoma occurs. The signs of glaucoma include congestion of conjunctival and episcleral vessels, dilated pupil (unless posterior synechiae and iris bombé are present), subluxation of the lens and buphthalmos. There are often only slight corneal changes. Treatment with carbonic anhydrase inhibitors (e.g. dichlorphenamide) may limit the rise in intraocular pressure but once the eye has become visibly enlarged, the prognosis for continued vision is poor.

LENS

Congenital conditions

Congenital lens malformations occur occasionally. Anterior capsular and subcapsular cataract may be associated with persistent pupillary membranes but other congenital cataracts are rarely encountered.

Acquired conditions

Cataract

Most cataracts develop secondary to penetrating wounds, blunt trauma or anterior uveitis.

Lens luxation and subluxation

Luxation of the lens results from rupture of its zonular attachments to the ciliary body. The luxated lens may move into the anterior chamber, or posteriorly into the vitreous. In subluxation, part of the zonule remains intact; the lens remains essentially in its normal plane but is displaced to one side, resulting in a gap or 'aphakic crescent' between the lens and pupil margin.

Luxation or subluxation of the lens can result from trauma or glaucoma, or can be associated with anterior uveitis or cataract formation. Primary lens luxation is not recognised in the cat but apparently spontaneous luxations are seen, particularly in older cats. Subluxated lenses and posteriorly luxated lenses do not require removal. Anterior luxations occasionally cause secondary glaucoma and should probably be removed.

POSTERIOR SEGMENT

Vitreous

A number of secondary vitreal changes can occur, e.g. chorioretinal disease may lead to the accumulation of inflammatory material or blood within the vitreous.

The choroid, retina and optic nerve

The normal feline fundus (Fig. 20.8).

The tapetum occupies roughly the dorsal half of the fundus and extends to just below the optic disc. It is typically a yellow-green colour but may be orange, red or occasionally blue. The optic disc is round and a grey-white colour. Retinal arteries and veins usually leave the edge of the disc in three main groups, with additional vessels in between. There may be a thin rim of pigment or hyper-reflectivity around the disc. The non-tapetal fundus is usually a dark grey-brown with retinal vessels visible on its surface. In white, cream or Siamese cats there may be a lack of pigment in the non-tapetal fundus exposing the choroid and its closely aligned, roughly parallel vessels. This gives a striped (tigroid) appearance. In more

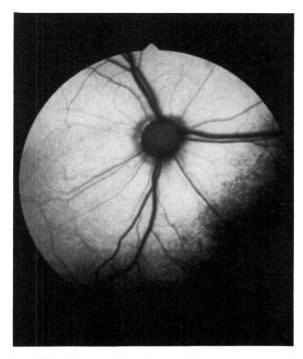

FIG. 20.8   Normal feline fundus. The tapetum extends well below the optic disc. The disc itself is typically circular with a slightly darker rim of retina. The arrangement of the blood vessels in three main groups, which do not anastomose, is also typical.

extreme cases, choroidal vessels may be exposed in the tapetum as red streaks or the tapetum may be absent and choroidal vessels visible over the entire fundus.

Congenital conditions

Retinal dysplasia

This is the most common congenital condition affecting the fundus. *In utero* infection with panleukopenia virus is a cause of retinal dysplasia. There may be large focal or multifocal areas of retinal degeneration across the tapetal and non-tapetal fundus. In the tapetal area these appear as sharply demarcated areas of increased reflectivity and colour change, whereas in the non-tapetal area, foci of pigmentary change are seen. Signs of cerebellar hypoplasia may also be present.

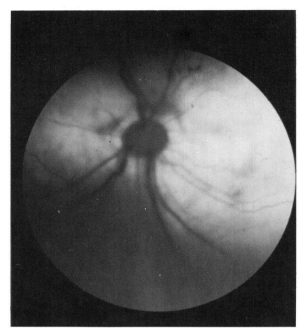

FIG. 20.9 Hypertensive retinopathy in an old cat with hyperthyroidism. There is exudate, haemorrhage and a shallow detachment above the optic disc. Below the disc there is a more extensive detachment with the retina appearing as a pale grey membrane.

Acquired conditions

Retinal haemorrhage

Retinal haemorrhage is often associated with systemic disease. It may be subretinal, intraretinal or vitreal. It may be caused by trauma, posterior uveitis, hypertension, coagulopathies, or severe anaemia (retinal blood vessels appear pale). Retinal detachment may also be present (Fig. 20.9). A full clinical and laboratory work-up of all cats with retinal haemorrhage should be performed.

Retinal detachments

Retinal detachments are often associated with systemic disease and frequently occur bilaterally. They may be accompanied by retinal and vitreal haemorrhages. The list of possible causes is similar to that for retinal haemorrhage. Re-attachment may occur if the underlying cause is treated successfully, although some retinal degeneration is likely.

Hypertension is the abnormal elevation of systemic blood pressure. Sustained hypertension damages the walls of aterioles resulting ultimately in vascular leakage and exudation, ischaemia and haemorrhage. When this occurs in the retinal and choroidal circulation the consequences are serious and the clinical signs may include irregularity in retinal blood vessels, grey areas of retinal exudation, retinal, vitreal and anterior chamber haemorrhage, retinal detachment and papilloedema. Early changes are not often seen as cats do not usually show visual deficits in the early stages. Most cats are seen, therefore, with advanced changes and many are presented because of sudden onset loss of vision. Hypertension is usually secondary in the cat and the two most common causes are chronic renal insufficiency and hyperthyroidism. Bilateral retinal haemorrhage and retinal detachment always suggests systemic disease and because of the range of possibilities comprehensive medical investigation is indicated. Where hypertension is diagnosed (or suspected on the basis of other findings) early in the course of the disease vigorous anti-hypertensive therapy may result in reattachment of the retina and partial restoration of vision. In the longstanding cases the prognosis for resolution of the retinal changes is guarded.

Retinal and choroidal inflammation (posterior uveitis)

Posterior uveitis may accompany anterior uveitis. Active lesions in the tapetal area have a dull, hazy appearance and the affected retina is oedematous. Active lesions in the non-tapetal area appear grey. There may be perivascular cuffing with or without retinal haemorrhage and detachment. Retinal and choroidal scars should be distinguished from active inflammation. Scars in the tapetal region are more clearly demarcated than active lesions. Tapetal hyper-reflectivity due to retinal thinning is readily detected, but note that hyper-reflective areas appear dull if the ophthalmoscope light is not perpendicular to the lesion because the light is not reflected directly back to the examiner. Affected areas of tapetum can undergo colour changes and pigment (melanin) deposition is often a feature. In the non-tapetal area, scars usually appear as areas of depigmentation with clumps of pigment within them. The aetiology of posterior uveitis is similar to that of anterior uveitis (see above). Treatment consists of identification and treatment of the cause, if possible, and symptomatic treatment with systemic corticosteroids.

Nutritional retinal degeneration

Cats fed on a low taurine diet (e.g. some commercial dog foods or inappropriate home-made diets) are at risk of developing feline central retinal degeneration (FCRD). The initial lesions are oval areas of hyper-reflectivity in the area centralis (the tapetal area dorso-lateral to the optic nerve head) of both eyes. As the condition progresses, a second lesion dorso-medial to the optic disc appears. The two areas eventually join to form a hyper-reflective band. Degeneration of the entire tapetal area may occur. Once the condition has been diagnosed, provision of adequate dietary taurine (e.g. reputable commercial cat food) will prevent further progression of the lesions.

Inherited retinal degeneration

Two forms of generalised progressive retinal atrophy (PRA) are known to occur in the Abyssinian cat. The first is a dominant early onset form which has a low incidence in the pet population. Early signs of retinal degeneration are visible at 8 weeks of age. The second form has a later onset and is inherited recessively. It has a high incidence in the pet population in Sweden but not in the UK. A late onset form may be present in the Siamese. Occasionally, a clinically similar condition of unknown aetiology may be seen in mixed breed cats (Fig. 20.10). The lesions of PRA are bilateral and symmetrical. Retinal thinning, resulting in the progressive development of tapetal hyper-reflectivity, is accompanied by attenuation of retinal blood vessels. Depigmentation and pigment clumping in the non-tapetal fundus develops as the condition progresses. In advanced cases there is extreme tapetal hyper-reflectivity and an apparent absence of retinal blood vessels. Pupillary light responses are reduced as the retinae degenerate. Secondary cataract formation is less common than in dogs with similar conditions.

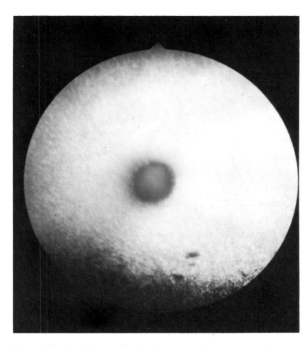

FIG. 20.10 Pan-retinal degeneration of unknown origin in a mixed breed cat. There is extreme hyper-reflectivity of the tapetum and attenuation of the retinal blood vessels (compare with the normal fundus in Fig. 20.8).

NEURO-OPHTHALMOLOGY

Anisocoria

Anisocoria is a difference in pupil size. It is one of the signs of Horner's syndrome. This syndrome is due to a lesion affecting the sympathetic nerve supply to the head, resulting in miosis, ptosis, third eyelid protrusion and enophthalmos. Lesions may occur at any site along the path of the sympathetic supply to the head (e.g. brachial plexus, musculature of the neck, middle ear cavity). Other causes of anisocoria include intraocular disease (glaucoma or uveitis), damage to the parasympathetic nerve supply to the iris, mid-brain lesions and lesions within the central visual pathways prior to the lateral geniculate nucleus. Cats with feline dysautonomia have dilated, poorly responsive pupils.

Nystagmus

Nystagmus is a spontaneous, rapid rhythmic movement of the eyes. Congenital nystagmus occurs in the Siamese. Affected animals have a fine, rapid, oscillatory nystagmus. Kittens with severe visual deficits may exhibit what is described as a 'searching' nystagmus. Nystagmus also results from peripheral and central vestibular disease and cerebellar disorders.

Lesions of the central visual pathways

The degree to which these affect vision depends on their extent and site. If lesions involve the optic nerves or optic tracts there will also be abnormalities of the pupillary light reflex. Lesions of the visual pathways central to the optic tracts spare the pupillary light reflex. Tumours such as lymphosarcoma are amongst the commoner causes of lesions of the central visual pathways. Central blindness (sometimes temporary) may occasionally occur following general anaesthesia if the patient has suffered a period of anoxia causing cerebral damage.

FURTHER READING

1. Barnett K.C., Ricketts J.D. (1985) The Eye. In: Chandler E.A., Gaskell C.J., Hilbery A.D.R. (eds) *Feline Medicine and Therapeutics*, pp 176–197. Blackwell Scientific Publications, Oxford.
2. Brightman A.H., Ogilvie G.K., Tompkins M. (1991) Ocular disease in FeLV-positive cats: 11 cases (1981–1986). *J. Am. Vet. Med. Ass.* **198**: 1049–1051.
3. Crispin S.M. (1987) Uveitis associated with systemic disease in cats. *Feline Practice* **17**: 16–24.
4. Davidson M.G., Nasisse M.P., English R.V., Wilcock B.P., Jamieson V.E. (1991) Feline anterior uveitis: A study of 53 cases. *J. Am. An. Hosp. Ass.* **27**: 77–83.
5. English R.V., Davidson M.G., Nasisse M.P., Jamieson V.E., Lappin M.R. (1990) Intraocular disease associated with feline immunodeficiency virus infection in cats. *J. Am. Vet. Med. Ass.* **196**: 1116–1119.
6. Martin C.L. (1981) Feline Ophthalmological Diseases. *Modern Veterinary Practice*.
   1. Diseases of the eyelids **62**: 865–870.
   2. Conjunctival diseases **62**: 929–933.
   3. The membrana nictitans and lacrimal apparatus **63**: 33–36.
   4. The cornea **63**: 115–122.
   5. The anterior chamber and glaucoma **63**: 209–213.
   6. The lens and anterior uvea **63**: 287–292.
   7. The choroid, retina and optic nerve **63**: 385–390.
   8. The globe and ocular neoplasm **63**: 449–452.
7. Nasisse M.P. (1991) Feline ophthalmology. In: Gelatt K.N. (ed.) *Veterinary Ophthalmology*, 2nd edn, pp 529–575. Lea and Febiger, Philadelphia.

21

Disorders of the Ear

CHRISTOPHER J.L. LITTLE

Aural disease is frequent in cats and a common reason for veterinary attention. Most of the conditions which commonly afflict the feline ear can be treated speedily and effectively provided the clinician has a thorough understanding of their causes and, from the outset, adopts a logical, diligent and careful approach to their diagnosis and management. Ancillary investigations will frequently contribute substantially to the problem-solving process. An ordered approach to the investigation of feline ear disease is presented in Fig. 21.1.

The ear is divided into three functional parts: external, middle and inner. The external ear consists of the pinna and the external auditory meatus (external ear canal). Diseases of clinical significance afflict the external ear much more frequently than the middle or inner ear.

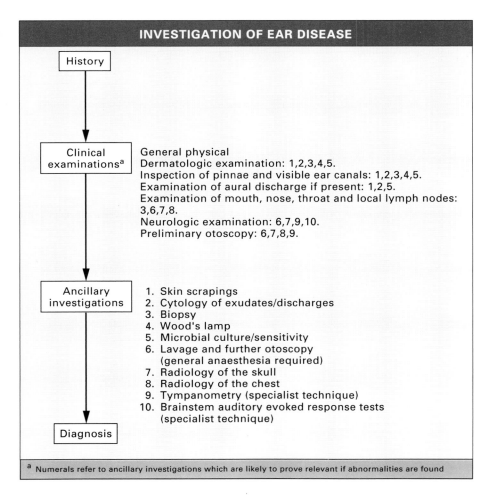

INVESTIGATION OF EAR DISEASE

History

Clinical examinations[a]

General physical
Dermatologic examination: 1,2,3,4,5.
Inspection of pinnae and visible ear canals: 1,2,3,4,5.
Examination of aural discharge if present: 1,2,5.
Examination of mouth, nose, throat and local lymph nodes: 3,6,7,8.
Neurologic examination: 6,7,9,10.
Preliminary otoscopy: 6,7,8,9.

Ancillary investigations

1. Skin scrapings
2. Cytology of exudates/discharges
3. Biopsy
4. Wood's lamp
5. Microbial culture/sensitivity
6. Lavage and further otoscopy (general anaesthesia required)
7. Radiology of the skull
8. Radiology of the chest
9. Tympanometry (specialist technique)
10. Brainstem auditory evoked response tests (specialist technique)

Diagnosis

[a] Numerals refer to ancillary investigations which are likely to prove relevant if abnormalities are found

FIG. 21.1 Investigation of ear disease in the cat.

DIFFERENTIAL DIAGNOSIS AND TREATMENT OF DISEASES MAINLY RESTRICTED TO THE FELINE PINNAE

Condition	Clinical findings	Diagnostic aids	Prevalence	Modes of treatment
Actinic dermatitis	Ear margin: Scaling Crusting Alopecia Ulceration Haemorrhage Distortion	Biopsy	Mainly white-eared cats. More common in sunny regions	Sharp surgery or cryosurgery Retinoids (see text)
Abscesses/ lacerations	Anorexia Dullness Pyrexia Haemorrhage Purulent discharge Swelling Lymphadenopathy (Also many other sites)	CBC	Common	Systemic antibiotics and surgical debridement and repair
Demodicosis[a]	Mild/moderate pruritus Pinnal alopecia Ceruminous otorrhoea (Also head, limbs or generalised)	Skin scraping Smear of otorrhoea	Uncommon	Topical miticides: pyrethrins or rotenone or amitraz or lime-sulphur
Dermatophytosis[b]	Pinnal alopecia Mild pruritus (Also head, limbs or generalised)	Wood's lamp Skin scraping Hair preparation	Common	May be self-limiting Griseofulvin or ketaconazole or topical imidazole
Frostbite	Ear tips: Pallor (initially) Erythema Scaling Distortion Necrosis (Also tail or scrotum)	-	Uncommon except in very cold regions	Bland protective ointments Cosmetic surgery Amputation
Haematoma	Sudden onset Fluctuant swelling of pinna	Otoscopy Full assessment of ear canals	Common Secondary to other ear diseases	Surgery
Idiopathic pinnal alopecia	Alopecia Slight scale	-	Common, especially Siamese	None
Notoedric mange[c]	Intense pruritus Alopecia Scaling Crusting Self-trauma (Also face, paws generalised)	Skin scraping	Rare in Europe Cluster outbreaks in North America	Rotenone or amitraz or ivermectin or lime-sulphur
Pemphigus foliaceus (PF) and Pemphigus erythematosus (PE)	Papules Crusting Scaling Alopecia	Impression smears Biopsy Immuno-histopathology	Uncommon	Gold salts or prednisolone + azathioprine or prednisolone + cyclophosphamide
Rabbit flea[d]	Pruritus Papules Nodules Excoriation Self-trauma	Close visual inspection of margins of pinnae	Common in Australia Recorded in Europe Hunting cats	None
Sarcoptic mange[e]	Intense pruritus Alopecia Papules Crusting Self-trauma Secondary pyoderma (Also elbows, back, chest, abdomen, hairless sites)	Numerous skin scrapings	Rare	As for Notoedric mange

continued

DIFFERENTIAL DIAGNOSIS AND TREATMENT OF DISEASES MAINLY RESTRICTED TO THE FELINE PINNAE				
Condition	**Clinical findings**	**Diagnostic aids**	**Prevalence**	**Modes of treatment**
Trombiculosis[f]	Alopecia Scaling Pustules Self-trauma	Visual inspection (Henry's pocket) Skin scraping	Common Seasonal Wooded regions	Self-limiting Pyrethrins or amitraz

[a] *Demodex cati* or unnamed *Demodex* species.
[b] *Microsporum canis, Trichophyton mentagrophytes*, occasionally other species.
[c] *Notoedres cati.*
[d] *Spilophyllus cuniculi*
[e] *Sarcoptes scabiei* var *canis*
[f] Numerous species including: *Trombicula (Eutrombicula) alfreddugesi* (North American chigger); *Trombicula (Neotrombicula) autumnalis.*

Therapeutic regimens are dealt with in detail in chapters 22 and 23.

FIG. 21.2   Differential diagnosis and treatment of diseases mainly restricted to the feline pinnae.

THE PINNA

A variety of diseases can present with lesions on the pinnae of cats. Lacerations and abscesses are probably the most frequent problems: they almost invariably result from fight wounds and are thus more common in entire males. Treatment with systemic antibiotics and surgical debridement offers an excellent prognosis. Reconstructive surgery to the pinna should not be attempted unless bacterial infection is under control.

Haematomas of the pinnae occur relatively frequently. They are associated with head-shaking and almost invariably indicate disease in the ear canal. The haematoma can be treated effectively by surgical means but thorough investigation and treatment of the underlying disease is also necessary if a satisfactory outcome is to be achieved.

Generalised and localised skin conditions may affect the pinnae. These include: actinic (solar) dermatitis, flea allergy, food allergy, trombicula infestation (chiggers), notoedric and sarcoptic mange, demodicosis, dermatophytosis, atopy, pemphigus foliaceus, pemphigus erythematosus, systemic lupus erythematosus and frostbite. In order to investigate these problems the veterinarian should follow the diagnostic protocols used elsewhere in dermatology. Actinic dermatitis is dealt with in more detail below.

Several rare congenital abnormalities of the pinnae have been reported in cats. These have included: complete absence, four ears, folded pinnae and non-symmetrical pinnae. Two forms of lysosomal storage disorder, mucopolysaccharidosis type I & VI, have been reported in this species; in each instance, presenting signs included small pinnae.

Fig. 21.2 details the differential diagnosis and treatment of some important conditions afflicting the feline pinnae.

Actinic dermatitis and squamous cell carcinoma of the pinna

Actinic (sunlight-induced) dermatitis frequently afflicts the ears tips of cats where the hair covering is thin. The lesions, which may be bilateral, are more common in white animals and those with white pinnae. The exact biologic behaviour of this condition is not understood. However the actinic lesion is precancerous, a precursor to squamous cell carcinoma, and the pathogenesis is thought to follow a similar course to bovine ocular squamous cell carcinoma.[8]

Hyperaemia of the tip and margins of the pinna is the earliest lesion which may be accompanied by scaling and oedema. Chronic localised dermatitis, with hair loss, ulceration and haemorrhage, occurs as the condition progresses; thickening and distortion of the pinna is frequent. Over a period of months or years the lesion may transform into an erosive squamous cell carcinoma. Such lesions are locally invasive. The regional lymph nodes may become involved late in the course of the disease but systemic metastasis is rare. Most animals with frank neoplasia are five years of age or older and the majority are male.[2,4]

Whenever this problem is suspected, evaluation of the patient must include careful palpation of the local lymph nodes. Lymph node biopsy or aspiration cytology and chest radiographs must also be considered. Sharp surgical excision is the treatment of choice for advanced actinic lesions and squamous cell carcinoma of the ear tip. To avoid recurrence, a margin of at least 5 mm of normal tissue should be removed; in this event prognosis is good. Histopathological assessment of the tissue is recommended. Cryosurgical management of the condition has also been attempted. Mild or early lesions are likely to progress unless steps are taken to reduce exposure to UV radiation from the sun. It may be practical to keep animals indoors during the day. The application of sunscreen cream to the pinnae has been widely recommended but most cats wash this off soon after it has been applied. Recently oral synthetic retinoids have been used in cats to treat these lesions, so far without success although trials are continuing.

THE EXTERNAL EAR CANAL

Ear mites: *Otodectes cynotis*

The psoroptid ear mite *Otodectes cynotis* is by far the commonest cause of otitis externa in the cat, accounting for 50–84% of cases.[12] Serological studies have shown that the overwhelming majority of cats have been exposed to this parasite, although only a proportion are infested at any one time. In clinical practice frank otitis associated with the presence of *Otodectes* is most frequently recognised in young cats.

The mite lives in the ear canal where it feeds on tissue fluids, including blood.[11] In response to the presence of the mite, there is an accumulation of cerumen, exfoliated skin debris and serum. This material forms a dark brown crust in the ear canal which is often said to resemble coffee grounds. Most of the mites live between the crust and the skin surface in a warm, moist environment protected from desiccation. The number of mites present in the ears of an afflicted cat varies. Moreover, the degree of aural irritation which

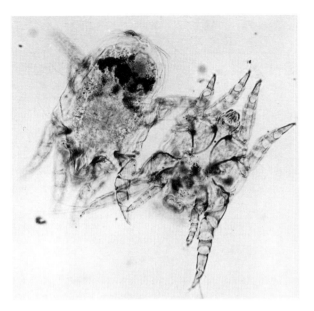

FIG. 21.3   Male and female adult ear mites *Otodectes cynotis*. In the female the fourth pair of legs is rudimentary.

this infestation provokes apparently bears little relationship to either the parasite burden or the amount of accumulated debris in the ear canals. A secondary bacterial infection may exacerbate otoacariasis.

The clinical signs typically associated with ear mite infestation include the presence of the characteristic crusty material in the ears, head shaking, and scratching of the ears with the hind feet; the claws are not sheathed during this action so that considerable excoriation of the ear canal and periaural tissues may ensue. Discomfort or aggression may be exhibited when the ears are examined; however, many cats harbouring ear mites show little sign of frank aural irritation or pain. Otoacariasis is virtually always bilateral. The presence of *Otodectes* can often be confirmed during otoscopic examination when the light-coloured mites may be seen moving against the dark-coloured background. Visual inspection of debris removed from the canals and placed on a dark surface may reveal the parasites crawling away (Fig. 21.3). A magnifying glass may be useful. Microscopic examination of mineral oil preparations of the cerumen is frequently not helpful.

Histological studies of affected cats have revealed epidermal and glandular hyperplasia in the integument of the ear canal together with an inflammatory infiltrate in the dermis. Mast cells and macrophages predominate although lymphocytes and plasma cells are also present. Neutrophils and eosinophils have not been observed in these tissues except where secondary bacterial infection has occurred. Hyperaemia and oedema of the tissues have also been recognised. Immediate and Arthus-type hypersensitivity reactions to mite antigens have been demonstrated in cats infested with *Otodectes* mites whereas delayed-type hypersensitivity has not been recognised.[11]

Otodectes cynotis is not host specific. The mite frequently affects dogs and may also cause lesions in people.[6] The life-cycle of the mite is completed in three to four weeks. Eggs are laid singly on the host. The larval stage is followed by protonymph and deutonymph stages before adulthood is attained. Adult mites live for about two months. The mites are not confined to the ears but may be found elsewhere on the body, especially the head, rump and paws.[12] Some controversy exists concerning the ability of *Otodectes* mites to survive in the environment but it seems clear that, when a cat is treated, normal cleaning of the home is all that is required to remove this reservoir of infestation.[6,12]

Most topical parasiticides are effective against Otodectes and it is wise to treat all cats and dogs in a household together because asymptomatic carrier animals are frequent. Treatment should aim to cleanse the ear canals of accumulated debris using mineral oil or a proprietary cerumenolytic, and kill the mites in the ears and elsewhere on the skin. Preparations for the ears combining mineral oil together with an acaricide are very effective; gamma BHC (lindane) has recently been withdrawn from use in the UK but rotenone may be used, although it must be employed with care in this species.[1] Proprietary ear drops containing pyrethroids, carbamates, or thiabendazole may also be used. The ears must be treated over a period of about three weeks to be effective. This may be because the mites are shielded from insecticide by debris, or the eggs are resistant to acaricides, or it may be due to the presence of wandering mites elsewhere on the body. In addi-

tion to local treatment, whole-body medication with an insecticide such as a pyrethroid is advisable. Oral cythionate has been used successfully to treat *Otodectes* infestation in fractious cats (1.5 mg/kg). Ivermectin (200–400µg/kg, as a single dose subcutaneously) and Amitraz (0.05% on the body, 0.5% diluted with 50% propylene glycol in the ear canals) have also been used with good results. Neither ivermectin nor Amitraz are licensed for use in cats.

Tumours of the external ear canal

Ceruminous gland tumours of the ear canal are relatively common in the cat. Many, perhaps the majority, are malignant. The tumours, which may be multiple, are usually bluish, pale pink or grey in colour and blister-like or pedunculated; they tend to occlude the lumen of the ear canal. The surface of these tumours is frequently ulcerated, predisposing to secondary bacterial infection. Unilateral haemorrhage or purulent otorrhoea accompanied by head shaking and scratching, are the usual presenting signs. Ceruminous gland tumours often arise in the horizontal portion of the canal close to the ear drum so that thorough otoscopic inspection of the ear may be necessary before the lesion is found. The condition afflicts older cats, aged seven years and upwards, predominantly males.

In the live animal, adenomas and adenocarcinomas of the ceruminous glands cannot be distinguished with accuracy from ceruminous gland hyperplasia. Histopathology of the tissue is the only sure way to reach a diagnosis. Malignant lesions may cross into the middle ear cavity or metastasise to involve the local lymph nodes; indeed these secondary tumour deposits can outgrow the primary lesion. A malignant ceruminous gland tumour should be suspected if an elderly cat is presented with a mass in the region of the parotid salivary gland or superficial cervical node. Ulceration or abscessation of this mass may occur. It can prove difficult to differentiate an anaplastic ceruminous gland tumour from a tumour of the parotid salivary gland even on histopathological grounds. Distant metastasis of ceruminous gland tumours can occur. In cases of doubt radiographs of the middle ear cavity and chest prove useful.

Other tumours have been reported in the feline ear canal, albeit rarely. Squamous cell carcinomas may spare the ear tips and affect the ear canal. There have also been sporadic reports of squamous papillomas, basal cell carcinomas, fibromas, melanomas and sebaceous gland tumours.[8] Occasionally an inflammatory polyp (see below) originating from the middle ear cavity is found in the external ear canal and may be mistaken for a tumour.

Wide surgical excision is the treatment of choice for tumours of the ear; in fact aural tumours are the most frequent indication for surgery to the feline ear canal. Access to the site of origin of the tumour is hampered by the anatomy of the ear so that in most instances a lateral wall resection or vertical canal ablation is a necessary part of this surgery. Prognosis is guarded. Where the middle ear cavity or other periaural tissues are involved, radical surgery is required if recurrence is to be avoided. Total ear canal ablation can be combined with bulla osteotomy and curettage of the middle ear cavity. However, surgery of this sort should not be undertaken unless the surgeon has a good working knowledge of the delicate anatomy of this region.[9]

Suppurative and mycotic otitis externa

Bacteria are not considered to be primary aetiological agents in feline otitis externa but may complicate the condition once it is established. Indeed it is reasonable to presume that virtually any lesion of the pinna or ear canal may predispose to secondary bacterial otitis. However, purulent otitis externa in the cat is usually unilateral and frequently results from one of three causes: a bite wound, an aural tumour, or a polyp which has arisen in the middle ear cavity. Where bilateral suppurative otitis externa occurs it most frequently arises as a result of self-inflicted trauma subsequent to severe otodectic mite infestation; in these circumstances the mites tend to evacuate the ear but are still likely to be present elsewhere in the coat.[12]

Where suppuration is present in the ear canal, systemic or local antibiotics are a useful part of the therapy irrespective of the primary cause.

The yeast *Malassezia pachydermatis* is often present in the ear canal of the healthy cat but is more frequent and more abundant in diseased ears. The exact contribution that this agent makes to otitis externa in this species is still uncertain. Treatment of the ears with antimycotic preparations is frequently advised but remains controversial.

THE MIDDLE EAR CAVITY

The middle ear cavity of the cat is divided into two compartments by an incomplete septum. The smaller compartment, which contains the auditory ossicles, lies dorsal and lateral to the larger compartment.[9] In addition to the three auditory ossicles found in other mammals the middle ear of the cat contains a conical cartilage, the precise function of which has not been established.

Inflammatory polyps

Inflammatory polyps are well known as a cause of aural disease in the cat. The condition, which usually occurs in young animals, is not uncommon. The pathogenesis is obscure and has provoked lively controversy. A review of this controversy has been published recently.[10]

The polyps are formed of granulation tissue rich in inflammatory cells and covered by an epithelium which is either stratified squamous or pseudo-stratified and ciliated. They originate in the dorsolateral compartment of the middle ear cavity and expand through the tympanic membrane to occupy the lumen of the ear canal. Secondary bacterial infection of the ear frequently occurs. Presenting signs are suggestive of unilateral otitis externa, typically otorrhoea and head shaking. Otoscopic examination should reveal the polyp. Radiographs of the head show evidence of middle ear disease.

Inflammatory polyps may also be found in the nasopharynx of young cats, emanating from the pharyngeal ostium of the Eustachian tube (Fig. 21.4). These lesions are indistinguishable from aural polyps on histological grounds. It seems certain that these masses also originate in the middle ear cavity; indeed polyps may be found in both the nasopharynx and ear canal concurrently. Cats with nasopharyngeal polyps typically have signs of upper respiratory obstruction such as nasal discharge, sneezing, stridor, dyspnoea, and

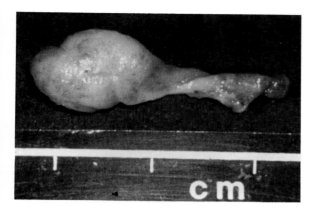

FIG. 21.4 A nasopharyngeal polyp from a cat. The pedicle emanated from the Eustachian tube.

dysphagia. Lateral radiographs of the nasopharynx and dorso-ventral or open-mouth views of the skull facilitate diagnosis but frequently the condition can be recognised from clinical signs and visual or digital inspection of the nasopharynx.

The treatment of both nasopharyngeal and aural polyps is straightforward. Both lesions may be removed successfully by traction under general anaesthesia. Endotracheal intubation is essential because of the dangers of airway obstruction. In animals with aural polyps, access to the mass will frequently be improved by performing a lateral wall resection to the ear. Access to nasopharyngeal polyps is made easy if the soft palate is reflected rostrally; rarely, it may be necessary to split the soft palate. Granulation tissue and thick mucus 'glue' is invariably present in the middle ear when either or both these polyps are found in a cat. Thus, ideally, ventral bulla osteotomy and curettage of both compartments of the ipsilateral middle ear cavity should be performed at the time the polyps are removed. Recurrence of the polyp(s) may frequently occur if this procedure is not performed.[5]

Otitis media

In a survey of post mortem material it was clearly established that otitis media is a common incidental finding in the cat,[7] and this has been confirmed by the author's observations. Inflammatory disease within the middle ear cavity may interfere with sound conduction through this region. However, in most cases where otitis media occurs it is likely to remain clinically silent unless the lesion extends to involve the external ear, inner ear, nasopharynx, or the nerves which pass through the middle ear cavity. Although there has been much written which implies that unrecognised otitis media is frequently responsible for chronic suppurative otorrhoea in both the cat and the dog, there is little firm evidence to support this allegation. The tympanic membrane of the cat, like that of other mammals, is resistant to rupture as a consequence of either otitis externa or otitis media and also heals rapidly following perforation. Thus, although inflammatory middle ear disease may be quite common in the cat, otitis media alone is very unlikely to be presented as a clinical problem to the practising veterinarian.

Tumours in the middle ear cavity

Tumours of the external ear canal may cross into the middle ear cavity, as already described. Squamous cell carcinoma of the middle ear has also been reported and may extend to involve the inner ear and other periaural tissues.

INNER EAR DISEASES

Deafness

Deafness is relatively rare in the cat and few aged or senile cats exhibit signs of it. However, it has long been recognised that a large proportion (around 20%) of white cats are deaf. Furthermore, blue-eyed white cats are more frequently deaf than yellow-eyed white cats. The condition, which is inherited as an autosomal dominant with incomplete penetrance, is due to cochleosaccular degeneration during the early post-natal period. Either unilateral or bilateral deafness may occur but in practice only those animals with bilateral deafness are likely to be presented for veterinary examination.

Deaf cats and kittens may be brought to the veterinarian because deafness is suspected or for apparent behavioural problems such as aggression or separation anxiety. The animal may be difficult to rouse from sleep but will be startled by touching. In practice, assessment of auditory function must usually rely on crude techniques but specialist assessment by brainstem auditory evoked potential testing is now practical and dependable. In view of the fact that deaf animals can be a danger to themselves and people, particularly on the roads, it may be wise to recommend that these animals are kept confined. This subject has been reviewed.[3]

Otitis interna

The most common cause of otitis interna or labyrinthitis is extension of otitis media to involve the structures of the inner ear housed in the petrous temporal bone. Clinical signs usually develop over a period of several days and will typically include head tilt, and leaning or stumbling to the affected side. The cat may circle towards this side. More rarely, horizontal nystagmus will be seen with the fast component directed away from the affected ear. Vomiting may be present and pyrexia should be expected. There may be pain around the tympanic bulla and when the jaw is opened. In some instances the submandibular lymph nodes will be enlarged or painful. Neuropathies such as facial nerve paralysis and Horner's syndrome confirm that the middle ear is involved, but are not found in the majority of cases. In many instances there will be evidence of otitis externa or a history suggestive of long-standing ear disease. Useful ancillary aids to confirm the diagnosis include: radiographs of the skull (Fig. 21.5), cytology and otoscopy of the external ear and a complete blood count. In some instances the condition extends to cause meningitis or a brain abscess. Where this occurs the clinical signs worsen progressively.

Conservative treatment of otitis interna is usually attempted with antibiotics such as chloramphenicol (50 mg/kg at eight-hour intervals). However, bactericidal antibiotics such as clavulanate-potentiated amoxicillin are likely to penetrate this site well when inflammation is present and can also be used. Concurrent corticosteroid therapy has been recommended but must be used with care. Prognosis is guarded. Where major soft-tissue and bony changes are recognised on skull radiographs, surgical exploration and debridement of the area is indicated but may be unrewarding.

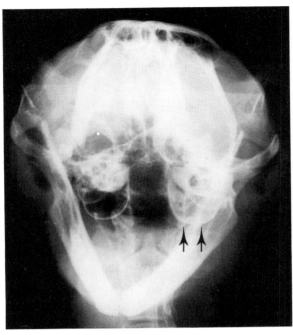

FIG. 21.5 Open-mouthed radiograph of a cat with unilateral (left) otitis externa, media and interna. Note the increased opacity of the affected middle ear (arrowed).

Feline peripheral vestibular syndrome

Labyrinthitis must be distinguished from idiopathic feline vestibular syndrome. This syndrome is common in cats and its onset is peracute. The vestibular signs in this disease tend to be more severe than those found in otitis interna. Systemic signs such as pyrexia are absent and there is no evidence of disease in the external ear, nasopharynx, middle ear cavity or the other nerves which pass through this region. Findings from ancillary tests such as radiography are normal. The cause of this condition is unknown but it rapidly improves without treatment, although a residual head tilt may remain for life.

REFERENCES

1. Chesney C.J. (1988) An unusual species of demodex mite in a cat. *Vet. Rec.* **123**, 671–673.
2. Cotchin E. (1961) Skin tumours of cats. *Res. Vet. Sci.* **2**, 353–361.
3. Delack J.B. (1984) Hereditary deafness in the white cat. *Compend. Contin. Educ. Pract. Vet.* **6**, 609–617.

4. Guaguere E., Guaguere-Lucas J. (1985) Pathologie tumorale de l'oreille des carnivores domestique. *Pratique medicale et chirurgicale de l'Anim. de Cie.* **20**, 87–93.

5. Kapatkin A.S., Matthiesen D.T., Noone K.E., Church E.M., Scavelli T.E., Patnai A.K. (1990). Results of surgery and long-term follow-up in 31 cats with nasopharyngeal polyps. *J. Am. Anim. Hosp. Ass.* **26**, 387–390.

6. Larkin A.D., Gaillard G.E. (1981) Mites in cats ears: A source of cross antigenicity with house dust mites. Preliminary report. *Ann. Allergy* **46**, 301–304.

7. Lawson D.D. (1957) Otitis media in the cat. *Vet Rec.* **69**, 643–647.

8. Legendre A.M., Krahwinkel D.J. (1981) Feline ear tumours. *J. Am. Anim. Hosp. Ass.* **17**, 1035–1037.

9. Little C.J.L., Lane J.G. (1986) The surgical anatomy of the feline bulla tympanica. *J. small Anim. Pract.* **27**, 371–378.

10. Pope E.R. (1989) Feline inflammatory polyps. *Companion Animal Practice* **19**, 33–35.

11. Powell M.B., Weisbroth S.H., Roth, L., Wilhelmsen C. (1980) Reaginic hypersensitivity in *Octodectes cynotis* infestation of cats and mode of mite feeding. *Am. J. Vet. Res.* **41**, 877–882.

12. Scott D.W. (1980) External ear disorders. *J. Am. Anim. Hosp. Ass.* **16**, 426–433.

FURTHER READING

Dorn R.C., Taylor D.O.N., Schneider R. (1971) Sunlight exposure and risk of developing cutaneous and oral squamous cell carcinoma in white cats. *J. Nat. Cancer Inst.* **46**, 1073–1078.

Evans A.G., Madewell B.R., Stannard A.A. (1985) A trial of 13-cis-retinoic acid for treatment of squamous cell carcinoma and paraneoplastic lesions of the head of cats. *Am. J. Vet. Res.* **46**, 2553–2557.

Gaag I. van der (1986) The pathology of the external ear canal in dogs and cats. *Veterinary Quarterly* **8**, 307–317.

Gibbs C. (1978) Radiological refresher 11: The head – part III: Ear disease. *J. small Anim. Pract.* **19**, 539–545.

Kirk B. (1990) Living with a deaf cat. *Bulletin of the Feline Advisory Bureau* **27**, 59.

Pearson G.R., Hart C.A. (1980) A case of otitis in a domestic cat. *J. small Anim. Pract.* **21**, 333–338.

Schneck G. (1988) Use of ivermectin against ear mites in cats. *Vet. Rec.* **123**, 599.

Scott D.W. (1984) Feline dermatology 1979–1982: Introspective retrospections. *J. Am. Anim. Hosp. Ass.* **20**, 537–564.

22

Disorders of the Skin

GAIL A. KUNKLE

A limited number of reaction patterns occur in the skin, and multiple symptoms are noted with each. This chapter takes a problem-solving approach to diseases of the skin, categorising them under five major problems:

1. Pruritus
2. Alopecia
3. Exudative, Crusting and Scaling Dermatitis
4. Erosive and Ulcerative Dermatitis
5. Nodules and Draining Tracts.

HISTORY

The history of the dermatological patient is of major importance in devising a list of differential diagnoses. Useful facts include how the lesion(s) started, what course it took, and prior response to any therapy. Are other animals or people in the household similarly affected? Do the owners perceive the patient to be pruritic or uncomfortable? Where does the cat live? What is its lifestyle and its diet? Are there any unusual details?

PHYSICAL EXAMINATION

A thorough general physical examination should be performed on all dermatological patients. It may be necessary to clip an area for optimum viewing of the cutaneous lesions. The ears, interdigital spaces, nail folds, mucocutaneous junctions and footpads should be examined as well as the haired skin. Peripheral lymph nodes should be palpated.

The examiner should note the presence or absence of primary cutaneous lesions and their location. If all lesions noted are secondary, the owner should be asked about the prior presence of pustules, bullae, vesicles or other primary eruptions. The degree of pruritus elicited by

CAUSES OF FELINE PODODERMATITIS
Bacterial
Paronychia
Fungal
Dermatophytosis
Sporotrichosis
Immune-mediated
Pemphigus foliaceus
Systemic lupus erythematosus
Plasma cell pododermatitis
Virus
Pox virus
Contact dermatitis
Parasitic
Notoedres
Ticks
Mosquito
Eosinophilic granuloma complex
Neoplasia
Metastatic bronchogenic carcinoma

FIG. 22.1   Causes of pododermatitis.

handling the cat during the physical examination should be noted. The distribution of lesions is very useful in narrowing the differential diagnoses (Figs 22.1 and 22.2).

PROBLEM AND DIFFERENTIAL DIAGNOSES

Once the history has been obtained and examination completed, the veterinarian can list the problems. By focusing on the major skin problem and referring to the figures in this chapter, a list of differential diagnoses can be developed. The clinical signs and history should enable the development of an abbreviated list of most likely differentials for the problem, and

CAUSES OF FELINE FACIAL DERMATOSES
Bacterial
Folliculitis Abscess Leprosy
Fungal
Dermatophytosis Sporotrichosis Cryptococcosis Mycetoma
Feline acne
Eosinophilic granuloma complex
Collagenolytic granuloma Indolent ulcer
Solar/actinic dermatosis/aquamous cell carcinoma
Parasite
Notoedres *Demodex* *Otodectes* Mosquito
Immune-mediated
Food allergy Pemphigus foliaceus/erythematosus Systemic lupus erythematosus
Viral
Herpes virus Calicivirus Pox virus
Drug eruption

FIG. 22.2   Causes of facial dermatoses.

diagnostic testing is then used as an aid in defining the disease.

DIAGNOSTIC AIDS

Skin scrapings

These are inexpensive and easy to perform, and they provide useful information. A skin scraping should be part of almost every dermatological case.

The hair should be clipped from the area. A dull, clean, No. 10 scalpel blade is used for the scraping, with a heavy grade, good quality mineral oil. Oil is placed on the skin and the slide. For deep skin scraping, the skin should be pinched and scraped until capillary oozing occurs. For superficial scrapings, the stratum corneum should be scraped. With a coverslip and 100X magnification, the entire slide should be examined under low lighting.

Direct examination of the hair and scales

This can be useful for identification of superficial fungi. A clearing agent such as 10–20% KOH can be used. At 400X magnification, hairs under the coverslip can be examined for arthrospores. As the spores are small, clear and somewhat refractile, this is not an easy diagnostic test and generally requires some prior experience.

Hair shafts can also be examined microscopically for morphology. The hairs should be plucked gently and laid in a small pool of mineral oil under the coverslip. The ends of the hairs, as well as the root and cuticle, can be evaluated.

Cytology

Cytology does not usually define the specific diagnosis but it can be very beneficial in suggesting the most likely path for pursuing diagnosis. It may also aid in the selection of therapeutic drugs while results of further diagnostic tests are pending.

Touch preparations of exudative lesions can be stained and examined microscopically for cell types and presence of organisms. An aspirate can be collected from intact primary lesions such as pustules or vesicles, and nodules can also be aspirated. A thin monolayer of cells or organic material is ideal on the slide.

A variety of stains can be used for cutaneous cytology. Wright's stain is useful for cell morphology. Gram stains are helpful in categorising and roughly quantifying pathogens. For wet mounts of exudate, new methylene blue is commonly selected. Various stains are available for fungi and for examination of tissues for acid-fast organisms.

Biopsy

Most cutaneous biopsies can be collected with the aid of a local anaesthetic agent, carefully introduced subcutaneously beneath the lesion. However, general anaesthesia is usually necessary if the head, ears, feet or mucous membranes require biopsy. In fractious cats, sedation may be required for other biopsies and even cytology in certain cases.

The lesion or area to be biopsied should not be scrubbed to remove scales or crust unless the biopsy is to be used for culture. Small lesions are biopsied with disposable biopsy punches, that are available in 4mm and 6mm diameter. Larger lesions should be excised completely or a wedge-shaped sample should be removed. It is often useful to allow small biopsies to dry on a piece of cardboard or tongue depressor before placing them in 10% buffered formalin, in order to prevent thin lesions from curling. If a biopsy is to be collected for culture, the site should be surgically scrubbed first. The sample may be divided, half for culture and half for histopathological examination.

The success of histopathological assessment depends on two important choices: careful selection of the biopsy site (collecting primary lesions whenever possible) and the crucially important selection of a veterinary pathologist with expertise in dermatology.

Intradermal skin testing

For this technique, very small amounts of dilute antigen preparations are injected intradermally. Antigens and dilutions useful for dogs have also been used successfully in cats.

Culture

Cultures are frequently necessary to aid diagnosis and treatment in feline dermatology. The tests are often expensive and require significant forethought. When possible, antimicrobial drugs should be withheld for 48 to 72 hours before materials are collected for culture. If a biopsy is used for culture, the tissue should be removed aseptically, placed in a sterile container and the biopsy kept moist and cool while it is being transported to the laboratory.

Routine microbiology laboratories are useful for common bacterial and fungal pathogen identification. For uncommon pathogens, specific techniques may be required and it is always best to check with the laboratory first.

Haematology and serology

In some cases, haematological and serological evaluations can be helpful in identifying the disease or aiding the selection of the appropriate therapeutic agent.

PRURITUS

Pruritus or itching is defined as 'an unpleasant cutaneous sensation that provokes the desire to scratch or rub the skin'. In most species this condition results in self-trauma to the skin. In the cat, perhaps due to behavioural differences, self-trauma to the haircoat or skin may occur. In fact, symmetrical hair loss may be the only presenting complaint. Whereas the dog often excoriates itself with scratching, the cat tends to groom and bite

CAUSES OF PRURITUS
Allergy
Food allergy Flea allergy Atopy Intestinal parasitism
Ectoparasites
Cheyletiella *Notoedres* *Otodectes* *Trombicula* Pediculosis
Infectious
Bacterial Fungal Viral
Miliary dermatitis
Allergy Ectoparasites Infectious
Eosinophilic granuloma complex (EGC)
Eosinophilic plaque Collagenolytic granuloma
Contact dermatitis (allergic or irritant)
Drug eruption
Systemic disease/neoplasia
Autoimmune disease
Pemphigus foliaceus/erythematosus Systemic lupus erythematosus

FIG. 22.3 Causes of pruritus.

in response to the itch sensation, as well as scratch. Scratching that results in obvious damage to the skin occurs in the cat only in more severe cases of itch.

The clinical signs of pruritus may be localised or generalised. The condition may be sporadic or continual, seasonal or non-seasonal. A cat with pruritus may present with alopecia, or be crusty, scabby, exudative, or ulcerated. Signs vary markedly with the cause of the pruritus. There may or may not be primary cutaneous lesions (see Figs 22.3, 22.4 and 22.5).

Allergy

The hallmark of allergy is pruritus.

Food allergy

Clinical signs

The cutaneous lesions of food allergy comprise all forms of self-trauma, including excoriations, lesions induced by licking and broken stubbly hairs secondary to excessive grooming. Licking, rubbing and scratching are the major clinical signs but removal of hair by pulling with the lips and teeth is seen occasionally.

Miliary dermatitis (see p. 336) with papules, crust and scabs may be the primary presentation. Head and neck lesions predominate in some cats with food allergies but not all signs of head and neck pruritus are due to food allergy. In other cats symmetrical self-induced hair loss is the major sign.

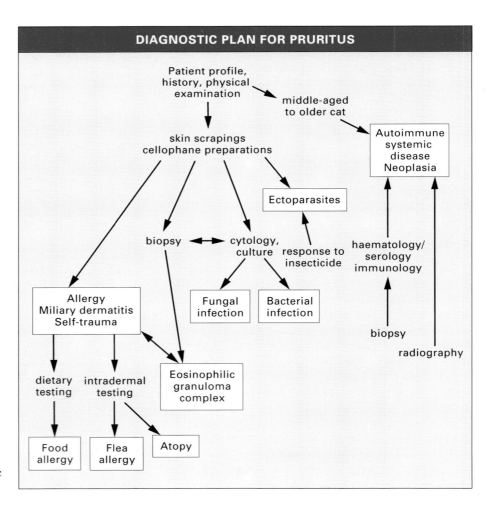

FIG. 22.4 Diagnostic plan for pruritus.

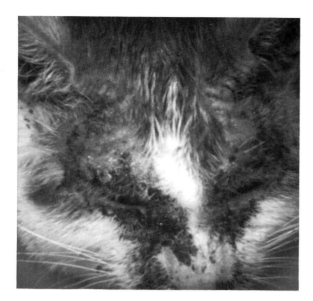

FIG. 22.5 This middle-aged neutered male cat has severely excoriated his face due to severe pruritus.

Signs of food allergy can occur at any age, and can be seen in young cats. Concurrent gastrointestinal signs are not noted in all cases. There is usually no history of recent change in diet (food allergy usually occurs after chronic exposure). Although food allergy is generally considered to be a perennial disease, signs may be sporadic because of the client's rotation of a variety of diets to feline pets. The history often includes a poor response to steroids.

Diagnosis

Intradermal skin testing with food allergens is inconsistent and unreliable as a method of diagnosis. The standard method of diagnosis uses an assessent of response to a restricted (hypoallergenic) diet, with confirmation by exacerbation of symptoms with provocative challenge with the original diet. The components of the restricted diet vary with geographical location, prior exposure to proteins, and availability, as well as owner and patient acceptance. A home-cooked diet with one carbohydrate and one protein source is ideal, as it eliminates the consideration of metal from the can and the constituents of prepared pet foods. A home-cooked diet aids in assessing food intolerances which may not be immunologically mediated, as well as restricting the food intake to one protein. In the cat, this protein is generally lamb, rabbit, chicken, egg or horsemeat. Fish and milk are probably best avoided as they seem to be over-represented as allergens responsible for cutaneous signs in the cat.

If there is more than one cat in the household it may be necessary to feed all of them the restricted diet to prevent the affected cat from eating other cat food. All treats should be discontinued.

The length of time a restricted diet should be fed is controversial. Most concur that a change in diet does not effect a rapid improvement. Generally, after 3–4 weeks, there should be notable improvement, with decrease in clinical signs. The diet can then be extended for an additional month or longer before attempting provocation. Owner compliance with a restricted diet after one month with no improvement in clinical signs is generally poor, so the number that would actually improve with longer diet trials has not been well defined.

If the pruritus is severe, an Elizabethan collar or some other mechanical barrier may be necessary for the first few weeks of the diet trial. In other cats, a short course of oral steroids or antihistamines may be useful in decreasing the severity of symptoms temporarily. Fatty acid supplements containing fish oils should not be given concurrently during a restricted diet trial for suspected food allergy.

Once a tentative diagnosis of food-responsive dermatosis has been made, the suspected food should be introduced as a provocation. The signs generally recur within 24 hours but in a few cases a gradual increase in signs may be noted over 5–7 days. A positive provocation test does not truly define that the food reaction is an allergic one, because current methodologies cannot confirm that this reaction is mediated immunologically. A positive provocation may occur with either true food hypersensitivity or food intolerance. For the patient's sake, defining the mechanism is not important: avoiding the offending food is the key to management.

Treatment

Medical management is generally not effective for long-term control of the food-sensitive cat.

Identification and avoidance of the offending foods is the ideal long-term treatment. In many cases, only certain types of commercial foods will be unacceptable and the specific substances inducing the signs will not be identified. In some cases a commercial balanced food can be identified that does not result in clinical signs; in others the cat may need to be fed a home-cooked diet indefinitely. Attempts should be made to balance the diet, perhaps with the advice of nutritional consultants from pet food companies.

In some diet-responsive patients, signs may reoccur after long-term control. It is possible for cats to become sensitised to their new diet and another restricted diet trial and challenge test may be warranted.

The prognosis for the food-sensitive cat is guarded. In most cases, diet manipulation is extremely rewarding. However, in a few instances cases can be difficult to manage in the long term, even with the most compliant clients. Subsequent diet changes or the use of an Elizabethan collar may be required to break the itch-scratch cycle.

Atopy

Although IgE has not been well-characterised in the cat to date, cats have been shown to have immediate intradermal skin test reactions to allergens that can be transferred to normal cats by serum. This is strong evidence for IgE mediated hypersensitivity in the cat. Several dermatologists have noted an association of positive antigen skin test reactions with clinical signs of pruritus in the cat and it is currently assumed that feline atopy mimics the pathomechanism of canine atopy.

Clinical signs

Feline atopic disease has not yet been characterised totally. Pruritus is the hallmark and primary lesions may or may not be present. Signs vary and include lesions of miliary dermatitis, self-induced symmetrical hair-loss, excoriations, broken hairs, crusts, scabs, and eosinophilic plaque lesions. Age, breed and other aspects are not well delineated. Signs may be seasonal or perennial. Usually there is a history of early response to corticosteroids.

Diagnosis

The diagnostic test of choice is intradermal skin testing. The same antigen concentrations that are used for the dog seem to be useful in diagnosis in the cat. The cat can be restrained minimally or a cat bag can be used. Ketamine hydrochloride has not been noted to cause obvious interference with skin testing. Interpreting the skin test in the cat is more difficult as positive wheal and flare reactions are not marked as in other species. Erythema is an uncommon factor and palpation plays a major role in evaluation of intradermal reactions.

An *in vitro* feline allergy test has recently been made available. No objective information is available yet on its usefulness for identifying and treating the suspect atopic cat. *In vitro* tests for dogs are not useful for diagnosis, as anti-feline IgE antibody must be used for the cat.

Treatment

Corticosteroid therapy in the cat is very useful and more practical for long-term management because cats tolerate glucocorticoids much better with fewer side effects than other species. Oral prednisone or prednisolone are preferable in cats where they are effective and owners can manage the daily or alternate day administration. Oral steroids also allow more careful management of the dose and reduction with improvement of clinical signs. Injectable methylprednisolone acetate is quite useful in most patients as long as the owner and veterinarian are aware that side effects may occur. There is wide variation in the side effects which may be noted with the same dosage of injectable steroid in different cats of the same size.

Antihistamine therapy is of benefit in some feline cases. Oral chlorpheniramine at 2–4 mg per cat bid will control clinical signs indefinitely in some cats.

Immunotherapy has been used in a small number of cats with reports of success varying from 50% to 100%.

Intestinal parasitism

Intestinal parasitism may occasionally result in pruritus, presumed to be mediated by IgE. Cats with generalised pruritus should be assessed for endoparasitism and treated if parasites are identified. This is a very rare cause of pruritus.

Ectoparasitism

Cheyletiella

Three species of *Cheyletiella* mites are known to infest the cat; *C. blakei* is the most common. The mites move about rapidly on the skin and have characteristic biting mouthparts that pierce the skin periodically. They are known to live off the animal for many days. Transmission may occur by direct contact, by fomites, or via other parasites such as fleas.

Clinical signs

The signs are extremely varied, even from cat to cat infected similarly in the same household. The most common presentation is that of noticeable dandruff with or without pruritus. Papules, crusts and generalised miliary dermatitis are seen in another presentation. Alopecia which is self-induced by excessive grooming can also be seen. Finally, some cats are asymptomatic, even with moderate infestations.

Young animals, especially those from kennels or pet shops, seem to be at high risk, and long-haired cats seem to be over-represented. There may be a history of onset of signs in relationship to acquisition of a new animal even if it is asymptomatic.

Occasionally, in-contact humans may be affected.

Diagnosis

The diagnosis of *Cheyletiella* infection is made by microscopic identification of the mite from superficial skin scraping or transparent adhesive tape collections. A fine-toothed comb can be useful in assessing a patient for the 'walking dandruff' mite. A large magnifying lens can be helpful in visualising the mites. In difficult cases, where mites are suspected but not identified, an extensive brushing and modified flotation technique sometimes allow definitive diagnosis.

Treatment

For adequate therapy, a parasiticidal shampoo (such as one containing pyrethrin) must be used weekly for 4–6 weeks on all in-contact pets. Dips and powders may also be effective: the active agent is not as important as repeated and thorough treatment. It is very important to treat the environment as well, by insecticidal fogging, spraying and vacuuming. Ivermectin (which is not licensed for use in the cat) has been used successfully to treat this condition in cats at 200 μg/kg body-weight SC.

Notoedres cati

This is the sarcoptid mite of the cat. It is smaller than the canine mite, and has a dorsal anus. Generally these mites are easier to find in scrapings than *Sarcoptes* sp. in the dog. The life cycle is spent entirely on the cat and the mite is highly contagious. The disease is rare.

Clinical signs

This mite causes pruritic head mange of cats. The lesions are usually noted around the ears and preauricular area, spreading to the head and neck. The perineum may be affected as well as the feet. Crusting and erythema are generally marked and pruritus with self-trauma is generally severe. Peripheral lymphadenopathy is common. The condition seems to be endemic in certain geographical areas and can affect large numbers of cats and kittens housed together.

Diagnosis

Mites are generally easily identified in skin scrapings from lesions.

Treatment

Gentle bathing to remove crusts and scale should precede treatment with a parasiticidal dip such as 2% lime sulphur. This is repeated every 5–7 days for 4–6 weeks. All in-contact cats should be treated and the environment should be thoroughly vacuumed. Neither amitraz nor ivermectin have been approved for use in the cat but amitraz dips have been used by some (toxicity is variable) and ivermectin has been used successfully at 100 µg/kg SC.

Otodectes

Otodectes cynotis most commonly causes otitis externa but occasionally cats will develop cutaneous lesions. It is a rare cause of dermatitis.

Clinical signs

Lesions are noted on the head and neck first and consist of signs of self-trauma as well as erythema, crusting and scaling. Pruritus is generally marked. Miliary dermatitis has also been attributed to *Otodectes* sp in rare instances.

Diagnosis

Diagnosis is made by finding the mite on superficial skin scrapings from affected areas.

Treatment

Most parasiticidal therapy will effectively kill these mites. Ears should be treated concurrently even if no mites are noted in the external ear canal. All dogs and cats in the household should be treated with parasiticides. Ivermectin (not licensed for the cat) has also been used effectively at 200 µg/kg body-weight SC, repeated after 3 weeks.

Trombicula autumnalis

This is the harvest mite or chigger and there are several species that may cause problems in outdoor cats, depending on the geographical location. The adult mite lives in decaying vegetation, fields and woods, with a presumed natural host of small rodents. The parasitic larvae emerge in late summer and autumn and may infest a variety of animals, including man.

Clinical signs

There may be intense pruritus on the edges of the pinnae, eyelids, feet and abdomen in some cats. In other animals there may be minimal pruritus and more crusting. The mites are easily identified as bright orange-red dots adhering tightly to the skin, where they may remain for up to 2 weeks.

Diagnosis

The visualisation of the mites as tiny orange bugs usually allows a tentative diagnosis. With gentle scraping, they can be collected and examined microscopically.

Treatment

Shampoo or dip with a parasiticide which is safe for the cat is usually effective. Treatment may be repeated if necessary. The important part of therapy is to prevent recurrence by restricting the cat from fields and woods during the parasite season.

Pediculosis

Lice are host-specific; the common feline louse is *Felicola subrostratus*, which is a biting louse. The life cycle is completed entirely on the host.

Clinical signs

Signs are highly variable. There may be pruritus as severe as that seen in flea allergy or miliary dermatitis; or there may be mild seborrhea or only mild pruritus or no lesions at all. Secondary lesions of self-trauma may be apparent if pruritus is severe.

Diagnosis

Diagnosis is by identification of the louse or its eggs on the skin and haircoat. A hand-held magnifying lens can be beneficial in searching the coat.

Treatment

Treatment generally consists of insecticidal shampoos repeated at intervals of 7–10 days. All pets should be treated and assessed for underlying disease or poor environmental husbandry.

Bacterial, fungal and viral infections

Pruritus may be mild to moderate in the case of bacterial infections but the major clinical signs, which may be focal or generalised, are usually crusting, scaling and exudative (see p. 334).

Intermediate and deep fungal infections are not usually pruritic; nor is dermatophytosis (see p. 335) except in young kittens and occasionally in an adult. More crusting and scaling are noted clinically if there is significant pruritus.

Cowpox virus infections commonly have pruritus as a feature. Infection is manifested as papular, ulcerated and scabbed lesions at the site of trauma, usually the head, neck or limbs, and they may progress to involve the entire body. This virus is discussed in detail on p. 343.

Eosinophilic granuloma complex (EGC)

Eosinophilic plaque

Eosinophilic plaque is the form of eosinophilic granuloma complex that is intensely pruritic in almost all cases. Its aetiology is most likely to be allergic, and cats with these lesions should be examined for an allergic disorder.

Clinical signs

Eosinophilic plaques are raised, usually well demarcated, roughened, glistening, erythematous lesions that are generally so pruritic that simply manipulating them will trigger rapid tongue movements in affected individuals. Lesions are found commonly on the ventral abdomen or other areas of the trunk. They may be focal and localised to one area; they may be multifocal and scattered over the body; or in rare instances they may become generalised. Pruritus is intense and the lesions are usually moist. Tissue and circulating eosinophilia are both frequent features. Associated peripheral lymphadenopathy is common.

Diagnosis

Diagnosis is by the clinical appearance of the lesion(s) supported by a finding of eosinophilia. Biopsies reveal a spongiotic epidermis with a perivascular eosinophilic dermatitis; these can be useful to rule out other differentials such as neoplasia. Because hypersensitivity has been identified as a responsible aetiological agent in many cases of eosinophilic plaque, allergies should be considered as potential underlying causes.

Treatment

Glucocorticoids are generally the most useful for the immediate relief of clinical signs of eosinophilic plaque. Interruption of the itch-scratch-lick cycle is important and trauma seems to play a role in the worsening of this lesion.

In lesions that are recurrent or multi-focal, an allergic aetiology (flea allergy, food allergy, or atopy) should be pursued. In severe, generalised cases of eosinophilic plaque, long term control of the patient can become quite frustrating. Some of these cats have very extensive circulating eosinophilia in conjunction with their skin lesions which may become resistant to the effects of systemic steroids.

Collagenolytic granuloma (linear form)

The linear form of the granuloma with collagen necrosis can sometimes be intensely pruritic. This lesion is asymptomatic in many cats.

Clinical signs

The linear form of the collagenolytic granuloma is usually noted as a firm, well-demarcated white to yellow-pink band of tissue extending down the caudal thigh(s) and occasionally noted in the axilla or on the trunk. In young kittens these are not usually a major problem but in some instances pruritus and self-trauma will become severe.

Diagnosis

Diagnosis is clinical and histopathological. Biopsy shows a true granuloma with collagen necrosis with or without eosinophils.

Treatment

In cases in which pruritus is severe, glucocorticoid therapy is indicated. If lesions are recurrent or refractory, hypersensitivity should be investigated.

Contact dermatitis (allergic or irritant)

Contact dermatitis is not recognised with any frequency in the cat. This is probably due to the characteristically intensive grooming, which removes most foreign materials from the skin and haircoat in a short time. Most contact lesions are believed to be due to irritation. Pruritus is variable and the lesion is usually exudative or ulcerative (see p. 341).

Autoimmune disease

When pruritus is one of the major features of autoimmune disease it is usually a more superficial disease that is exudative or crusting (see p. 337).

Systemic disease/neoplasia

On rare occasions pruritus can be caused by systemic disease. Hepatic or renal disease may result in increased circulating factors that have not been characterised but may result in pruritus. Mast cell tumours (systemic or cutaneous) may also cause generalised itch.

ALOPECIA

Alopecia, or loss of hair, can occur in a variety of clinical conditions. It may be localised or generalised, with or without a symmetrical distribution. The most important clinical aspect is to differentiate if the hair is being shed or is breaking off, or if the cat is removing or breaking the hair by grooming. This can be a difficult task. Cats that are shedding excessively for physiological reasons will also groom to remove loose hair so that the increased consumption of hair does not necessitate a diagnosis of self-induced alopecia. The use of an Elizabethan collar for assessing the origin of hair loss is helpful, but circumstances do not always allow its use.

Alopecia can be present with or without dermatitis. It may be helpful to assess this before narrowing the list of differentials to be pursued (see Figs 22.6 and 22.7).

Dermatophytosis

Dermatophytosis is a very common cause of alopecia in the cat. Kittens and adult long-haired cats are most at risk. The causal agent is generally *Microsporum canis*.

Clinical signs

There is considerable variation of clinical signs with dermatophytosis infection. Focal alopecia is most commonly noted, with or without crusting. The hairs often appear broken on microscopic examination. In adult cats, especially those with long hair, there may be a diffuse thinning of the entire haircoat. Miliary lesions may be seen but alopecia is the major complaint in most cases. Pruritus is generally not a major complaint. Humans in the household may also be affected.

Diagnosis

The diagnosis is made conclusively from positive fungal culture. Other helpful diagnostic tools include examination of the haircoat with a Wood's

CAUSES OF ALOPECIA
Dermatophytosis
Demodicosis
Endocrinopathy
Feline endocrine alopecia Hyperthyroidism Hypothyroidism Hyperadrenocorticism
Idiopathic feline symmetrical alopecia
Self-induced alopecia
Allergy Parasite Behaviour Combination
Miliary dermatitis
Allergy Parasite Infectious
Telogen effluvium
Drug-induced alopecia
Autoimmune disease

FIG. 22.6   Causes of alopecia.

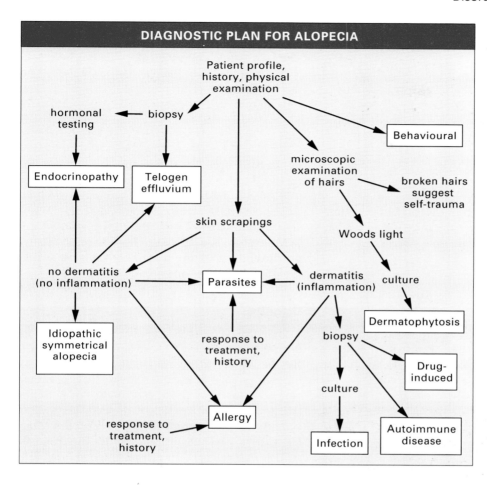

DIAGNOSTIC PLAN FOR ALOPECIA

Patient profile, history, physical examination

hormonal testing ← biopsy

Behavioural

Endocrinopathy

Telogen effluvium

microscopic examination of hairs

broken hairs suggest self-trauma

skin scrapings

Woods light

no dermatitis (no inflammation)

Parasites

dermatitis (inflammation)

culture

Idiopathic symmetrical alopecia

response to treatment, history

biopsy

Dermatophytosis

Drug-induced

culture

response to treatment, history

Allergy

Infection

Autoimmune disease

FIG. 22.7 Diagnostic plan for alopecia.

light for the presence of positive yellow-green fluorescence. Microscopic examination of broken hairs can lead to identification of ectothrix spores and this is highly suggestive of fungal invasion of the hair.

Treatment

The clinical management of dermatophytosis varies according to the age of the affected animal and the availability of different fungicidal drugs (there is significant geographical variation). Minimal therapy consists of clipping the hair from all affected lesions and application of a topical fungicidal agent until they have cleared. In healthy, young animals with normal immunological responses, dermatophytosis is a self-limiting disease.

Attempts should always be made to decrease environmental contamination even if the lesion is small.

For cats with multiple lesions or generalised infection, both topical and systemic drug therapy are indicated. A whole-body clipping of the haircoat is recommended to decrease reinfection rates. Topical shampoos or dips with fungicidal products should be repeated frequently. Systemic therapy with griseofulvin or ketoconazole can be used. Griseofulvin (40–110 mg/kg/day PO) can be given to nonpregnant cats but they should be tested for feline immunodeficiency virus (FIV) before this therapy is instituted, as neutropenia has been reported. Griseofulvin can also induce anaemia, although it is uncommon and likely to be idiosyncratic in origin. Ketoconazole (10-15 mg/kg/day) can also be used to treat generalised dermatophytosis but it can cause hepatotoxicity and anorexia in cats.

Patients should be treated until fungal cultures are negative. In multi-cat households or in catteries, management of generalised dermatophytosis can be quite challenging and somewhat discouraging. Several texts have outlined appropriate steps for cattery management.

Demodicosis

This is a rare condition in the cat but one that results in alopecia because the mite is a follicular pathogen which resides in the hair follicle, resulting in the loss of the hair.

Clinical signs

Affected cats are generally older adults with focal or multi-focal areas of alopecia, follicular plugging and a greying appearance to the skin. Other signs of systemic illness may be apparent. Secondary bacterial infection may occur.

Diagnosis

Diagnosis is by positive identification of the *Demodex cati* mite upon deep skin scrapings or via biopsy of lesions.

Treatment

In most cases, an intensive search should be made for underlying, predisposing diseases such as neoplasia, diabetes mellitus and viral infections. There are no specific approved drugs for the treatment of demodicosis in the cat. Amitraz dips have been used but there is greater toxicity for this drug in the cat and it must be used at a reduced dosage. Some success has been achieved with lime sulphur dips.

Endocrine

Feline endocrine alopecia

The incidence of this condition is controversial. Because endocrine imbalances have a significant

effect on hair growth, it is likely that some haircoat changes are manifest with feline endocrinopathies. The term feline endocrine alopecia has been used to describe a specific clinical picture in the cat but the specific endocrine abnormality has not been well identified.

Clinical signs

The condition occurs in neutered cats (males are reported to be over-represented) and is exhibited as diffuse thinning of the hair primarily affecting the anogenital region, caudomedial thighs and ventral abdomen. Hairs are easily epilated and there are no skin lesions. There is no history of pruritus and there are no clinical signs other than the dermatological ones.

Diagnosis

Diagnosis is by exclusion of other aetiologies for diffuse hair thinning. These include behavioural factors that might result in trichotillomania. Causes of pruritus such as the allergic diseases, as well as ectoparasites should be evaluated. Most of the differentials mentioned for alopecia (Fig. 22.6) should be considered. Biopsies are not diagnostic and, after exclusion of other differentials, a diagnosis is based on response to therapy.

Treatment

In the past, the standard therapy for suspected feline endocrine alopecia has been combined androgen-oestrogen therapy. Others have reported that this condition responds to progestational compounds as well as thyroid supplementation.

It is important to decide if drug therapy is indicated. In some individuals, hair will regrow spontaneously. Hormone therapy is not without risk and when a true deficient state cannot be identified, use of drug therapy should receive careful consideration.

Hyperthyroidism

Feline hyperthyroidism is usually due to chronic intrinsic thyroid disease and the major signs are not dermatological but systemic due to the resultant increased metabolic rate. Alopecia can be seen with hyperthyroidism for a variety of reasons. There may simply be excessive shedding. In other cases affected cats may pull hair for unknown reasons (probably related to their physiological state).

Hypothyroidism

Spontaneous hypothyroidism is rare in the cat although it sometimes occurs after thyroidectomy. Regardless of cause, there is an easily epilated dry haircoat with features of bilateral symmetry. The skin may feel thickened. Clinical signs are not easily distinguishable from other feline endocrinopathies. The diagnosis may be difficult because many commercial laboratories do not have normal values for the cat. A trial of response to therapy is not without concern because of the cardiac effects of thyrotoxicosis. Also, normal animals are known to have increased numbers of anagen hairs after supplementation with thyroid hormone and so a temporary response to treatment may occur even when the aetiology is not true hypothyroidism. This diagnosis should be made with care and thyroid function evaluated on several occasions or by more than one method.

Hyperadrenocorticism

This is a poorly defined disorder in the cat but can be iatrogenic, pituitary dependent, or adrenal in origin. The skin may become thin and tear easily. There may be symmetrical truncal hair loss. Adrenocorticotropin hormone stimulation tests can be helpful in making the diagnosis but it is important to remember that the stress associated with chronic illness in older cats can also lead to exaggerated response testing. Therapy is directed at restoring circulating steroid levels to normal.

Idiopathic feline symmetrical alopecia

This term has been used recently to describe cases of symmetrical hair loss for which a defined cause cannot be found, even after extensive diagnostic tests (some probable cross-over with feline endocrine alopecia?). Some cats respond to supplementation with triiodothyronine therapy.

For clients who are interested in identifying an aetiology, a number of diagnostic tests and possible elimination therapies can be carried out. One should also discuss the option of not treating these patients, as the condition is merely cosmetic in most cases.

Self-induced alopecia

Alopecia/allergy

As mentioned under the section on Pruritus, hypersensitivity reactions can manifest in the cat as increased hair loss due to grooming behaviour. It is not clear why some cats with itchy skin will develop primary cutaneous eruptions and have significant self-traumatic lesions whereas others with pruritus from the same aetiology will simply sit and lick, breaking the hairs and physically removing them with no signs of primary lesions or self-trauma to the skin itself. It is difficult to clinically differentiate between self-induced alopecia and increased hair loss. Any suspicion of pruritus as perceived by the owner should suggest that a diagnosis of allergy be pursued. A historical response to glucocorticoid therapy should suggest that allergy may be implicated.

Clinical signs

Cats with alopecia as the primary sign of allergy generally have symmetrical hair thinning or total loss of hair on the trunk (Fig. 22.8). The area may be diffuse or well-delineated. Anatomical areas reached by mouth are affected. The remaining hairs may be broken and stubbly if the cat is chewing or pulling and breaking them. In other cats no broken hairs remain and only new hair growth is palpable.

Diagnosis and treatment

These are the same as for Allergy (see above).

Ectoparasites

Cats with ectoparasitism may develop bilaterally symmetrical alopecia without sign of primary lesions. This can occur with *Cheyletiella* infestations

FIG. 22.8 Symmetrical alopecia due to excessive grooming behaviour.

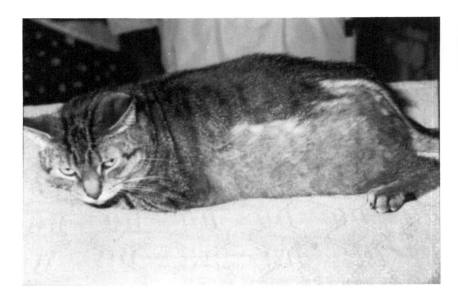

or with fleas (usually when accompanied by flea allergy) – see p. 325 for details.

Behavioural alopecia (psychogenic alopecia, trichotillomania)

The incidence of this condition is not known. Some cats with no signs of pruritus will begin excessive grooming and hair-pulling coincident with a stressful event. This can occur in any age or breed of cat but seems to be more common in housecats.

Clinical signs

The signs are similar to other causes of self-induced alopecia. These cats will often have alopecia on the dorsal and lateral aspects of the forelimb, which they can easily groom from a normal sitting position, and these focal lesions of hair loss are often very well demarcated. Sometimes the temperament changes of the cat suggests that it becomes easily excited or stressed.

Diagnosis

The diagnosis is difficult. Microscopic examination of hairs can sometimes be helpful if the cat is actually breaking the hairs. However, if the cat is removing the entire hair from the follicle, behaviour-induced trichotillomania cannot be differentiated easily from pruritus. If a good history can be obtained for a marked change in behaviour or environment, this is helpful. A response to therapy is useful but does not prove a definitive behavioural aetiology.

Treatment

The major tools of treatment in these cases are either behavioural modification therapy or pharmacological behaviour-altering drugs or a combination of both.

If the owner can correct the inciting problem, by altering the environment (for example, removing a threatening cat from the household), then this should be attempted. Increasing the amount of positive attention received by the affected patient is another aspect of behaviour modification therapy.

Drug therapy is another adjunct in the treatment of these cases. Some prefer to use tranquilising drugs such as phenobarbital or valium whereas others have better success with mood-altering drugs such as progestational compounds or tricyclic antidepressants. These are best used in conjunction with environmental changes and they should be used for short periods while the habitual behaviour is being altered. There seems little justification for long-term drug therapy in these cats. The clinical signs are unsightly but not harmful to the patient. Most patients have a waxing and waning of clinical signs and the alopecia generally stays restricted to areas easily reached by the cat.

Combination self-induced alopecias

In some cases, a combination of pathology and habitual excessive grooming develops. What begins as a mild pruritus or the discovery of a few fleas can develop into obsessive grooming behaviour. In these cases, the aetiology of the clinical lesions may thus be multifactorial and the treatment plan may need to use a variety of approaches.

Miliary dermatitis

There may be significant alopecia associated with the self-trauma of a cat with miliary dermatitis. This crusting, scabbing disease may be due to a variety of causes and is discussed in detail on p. 336.

Telogen effluvium

This may occur in any age, breed or sex of cat. It may occur after systemic disease, after drug therapy, gestation or lactation.

Clinical signs

The signs are excessive shedding of hair. The condition is usually generalised and in the owner's history, the onset is rather sudden. It may be accompanied by increased trichobezoar production as large quantities of hair are ingested by the cat as it attempts to groom away all the loose hair. The signs may occur up to three months after the initiating event, sometimes making it difficult to pinpoint the cause.

Diagnosis

The diagnosis is a clinical one although it can be confirmed by examination of easily epilating hairs that are shown to have glistening white bulbs. Histopathological examination of tissue shows large numbers of telogen hair follicles.

Treatment

The treatment is conservative as new anagen hairs will replace the thinning haircoat within three months in most cases. If hair regrowth does not occur and an endocrinopathy cannot be defined, a short course of thyroid supplementation may induce production of anagen hairs. The therapy is discontinued once hair regrowth is initiated.

Drug-induced alopecia

Focal alopecia can be seen at the site of a topically administered drug or at the site of an injection. Corticosteroids and repositol progestational compounds are the more commonly implicated drugs. Hair loss is noted first, followed by thinning of the skin, depigmentation and, in some cases, ulceration or tearing of skin.

Autoimmune diseases

It is possible, although unlikely, that hair loss may be the presenting sign with cutaneous manifestations of autoimmune disease. When this occurs, it is usually seen in chronic cases and the primary bullous or pustular lesions have been overlooked by the owner (see p. 337).

SCALING/CRUSTING/EXUDATIVE DERMATITIS

This grouping encompasses the more common presenting feline dermatitis cases (Fig. 22.9). It is a rather broad classification because many diseases and secondary self-trauma will lead to crusting. Likewise these problems are not always seen together; for example, fine scale may be the only finding in a primary abnormality of keratinisation. However, the signs are found together with some frequency and can be most challenging (Fig. 22.10).

CAUSES OF SCALE/CRUSTS/EXUDATES
Infectious
Bacterial: folliculitis/furunculosis, paronychia Fungal: dermatophytosis Viral
Miliary dermatitis
Allergy: flea allergy, atopy, food allergy Infectious Ectoparasites
Autoimmune disease
Pemphigus foliaceus and Pemphigus erythematosus Systemic lupus erythematosus
Parasitic
Notoedres *Cheyletiella* *Lynxacarus* *Demodex*
Drug eruption
Actinic (solar) dermatitis
Feline acne
Stud tail
Mycosis fungoides

FIG. 22.9   Causes of scale, crusts and exudates.

Infections

Superficial lesions with infectious aetiologies would be most likely to lead to small quantities of exudate followed by crusting.

Bacterial folliculitis

Clinical signs

Hair follicle infections due to bacterial invasion are uncommon in the cat but the reason for this is not clear. When noted, lesions are follicular-oriented papules, rare pustules, and predominantly crusts and small scabs. Exudate with folliculitis is not a major feature. There is no age or breed predilection. Lesions may occur on the head, neck or trunk.

Diagnosis

The usual diagnosis of bacterial folliculitis is made by a favourable response to antibiotic

therapy. Biopsies may indicate a neutrophilic dermatitis and cytology of exudate will usually reveal degenerative neutrophils and bacteria.

Treatment

Treatment consists of topical cleaning and removal of the crusts and exudate in conjunction with oral antibiotic therapy. Lincomycin, oxacillin and cephalosporins are drugs useful in treatment. Long-term therapy or recurrences have been noted in some cases.

Bacterial paronychia

Clinical signs

This rare condition occurs in older cats. Swelling, pain, erythema, crusting, and purulent or serous exudate of the nail bed are among the presenting signs. The claws may be cracked and split.

Diagnosis

Bacterial infection in this area is usually secondary and a search should be made for an underlying cause. Diagnosis is by ruling out other differentials, by identifying pathogenic bacteria, and by a favourable response to antibiotic therapy.

A major differential would be autoimmune disease such as pemphigus foliaceus, which can result in a caseous nail bed exudate with neutrophils and acanthocytes. Neoplasia should be considered and biopsies will be helpful in evaluation. Contact dermatitis, dermatophytosis, trauma, and the eosinophilic granuloma complex are among other differentials.

Treatment

Look for and treat the underlying cause. Soaking can be helpful. Antibiotic therapy for 6–8 weeks is advocated. Environmental changes (in type of cat litter, for example) may be beneficial. In particularly refractory cases, surgical removal of the claws may be the only effective treatment.

Dermatophytosis

The major sign of dermatophytosis is alopecia and the problem is therefore discussed in detail on pp 329–330. However, since fungal invasion of the hair occurs in the follicle, cats with dermatophytosis may have crusting and scaling as primary clinical signs. These can present as focal crusting and somewhat exudative lesions, often found on the head and extremities. Generalised dermato-phytosis can result occasionally in miliary dermatitis rather than primary alopecia.

Viral infections

With the systemic viral diseases of feline immunodeficiency virus (FIV), feline infectious peritonitis (FIP) or feline leukaemia virus (FeLV), it is possible to see generalised scaling of the skin. This seborrhoeic condition is not diagnostic of viral

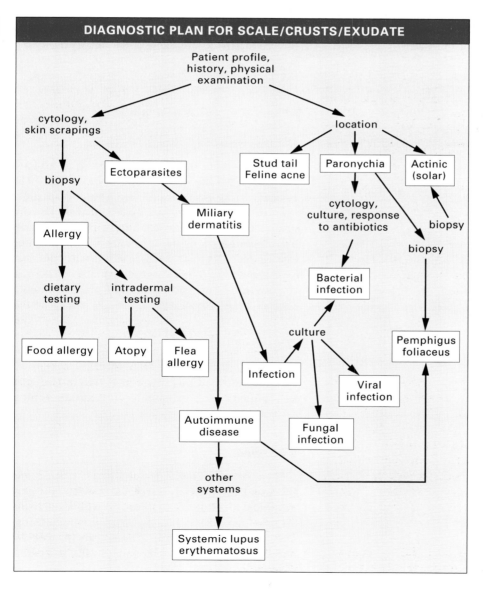

FIG. 22.10 Diagnostic plan for scales, crusts and exudates

infection but it is seen with a variety of systemic illnesses in the cat.

Miliary dermatitis

Clinical signs

Rather than being a definitive diagnosis, miliary dermatitis is a descriptive term for tiny focal crusts scattered generally over the dorsal and, in later stages, over the ventral trunk (Fig. 22.11). The dorsal neck is frequently the site of early lesions. It can occur in any age, breed or sex of cat, and may be seasonal or year-round. Pruritus is usually present but not always to the degree one would expect for the quantity of dermatitis.

Diagnosis

There are many causes of miliary dermatitis in the cat, including the allergic diseases of flea

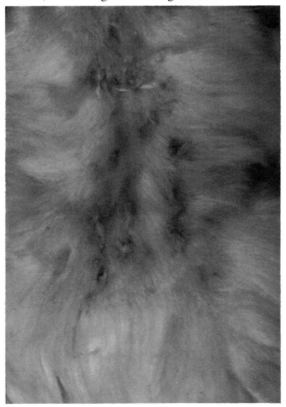

FIG. 22.11 Exudative, crusting and scaling dermatitis on ventral neck of cat with concurrent dorsal miliary dermatitis.

allergy, food allergy and atopy, as well as the ectoparasites and infectious causes of folliculitis. The literature suggests some much less common aetiologies as well. In geographical areas where fleas occur, many cases of miliary dermatitis are due to flea allergy. An attempt to identify the cause of miliary dermatitis should be made by use of skin scrapings, fungal culture, allergy testing, distribution and history of clinical signs, and prior response to therapy.

Treatment

Treatment should be directed towards the identified underlying aetiology. When miliary dermatitis is idiopathic in origin, the response to corticosteroid therapy is usually favourable.

Miliary dermatitis in flea allergy

Clinical signs

The lesions of flea allergy can occur at any age but are generally seen in the young adult. The primary locations of lesions are the dorsal trunk, tailroot, caudal thighs and the dorsal neck. Lesions are bilaterally symmetrical and pruritus is usually accompanied by signs of licking, scratching and loss of hair. The signs correspond with the presence of fleas or flea excrement on the cat or in the environment, and generally worsen with each season of flea exposure.

Diagnosis

The diagnosis is made from the clinical signs. It can be confirmed by intradermal skin testing with flea antigen and is usually substantiated by a favourable response to flea control.

Treatment

Flea control is the treatment of choice and the ideal methodology will vary from one geographical location to another. As well as environmental control, treatment of all in-contact dogs and cats is advocated. Choice of insecticides and cleaning regimens depends on the individual case.

Autoimmune skin disease

Autoimmune skin disease can result in superficial or deep lesions. Diseases with lesions in the upper layers of the epidermis are most likely to present with crusting or exudative lesions.

Pemphigus foliaceus/erythematosus

Clinical signs

Pustules, vesicles, and crusts with serocellular or purulent exudate characterise the lesions of pemphigus foliaceus and pemphigus erythematosus. In pemphigus foliaceus, the lesions specifically affect the face, ears, extremities and ventral abdomen. In severe cases the lesions may be generalised. In pemphigus erythematosus, similar signs occur but the lesions are confined to the head. Cats are generally but not exclusively middle-aged to older. They may be depressed, febrile and have peripheral lymphadenopathy. Pruritus and excessive licking may be features.

Diagnosis

Diagnosis is based on the history, physical examination, cytology of pustules, histopathological examination of primary lesions, and immunopathology findings. Biopsies indicate subcorneal or intragranular pustules containing neutrophils, eosinophils and acanthocytes. Secondary bacterial infection may occur, in which case an attempt should be made to assess bacterial involvement. This can be done by cultures and by response to antibiotic therapy.

Treatment

Treatment for the pemphigus complex can be difficult and requires immunosuppressive therapy. It can be accomplished with glucocorticoids in some cats, although a variety of steroids may be necessary for control in different patients. Other potent immunomodulating drugs (such as chlorambucil) or chrysotherapy, may be necessary. A significant amount of time and financial commitment are necessary from the owner before long-term therapy is undertaken.

Lupus erythematosus

Pustules may be present in the systemic form of lupus erythematosus in cats and there are many similarities with the pemphigus complex. In other lupus cases the presenting lesions are erosive and ulcerative, which is more indicative of the immunological reaction directed toward the basement membrane area (see p. 340).

Parasites

Infestation by any of the ectoparasites (see pp 325–326) can result in crusting and scaling. The *Notoedres cati* mite is often responsible for excessive crusting and scaling, especially of the head and neck region, and the *Cheyletiella* mite can produce a variety of clinical lesions, including a fine scaling which has inspired the term 'walking dandruff' for this parasite and its clinical sequelae. Any case of feline seborrhoea should be examined for possible *Cheyletiella* infestation.

Lynxacariasis is an uncommon disease caused by *Lynxacarus radovskyi*, which attaches to the hair shafts. The patient may have small scales or miliary dermatitis. The diagnosis is made by identification of the mite from scraping, tape preparations or combings. Insecticidal therapy weekly for several treatments generally eliminates the problem.

The *Demodex* mite can inhabit the hair follicle, resulting in alopecia, but one species noted in cats has been reported to result in crusting and superficial scaling.

Drug eruption

Eruptions due to drugs can be extremely variable in clinical presentation. Crusts, scale, and even miliary dermatitis can be manifestations and the subject is discussed further on p. 340.

Solar lesions

Clinical signs

Older cats with significant sun exposure are most commonly affected by solar lesions, which are noted in white or light-coloured areas of the haircoat. Lesions include erythema, hair loss, and scaling of affected areas. Crusts and ulceration may follow months of redness and scale. Ears, preauricular areas and the nose are usually affected. Pruritus is not severe.

Diagnosis

The diagnosis is by clinical appearance and distribution of the lesions, and by histopathological findings. Atypia and dysplasia of the epidermis are the more commonly recognised histopathological occurrences. Changes in the dermis may occur.

Treatment

Removal of the cat from the sun or protection from further solar damage is important in preventing the development of squamous cell carcinoma.

Feline acne

Clinical signs

Feline acne is a well-recognised clinical entity in the cat and can occur at any age. However, the pathological mechanism and actual aetiology are unclear. Lesions consist of comedones, papules, erythema, crusts, and exudation on the chin. Pustules are noted occasionally and there may also be swelling. Pruritus may be marked to minimal.

Diagnosis

Diagnosis is from the clinical appearance of the lesions. Histopathological findings may include follicular plugging, hyperkeratosis, perifolliculitis, folliculitis and furunculosis.

Treatment

Secondary bacterial involvement in feline acne is common and most treatment regimens suggest antibiotic therapy initially. Topical cleansing of the area with follicular flushing agents such as benzoyl peroxide are beneficial. Some cats with minor signs are much better treated with 'benign neglect' rather than aggressive therapy.

Stud tail

This somewhat greasy, sometimes scaly, localised seborrhoea is found on the dorsal area of the tail approximately one third of the area distal to the body. There may be matting of the hairs. Stud tail occurs primarily in intact breeding male cats in confined circumstances but has been noted in females and neutered as well as intact animals. The aetiology is unknown; the diagnosis is based on the clinical appearance of the lesions and treatment is managerial but not always totally successful.

CAUSES OF EROSION/ULCERATION
Autoimmune
Pemphigus vulgaris Bullous pemphigoid Lupus erythematosus Cold haemagglutinins
Drug eruption
Erythema multiforme Toxic epidermal necrolysis
Contact irritant
Toxicosis
Eosinophilic granuloma complex
Ulcer
Plasma cell pododermatitis
Infectious
Bacterial Fungal Viral Herpes Calicivirus Poxvirus Leishmaniasis
Neoplasia
Mast cell tumour Basal cell tumour Squamous cell carcinoma Cutaneous lymphoma
Temperature-dependent lesions
Burn Frostbite
Snake bite/Arthropod bite
Thromboembolic disease
Non-healing wounds of hyperadrenocorticism

FIG. 22.12   Causes of erosion and ulceration.

Mycosis fungoides

This is an epidermotrophic form of lymphoma and is seen rarely in the cat. Lesions can be multifocal or generalised with erythema, plaques, crust, scale, exfoliation and even nodules and ulceration. Older animals are more likely to develop neoplasia. Histopathological examination should be diagnostic.

EROSION/ULCERATION

Lesions which are erosive involve the deeper layers of the epidermis and when healing occurs there is no scarring. Ulceration is a deeper lesion extending to the bottom of the epidermis and scarring may occur. Clinically it is unlikely that one can appreciate a difference between erosive and ulcerated lesions unless there is extensive full thickness necrosis as occurs in a burn. Erosion and ulceration represent another problem in feline dermatology (see Figs 22.12 and 22.13).

Autoimmune disease

The autoimmune diseases listed in Fig. 22.12 have rarely been diagnosed in the cat. Because of this, they are discussed together.

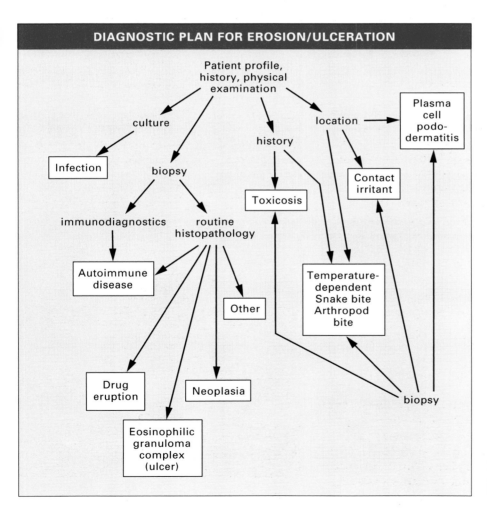

FIG. 22.13 Diagnostic plan for erosion and ulceration.

Clinical signs

Middle-aged to older cats are more likely to develop autoimmune skin diseases. Those which may result in erosive or ulcerative lesions will usually involve the mucocutaneous areas. Lesions may also be noted inside the oral cavity and, depending on the disease, on the trunk or extremities as well. Vesicles and blisters may be apparent, although they are usually short-lived. In lupus and cold agglutinin disease, compromised cutaneous blood supply may create lesions of discoloration, swelling and necrosis. Systemic signs such as depression, fever, anorexia and lymphadenopathy may be seen with any of the ulcerative forms of autoimmune skin disease.

Diagnosis

The diagnosis is made by clinical and histopathological findings, the latter differing somewhat in the different diseases. In lupus, the presence of antinuclear antibodies in significant titre are useful in the diagnosis. Other immunodiagnostics can be of benefit as well.

It is important to consider carefully the other differentials for ulceration and erosion before making a diagnosis of autoimmune skin disease. Infectious causes of ulceration should be assessed so that aetiologies such as candidiasis, viruses, and bacteria have been eliminated.

Treatment

Therapy is specifically aimed at immunosuppression with drug protocols that are designed for individual patients under evaluation. The prognosis for these ulcerative autoimmune diseases is usually guarded. Controlling these patients in the long term without progression of the disease or serious side effects from the medication is difficult to attain, and only dedicated owners should attempt treatment.

Drug eruptions

Eruptions due to drugs are rarely reported in the cat and have a wide variety of clinical manifestations. Any of the problems presented in this chapter may be primary presenting complaints for a drug eruption. The following lesions have been noted as caused by drugs in certain situations: urticaria, photosensitivity reactions, morbilliform eruptions, fixed drug eruptions, lichenoid drug eruptions, generalised erythroderma, vasculitis, erythema multiforme, and toxic epidermal necrolysis (Fig. 22.14). Drug eruptions may occur from drugs administered topically or systemically. Drug reactions likely to result in ulcerative or erosive lesions will generally be either erythema multiforme or toxic epidermal necrolysis.

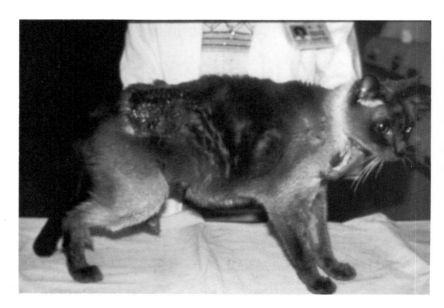

FIG. 22.14   Erosive and ulcerative dermatitis due to drug eruption (case of Dr Mary Pichler).

Erythema multiforme

Not all lesions of erythema multiforme are due to reactions to drugs. In veterinary medicine drugs are more commonly identified as the underlying aetiology. Erythema multiforme may also be seen with systemic illness or neoplasia and it may also be of unknown aetiology. The exact mechanism of development of most drug eruptions is not well known. An immunologically-mediated reaction is the most accepted proposed pathological mechanism.

Clinical signs

Lesions are usually acute in onset and include vesiculobullous lesions, erosions, ulceration, papules and plaques. They may be focal or multifocal in distribution and may involve mucocutaneous sites as well as the haired skin. Constitutional signs may occur, depending on the extent of the lesions.

Diagnosis

The diagnosis is made from the clinical signs in conjunction with histopathological findings, which include single cell necrosis of keratinocytes with an interface dermatitis. The differentials should include autoimmune diseases and infectious causes.

Treatment

The primary treatment is identification and cessation of the offending drug, along with secondary supportive care for the lesions.

Toxic epidermal necrolysis

Toxic epidermal necrolysis is not always the result of a drug and can be due to systemic illness or neoplasia, or idiopathic in origin. It is a much more serious disease.

Clinical signs

There is an acute onset of focal areas of full thickness necrosis and sloughing of the skin. This may progress rapidly and generalise. The lesions look like severe burns. The skin and oral mucosa may be involved. There are often concurrent systemic signs.

Diagnosis

The diagnosis is based on the history, clinical signs, and skin biopsy which indicates full thickness coagulation necrosis of the epidermis. Early in the process, inflammatory infiltrates should be minimal, but a marked interface dermatitis may occur in the later stages.

Treatment

The prognosis for this disease is guarded, even if the offending drug is identified and discontinued early on. Supportive care similar to that needed for a severe burn constitutes the primary treatment. Corticosteroid therapy for drug reactions is controversial.

Contact irritant

Clinical signs

Signs are acute in onset and occur usually at points of anatomical contact with the offending agent. The extremities, the perineum, the face and ears would be likely areas for an environmental irritant to initiate an inflammatory reaction. Lesions may be pruritic or painful, depending on the depth of the lesion. Lesions are usually focal because of the nature of the contactant but they can be generalised if an irritant solution has been applied to most of the cat.

Diagnosis

The diagnosis is primarily a clinical one based on history in conjunction with the physical findings. A response to symptomatic therapy after rinsing away the offending agent is usually the manner in which the diagnosis is supported. Histopathological findings include neutrophilic inflammation.

Treatment

Therapy centres around symptomatic care once the irritant has been removed. The lesions should heal with supportive care.

Toxicosis

Toxicity, such as that seen with thallium, can result in ulceration. These conditions are rare, but depending on the history, one should keep an open mind about their inclusion in the differential diagnosis. With certain toxicities (e.g. thallium or hypervitaminosis A) there are somewhat characteristic histopathological findings.

Eosinophilic granuloma complex/indolent ulcer

Clinical signs

The indolent ulcer is a well circumscribed, ulcerated lesion seen unilaterally or bilaterally on the upper lip. It is usually raised peripherally with a clear firm pink to white border and a concave central ulcer, although patients do not usually exhibit discomfort. Lesions may occur in animals of any age and oral collagenolytic granulomas or eosinophilic plaque lesions may occur concurrently.

Diagnosis

The diagnosis is made from the clinical appearance of the lesion. There is no tissue or blood eosinophilia with this disease. Histopathological findings are those of a non-specific chronic ulcerative dermatitis.

Treatment

Some lesions respond to antibiotic therapy with significant reduction or resolution of lesions. Because the aetiology of this lesion is not known, it is unclear why some of these lesions respond to antibiotics.

Most veterinarians find that corticosteroid therapy, especially injectable methylprednisolone acetate, is beneficial in the treatment of this entity. Surgical excision, cryosurgery and radiation therapy have been useful in individual cases. Most recently laser therapy and chrysotherapy have been used in a few refractory cases. Progestational compounds are beneficial in some cases but the potential side effects of treatment must be considered.

Plasma cell pododermatitis

Clinical signs

Cats may have lesions on one or more feet. Primary lesions are swollen, often ulcerated metacarpal or metatarsal foot pads. There may be pain and lameness.

Diagnosis

Cytology of deeper lesions may be useful in revealing large numbers of plasma cells. Histopathological examination of tissue reveals superficial and deep perivascular or diffuse plasma cell dermatitis. A small number of cases have positive antinuclear antibody tests as well as immune-mediated glomerulonephritis.

Treatment

Since the aetiology is unknown, specific therapy is difficult. There is some evidence that this condition is immune-mediated and therapy has thus been directed at immunosuppression with corticosteroids. Radical surgical excision of affected tissue may give temporary relief.

Bacterial furunculosis

Bacterial furunculosis may result in multiple ulcerated cutaneous lesions. These are rare in the cat and are most likely to occur secondarily in feline acne. Furunculosis should be managed similarly to folliculitis (see p. 334) but for a longer duration.

Fungal infections

It is possible for furunculosis to occur when a hair follicle ruptures due to infection of the hair with *Microsporum canis*. This is not a common form of dermatophytosis (see p. 328) but when it is present there will be multifocal ulcerative or draining lesions. Sporotrichosis and systemic fungal infection can have primary ulcerative dermatological lesions.

Candidiasis can result in ulcerative mucocutaneous lesions in immunocompromised individuals, though this is rare.

Viral infections

Herpes virus and calicivirus

Both these viruses have been noted to cause ulcers and blisters in the oral cavity and occasionally on the feet. This is generally in association with other systemic signs of viral infection. Diagnosis is based on the concurrent clinical findings and a strong suggestion of viral aetiology based on the histopathology. Isolation of the viral agent may be possible. Primary therapy is directed against secondary bacterial invaders, in conjunction with optimum nursing care.

Cowpox virus

Lesions have been described in the United Kingdom and continental Europe and systemic signs may precede the development of well demarcated nodules, plaques and ulcers in the skin. Sloughs and subsequent scarring may occur. Lesions may occur in adult cats or kittens and are found on the face, ears and extremities. The diagnosis is made by histopathology, serology and virus isolation. Most affected cats will recover spontaneously, but it may take several months. For further details, see chapter 23.

Leishmaniasis

Leishmaniasis is caused by a protozoan, *Leishmania donovani*, transmitted by bloodsucking sandflies and is endemic in certain areas of the world. In the cat, ulcerated lesions usually occur on the head. The diagnosis is made by histopathological examination of tissue and the presence of intra- and extracellular organisms of *Leishmania*. Successful drug treatment regimens for the cat are not well elucidated.

NODULES AND DRAINING TRACTS

These two problems may be seen separately or together; they are often noted concurrently, or the nodule later ruptures and reveals a draining tract. Lesions may be single or multiple. As part of the diagnostic plan for nodules and draining tracts, it important to record a complete history that includes the location of the lesion(s), the environment, the geographical area and any prior response to therapy. The physical examination should include palpation of lymph nodes and retinal examination, as well as radiography in specific cases. Serology, cytology, culture and histopathological examination of tissues are all important aspects for diagnosis and definition of optimum therapy (see Figs 22.15 and 22.16).

Cat-bite abscess

Clinical signs

Signs are very common in cats and usually include pain, swelling, fever, depression and sometimes lameness. Swelling usually occurs after bite wounds or other trauma introduce bacteria into soft tissues. Eventually the abscess may rupture and drain a purulent or serosanguinous exudate. Common locations are the extremities, head, tail and back. Intact male cats are most frequently affected but either sex may be involved. Signs vary depending on the location of lesions, severity, and individual response.

Diagnosis

The diagnosis is based on the history, physical findings, cytology and response to therapy.

Treatment

Establishing effective drainage of the lesion and flushing it to remove exudate and debris are important aspects of therapy. Drains are necessary in some cases, depending on the anatomical location. Systemic antibiotic therapy is usually indicated. If the lesion has not localised, hot compresses may hasten the rupture and drainage.

Most cat-bite abscesses are caused by *Pasteurella* organisms and respond well to therapy. If lesions do not improve with supportive care, other causes of draining tracts (Fig. 22.15) should be considered.

Botryomycosis

In this rare condition, bacteria which are usually coagulase positive *Staphylococcus* form 'grains'

CAUSES OF NODULES AND DRAINING TRACTS
Infectious
Bacterial
Abscess/cellulitis Botryomycosis (bacterial pseudomycetoma) Nocardiosis Dermatophilosis Mycobacterial granulomas: tuberculosis, feline leprosy, atypical mycobacteriosis *Rhodococcus equi* Feline plague
Fungal
Subcutaneous dermatophytosis (pseudomycetoma) Eumycotic mycetomas Phaeohyphomycosis Zygomycosis Hyalohyphomycosis Sporotrichosis Cryptococcosis Other systemic fungi
Protothecosis
Parasites
Cuterebriasis
Foreign bodies
Eosinophilic granuloma complex
Collagenolytic granuloma Eosinophilic plaque
Xanthomatosis
Panniculitis
Neoplasia

FIG. 22.15   Causes of nodules and draining tracts.

surrounded centrally by pyogranulomatous inflammation. Single or multiple nodules may be present. Granules are usually small. The diagnosis is made by cytology, culture and histopathological examination. Treatment is by excision of the lesion and post-surgical antibiotic therapy selected from sensitivity data.

Nocardia

Clinical signs

This uncommon infection is usually contracted by trauma and contamination with infected soil. Cellulitis is the presenting problem. Ulcers, nodules and draining tracts are usually noted on the limbs.

The exudate is brownish red and may contain granules. The patient may have concurrent systemic illness or appear unwell as there may be underlying conditions which are immunosuppressive.

Diagnosis

The history, physical examination findings and cytological examination of exudate are useful in reaching a diagnosis. Organisms are partially acid-fast filamentous bacteria. Biopsy generally indicates a pyogranulomatous inflammation with or without panniculitis and rarely with granules. The organism can be cultured aerobically.

Treatment

This can be a difficult infection to treat. Long-term antibiotic therapy with penicillin or ampicillin in combination with sulphonamides are recommended. It may be best to remove surgically as much of the lesion as possible. The prognosis for long-term cure is guarded.

Mycobacterial granulomas

Tuberculosis

Single to multiple nodules or abscesses may develop when a cat is exposed to animals or man infected with *Mycobacterium tuberculi*. The condition is rare but warrants serious consideration if the history suggests its possibility.

Feline leprosy

Clinical signs

This disease is seen primarily in specific geographical regions such as the Northwestern United States, Canada and certain regions of New Zealand. The likely aetiological agent is *Mycobacterium lepraemurium*, which causes rat leprosy. Clinical lesions are usually single to multiple nodules, with or without ulceration and drainage. Lesions are noted on the head and extremities.

Diagnosis

The diagnosis is based on clinical findings plus the presence of many intracellular acid-fast

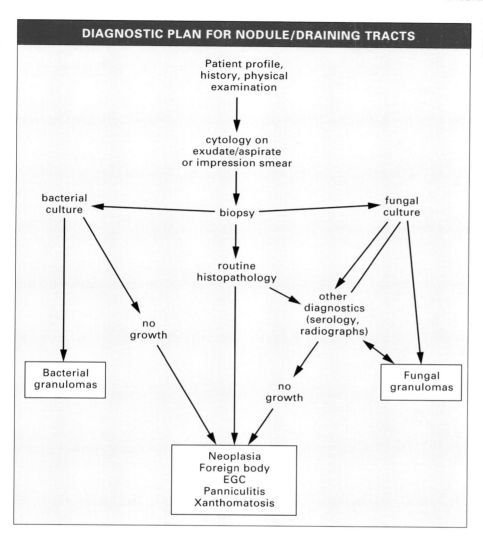

FIG. 22.16 Diagnostic plan for nodules and draining tracts.

organisms noted within macrophages. This organism is unlikely to be grown in culture.

Treatment

If possible, the lesion should be removed surgically. There are occasional reports in the literature of success with medical treatment but most of the drugs that have been used have serious toxicities.

Atypical mycobacteriosis

Clinical signs

Lesions are small nodules or multifocal draining tracts involving the subcutaneous fat. Fistulas and dehiscence from biopsy sites are common. Small punctate ulcers which heal with thin skin overlying cutaneous defects are seen frequently. In general, patients are not systemically ill but may present aesthetic problems with the drainage of exudate. The inguinal fat pad area is affected commonly. The lesions can resemble other abscesses in the early stages but they do not respond to therapy in the same manner.

Diagnosis

Diagnosis is by direct cytology, histopathological examination of tissue, and culture. Direct cytology may reveal an occasional acid-fast rod but organisms are difficult to identify. Histopathology reveals a pyogranulomatous panniculitis with occasional organisms. Culture may allow identification of the offending agent after 5–7 days.

Treatment

The treatment is frustrating. Antibiotics suggested by culture and sensitivity results are helpful in selection of optimum drugs for management. If lesions are small, surgical excision may be rewarding but most surgical interventions in these cases become 'nightmares' of dehiscence. Some lesions may regress spontaneously. Quinolones and synthetic tetracyclines have been useful in some cases. The prognosis is guarded.

Rhodococcus equi

This bacterial infection, rarely recorded in the cat, occurs when *Rhodococcus equi* invade and proliferate in the dermis or subcutaneous tissues. Affected cats should have a history of exposure to horses. The lesions are generally non-healing progressive abscesses, that may result in systemic signs, and the agent is identified by culture.

Feline plague

Clinical signs

This disease has been reported occasionally in the Southwestern United States and can affect any age, breed or sex. Lesions are cutaneous abscesses; lymphadenopathy, depression and fever occur. The plague organism is transmitted by fleas and these parasites have usually fed on wild rodents.

Diagnosis

The aetiological agent is *Yersinia pestis*. The diagnosis is made by compatible history and clinical findings, and confirmed by culture.

Treatment

Therapy involves systemic antibiotic care and establishing drainage. Recovery usually occurs after one week of tetracycline, chloramphenicol or other antimicrobials.

It is important to note the potential for human infection. In suspect areas, precautions should be taken to protect the veterinarian and others handling a cat with suspected infection.

Fungal infections

Subcutaneous dermatophytosis (pseudomycetoma)

Clinical signs

Signs are generally seen in long-haired cats. They present as solitary or multiple cutaneous or subcutaneous nodules, with or without draining tracts.

Diagnosis

The diagnosis is made by histopathological examination and by culture from the lesion. Isolates may be *Microsporum canis* or *Trichophyton mentagrophytes* (Fig. 22.17).

Treatment

The optimum therapy is to remove the lesions surgically. If the cat has concurrent generalised dermatophytosis or the lesion is not resectable, systemic antifungal drugs such as griseofulvin or ketoconazole are indicated as well.

Eumycotic mycetomas

These lesions are generally solitary and present with drainage, swelling and granules. These

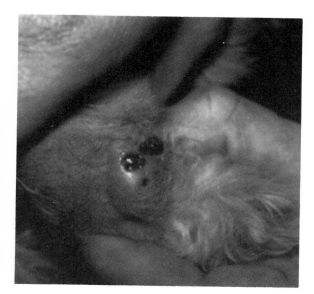

FIG. 22.17   Nodule with ulceration and granular exudate noted on extremity of Persian cat. The lesion was due to *Microsporum canis.*

tumour-like lesions can result from a variety of organisms which are organised into granules in the central portions. The treatment of choice is surgical excision.

Sporotrichosis

Clinical signs

Lesions consist of ulcerated, draining nodules or crusted lesions commonly noted on the head or extremities. Infection occurs when soil-borne organisms enter the skin through trauma. There are usually multiple lesions and associated lymphadenopathy. In the cat, infection often spreads to other organs.

Diagnosis

The diagnosis is made by culture, cytology, histopathology and immunofluorescent antibody testing of skin biopsy specimens.

Treatment

The treatment is sodium iodide or ketoconazole. The prognosis is guarded in cats because

they do not tolerate the drugs well and progression may occur in spite of treatment. Most important is the potential transmission to man; precautions should be taken as spread has occurred even when gloves have been worn by animal handlers.

Cryptococcosis

The lesions include swelling, nasal discharge, draining tracts, and ulcerated and crusted cutaneous lesions. Systemic disease is most common. The organism is *C. neoformans* and the diagnosis is made by cytology, biopsy, culture and serology. Therapy is with ketoconazole, fluconazole or itraconazole but the prognosis is guarded.

Cuterebriasis

This is usually easily diagnosed because the clinical lesions include a nodule with a breathing pore on the head or extremities. It is most often seen in kittens but can affect cats of any age. The problem occurs when the larva of the *Cuterebra* fly burrows into the skin and a foreign-body granuloma develops. Treatment is the removal of the larva.

Foreign bodies

Lesions develop in the subcutaneous tissues when foreign material such as hair, keratin, plant, wood or other matter incites a granulomatous inflammatory process in an attempt by the body to reject the material. Drainage often results. Excision or total removal of the foreign material is appropriate.

Eosinophilic granuloma complex: collagenolytic granuloma

These often occur as pink to yellow-pink nodules in the pharynx or on the tongue. They may be present on the ventral chin, lower or upper lip and, rarely, on the feet. They may be firm and linear, in some instances extending down the rear legs. They have been noted on the nose, ears and feet in association with insect bites. The diagnosis is made by histopathological examination of the tissues and treatment is glucocorticoid therapy in most cases. If insect-bite is suspected as the cause, this should be investigated.

Xanthomatosis

This rare condition is characterised by granulomatous lesions associated with altered systemic lipid metabolism and in some cases associated with diabetes mellitus. Diagnosis is by biopsy in conjunction with systemic findings.

Panniculitis

There are a variety of aetiologies for panniculitis, including nutritional, infectious and idiopathic causes. The lesions are deep nodules which periodically drain a greasy serosanguinous exudate. Treatment varies according to the cause.

Neoplasia

Neoplasia should be considered in many cases which present with nodules. This is especially true if the lesion is not draining or the cat is middle-aged to older. It is beyond the scope of this chapter to discuss cutaneous feline neoplasias. Basal cell tumours, mast cell tumours, fibrosarcoma and squamous cell carcinomas are among the more common skin tumours in the cat.

FURTHER READING

Greene C., (ed) (1990) *Infectious Diseases of the Dog and Cat*. W.B. Saunders Co., Philadelphia.

Grant D.I. (1986) *Skin Diseases in the Dog and Cat*. Blackwell Scientific Publications, Oxford.

Muller G., Kirk R., Scott D.W. (1989) *Small Animal Dermatology*, 4th edn. W.B. Saunders, Philadelphia.

Scott D.W. (1989) Diseases of the Skin. In: Sherding R.G. (ed) *The Cat, Diseases and Clinical Management*, Vol 2, pp 1529–1600. Churchill Livingstone, New York.

Scott D.W. (1990) Feline Dermatology 1986 to 1988; Looking to the 1990s through the eyes of many counsellors. *J. Am. An. Hosp. Ass.* **26**: 515–543.

Thoday K.L. (1990) Aspects of Feline Symmetric Alopecia. In: von Tscharner C., Halliwell R.E.W., (eds) *Advances in Veterinary Dermatology* Vol 1, Ballière Tindall, London.

Willemse T. (1991) *Clinical Dermatology of Dogs and Cats* Lea & Febiger, Philadelphia.

23

Infectious Diseases

ANDREW H. SPARKES, ALICE WOLF and JOSEPHINE M. WILLS

VIRAL DISEASES

Feline parvovirus (panleukopenia, feline infectious enteritis, cat distemper)

Feline panleukopenia, feline infectious enteritis (FIE) and cat distemper are all synonyms for disease caused by feline parvovirus infection. Feline parvovirus is found worldwide and is closely related to the parvoviruses infecting mink, raccoons and dogs. Large quantities of virus are shed in the faeces of acutely infected animals; low grade shedding may occur from the oropharynx of asymptomatic carriers. Infection is usually acquired by the oral route. The virus is very resistant to environmental degradation and may remain infectious for months or years under favourable conditions. Serious epidemics of disease can occur where large numbers of susceptible cats are housed together with ill or carrier cats in catteries, multiple cat households and rescue centres.

Feline parvovirus prefers to replicate in rapidly dividing cells, particularly the intestinal epithelium, bone marrow, and lymphoid cells. Two distinct syndromes of disease result, depending on whether the infection is acquired pre- or postnatally. 'Classic' feline panleukopenia occurs in cats over 6 weeks of age. Young kittens may develop peracute disease and die suddenly with few premonitory signs of illness. Clinical signs in older kittens or adults with acute disease include anorexia, vomiting, diarrhoea and fever. Abdominal palpation may trigger retching because of abdominal pain. Affected cats may assume a characteristic posture of 'drooping over the water bowl', presumably because they are thirsty but resist drinking because of nausea and abdominal pain. Haemograms performed at this time demonstrate severe leukopenia, particularly neutropenia.

Diagnosis of feline parvovirus infection is usu-ally based on the appearance of classical clinical signs and haematological findings in an unvaccinated cat. The differential diagnosis should also include salmonellosis and a panleukopenia-like syndrome caused by feline leukemia virus infection. Faeces can be examined for parvoviral particles if a definitive diagnosis is required.

Treatment includes supportive parenteral fluid therapy to reverse dehydration and maintain fluid and electrolyte balance. Broad-spectrum parenteral bactericidal antibiotic therapy is given to combat bacterial invasion resulting from intestinal damage and immunodeficiency due to leukopenia. Oral fluids and food should be withheld until vomiting ceases. Many cats will recover from feline parvovirus enteritis if given prompt and aggressive therapy. Diarrhoea may persist in some cats for several weeks after apparent clinical recovery because of severe intestinal damage.

Prenatal and perinatal (up to two weeks postnatal) feline parvovirus infection produces a unique syndrome of cerebellar hypoplasia, rather than gastrointestinal disease. Affected kittens are usually identified because ataxia, dysmetria and hypermetria are observed when they begin to walk. Cerebral function is unaffected and these 'shaky' kittens may make suitable pets if their gait deficit is not too debilitating.

Both killed and modified live-virus feline parvovirus vaccines are very effective in protecting cats against infection. Kittens should receive their first vaccination when they are between 6 and 8 weeks of age and this should be repeated every 3–4 weeks until 12–16 weeks of age. Adult cats should receive a total of two vaccinations, 3–4 weeks apart. Most veterinarians recommend yearly booster vaccinations to assure continued protection. Environmental contamination should be reduced by cleaning with a 1:30 hypochlorite solution and improving husbandry conditions.

Feline leukaemia virus

Feline leukaemia virus (FeLV) is a type-C oncornavirus in the family Retroviridae. It can be found worldwide and its host range includes both wild and domestic cats. Infection may be transmitted vertically from a queen to her kittens *in utero* or in milk, or horizontally from cat to cat. Saliva from FeLV infected cats often contains large amounts of virus; smaller but significant amounts are also found in other secretions and excretions. The virus is very fragile in the environment and close contact between cats is usually required for its transmission. Infection is usually acquired by the oral route; however, bite wounds may directly inoculate salivary virus. It can also be transmitted by blood transfusion but haematophagous arthropods have not been shown to transmit the disease. The incidence of FeLV infection in cat populations varies, depending on husbandry conditions; it may be 0% in closed, FeLV-negative catteries or confined households, 1–3% in free-roaming suburban cats, and up to 30% in FeLV infected multi-cat households.

Following oral exposure, FeLV replicates in the local oropharyngeal lymphoid tissue. Primary viraemia carries virus to distant lymph nodes and bone marrow where further replication occurs. A secondary viraemia then carries virus to the internal organs and epithelial tissues. The course of FeLV infection can be aborted by the cat's immune system at any point in this sequence but complete recovery is unlikely once bone marrow infection has been well established.

Susceptibility to FeLV is also age-dependent. Approximately 70% of kittens exposed to FeLV before they are 8 weeks old will become persistently viraemic. Kittens 8–12 weeks of age have a 30–50% rate of viral persistence. Adolescents and adult cats are very resistant to infection with a 10–20% rate of persistent infection following FeLV exposure.

During FeLV virus replication, proviral DNA is inserted into the genome of host cells. Some host cells may contain latent, non-replicating virus after apparent recovery from infection. These latently infected cells are removed by the immune system over the course of weeks to years. Until all virus-infected cells are cleared, FeLV replication can be reactivated by stress, concurrent disease or corticosteroid administration. Because latently infected cats are not actively producing virus, they cannot be identified by routine tests that detect FeLV antigen.

Affected cats can remain asymptomatic for months or years following infection. Clinical signs include both neoplastic and non-neoplastic disorders. Neoplastic syndromes include lymphosarcoma (multicentric, thymic, alimentary and miscellaneous) and myeloproliferative diseases (true leukaemia). Non-neoplastic disorders include haematological abnormalities (aplastic or hypoplastic anaemia, pancytopenia), neurological disorders (anisocoria, urinary incontinence, neuropathies, myelopathies), multiple cartilaginous exostoses and other benign hyperplastic syndromes, as well as FeLV-induced immunosuppression and immune-complex disease. Immunosuppression, which is responsible for much of the morbidity and mortality associated with FeLV infection, predisposes affected cats to chronic secondary viral, bacterial, fungal and parasitic infections that respond poorly to appropriate treatment. Immune-complex diseases associated with FeLV include autoimmune haemolytic anaemia, glomerulonephritis, polyneuritis, myositis, and chronic progressive polyarthritis.

The diagnosis of FeLV infection is made by identifying p27 viral core protein in serum, tears, or saliva (ELISA test), or in infected peripheral or bone marrow white blood cells and platelets (IFA test). There is at present no effective specific treatment and therapy is therefore directed at treating symptoms and secondary infections. The prognosis for FeLV infected cats depends on the status of their immune system and husbandry conditions. In multiple cat households, where they are subject to high levels of stress, crowding and concurrent disease, the mortality rate for these individuals is approximately 85% within 3 years of diagnosis. Alternatively, affected cats confined indoors in a low stress environment may live relatively symptom-free for many years.

Control of FeLV in closed feline populations is best achieved by 'test and removal' procedures. All cats in the population are tested and affected individuals are removed. This procedure is repeated until all remaining cats test negative on two sequential tests administered 3 months apart. New cats should be isolated and have two negative FeLV tests, 3 months apart, before being allowed to mingle with the remainder of the population. Free-roaming cats and cats in FeLV infected households are at the greatest risk of exposure and vaccination should be considered for these individuals. Five commercial feline leukaemia virus vaccines have been produced and a number of others are in various stages of development. None of these vaccines has provided complete protection against FeLV challenge infection but they may provide some cats with some protection. Confinement of cats to prevent exposure to FeLV carriers will also significantly reduce the risk of contracting this disease.

There is some controversy regarding the potential transmission of FeLV to humans. Although FeLV will grow in human cells in tissue culture under laboratory conditions, there is no serological or epidemiological evidence that it can infect humans or is associated with any human disease condition. Nevertheless, it is probably wise for immunoincompetent individuals (children less than 3 years of age) or immunosuppressed persons (pregnant women, people undergoing immunosuppressive cancer or organ transplant chemotherapy, and individuals infected with human immunodeficiency virus) to limit their exposure to FeLV infected cats.

Feline sarcoma virus

Feline sarcoma virus (FeSV) is a recombinant form of FeLV. It is generated *in vivo* in persistently FeLV-infected cats by rare, random integration of a host *sarc* gene into proviral DNA during replication. Each feline sarcoma virus is genetically unique, replication defective, and cannot be transmitted horizontally. Feline sarcoma virus induces the formation of single or, more commonly, multicentric fibrosarcomas in cats less than 7 years old. Diagnosis is usually based on history, physical findings, and biopsy diagnosis of fibrosarcoma in a young FeLV-positive cat. FeSV-induced fibrosarcomas, like other fibrosarcomas, respond poorly to all forms of therapy. These cats have the additional disadvantage of suffering concurrently from other forms of disease associated with FeLV. The prognosis for patients with FeSV-induced tumours is grave. Most affected cats survive less than 4 months following diagnosis.

Feline immunodeficiency virus

Feline immunodeficiency virus (FIV) is a recently discovered lentivirus infection which has rapidly become recognised as an important and prevalent disease of cats.[28] In addition to its significance as a feline pathogen, FIV is also important as a model for human immunodeficiency virus (HIV) infection. Lentiviruses are a subfamily of the retroviridae (RNA viruses) and, in common with all members of this family, FIV possesses a reverse transcriptase enzyme enabling a DNA copy of the viral genome to be made and incorporated into the chromosomal DNA of the host cell. Although FIV is a newly identified virus, retrospective serological studies have shown that it was present in domestic cat populations in the UK in 1975 and the USA in 1968, and it has probably been in existence for many centuries.

Feline immunodeficiency virus infection is endemic in domestic cat populations in most countries throughout the world, and there is also evidence of infection in wild felidae. Some variation is seen in the prevalence of infection between different countries, which may reflect differences in the cat populations studied. However, several common trends are found. Its prevalence is higher in sick cats (typically 15–20% in the UK and USA) than in healthy cats (typically 1–5% in the UK and USA), and also much higher amongst male, free-roaming and non-pedigree cats.[19] Infection is uncommon in cats less than a year old but the prevalence rises steadily with age to a peak in cats 6–10 years old.

These epidemiological findings confirm other studies which suggest that biting is the primary route of transmission for FIV. Parenteral inoculation of FIV is an efficient means of transmitting infection experimentally, and virus is known to be shed, often in high quantities, in the saliva of infected cats. It therefore appears that the cats most at risk of contracting FIV are those which roam freely, and fight frequently with other cats – behaviour which is often associated with mature male cats. Other routes of transmission are possible but probably much less important. The virus is considered to be labile and so environmental contamination is unlikely to be a major problem, although prolonged close contact between cats (including mutual grooming and sharing of feed bowls) may result in direct or indirect transmission on occasions. This is not a very efficient means of transmission, however: spread of infection in closed colonies of cats, without evidence of biting or scratching, is rare. There is no evidence of sexual transmission but vertical transmission has been observed both pre- and post-natally. Further investigation is necessary to determine how important this mode of transmission might be.

As normal immune responses are unable to eliminate FIV infection, cats develop a permanent infection. Shortly after inoculation with the virus, many infected cats undergo a distinct primary phase of infection which has several characteristic features.[35] Seroconversion occurs 2 weeks or more after infection, at which time virus may also be recovered from circulating lymphocytes. Around 5 weeks post-infection some cats show mild to moderate pyrexia lasting several days, and most develop generalised lymphadenopathy which may last for several months. Transient or prolonged haematological abnormalities, most notably neutropenia and leucopenia, also develop in some cats. Following the primary phase of infection, most or all infected cats probably go through an intermediate asymptomatic phase, which is likely to last several months to years. The exact duration of this phase is highly variable and dependent on many factors such as the age of the cat, route of infection, and perhaps pathogenic variations in viral strains of FIV. Feline immunodeficiency virus was shown early on to have a tropism for T-lymphocytes, and progressive deterioration in immune function has been documented in cats infected with FIV along with depletion of CD4+ (T-helper) lymphocytes. These features are also typical of HIV infection in humans.

The later stages of FIV infection are characterised by the development of clinical signs related to the immunodeficiency syndrome, and are similar to those which may occur following FeLV-induced immunosuppression. It is unclear whether all infected cats progress inevitably to this stage of the disease but it is probable that most do, given enough time. Clinical signs are frequently associated with secondary or opportunistic infections but the course of the disease and the signs exhibited show tremendous variation between individuals.

The major clinical signs noted in FIV-infected cats include:

- Malaise/lethargy
- Chronic stomatitis
- Weight loss
- Chronic rhinitis
- Lymphadenopathy
- Neurological disorders
- Chronic dermatoses
- Chronic gingivitis
- Inappetence
- Pyrexia
- Chronic diarrhoea
- Conjunctivitis/epiphora
- Uveitis
- Neoplasia

Diseases of the oral cavity, respiratory tract and gastrointestinal tract are most commonly encountered, in addition to non-specific signs of illness such as pyrexia, lethargy and weight loss. Some cases of severe purulent necrotising gingivitis (Fig. 23.1) have been seen in cats infected with FIV, and have also been described in severely immunosuppressed cats infected with FeLV. Although FIV is not regarded as an oncogenic virus, a high prevalence of tumours has been observed in infected cats, and a correlation has been shown between FIV infection and the occurrence of

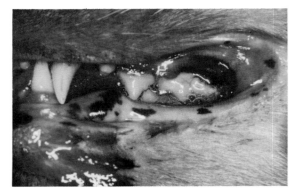

FIG. 23.1 Acute necrotising gingivitis in an FIV-infected cat.

lymphoid malignancies independent of FeLV infection. These findings may represent another aspect of the immunodeficiency syndrome associated with FIV infection. Like HIV, FIV has been shown to be neurotropic and, although not common, a variety of neurological signs have also been observed in infected cats, including behavioural abnormalities, anisocoria and convulsions.

Specific secondary or opportunistic infections identified in FIV infected cats have included:

- *Haemobartonella felis*
- Notoedric mange
- Pox virus infection
- Systemic candidiasis
- FIP
- Pyothorax
- Demodicosis
- Toxoplasmosis
- Bacterial cystitis
- Cryptococcosis
- Pyoderma
- Bacterial pneumonia

The occurrence of some of these infections would immediately raise suspicion of an underlying immunosuppression, whereas the role of FIV infection in others is uncertain.

In many cats where FIV infection is diagnosed, there is a history of chronic illness. This may start as episodes of mild recurrent disease but generally a progressive deterioration is seen, with signs becoming more persistent and more severe, although the time course for this is highly variable. In the latter stages there are often multiple severe clinical signs, which may require euthanasia or result in death. None of the clinical signs encountered are diagnostic for FIV, although the clinical picture often suggests an underlying immunodeficient state. Where the significance of finding FIV is difficult to assess, the establishment of an accurate staging system based on clinical and laboratory findings will be useful and will provide important prognostic information.

Clinicopathological abnormalities are common in cats infected with FIV, but again a diversity of changes are seen (Fig. 23.2). In general cytopenias are more common and more severe in cats with advanced clinical disease.

Routine diagnosis of FIV infection relies on the

CLINICOPATHOLOGICAL ABNORMALITIES IN FIV	
Lymphopenia	29%
Neutrophilia	27%
Anaemia	18%
Leukocytosis	13%
Leukopenia	13%
Neutropenia	11%
Hyperglobulinaemia	25%

FIG. 23.2   Common clinicopathological abnormalities in 90 cases of FIV infection.

permanent nature of the infection, and is based on the detection of serum antibodies to viral proteins in infected cats. Commercial ELISA serological tests are available in a microtitre plate form (used by many commercial laboratories) and an 'in-house' membrane ELISA (CITE®-IDEXX) form. The latter is also available as a combined test for FeLV and FIV. These tests are simple, readily available and reported to have a high sensitivity and specificity. Generally there is fairly good agreement between the different commercial and research serological tests available, although discrepancies do occur and occasional false positive or false negative results can be obtained.[3, 18] In addition to rare false negative serological results, a study employing virus isolation in conjunction with serology for FIV diagnosis has revealed that up to 20% of infected cats may be seronegative, probably for a variety of different reasons.[16, 17] A negative serological test therefore does not preclude the possibility of FIV infection. Further work is necessary to confirm the proportion of infected cats not detected by the current commercial assays and to develop more sensitive tests.

Treatment for FIV infected cats is largely symptomatic and supportive, based on clinical findings. Many of the drugs known to inhibit HIV replication are also effective against FIV, and agents such as 3-azido-3-deoxythymidine (AZT) and 9-(2-phosphonomethoxyethyl)adenine (PMEA) have been shown to have *in vitro* activity against FIV and also the potential to result in clinical improvement when administered to symptomatic cats. Nevertheless, such drugs are not without side effects and, as in humans, bone marrow suppression appears to be a frequent complication. Further trials are necessary to establish the efficacy and safety of these and other drugs for long-term use in cats, and even with this knowledge it is unlikely that widespread use of antiviral agents will be economically viable.

As many concurrent diseases are seen in FIV infected cats, it is important to continue appropriate investigations after the diagnosis of FIV to establish specific diagnoses where possible, and to institute appropriate therapy for these. In the absence of further specific diagnoses, symptomatic treatment with, for example, antibiotics is often rewarding. The use of glucocorticoids (usually daily or alternate daily prednisolone) is beneficial in some cases, probably through their potent anti-inflammatory activity. However, as these agents are themselves immunosuppressive they should be used with caution, and in the long term their use may be deleterious.

As with HIV, development of a vaccine for FIV is problematic and it is unlikely that one will be available in the near future. Present control of FIV is therefore aimed at preventing exposure of susceptible cats to the agent. The risks of a cat contracting FIV can be minimised by avoiding contact with other cats, particularly strays and ferals. Consideration should be given to keeping the cat indoors, allowing only supervised access outdoors, restricting outdoor access to the garden only or limiting outdoor access by, for example, keeping the cat in at night. Castration of male cats at an early age will reduce the desire to wander and reduce sexually motivated aggression. Control of roaming and aggressive behaviour of cats in which FIV infection has been diagnosed is also important, in order to reduce the possibility of transmitting the infection to others.

In a multi-cat household where only a proportion of the cats are infected with FIV, the risk of transmission appears low if there is no aggressive behaviour between them. Separation of infected and non-infected cats may be desirable in some situations but, in view of the problems with serological diagnosis, not all seronegative cats will necessarily be free from infection.

Viral-induced upper respiratory tract disease

Three viruses have been implicated in respiratory tract disease, (which is often described by owners as cat 'flu). The majority of cases of infectious respiratory disease are caused by either felid herpesvirus 1 (FHV 1) or feline calicivirus (FCV). Felid herpesvirus 1 was originally called feline rhinotracheitis virus, referring to the disease it causes. It is a double-stranded DNA virus and there is a single serotype. Feline calicivirus is a single-stranded RNA virus, with considerable antigenic variation. This leads to variation in virulence and pathogenicity and therefore clinical signs may be subclinical, mild or severe. The third virus, feline reovirus, is unlikely to be important clinically. It is a double-stranded RNA virus and there are three serotypes, which are present in cats worldwide. It was originally isolated from the intestine of a cat which on experimental challenge produced a mild and self-limiting syndrome of conjunctivitis, serous ocular discharge and photophobia. The clinical signs are not severe enough to warrant treatment and the condition will not be considered further.

Clinical signs

The clinical presentation of viral-induced upper respiratory tract disease is familiar to the veterinarian. The first indication of infection is often paroxysmal episodes of sneezing. This is followed by serous oculonasal discharge, becoming mucopurulent, and conjunctivitis. The cat is often pyrexic, and is depressed and inappetent. Laryngotracheitis may occur with FHV, and there may be hypersalivation, cough and voice changes or loss of voice. In severely affected cats, particularly kittens, the nasal passages can be completely blocked with mucopurulent discharge and the cat has to resort to open-mouth breathing. Bronchopneumonia or pneumonia may occur if there is secondary bacterial involvement, or if a severe pneumotropic variant of FCV is involved.

With some variants of calicivirus, small vesicles occur on the tongue, palate or median cleft of the nostrils which rapidly rupture, leaving ulcers. Ulcerative glossitis may be the only clinical sign. With FHV 1 infection, tongue ulcers sometimes occur; and occasionally there is severe eye involvement, with interstitial keratitis and corneal ulceration, which can lead to perforation of the eyeball, and adhesions of the nictitating membrane to the conjunctivae.

Ulceration of the skin has been reported rarely with both viruses, but particularly with FHV. The skin lesions vary in distribution and appearance. They can be located at the mucocutaneous junctions, around the pads, or on the medial aspect of the front legs, where the cat uses its front paws to groom its face. The lesions may be dry and crusty, or moist and granulomatous.

Abortion has been reported in cats infected with FHV experimentally. However, the abortion may have been due to the non-specific debilitating effects of the disease, rather than the virus. The role of FHV in naturally-occurring abortions is not known.

Clinical signs tend to resolve in 7–20 days. Mortality rate is not high, except in very young kittens, where dehydration can be a problem, or with particularly pathogenic variants of FCV causing pneumonia. One of the most serious consequences of FHV infection in particular is the development of chronic rhinitis and secondary sinusitis, and these cats are often referred to as 'snufflers'. This syndrome usually follows severe infection, and is extremely persistent and refractory to treatment. The virus may permanently damage the epithelial lining of the mucosae, so that persistent secondary bacterial infection can occur. These cats show recurrent signs of upper respiratory noise, nasal discharges, sneezing and occasionally chronic conjunctivitis, but are otherwise normal.

In recent years, syndromes other than respiratory tract disease have been associated with FCV. However, when susceptible cats have been infected experimentally with isolates from these syndromes, the 'classic' disease caused by FCV has been produced rather than the expected new clinical syndrome. In particular, chronic stomatitis/gingivitis and polyarthritis/transient limping syndrome are often associated with FCV. In cases of chronic stomatitis and gingivitis, FCV can often be isolated from oropharyngeal swabs, although the precise relationship is still unclear. The limping syndrome may result from natural infection with FCV but it may also follow a primary vaccination course with a live calicivirus component, after either the first or second vaccination. Signs develop within 2 days of vaccination and consist of pyrexia, depression and rapidly shifting lameness. The syndrome re-

solves in a few days. The pathogenesis is unclear, although viral antigen has been demonstrated in articular cartilage (see Chapter 17).

Diagnosis

Diagnosis of acute viral-induced upper respiratory tract disease is based on the history and the clinical signs. Some distinction can be made between FHV and FCV from the presenting signs, such as prominent ulceration of mucous membranes with FCV, or hypersalivation with FHV. In most situations, it is not necessary to confirm which pathogen is present, particularly in a single non-breeding cat, as treatment is symptomatic. However, if a breeding colony is infected endemically, then accurate diagnosis of the aetiological agent will enable the correct control policies to be implemented, to prevent further litters from becoming infected. Confirmation of infection is carried out by virus isolation in cell culture. Oropharyngeal swabs should be taken, preferably in the acute stages of the disease, ensuring the swab is moist with the cat's saliva. The swab should be sent to an appropriate laboratory, in the virus transport medium they have provided. Some transport media will maintain viability of chlamydia as well as viruses and can be stored in a freezer for at least 6 months, to be thawed when needed.

Samples should be kept cold until transported to the laboratory within 24–48 hours. If FHV is confirmed, it is a significant pathogen and other in-contact cats with the same clinical signs are likely to be infected also. If FCV is isolated, it is likely to be the cause in a cat with signs of respiratory disease, but a large percentage of clinically healthy cats carry the virus, which could be a non-pathogenic variant.

Treatment

Treatment of viral-induced upper respiratory disease is mainly supportive and designed to counter the effects of dehydration, inanition, respiratory distress and secondary bacterial infection. Nursing of the cat is very important and is best carried out by the owner in the home. The cat will be less stressed than if hospitalised, and there is less chance of cross-infection of other cats in the hospital.

Conjunctival and nasal exudates should be wiped away regularly and topical antibacterial therapy applied. If the airways are blocked, some cats may tolerate mucolytics or steam inhalation. Strong smelling foods should be offered, such as pilchards or sardines. If eating is painful due to ulceration, then soft or liquidised foods should be offered. Fluid therapy and nutritional support are indicated in those cats that are unable to sustain themselves. Liquid nutrition and fluid replacement should either be force fed, or given by nasogastric tube, at least three or four times daily.

Broad spectrum antibiotics should be given for 10 days to counter secondary bacterial infection. If swallowing is painful, paediatric syrup can be given by the owner. Specific anti-herpetic eye medications (e.g. acyclovir) can be used to treat keratitis associated with FHV.

Treatment of chronic snufflers is limited to palliative therapy with oral broad spectrum antibiotics to control bacterial infection. However, the clinical signs often recur after the antibiotics have stopped. Treatment of chronic ulcerative gingivitis associated with FCV is very disappointing. General management includes oral hygiene and broad spectrum antibiotics in conjunction with metronidazole. Corticosteroid therapy is advocated by some clinicians but their potential impact on the chronic virus carrier state should be considered.

Epidemiology

The feline respiratory viruses are maintained in cat populations in three ways. They can be transmitted from an acutely infected cat to a susceptible one, through infectious conjunctival or nasal discharges or oropharyngeal secretions. Natural transmission is via oral, nasal or conjunctival routes. High numbers of viral particles are excreted in the first 3 weeks of infection, and macrodroplets from a cat's sneeze can travel over a metre. The viruses can also persist in the environment for short periods, so fomite transmission is possible, as well as via personnel.

A more significant source of infection is the asymptomatic carrier cat. A chronic carrier state may develop subsequent to infection with either FHV or FCV. In the acute phase of disease, virus shedding stops after 10–30 days. After this time,

any cat that is persistently infected with virus is a carrier. However, there are important differences in the carrier status of the two viruses. The most significant difference is that the carrier state for FHV is characterised by a latent phase with only intermittent periods of virus shedding, whilst FCV carriers excrete virus continuously for prolonged periods. The carrier status with FHV is similar to the latency shown by herpes viruses in other species. Re-activation and re-excretion can be induced by stress such as rehousing, boarding, kittening, or corticosteroid administration. Carriers of FHV shed virus for 1–13 days about one week after the stress.

Identification of carrier cats can be difficult, and can only be confirmed by virus isolation from oropharyngeal swabs. Carriers of FHV are difficult to identify because of the intermittent pattern of shedding. Most success has been achieved by taking a series of swabs, 4–13 days after a period of stress. Re-excretion of virus may lead to recrudescence of clinical signs. These are likely to be mild, such as conjunctivitis with slight serous discharge, often unilateral. It is worth taking an oropharyngeal swab at this stage.

Viral-induced upper respiratory disease is most often a problem in kittens, particularly those in multi-cat households and breeding colonies. Re-activation of FHV occurs in queens from stress of parturition and lactation, and this is an important source of infection for kittens. Maternally derived antibody (MDA) in kittens may persist for 2–10 weeks for FHV, and for 10–14 weeks for FCV. However, the relationship between these antibody levels and actual protection against challenge is not established. Infection can take place at an early age, even in the presence of high levels of MDA. This may allow the virus to establish itself without clinical illness; if disease does occur, it is usually milder.

The clinical and epidemiological features of these diseases are summarised in Fig. 23.3.

Prevention, control and management

Vaccination against FHV and FCV is an important part of control of the disease but it should not be considered as the sole means of disease prevention. A combination of good husbandry practices,

EPIPEMIOLOGICAL FEATURES OF FELINE VIRAL UPPER RESPIRATORY TRACT DISEASE		
Factors	**Herpesvirus**	**Calicivirus**
Virus		
Isolates	Antigenically similar	Many variants
Serotype	One	Many
Virulence	Highly virulent	Varies with strain
Stability outside host	<24 hours	8-10 days
Susceptability to disinfectants	Hypochlorite, quaternary ammonium compounds, alcohol 1 in 32 dilution of household bleach is effective for catteries	Same
Route of infection	Intranasal, oral, conjunctival	Same
Site of replication	Nasal mucosa, trachea, conjunctiva	Lung, conjunctiva, nasal and oral mucosa
Clinical disease		
Incubation period	2-17 days	2-10 days
Transmission	Cat-to-cat, indirect, aerosol	Same
Course	2-4 weeks	1-2 weeks
Signs	Sneezing, nasal discharge, hypersalivation, conjunctivitis, ocular discharge, blepharospasm, coughing, pyrexia, inappetence. Occasionally ulcerative keratitis Chronic snufflers	Sneezing, nasal discharge, conjunctivitis, ocular discharge, blepharospasm, chemosis. Occasionally pneumonia, ulcers on tongue, palate, nares Ulcerative gingivitis Chronic snufflers
Morbidity	High	High
Mortality	Variable, low in adults	Variable, depends on variant
Carrier	Common (80% infected cats) Clinical signs mild to absent Latent infection - virus excreted intermittently Excretion precipitated by stress Virus shed up to 14 days following stress	Common (50% infected cats) Clinical signs mild to absent Virus excreted continuously, not specifically activated by stress Low medium and high level excretors

FIG. 23.3   Summary of the clinical and epidemiological features of feline virus-induced upper respiratory tract disease.

appropriate hygiene measures and an understanding and application of the epidemiology of the viruses, as well as vaccination, should be modified according to housing situations and disease status. Vaccinated cats are not totally protected from disease. If the cat meets a vigorous challenge with virulent virus, mild upper respiratory signs may occur, although severe disease is unlikely.

Three types of vaccine are available: modified live systemic, modified live intranasal and killed systemic. Parenteral vaccination gives good systemic immunity but weak local immunity. Most manufacturers recommend vaccination at 9 weeks and 12 weeks, followed by annual boosters. Cats at risk of exposure to high doses of viral particles could be vaccinated every 6 months. Modified live systemic vaccines produce good protection, and are safe, but care should be taken to ensure they are administered by the intended route. Infection,

and possibly the development of disease, can be produced by the cat inhaling an aerosol of a modified live parenteral vaccine, or if vaccine is left on the coat or skin for the cat to groom. The modified intranasal vaccine provides some specific advantages over systemic vaccines. It stimulates local immunity within the nasal cavity, which provides protection at the usual point of entry of the virus. This immunity is induced more rapidly than that from systemic vaccines, with protection against FHV within 5 days and partial protection at 2 days. This can be useful if a cat is due to enter a high risk area, such as a boarding cattery, and there is insufficient time available to carry out a complete vaccination course with a systemic vaccine. Vaccination in young kittens is also possible, and is not blocked by the presence of MDA. However, mild signs of upper respiratory disease, including sneezing and nasal ulcers, may occur following the use of intranasal vaccines.

Apart from the vaccine reactions described, there may be other reasons for apparent vaccine breakdowns. The cat may already be incubating the disease, or may be a carrier. Vaccinating a carrier cat will not eliminate infection, and if FHV is already present the stress of vaccination may be sufficient to reactivate latent virus and initiate clinical signs. Other factors may be involved, such as intercurrent disease (particularly immunosuppressant viruses, FeLV and FIV), infection with other respiratory pathogens or a virulent variant of FCV not protected against by the vaccine. Also, there is little information available to assess the likelihood of a vaccinated cat which meets field virus becoming subclinically infected and subsequently a carrier.

Management of virus-induced respiratory disease

Virus-induced respiratory disease is a common problem, particularly in breeding catteries, for which the veterinarian is often called upon to recommend control regimens. The appropriate advice depends on circumstances and disease status.

1. Single-cat household pet

Pet cats with access to outdoors and therefore to other cats, or those likely to enter a boarding cattery or veterinary hospital, should be vaccinated routinely. If the cat had severe respiratory disease as a kitten, it may be a carrier and periods of stress should be avoided. Rather than entering a boarding cattery at holiday time, it is less stressful for the cat if a neighbour feeds it at its home.

2. Breeding catteries

If a breeding cattery is free from respiratory virus in terms of both disease and carriers, such an ideal situation should be maintained. This is usually possible in a closed colony, but maintaining a closed colony is not practical when cats are taken to shows or to stud cats, or queens are taken in for mating, or new stock is introduced. Attempts to keep a colony virus-free include using a killed systemic vaccine, boosting cats prior to exposure to strange cats, and quarantining and swabbing any new additions to the colony.

In breeding catteries where the disease is already present, the owner may wish to eliminate the virus completely and establish a virus-free colony, or accept that the virus is present and manage the disease situation as best as possible. To eliminate the virus completely, carrier cats should be identified by virus isolation as described earlier, or through a history of queens that regularly have infected litters. These cats can be rehomed to single-cat households, or disposed of. In most cases, the disease situation is managed. A number of points can be adopted:

- Regular vaccination of adults, with boosters prior to situations of high risk exposure. Vaccination prior to mating, or during pregnancy with a killed vaccine, will help boost maternal antibodies and therefore MDA in kittens.
- Kittening and rearing in isolation. This reduces the chance of exposure of the kittens to shedding carrier cats, and is a practical method of identifying carrier queens that pass infection on to their kittens.
- If the queen is suspected to be a carrier, the kittens should be weaned into isolation, away from the dam, as soon as possible (by 4 weeks).
- If this is not possible, the cats should be protected from infection from the queen by early vaccination. Intranasal vaccination will not be blocked by MDA in the same way as the systemic vaccines. A vial of vaccine can be divided between a litter of kittens at 3 weeks old. If a systemic vaccine is to be used, repeated doses should be given every 2–3 weeks from 3 weeks until the normal time for primary vaccination.

3. Boarding catteries

Cats should be fully vaccinated prior to entering a boarding cattery. However, some cats will invariably be carriers and hygienic measures should be adopted to prevent cross-infection (Fig. 23.4).

Feline rabies

The aetiological agent of rabies is an enveloped RNA virus of the family Rhabdoviridae. The disease is found in most parts of the world except Antarctica, Australia, New Zealand, Hawaii, England, Scandinavia, Iceland and Japan. Wildlife

RECOMMENDATIONS TO PREVENT SPREAD OF THE RESPIRATORY VIRUSES IN A BOARDING CATTERY

1. Make sure all incoming cats are fully vaccinated.
2. House cats individually, unless from same household.
3. Build cattery with solid partitions between pens. Ensure frontages are at least 1 m apart, and the surface of the pen is easily washable.
4. Arrange pen so food bowl and litter tray may be removed routinely without entering the pen, i.e. do not handle cats more than necessary.
5. Either wash hands in disinfectant bucket between visiting each pen; or have a pair of rubber gloves on a peg by each pen for use only with that pen. Disinfect thoroughly before use with a new boarder.
6. Wear rubber boots and, if it is necessary to enter the pen, step into a disinfectant bath.
7. Either use disposable food trays; or have two sets of feed bowls used on alternate days. Soak used set in 1 in 32 bleach/detergent solution for several hours, and then leave thoroughly rinsed and dried until re use 24 hours later.
8. Prepare food in central area.
9. Replace badly soiled litter trays with another previously disinfected and prefilled in a central area, i.e. a similar system to the feed bowls.
10. When cat goes home, thoroughly disinfect cage, allow to dry, and preferably leave empty for 2 days before re-using.
11. Put cats with any signs of a previous respiratory infection (e.g. ocular discharge, chronic rhinitis), cats known to have had respiratory disease, and any suspect carrier cats from past experience in one section, or at one end of the cattery, and feed last.
12. Feed cats in same order every day and attend to each pen completely before moving onto the next.
13. Reduce concentration of virus in environment by adequate ventilation, low relative humidity, and optimum environmental temperature.

FIG. 23.4   Recommendations to prevent the spread of respiratory viruses in a boarding cattery. Chandler, Gaskell and Hilbery (1985) *Feline Medicine and Therapeutics* Blackwell Scientific, Oxford.

serves as the principal environmental reservoir for rabies virus in enzootic areas. Major reservoir animals include fox, raccoon, skunk and bats.[29] Transmission to cats occurs from bites of infected animals. Another source of feline rabies has been insufficiently attenuated, modified live virus rabies vaccines. This problem has been eliminated with the introduction of efficacious killed virus vaccines.

Domestic cats are more resistant than dogs to 'street' (virulent) strains of rabies virus. The incubation period following infection is highly variable and depends on the site of virus inoculation. The median incubation period in one experimental study was 42 days.[32] Virus first replicates at the inoculation site then spreads proximally via peripheral nerves to reach the central nervous system (CNS). Usually, initial clinical signs are present for only 24 hours; they include low grade fever and behavioural changes such as restlessness, irritability, hiding or increased affection. The excitatory stage ('furious' rabies) may last 2–4 days and is not exhibited by all cats. Signs during this stage include muscle fasciculations, weakness, ptyalism, ataxia and incoordination, with increased irritability and aggressiveness. The final stage ('dumb' or 'paralytic' rabies) lasts 1–4 days. Progressive neurological dysfunction during this time causes generalised paresis, paralysis and convulsions, and leads to death.

Vaccine-associated rabies has been documented in several FeLV-infected cats. Testing for FIV was not available at the time these reports were published and it is possible that other affected cats were infected with this retrovirus. Retroviral immunosuppression may have contributed to the apparent virulence of the vaccine virus in these patients. Clinical signs in cats with vaccine-induced rabies were highly variable. In some, paresis or paralysis was localised to hind limbs (the site of vaccine inoculation); in others the disease progressed to produce signs of 'classical' rabies.[8]

The clinical diagnosis of rabies infection should be suspected in a patient that develops typical clinical signs if there is possible or known exposure to a reservoir host. However, a confirmed history of appropriate pre-exposure vaccination with an approved killed rabies vaccine is usually sufficient to place rabies low on the differential diagnosis list. Alternatively, because of the serious nature of this zoonosis, it is best to assume that any unvaccinated cat with unexplained neurological or behavioural abnormalities residing in an enzootic area has rabies until proven otherwise. Appropriate precautions should be used in handling suspects.

The diagnosis can be confirmed with the histological finding of Negri bodies (accumulations of intracytoplasmic budding virus in protein matrix) within the CNS. Immunofluorescent antibody testing for virus is also a highly accurate method to detect affected animals.

Although a few clinically affected cats infected with rabies may recover, treatment is not recommended because of the risk of handling such patients. Prevention of feline rabies is becoming increasingly important because cats are now the most common rabies-infected domestic animal in the United States[29] and in some areas of Europe. A number of highly efficacious, killed virus rabies vaccines are now available and all cats in enzootic areas should be vaccinated according to local public health regulations. Cat-to-cat transmission of rabies is unusual but feral cat populations should also be controlled to reduce the risk of human exposure to rabid cats.

Feline coronavirus infections

Coronaviridae are a family of enveloped RNA viruses, which include important feline pathogens. Many different strains of coronaviruses have been isolated from cats, varying both in their virulence and their infectivity. The isolates are generally designated as one of two types:

- Feline infectious peritonitis virus (FIPV) strains, which are responsible for a fatal systemic immune-mediated disease.
- Feline enteric coronavirus (FECV) strains, which may cause subclinical disease, or mild to moderate diarrhoea in infected individuals.

The different strains of FIPV and FECV are very closely related and form a distinct antigenic cluster together with certain other coronaviruses, including transmissible gastroenteritis virus (TGEV) and canine coronavirus (CCV). The precise relationship between these viruses is not yet clear and this contributes to poor understanding of a number of aspects of feline coronavirus infections.

Feline enteric coronavirus

Feline enteric coronavirus has a tropism for the mature columnar epithelial cells of the small intestine, within which it replicates. Infection rarely results in severe disease and the virus generally causes subclinical infections, or mild to moderate diarrhoea lasting a few days, with clinical signs most likely to be seen in young kittens.[27] In colonies where FECV is endemic, it appears that some cats may remain carriers of the virus for prolonged periods (perhaps months or years) and others may have recurrent, inapparent infections.

The major significance of FECV is its close antigenic relationship to FIPV, and as a result of this antibodies induced by FECV are cross-reactive with those induced by FIPV, making interpretation of serological data problematic. Serosurveys indicate that infections with coronaviruses are endemic in most domestic cat populations throughout the world. In the USA and Europe the prevalence of seropositivity in the pet cat population is generally between 10% and 40%, but in multi-cat households or catteries the prevalence of positive titres is either zero or, more often, 80–90% or greater. It is generally thought that most seropositive cats have been exposed to FECV, and that only a small proportion have been exposed to an FIPV strain. Substantial evidence to support this theory is not yet available and it is possible that infections with strains of FIPV possessing low pathogenicity may also be prevalent.

Feline infectious peritonitis

The first descriptions of feline infectious peritonitis (FIP) in domestic cats were in the early 1960s, and it is now recognised as one of the most important of the feline viral infections. Several aspects of FIP are poorly understood at present, including the epidemiology and pathogenesis of the disease and the relationship between FIPV and FECV and other related coronaviruses.

The annual incidence of clinical FIP is probably considerably less than 1% in the general cat population. In catteries where FIP is endemic, the disease is sporadic with an annual incidence usually no greater than 5–10%. Although the incidence of FIP is low, the disease is almost invariably fatal once clinical signs develop. It is more prevalent in multi-cat households, which largely explains why pedigree cats are more commonly affected than non-pedigrees, but there is some evidence of specific breed predilections (e.g. the Burmese in the UK) which may indicate inherited predisposing factors (Fig. 23.5). There is no sex predilection with FIP. Although any age of cat can develop the disease, it is primarily a disease of young cats with most affected cats being under 2 years of age.

Cats may be exposed to FIPV from one of a number of possible sources but it is not yet possible to determine which are the most important. Environmental contamination with virus is unlikely to be of great significance as FIPV strains generally appear to be quite labile, and are susceptible to most commonly used disinfectants. Diseased cats are probably not a major source of virus: significant quantities of virus may be shed only for a short period following infection and there may be very little viral excretion by the time clinical signs develop. Furthermore, many cats that develop FIP have no known contact with other clinical cases.

Observations such as this led to the belief that carrier cats may be important in the epidemiology of FIP, and direct evidence of such a status is now available. It may be common for cats that resist challenge with FIPV to become carriers of the virus for a variable period afterwards, which may be prolonged (perhaps many months or years) in some cats. It is not known to what extent or under what conditions such cats may shed virus but it has been shown that carrier queens can sometimes pass the infection to their kittens (either *in utero* or post-natally), some of which may then develop the disease. Recently it has been suggested that FIPV strains may arise as sporadic mutations from less virulent viruses such as FECV, and that this could be a major source of virulent virus. There is some circumstantial evidence to support this hypothesis, but further studies are necessary to confirm that this does occur and to assess its potential importance in the epidemiology of FIP.

Most cats are probably exposed to FIPV by the oronasal route with initial replication of the virus in the mucosa of the gastrointestinal tract. Systemic infection occurs when the virus infects macrophages (the target cell for FIPV), within which it replicates and a cell-associated viraemia develops, resulting in widespread dissemination of the virus. The outcome following exposure to FIPV is dependent on many factors including the virulence of the infecting strain, the magnitude of viral challenge, the age of the cat, the immune response of the cat, and the route of infection. The cell-mediated immune (CMI) response to FIPV infection is thought to be a crucial factor so that a cat which develops a strong CMI response is probably able to resist challenge and become immune, whereas inadequate CMI responses allow the development of disease. The quality of the CMI response may also determine the type of disease that develops, with a poor CMI response allowing the development of effusive FIP, and an intermediate CMI response resulting in non-effusive disease – effectively a stage between effusive FIP and resistance to disease. In effusive FIP, pyogranulomatous vasculitis lesions develop in the serosal surfaces of the body cavities which lead to the development of effusions within the cavities, while in non-effusive cases the lesions are more typically granulomatous. Feline infectious peritonitis is an immune-mediated disease. A humoral immune response develops but the antibodies induced by the virus form immune complexes which contribute to the disease rather than result in a protective immunity.

The incubation period following experimental infection is short (typically 2–14 days) but under natural conditions it is extremely variable.[11] In the early stages, clinical signs may be non-specific with fluctuating pyrexia, lethargy, inappetence, weight

BREED DISTRIBUTION OF FIP		
Breed	**FIP cases (*n* =65)**	**Clinic population (*n* =1537)**
DSH	34%	49%
Burmese	20%	6%
Siamese	17%	20%
Others	29%	25%

FIG. 23.5 Breed distribution of 65 cases of FIP diagnosed at Bristol University's Feline Centre, compared to representative figures for the clinic population.

loss, and sometimes diarrhoea, but more specific signs develop as the disease progresses. They are usually classified into effusive ('wet') or non-effusive ('dry') forms of the disease, with effusive disease probably accounting for around 60–80% of cases. The duration of disease following appearance of clinical signs is variable and may last from a week to two or three months.

Effusive disease tends to have a shorter clinical course and is characterised by the accumulation of a variable amount of serous exudate within body cavities. Most commonly this involves the abdomen but involvement of the thoracic cavity is also seen, either alone or in combination with ascites. Occasionally a unilateral thoracic effusion is encountered. Accumulation of pericardial fluid is not uncommon, but the quantity is usually small.

The granulomas characteristic of non-effusive disease may occur in virtually any organs or tissues of the body but abdominal involvement is most common, with lesions developing in a variety of tissues including kidneys, liver, spleen and lymph nodes. The granulomas can be quite large, leading to palpable abnormalities in some cases, and clinical signs may develop specific to the organ(s) involved. In around 50% of non-effusive cases, there is involvement of either the central nervous system or the eyes. Neurological signs are usually multifocal and progressive, and the lesions may develop in the brain and the spinal cord. Ocular signs may be unilateral or bilateral and include retinitis, uveitis, and hyphaema (Fig. 23.6). The classification of FIP cases as either effusive or non-effusive is often arbitrary, and in many cases

CLINICOPATHOLOGICAL ABNORMALITIES IN FIP	
Lymphopenia	77%
Neutrophilia	45%
Anaemia	37%
Hyperproteinaemia	39%
Hyperglobulinaemia	39%
Hyperbilirubinaemia	25%
Azotaemia	17%

Fig. 23.7 Major clinicopathological abnormalities in 65 cases of FIP.

lesions develop typical of both forms of the disease, which may aid in the diagnosis.

Haematological and serum biochemical abnormalities are common in cases of FIP (Fig. 23.7). Hyperproteinaemia and hyperglobulinaemia have been reported in around 40–70% of FIP cases, and although this can be a dramatic finding, clearly in many cases serum protein concentrations are normal.[31] Other findings include elevations of alpha$_2$globulins and gamma globulins on serum protein electrophoresis, and other biochemical changes reflecting disease involvement of specific organs. Unfortunately, none of these laboratory findings are sensitive and specific indicators of FIP and therefore clinicopathological data need to be interpreted with care. Analysis of effusions can be particularly valuable, and in cases where non-effusive disease is suspected careful assessment should be made for the possible presence of small quantities of effusions that could be aspirated for laboratory analysis. The gross appearance of FIP effusions can be variable but the fluid is usually clear, straw-coloured and tacky (due to the high protein content), and fibrin clots may form if the fluid is left to stand. The total protein content of the fluid is in excess of 35 g/1 (and often in excess of 50 g/1), with globulins comprising at least 50% of the total protein. If a fluid does not fulfil these criteria, FIP is highly unlikely. However, these laboratory findings are not specific to FIP as some of the important differential diagnoses may produce effusions with similar protein levels. Most notable amongst these is lymphocytic cholangitis, which can result in an abdominal effusion indistinguishable from that seen with FIP (Fig. 23.8).

Coronavirus serology has been used extensively in the past as a diagnostic tool for FIP, but the

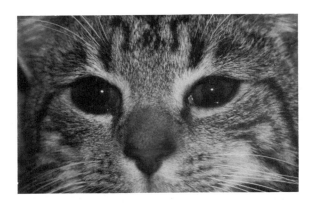

Fig. 23.6 Bilateral hyphaema in FIP.

PROTEIN ANALYSIS OF FIP AND LYMPHOCYTIC CHOLANGITIS EFFUSIONS		
	FIP	**Lym. Chol.**
Total protein (g/l)	39-98 (65)	28-109 (56)
Globulins (g/l)	23-80 (45)	7-91 (39)
Globulins as % of total	50-82 (68)	25*-83 (65)
* Only one case <50%		

FIG. 23.8 Protein analysis (range and mean) of 24 FIP effusions and 8 lymphocytic cholangitis effusions.

serological tests used currently are of limited value. As noted above, FIPV belongs to a group of related coronaviruses, and the current assays which are generally available cannot distinguish between antibodies induced by FIPV and other members of this group – most notably FECV, but CCV and TGEV may also cause asymptomatic infections in cats.[2] A large proportion of healthy cats and non-FIP diseased cats are coronavirus seropositive and a wide range of titres is observed in both these groups, although in general antibody titres tend to be higher in cats with FIP than those without FIP. While some FIP cases have low or negative titres, some cats without FIP (particularly those from multi-cat households) may have very high titres. A diagnosis of FIP cannot, therefore, be made on the basis of a high antibody titre and similarly FIP cannot be excluded in cases with low or negative titres. As with other clinicopathological data, it is essential to interpret coronavirus antibody titres critically and not to place undue emphasis on their significance. Currently a diagnosis of FIP can only be confirmed by demonstration of the typical histopathological lesions at post-mortem examination or in biopsy samples.

Once clinical signs of FIP develop, it is almost invariably a fatal disease. Symptomatic and supportive treatment (e.g. corticosteroids and antibiotics) may be palliative for a short while but deterioration will occur, necessitating euthanasia. Specific antiviral therapy may become available in the future but its value will depend on the development of improved diagnostic tests.

Control of FIP is dependent on a clearer understanding of the epidemiology of the disease and the development of an effective vaccine. Attempts at vaccine production in the past have been unsuccessful, largely due to the immune-mediated nature of the infection; antibodies induced by the vaccines have often exacerbated the disease when cats have been subsequently challenged with FIPV. Recently the first commercial FIP vaccine has been released in the USA: it is a modified live temperature-sensitive intranasal vaccine that apparently induces a strong local mucosal immunity. Experimental studies have demonstrated quite good efficacy with this vaccine, although limited reports of field use have not been so encouraging and there is some concern over the use of live coronavirus vaccines, particularly with regard to the possibility of recombination and thereby reversion to virulence.[26] No adverse effects have been reported with the modified live vaccine but development of an inactivated vaccine would be attractive.

Pox virus

The pox viruses are enveloped DNA viruses belonging to the genus orthopoxviruses of the family poxviridae. Viruses in this group include smallpox (now eradicated), vaccinia, and mouse pox virus. The virus infecting cats is identical to cowpox virus.

Pox virus infection of domestic cats and other Felidae has been described in Britain and other parts of Europe, and the condition appears to be relatively common. It is widely accepted that there is a natural reservoir host for the virus in which infection is endemic, and that cats become infected 'accidentally'. Direct and circumstantial evidence implicates small rodents as the most likely reservoir host. Most infected cats are young adults and active hunters, often (though not always) from a rural environment. Infection is usually thought to be acquired during hunting and lesions often develop at the site of a bite wound, presumably inflicted by the prey animal carrying

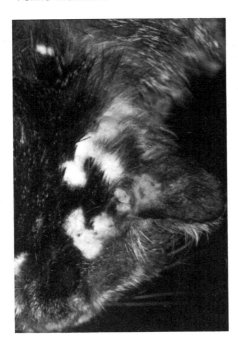

FIG. 23.9 Nodular lesions on head in pox virus infection.

the virus. Cat-to-cat transmission of pox virus has been shown to occur but is apparently rare.

Skin lesions are the dominant feature of feline pox virus infections.[24] Primary lesions may be papules, nodules (which may be crusted), or areas of cellulitis/abscessation, and usually develop on the head, neck or forelimbs (Fig. 23.9). Secondary lesions are often widespread, developing after several days to weeks; they are typically erythematous nodules, often several millimetres in diameter, which ulcerate and crust. Over several weeks the crusts separate and are shed, and the lesions regress. Healing may be considerably delayed by secondary bacterial skin infection. Pruritus is very variable and may be severe or absent.

In up to 20% of cats, systemic signs also develop which include oculo-nasal discharge, conjunctivitis, diarrhoea, anorexia and pneumonia. Severe cutaneous and systemic signs are frequently associated with immunosuppression, either iatrogenic (corticosteroids, megestrol acetate) or due to co-infections with agents such as FeLV and FIV, and in these cases the prognosis is poor.

The diagnosis may be confirmed by virus isolation performed on scab material or skin biopsies. Serology is also available but titres may remain high for months or years so that, unless a rising titre is demonstrated, recent infection cannot be confirmed.

There is no specific treatment for pox virus infection in cats and recovery is usually uneventful, although it may be prolonged. Antibiotics are routinely given until lesions have healed to prevent secondary infections but the use of any immunosuppressive agent (e.g. megestrol acetate or glucocorticoids) is absolutely contra-indicated in pox virus infections as these can induce fatal systemic disease. An Elizabethan collar may be necessary to prevent self-inflicted damage.

Rare cases of human pox virus infection have been linked to contact with infected cats, with skin lesions and 'flu type signs being reported. Pox virus infection is unlikely to be acquired from a cat if sensible hygiene precautions are taken, including the use of disposable gloves when handling infected cats.

Other viruses

Feline syncytium-forming virus

Feline syncytium-forming virus (FeSFV) belongs to the spumavirus subfamily of Retroviridae, and has a world-wide distribution. Known routes of transmission include biting (the virus is shed in saliva) and *in utero* infection of kittens, but other sources of infection may also be important and blood-sucking arthropods have been suggested as possible transmitters of the virus. Cat bites are considered important in the spread of infection, and the disease is therefore more prevalent in free roaming cats.

The virus may be recovered from many different tissues of infected cats where it is maintained as a latent infection, replication being suppressed by an immune response. Active replication occurs in the oropharyngeal region, resulting in shed of virus into the saliva. Despite the development of an immune response, infection is permanent. Whether FeSFV is a cause of disease in cats is speculative; whilst a statistical association has been demonstrated between the presence of FeSFV and the occurrence of certain diseases including proliferative polyarthritis, myeloproliferative diseases and lymphomas, experimental infections have failed to result in disease. FeSFV may serve as an indirect marker of other aetiological agents in the epidemiological studies as, for example, cats with FeSFV infection are often co-infected with FIV or FeLV due to common modes of transmission. Further studies are necessary to determine whether FeSFV is a pathogenic virus.

Herpes virus suis

Herpes virus suis is the agent responsible for Aujeszky's disease or pseudorabies. The disease has a world-wide distribution, with pigs being the natural host and reservoir for the virus. Other species can also be infected, including cats and dogs. Infection of cats occurs by direct contact with pigs, or through ingestion of infected meat. Cats are relatively resistant to infection with the virus but the condition is invariably fatal once disease develops. Virus rapidly spreads to the cranial nerves and central nervous system leading to clinical signs which include dysphagia, vomiting, hypersalivation, depression, vestibular signs, ataxia/paralysis, coma and death. Intense pruritus may also develop, usually around the face. Death is usually within 48 hours of the onset of signs. Diagnosis is based on clinical signs, histopathology, and immunofluorescent identification of the virus in tissues. The disease is highly unlikely to be encountered in Britain as an Aujeszky's disease eradication scheme has been in existence for several years.

Feline herpesvirus 2

Feline herpesvirus 2 or feline cell-associated herpes virus (FeCAHV) is closely related to bovine herpesvirus 4. The virus has been isolated from a cat suffering from feline urological syndrome (FUS), and was suggested as a possible aetiological agent in this disease. Further isolations of this virus from naturally occurring cases of FUS have not been made but it has been suggested this could be due in part to difficulties in recovering this highly cell-associated virus. Recently, experimen-

tal inoculations with FHV 2 have led to prolonged urinary tract infections but with no associated signs of lower urinary tract disease. The role of this and other viruses in the pathogenesis of FUS is still uncertain but there is no substantial evidence to date to implicate them as important pathogens.[21]

Astrovirus

Astroviruses are small RNA viruses which have been implicated as enteric pathogens in many species. They have been isolated from the faeces of cats in the USA, Britain and Australia. Although the virus can be recovered from normal as well as diarrhoeic faeces, experimental infection in kittens has resulted in mild, transient diarrhoea accompanied by pyrexia.[13] Astroviruses appear to be of low pathogenicity to cats.

Rotavirus

Rotaviruses are enveloped RNA viruses which have been isolated from kittens with diarrhoea. They have also been shown to cause mild, transient diarrhoea in experimentally infected kittens. Limited studies indicate widespread infection with rotaviruses in cat populations but, like astroviruses, they appear to be of low pathogenicity.

Reovirus

Reoviruses are non-enveloped RNA viruses which have been isolated from feline faecal samples and a wide range of body tissues. Based on limited serological studies, it appears that infection with reoviruses is widespread in cats but they are probably of low pathogenicity. In other species reoviruses may be primary or secondary pathogens in respiratory or intestinal tract diseases, and experimental infections with a reovirus isolate in cats led to a transient serous conjunctivitis.

Other enteric viruses

A variety of other viruses and virus-like particles have been isolated from the faeces of cats with or without diarrhoea, but their pathogenic potential is uncertain.[23] The isolates have included caliciviruses, picornavirus-like particles, coronavirus-like particles (morphologically distinct from FIPV and FECV), togavirus-like particles, and parvovirus particles unrelated to feline panleukopenia virus. Recently another novel agent which had characteristics of a torovirus was described in the faeces of cats. The presence of this agent was linked to the widely recognised syndrome of chronic diarrhoea accompanied by prolapse of the nictitating membranes.[25]

CHLAMYDIA

Chlamydia form an unusual group of organisms that used to be regarded as viruses. However, they are now generally regarded as highly specialised obligate intracytoplasmic bacteria.

Chlamydiosis

Chlamydiosis, or feline pneumonitis, is infection with a feline strain of *Chlamydia psittaci*, one of the most common causes of conjunctivitis in cats. In the United States it has been estimated to account for 5–10% of all feline respiratory illnesses; in the UK, chlamydia were isolated from 30% of conjunctival swabs from domestic cats with conjunctivitis.[34] The organism has also been isolated from cats in continental Europe, Canada, Japan and Australia, and it is likely to be found world-wide. The prevalence of chlamydial infection is highest in young cats and the disease tends to be more severe in kittens, often presenting with 'sticky eyes'.

Clinical signs

The organism is primarily a conjunctival pathogen, and in the early stage of the disease there is serous ocular discharge, blepharospasm, chemosis and hyperaemia of the palpebral conjunctivae. As the disease progresses, the conjunctivae become more hyperaemic and discharges become mucopurulent. The infection can be unilateral initially but soon becomes bilateral. Mild nasal discharge and sneezing may also occur, and there may be mild pyrexia at first in young kittens. However, affected cats usually continue to eat and are generally bright. More severe upper respiratory tract signs may be present but this generally reflects concurrent infection with either FCV or FHV. Clinical signs usually improve within a few weeks but mild conjunctivitis with occasional mucopurulent discharge may persist for months.

Chlamydia spp are important genital pathogens in other species and can cause infertility. However, their role in reproductive failure in cats is uncertain. They can infect the cat's genital and gastrointestinal tracts, and can be readily isolated from vaginal and rectal swabs of acutely infected cats. Abortion has been noted in some infected cats. But infertility has not been demonstrated in experimentally infected cats. The genital and gastrointestinal tracts may act as a reservoir of infection, and may be important epidemiologically.

Diagnosis

The most reliable methods of diagnosing chlamydial infection are by isolation from conjunctival swabs, or demonstration of a significant antibody titre. Conjunctival swabs should be rotated firmly over the palpebral conjunctiva, to desquamate epithelial cells to enable isolation of the organism. Conjunctival scrapings or smears taken in the first week of disease can be stained with Giemsa, and examined for intracytoplasmic chlamydial inclusions. However, this technique is unreliable, particularly after the first week. The diagnostic laboratory used by the veterinarian should be consulted prior to submission of material. If cell culture is used, then special medium is required to transport conjunctival swabs to the laboratory within 48 hours, as the organism has poor viability. There are also a number of non-cultural diagnostic methods available for identification. Chlamydial serology is useful to confirm endemic infection in a cattery; either high antibody titres or the demonstration of a rising titre. Indirect immunofluorescence (immunofluorescent antibody, IFA) is commonly used; however, high immunofluorescence titres to chlamydia will persist for over a year in cats that have apparently cleared the infection, and therefore do not necessarily indicate current infection.

Treatment

Tetracyclines are the treatment of choice for chlamydiosis in cats and it is advisable to treat both topically and systemically. Ophthalmic preparations containing tetracycline or oxytetracycline can be applied 3–4 times daily, or chlortetracycline 12 times a day. Oxytetracycline or doxycycline can be given orally, oxytetracycline up to 50 mg/kg/day, in 3 divided oral doses, or doxycycline at 5 mg/kg/day. Doxycycline, which has fewer side effects than oxytetracycline, needs only to be given once daily, and can be mixed in food with no adverse effect on absorption; however, it is more expensive. All cats in an infected household should be treated simultaneously for 4 weeks, or for at least 2 weeks after clinical signs have resolved. There is little evidence that long-term administration of doxycycline to kittens discolours their teeth or causes gastrointestinal upsets, although a yellow discoloration has been reported with oxytetracycline. *C. psittaci* is not sensitive to sulphonamides or neomycin, and only slightly sensitive to penicillin and chloramphenicol. The quinolones are effective against *Chlamydia* in other species, but they have not been evaluated in cats.

Transmission

The natural route of transmission of *C. psittaci* in cats is not clear. It is probably transmitted by close contact with infectious conjunctival and nasal secretions. The importance of infection of other sites (gastrointestinal and genital tracts) in transmission and perpetuation of the organism is not known. A 1:32 dilution of sodium hypochlorite is a suitable disinfectant to clean surfaces.

Although little is known, it is likely that a 'carrier' status exists with feline chlamydiosis. Excretion of the organism can continue for weeks or months following resolution of clinical signs. Chlamydia may persist and undergo slow replication with low numbers of organisms disseminated continuously, or it may be a true latent infection that requires activation before further excretion. Recurrent episodes of excretion may be hormonally induced, and stress factors may be involved.

Immunity

Kittens born to previously infected queens have maternally derived colostral antibodies against chlamydia, which provide reasonable protection from infection from the queen until they are about 5–8 weeks old. After this age, the kittens are susceptible to infection and disease; therefore in an endemically infected colony they should be weaned by 5–6 weeks and kept away from potentially infectious adults.

A modified live vaccine against feline chlamydiosis is available in many countries. Vaccination reduces the severity of clinical signs but does not prevent infection or excretion.[33]

Once chlamydia are endemic in a cat colony, elimination of the organisms is time-consuming, labour-intensive and expensive. Breeding should be stopped temporarily and a prolonged course of tetracyclines given to all the cats. To prevent introduction into a chlamydia-free colony, all new additions should be screened; serum that contains no chlamydial antibodies indicates that the cat has never been exposed to the organism.

There is limited evidence of feline *C. psittaci* causing disease in man. Reported cases describe a follicular conjunctivitis. In the absence of conclusive evidence, owners should be advised to maintain hygienic precautions when handling cats that are actively infected.

BACTERIAL DISEASES

Salmonellosis

Salmonella spp are motile, Gram-negative bacteria that can be isolated from the intestinal tract of a wide range of animal species. The organisms can survive for long periods outside the host and infection usually occurs by the faecal-oral route. *Salmonella* isolation rates in normal cats range from 0 to 44%. Infection and disease associated with *Salmonella* spp are most common in cats housed in groups under conditions of poor sanitation. Diseased migratory birds may also be a source of infection in individual cats that are allowed to hunt.

Most *Salmonella* infections in cats are inapparent. Clinical signs are more likely to occur in kittens than adult cats, the most common presentation being acute gastroenteritis with fever, vomiting and diarrhoea. Haematological evaluation often demonstrates severe leukopenia. Because of the similarity in clinical signs and haematological findings, salmonellosis can be difficult to differentiate clinically from feline parvovirus infection or panleukopenia-like syndrome associated with feline leukaemia virus infection. The diagnosis of salmonellosis is confirmed by ruling out the presence of other viral diseases and by isolation of *Salmonella* from the faeces.

Most *Salmonella* infections in otherwise healthy, adult cats are self-limiting within 7 days. Cats that are immunosuppressed due to concurrent retroviral infections, stress, corticosteroid treatment or other disorders are more likely to develop fatal *Salmonella* bacteraemia. Treatment includes fluid replacement and good nursing care. Chloramphenicol or trimethoprim-sulphonamide antibiotics are reported to be the drugs of choice in treating salmonellosis but their use is controversial. Antibiotic therapy may induce bacterial resistance, inhibit normal gastrointestinal flora and prolong faecal shedding of *Salmonella*. Although *Salmonella* serotypes isolated from cats can be pathogenic for human beings, cats are not considered a major source of infection for people.

Campylobacteriosis

Campylobacter jejuni is a Gram-negative, curved rod bacterium found in the intestinal tract of a variety of animal species throughout the world. Infection occurs by the faecal-oral route. Isolation rates of *C. jejuni* from normal cats range from 2–45%. The highest isolation rates come from young animals kept in high population density environments with poor husbandry conditions. The association of *C. jejuni* with disease is controversial because some studies have demonstrated identical isolation rates in clinically normal animals and those with diarrhoea.

Clinical signs reported from affected kittens include diarrhoea that may be soft and mucoid or profuse and watery, mild anorexia, dehydration, vomiting, and abdominal pain. Haematological and serum biochemistry findings are usually normal. Isolation of *C. jejuni* must be performed on specific culture media. Although the presence of *Campylobacter* in association with clinical signs of gastrointestinal illness is suggestive of a causal relationship, care must be taken not to overinterpret these findings. Healthy kittens may shed *C.*

jejuni and many other infectious agents and parasites cause diarrhoea in kittens. Most clinical signs caused by *Campylobacter* infection in older cats resolve within 7 days, though soft stools may persist for several weeks.

Kittens with severe, watery diarrhoea are subject to rapid dehydration. Treatment should include withholding oral food and water for up to 72 hours and parenteral replacement of fluids and electrolytes. Erythromycin is the antibiotic of choice for treating campylobacteriosis and is given at a dose of 10 mg/kg PO tid for 5–7 days. The clinical response to antibiotic therapy is often used to confirm *C. jejuni* as the cause of the observed clinical signs.

C. jejuni causes acute enterocolitis in human beings, particularly children. Persons should wash their hands thoroughly after handling infected cats. However cats are not considered to be a significant source of infection for people.

Escherichia coli

Escherichia coli is a variably motile, Gram-negative bacillus that is a normal inhabitant of the lower intestinal tract of a variety of animal species. A number of different serotypes of *E. coli* have been isolated; haemolytic strains are believed to be more pathogenic than non-haemolytic strains. *E. coli* organisms are relatively persistent in the environment and infection usually occurs by faecal contamination.

E. coli infection may cause a wide spectrum of clinical signs in a broad variety of organs and tissues. Infection of young animals with enterotoxigenic strains may cause severe gastroenteritis. Neonatal septicaemia resulting from infection at the time of parturition can result in pyelonephritis, pneumonia, or generalised bacteraemia. Immunocompromised cats are also susceptible to *E. coli* septicaemia and enterocolitis. Localised infections can be found in any cat and include (but are not limited to) pyelonephritis, endometritis, cutaneous abscesses, necrotic colitis, and endocarditis. *E. coli* can be isolated readily from infected tissues on routine bacteriological culture media.

Selection of a treatment regimen depends on the organs or tissues affected and the severity of infection. Antibiotic therapy should be selected on the basis of culture and sensitivity testing of the *E. coli* isolate. In general, most pathogenic isolates are susceptible to cephalosporins and aminoglycosides. Additional topical or systemic supportive care may be needed in some cats.

Mycobacteriosis

Systemic mycobacteriosis (tuberculosis)

Systemic mycobacteriosis in cats is usually caused by *Mycobacterium bovis*. Cats usually become infected by being fed untreated milk from infected dairy cattle. This infection is rarely seen in developed countries because of effective tuberculosis eradication programmes in cattle. Cats are much less susceptible to infection by *M. tuberculosis* (the tubercle bacillus of human beings), *M. avium* (causative agent of avian tuberculosis), and *M. microti* (vole bacillus). However, occasional feline cases have been described in the literature. Infection with *M. bovis* is usually acquired by ingestion; infection by inhalation or direct inoculation through the skin or mucous membranes has been documented in some cats. Systemic mycobacteriosis occurs most commonly in cats less than 5 years old. Most affected cats develop signs of chronic illness and wasting. Gastrointestinal signs are usually present and include vomiting, diarrhoea, inappetence, and abdominal mass lesions (granulomas) associated with intra-abdominal parenchymal organs. Pulmonary lesions are present in approximately 40% of affected cats and cause dyspnoea, pleural effusion, and in some cases coughing. Unifocal cervical or submandibular lymphadenopathy is an occasional sign; cutaneous lesions may arise from extension of infection from the underlying lymph nodes. Nasal cavity infection may cause nasal discharge and facial distortion. Tubercular metritis has been reported in a few queens. Rarely observed clinical signs include ocular disease and infection of the central nervous system, bones or joints. The results of haematological and serum biochemistry profiles are usually nonspecific and reflect the chronic, inflammatory character of the disease. Findings can include normocytic, normochromic, nonresponsive anaemia, leukocytosis, and hyperglobulinaemia. The diagnosis of systemic mycobacteriosis in confirmed by finding typical acid-fast bacilli in exudates or biopsy specimens from affected tissues.

Unfortunately, the diagnosis of systemic mycobacteriosis is not confirmed in most cats until late in the course of debilitating illness or post-mortem. Even if mycobacteriosis is recognised early, effective chemotherapeutic protocols have not been reported. Additionally, there may be a significant public health hazard to owners and veterinary personnel handling an affected cat. Therefore, because of the grave prognosis for the cat and the human health risk, euthanasia of the *M. bovis* infected cat is usually the kindest and wisest course.

Feline leprosy

Feline leprosy is caused by the acid-fast bacillus *Mycobacterium lepraemurium*, or a closely related species. The organism is ubiquitous; affected cats have been identified in many parts of the world. *M. lepraemurium* infection is probably acquired from rodent carriers and is more common in coastal areas than inland. Young cats less than 5 years old are most frequently affected.

Clinical signs consist of single or multiple skin lesions which are plaque-like and painless. The surface of the lesions may be ulcerated but discharge is not usually noticed. Lymph nodes draining the affected area are usually enlarged but *M. lepraemurium* organisms are difficult to find within them. The diagnosis of feline leprosy is confirmed by finding acid-fast bacilli within biopsy specimens from the skin lesions.

Complete surgical excision of the lesions is the treatment of choice but recurrence following surgery is common. Medical therapy following surgical removal consists of dapsone at 1 mg/kg PO tid for 2–4 weeks or clofazimine at 2–8 mg/kg sid for 6 weeks, then q72h for 4–8 additional weeks. There is no reported public health risk associated with feline *M. lepraemurium* infection.

Atypical mycobacteriosis

Atypical mycobacteriosis is caused by infection by a number of different *Mycobacterium* spp. The organisms are soil-borne and infection usually occurs by direct inoculation (trauma) or contamination of pre-existing wounds. Atypical mycobacteria are found world-wide but are more commonly isolated in humid, tropical climates.

These mycobacteria usually cause chronic cutaneous or subcutaneous fistulae and abscesses, or granulomatous panniculitis. Regional lymphadenopathy is present in some affected cats but systemic dissemination is rare. The atypical organisms may not be numerous in affected tissues and acid-fast stains should be performed on biopsy specimens taken from several sites. Most of them are reported to grow well on blood plates incubated at 37°C.

Surgical removal of affected tissues is often unsuccessful and incomplete excision usually results in wound dehiscence. Antibiotic therapy can be based on culture and sensitivity testing of the mycobacterial isolate; however, *in vivo* therapeutic results may not correlate well with apparent *in vitro* sensitivity. A recent report suggests that medical therapy with norfloxacin at 22 mg/kg PO bid, or (by extrapolation) enrofloxacin at 2.5 mg/kg PO bid, may be useful in the treatment of some of these atypical mycobacteria.

There is no known public health risk associated with feline atypical mycobacteriosis.

Pseudotuberculosis (*Yersinia pseudotuberculosis*)

Pseudotuberculosis is caused by the Gram-negative bacillus *Yersinia pseudotuberculosis*. This organism has been isolated from healthy cats and from a number of mammalian, avian and reptilian species. Cats usually become infected by ingesting infected rodents or birds. Immunosuppression may play a role in the development of illness in infected cats.

Clinical signs of pseudotuberculosis are usually referable to the gastrointestinal tract or abdomen and include fever, anorexia, vomiting, diarrhoea, abdominal pain, icterus, depression, and weight loss. Hepatosplenomegaly and peritoneal effusion are present in some cats. Lung involvement has been reported in a few cats but is rare. A definitive diagnosis can be made by identification of *Y. pseudotuberculosis* organisms in biopsy specimens from the liver or other affected tissues.

Antibiotic therapy with tetracycline, penicillin, chloramphenicol, or streptomycin may be successful if the disease is recognised early. As *Y. pseudotuberculosis* has reportedly been transmitted from cats to humans, affected cats should be handled with caution.

Plague

The causative agent of plague is *Yersinia pestis*, a small, Gram-negative bacillus. Plague occurs worldwide as an enzootic infection transmitted by flea bites in localised rodent populations. Cats become accidental hosts by ingesting infected rodents or being bitten by infected rodent fleas.

Following infection, the *Yersinia* organisms multiply rapidly regionally, and then disseminate haematogenously to internal organs and tissues. The bubonic form is most common and is characterised by regional lymphadenitis near the site of bacterial entry, which is usually the head and neck. The less common pneumonic form produces rapidly progressive pneumonia and overwhelming bacteraemia. Occasionally, both forms are found in the same animal. Diagnosis of plague is confirmed by identifying *Yersinia* organisms in exudate draining from or aspirated from affected lymph nodes, or cultured from blood.

Tetracycline is the antibiotic of choice for the treatment of *Y. pestis* infection; streptomycin and chloramphenicol are also reported to be effective. *Y. pestis* is a significant pathogen for humans and affected animals must be handled with caution. Contact with infectious exudates spontaneously draining or released from lymph nodes by surgical drainage is particularly hazardous. Public health officials should be notified if an affected cat is identified and prophylactic antibiotic therapy may be recommended for the attending veterinarian(s) and the cat's owners.

Leptospirosis

Cats are susceptible to infection with a number of different *Leptospira* spp. *Leptospira* are spirochaete-like bacilli that are commensal parasites found in the renal tubules of carrier host mammals. The organism is relatively sensitive to environmental degradation but may persist for a considerable time under warm, moist conditions. Following oral ingestion, the organism spreads haematogenously and rapidly localises in the kidneys and liver.

Feline *Leptospira* infections are usually asymptomatic and self-limiting within 7 days; the occurrence of clinical signs of leptospiral nephritis is rare. Confirming the diagnosis of leptospirosis is difficult because serological tests for anti-leptospiral antibodies do not correlate with *Leptospira* isolation in most cats. Leptospiral organisms may be identified on histological examination of kidney tissue or in bacteriological cultures of urine or affected organs.

Because few cases of clinical feline leptospirosis have been reported, little information is available regarding effective treatment. Combination therapy with penicillin and streptomycin has been used to eliminate *Leptospira* infection successfully in dogs. Some strains of *Leptospira* capable of infecting cats are pathogenic for humans. However, because of the rarity and self-limiting nature of leptospiral infections in cats, they are not considered a significant source of human exposure.

Septic infections

Pasteurellosis

Pasteurella multocida is a small, Gram-negative, facultative anaerobic bacillus that inhabits the oral cavity of cats and many other species. It is frequently isolated from infected cutaneous wounds and abscesses and is most likely introduced by bite wounds or licking.

Most *Pasteurella* infections in cats are superficial and well localised. The organism may be a secondary invader following viral respiratory infection and is often isolated from pleural exudates in cats with pyothorax. Septicaemia associated with pasteurellosis in cats is rare. Diagnosis is made by isolation of the organism from affected tissues.

Cutaneous *Pasteurella* infections are best treated by incisional drainage (for abscesses) and thorough topical cleansing. Systemic therapy with chloramphenicol, tetracycline, trimethoprim-sulphonamide or penicillin may be used to treat deeper infections or as an adjunct to topical therapy. Humans are susceptible to *Pasteurella* infections resulting from cat bite wounds.

Staphylococcus infections

Staphylococcus spp are small, Gram-positive, coccoid bacteria that are found in the environment, and on the skin and mucous membranes of the upper respiratory tract of mammals. Most of the organisms in this group are opportunistic pathogens and secondary invaders.

Staphylococci cause both deep and superficial infections that have no unique characteristics. Definitive diagnosis is made by isolation of the organism from infected tissues. Antibiotics should be selected by sensitivity testing because *Staphylococcus* spp are noted for their ability to develop resistance to penicillin and beta-lactam antibiotics. There is no public health hazard associated with feline staphylococcal infections.

Streptococcosis

Streptococcus spp are small, Gram-positive, coccoid, chain-forming bacteria that are normal inhabitants of the mucous membranes of the oral, respiratory and genitourinary tract and lower gastrointestinal tract. Outbreaks of disease in catteries caused by streptococci are often associated with poor husbandry conditions.

Streptococci can cause deep or superficial pyogenic infections that are indistinguishable from other bacterial infections. Cattery populations may be affected by epizootic streptococcosis, a specific syndrome that includes fever, mandibular lymphadenopathy with suppuration, conjunctivitis, sinusitis, cutaneous abscesses, and septic pleuritis. Neonatal streptococcosis is also a cattery problem, resulting from infection of kittens at the time of parturition. Affected kittens fail to thrive and necropsy examination demonstrates omphalophlebitis, peritonitis, thromboembolic hepatitis, myocardial necrosis, and pneumonia. Neonatal streptococcosis usually affects the kittens of primiparous queens; subsequent litters produced by these animals are usually normal.

Penicillin antibiotics are the drugs of choice for the treatment of streptococcal infections. Local incision, drainage and topical therapy may be indicated in some cats. Improved husbandry conditions will also decrease the occurrence of epizootic streptococcosis in cattery populations. Neonatal streptococcal septicaemia can be controlled by dipping the kittens' umbilical remnant in tincture of iodine and by administering benzathine and procaine penicillin at a dose of 150,000 IU SC of each compound to the queen and 7,500 IU SC of each to kittens at the time of parturition. It has been suggested that cats are reservoirs for group-A streptococci affecting humans; however, there is some evidence that humans may transmit this agent to cats, rather than the reverse.

Other miscellaneous bacterial diseases

Borrelia burgdorferi

The spirochaete *Borrelia burgdorfei* is the causative agent of Lyme disease, a condition recognised in humans and dogs, with a variety of clinical signs including arthritis in many cases (see Chapter 17). Ticks are considered to be a major vector of the organism. There is little information regarding *B. burgdorfei* infection in cats, but serological studies in the USA indicate a lower prevalence of antibodies in cat populations than in comparable dog populations. Initial studies have failed to demonstrate a clear association between seropositivity and clinical signs of Lyme disease, and it is uncertain whether the organism is a cause of disease in cats. The organism is susceptible to a wide range of antibiotics, including tetracyclines.

Tyzzer's disease

Tyzzer's disease is caused by the Gram-negative, spore-forming *Bacillus piliformis*. Feline disease associated with this agent is rare and occurs almost exclusively under conditions of poor husbandry and immunosuppression. Clinical signs include anorexia, depression, and diarrhoea. No effective treatment has been described because the diagnosis is usually confirmed by necropsy examination.

Brucellosis

Experimental infection of cats with *Brucella canis* produces transient bacteraemia but no clinical signs of disease. *Brucella* spp are not considered to be significant pathogens of the cat.

Tetanus

Clostridium tetani, a ubiquitous soil-borne bacillus, is Gram-positive, spore-forming and anaerobic. Disease results from inoculation of infectious spores into areas of hypoxaemic tissue. Clinical signs are similar to those in the dog and include spastic extensor rigidity of the limbs, prolapse of the nictitating membrane, and facial trismus. Tactile or auditory stimulation often aggravates extensor hypertonus. Treatment includes wound debridement, penicillin therapy, provision of a quiet environment, and supportive nursing care to maintain hydration and nutritional status. Muscle relaxants and tranquillisers may be used to reduce muscle tone. With prompt recognition and proper care, complete recovery is usual but may take as long as 4–6 weeks. Cats are relatively resistant to tetanus and prophylactic vaccination with tetanus toxoid is not recommended.

Actinomycosis

The Gram-positive *Actinomyces* spp are coccobacillary to filamentous bacteria. They occur worldwide and several species are normal inhabitants of the oral cavity and gastrointestinal tract of animals. *Actinomyces* infections are uncommon in cats and usually produce pyogenic or pyogranulomatous lesions in cutaneous or deeper tissues. The 'sulphur granules' seen classically in actinomycotic exudates are clusters of interwoven bacterial filaments. A definitive diagnosis of actinomycosis is made by identifying *Actinomyces* in exudates or bacterial culture. Treatment consists of surgical drainage of deep lesions combined with long-term (months) antibiotic therapy with penicillin. Tetracycline, erythromycin, cephalosporins, lincomycin, and clindamycin may also be effective.

Bordetellosis

Bordetella bronchiseptica, a small, Gram-negative coccobacillus, is a normal inhabitant of the upper respiratory tract of animals. Clinical disease caused by *Bordetella* is unusual in cats but this organism has been identified as a cause of bronchopneumonia in catteries. As with many other bacterial disorders, stress, crowding and poor husbandry conditions contribute to the incidence of disease in these environments. Tetracycline, chloramphenicol, aminoglycosides, cephalosporins or trimethoprim-sulphonamide can be used to treat *Bordetella* bronchopneumonia. Some cat breeders have used canine *Bordetella* bacterins in an attempt to prevent bordetellosis; however, these products have not been tested in cats for efficacy or safety and cannot be recommended. Improved cattery husbandry, including control of viral upper respiratory disease, is the best method of preventing feline bordetellosis.

Miscellaneous anaerobic bacterial infections

Anaerobic bacteria, including several species of *Bacteroides*, *Fusobacterium* and *Clostridium*, are frequently isolated from pyogenic infections in cats. Many of these organisms are normal inhabitants of the mouth and the distal genitourinary and gastrointestinal tract of animals. Following inoculation by means of bite wounds or trauma, anaerobic bacteria may cause infection in any tissue, organ or body site. Exudates produced by these bacteria are often tenacious, malodorous and highly suppurative. Definitive diagnosis is made by identification of the causative organism(s) in anaerobic culture. Most anaerobic organisms are susceptible to treatment with the penicillins, cephalosporins, clindamycin and metronidazole. Surgical curettage to remove necrotic tissue and improve tissue oxygenation will enhance healing.

Anthrax

Bacillus anthracis is a large, Gram-positive, spore-forming bacillus. Anthrax is most common in cattle and sheep. Cats are rare, accidental hosts and usually contract the disease by ingestion of infected meat. *Bacillus anthracis* is rapidly invasive producing overwhelming bacteraemia that results in acute death. A definitive diagnosis is made by identifying anthrax bacilli in post-mortem blood smears. The disease is not treatable once bacteraemia has ensued. Prevention is achieved by avoiding feeding raw meat. *Bacillus anthracis* is a significant human health hazard. Infected carcases should be handled with caution and incinerated or chemically decomposed to prevent further environmental contamination.

Listeriosis

Listeria monocytogenes, a small, Gram-positive coccobacillus, is environmentally hardy and resides in soil, water and sewage. Cats apparently possess a high degree of natural resistance to listeriosis. Clinical signs attributed to feline listeriosis include a rapidly fatal septicaemic syndrome that consists of fever, gastrointestinal colic, vomiting and diarrhoea, and an encephalitic syndrome that has not been well described. Most diagnoses are confirmed by bacterial culture obtained during post-mortem examination. Combination antibiotic therapy with ampicillin and gentamicin is recommended if the disease is recognised early. Trimethoprim-sulphonamide may also be effective and is preferred for central nervous system infection.

Moraxella

Moraxella lacunata is a small, Gram-negative coccobacillus that causes conjunctivitis in human beings and is related to *M. bovis*, the causative agent of bovine 'pinkeye'. *Moraxella lacunata* has been identified as the cause of an outbreak of conjunctivitis in a cattery, where treatment with tetracycline was curative.

Nocardiosis

Nocardia spp are aerobic, filamentous bacteria found in soil, straw, decaying vegetation and grasses. Nocardial infections are often opportunistic and may be associated with immunosuppression. Traumatic cutaneous inoculation of the organism results in progressive subcutaneous abscessation, most commonly on the distal limbs. Inhalation of *Nocardia* results in pneumonia and exudative pleuritis that is clinically indistinguishable from other forms of septic pleuritis. As the disease progresses, there may be systemic illness, wasting and dissemination of nocardial infection to other tissues. Definitive diagnosis is based on identification of the filamentous organism in cytological preparations or biopsy specimens. Affected cats should be tested for the presence of FeLV and FIV, because treatment of cats with concurrent retroviral infections is unlikely to be successful. Antibiotic therapy should be selected on the basis of culture and sensitivity testing if available. Trimethoprim-sulphonamide is usually the drug of choice for the treatment of nocardiosis. Because treatment with this agent is often needed for 4–6 months, folic acid should be given concurrently at a dose of 5 mg PO sid to prevent deficiency. Alternative drugs include amikacin, minocycline or chloramphenicol. Thoracic drainage and pleural lavage should be performed in patients with nocardial pleuritis. Nocardiosis is often extremely resistant to treatment and the prognosis for affected cats is guarded.

Dermatophilosis

Dermatophilus congolensis is a Gram-positive, filamentous, septate bacillus. It is a normal inhabitant of the skin of mammals and usually causes a superficial infection of the skin of larger mammals; infection of cats is rare.

Feline dermatophilosis occurs as a subcutaneous infection because of deep inoculation of the organism through open wounds or by trauma. *Dermatophilus* lesions may occur as granulomas in the mouth or tonsils, granulomatous lymphadenitis (usually of the popliteal lymph nodes) with fistulation, cutaneous lesions, or subcutaneous lesions in miscellaneous sites. Diagnosis is made by the identification of the organism on cytological examination of, or bacteriological culture from, exudates or tissue scrapings, or during histopathological examination of biopsy specimens.

Treatment consists of local excision of the lesions followed by several weeks of antibiotic therapy with penicillin. The prognosis for affected cats is good.

MYCOPLASMA

Mycoplasmas are small, coccoid, bacteria-like organisms lacking cell walls. In the cat, they are ubiquitous and are divided into three groups: Mycoplasma, Ureaplasma or T-mycoplasma, and Acholeplasma. Numerous species or strains have been isolated, including *Mycoplasma felis, M.*

gateae, M. feliminutum, M. arginini, Acholeplasma laidlawi, and ureaplasmas. However, their pathogenic role in disease is controversial. A number of studies looking at the frequency of isolation from healthy and sick cats demonstrate conflicting results: some show comparable isolation rates whilst others show significant differences. *M. felis* is the most commonly isolated species, followed by *M. gateae.*

Mycoplasmal conjunctivitis is caused predominantly by *M. felis.* Clinical signs and pattern of disease are similar to those caused by *Chlamydia psittaci,* with blepharospasm, chemosis, conjunctival hyperaemia and serous ocular discharge. A mild rhinitis and sneezing may occur. Infection can be unilateral initially, but can become bilateral. Clinical signs resolve after two to six weeks, although the organism can persist, and recurrent milder bouts of conjunctivitis may occur. More severe upper respiratory tract signs may be present, if other pathogens are involved, particularly Chlamydia or the respiratory viruses. Young kittens are more susceptible than adults, and it is a disease of multiple-cat households as well as single cats.

Diagnosis is based on isolation of *Mycoplasma* spp. from the conjunctival sac, for which specialist medium is required. Occasionally *M. felis* can be cultured on blood agar. Conjunctival smears stained with Giemsa may show numerous small coccoid rods on the surface of conjunctival epithelial cells or free. However, care should be taken to differentiate them from melanin granules, which are often present in the cytoplasm of conjunctival epithelial cells.

Mycoplasmal conjunctivitis can be treated effectively with topical tetracycline or oxytetracycline eye preparations, which are also effective against chlamydial conjunctivitis. Systemic treatment is not necessary, as cats appear to be resistant to developing systemic mycoplasmosis. Clinical signs will improve rapidly, within 5 days.

Mycoplasmas do not seem to be an important cause of respiratory disease in cats, though they may be secondary opportunist agents in acute upper respiratory tract disease and occasional reports of mycoplasmal pneumonia and pulmonary abscessation appear in the literature. The organisms have been isolated from the urinary tract of normal cats, and they have been implicated in feline lower urinary tract disease (formerly FUS), but attempts to isolate mycoplasmas from the urine of diseased cats has been unsuccessful. Ureaplasmas and *M. gateae* have been associated with spontaneous and experimentally induced abortions, foetal deaths and poor kitten survival. *M. gateae* has also been linked to a syndrome of arthritis and tenosynovitis in older cats; this is likely to be an opportunist infection in immunocompromised cats and the condition responds well to systemic tetracyclines. Mycoplasma-like organisms have been isolated from chronic, antibiotic-resistant cutaneous abscesses, for which treatment with tetracycline was successful.

FUNGAL DISEASES

The major systemic mycoses that affect cats are the dimorphic fungi *Histoplasma capsulatum*, *Blastomyces dermatitis* and *Coccidioides immitis*, all of which exist as free-living organisms in the soil. They have relatively well defined geographic distributions, based on their growth requirements for moisture and soil enrichment, and cats may become exposed while travelling through endemic areas. Alterations in the local environment, such as irrigation or drainage, can change a formerly unsuitable habitat into a site that favours fungal growth.

Mammals become infected by inhalation of infectious fungal particles from the environment. The dimorphic fungi convert from a mycelial to a parasitic phase at body temperature. Failure of the immune system to contain the infection in the pulmonary system results in general dissemination to other body organs via blood or lymphatics. Rare infection by direct cutaneous inoculation has been reported with *Coccidioides*.

Cats are very susceptible to infection with *Histoplasma*, moderately susceptible to *Blastomyces*, and highly resistant to infection by *Coccidioides*.

Histoplasmosis

Affected cats range in age from 4 months to 13.5 years, with the majority of cases occurring in cats less than 4 years of age. There is no known breed or sex predilection for this disease.

Signs of pulmonary disease are present in approximately 50% of affected cats and include dyspnoea, tachypnoea, and abnormal lung sounds. Non-specific signs of illness are also present including depression, fever, anorexia, weight loss, and pale mucous membranes. Dissemination of the infection occurs in most cats and other common findings include peripheral and visceral lymphadenopathy, hepatomegaly, granulomatous chorioretinitis, and lameness due to osseous involvement. Rare signs include skin lesions, oral ulcers, splenomegaly, nasal polyps, vomiting, and diarrhoea.

Normocytic, normochromic, non-regenerative anaemia is the most common clinical pathological abnormality. Leukocyte counts are often normal but some cats have developed leukopenia, lymphopenia, or severe pancytopenia. *Histoplasma* organisms can occasionally be found in circulating monocytes or neutrophils during routine blood film examination. Biochemistry profiles may reveal non-specific changes including hypoalbuminaemia, hyperproteinaemia and hyperglobulinaemia, or mild elevations of serum ALT activity and serum glucose levels. Urinalyses are usually normal. Most cats are not concurrently infected with feline leukaemia virus (FeLV) or feline immunodeficiency virus (FIV).

Thoracic radiographs reveal a linear or diffuse interstitial pattern that may be miliary or patchy. Affected bones are usually those of and surrounding the carpus and tarsus. Radiographic lesions in bone include osteolysis and osseous or periosteal proliferation.

Diagnosis is usually made by demonstration of the *Histoplasma* organisms in fine needle aspirates or biopsy specimens of affected tissues. Because most systemic mycotic agents affect the interstitium rather than the alveoli, transtracheal wash and bronchoalveolar lavage are less likely to recover organisms from the pulmonary tree. *Histoplasma* organisms are usually contained within cells of the mononuclear phagocyte system and are small (2–4 µm), single or multiple round bodies with a basophilic centre and lighter halo when stained with Wright's type haematological stains. Organisms are most easily discovered in lung and lymph node aspirates, and in bone marrow. Other tissues can be examined as directed by the clinical findings in each patient. Tissue biopsy can also be used to confirm a diagnosis of histoplasmosis. However, *Histoplasma* organisms do not stain well with H&E stains and special fungal stains are usually necessary to detect them in histopathological sections. Unfortunately, serological tests to detect antibody against *Histoplasma* are usually falsely negative in most cats with naturally occurring histoplasmosis.

Treatment should be instituted promptly because feline histoplasmosis progresses rapidly and the prognosis for all cats is guarded. The treatment of choice for most cats is combination therapy with amphotericin B and ketoconazole (KTZ). Amphotericin B is given intravenously by slow infusion at a dose of 0.25–0.50 mg/kg in 80 ml/kg of 5% dextrose solution. Treatments are given q48–72h until a total cumulative dose of 5.0–10.0 mg/kg is reached or drug-associated nephrotoxicity occurs. Nephrotoxicity may be reduced by adding 2 g/kg of mannitol to the amphotericin B infusion, or by prior saline loading or furosemide treatment. Renal function should be closely monitored during the course of treatment. If the blood urea nitrogen (BUN) level is 40–60 mg/dl, treatment should be suspended until the BUN values are normal. If the BUN value is greater than 60 mg/dl, amphotericin B treatment should be completely discontinued. Recently, it has been shown that liposomal encapsulation or lipid association of amphotericin B greatly reduces its toxicity without loss of therapeutic effects. This strategy may greatly enhance the ability to treat these systemic mycoses effectively.

KTZ therapy is initiated at 10–15 mg/kg PO bid concurrently with the above and is continued for 4–6 months after amphotericin B treatment is terminated. The acute adverse effects of KTZ include anorexia and vomiting. These signs will usually subside if the administration of KTZ is stopped for a few days, reinstated at a lower dose, and then slowly increased back into the therapeutic range over 10–14 days. Chronic side-effects of KTZ therapy include hepatotoxicity and lightening of the hair coat colour. These changes are usually reversible when KTZ administration is discontinued.

Itraconazole (ITZ) is another triazole that has shown good efficacy against *Histoplasma* in experimental animals and in clinical studies in dogs and cats. ITZ is given orally at a dose of 10 mg/kg sid and has fewer adverse effects than KTZ. This drug is currently under experimental new drug status but may soon be available on the human market. All of the azole drugs are teratogenic and embryotoxic and should not be given to pregnant animals.

Blastomycosis

Cats affected with blastomycosis range in age from 6 months to 18 years; however, approximately two-thirds of affected cats are less than 4 years of age. Male cats and Siamese or Siamese crossbreed cats may be at higher risk for infection.

Most of the clinical signs of feline blastomycosis relate to the respiratory system and include dyspnoea, tachypnoea, and cough. Fever, anorexia and weight loss commonly accompany these signs. Other systems may be affected causing central nervous system signs (ataxia, blindness, seizures), ocular lesions (anterior uveitis, retinitis, chorioretinitis), peripheral lymphadenopathy, skin lesions, vomiting and diarrhoea, and renal insufficiency. Pleural or peritoneal effusion has been reported in a few cats.

The haematological findings in feline blastomycosis are similar to those previously described for histoplasmosis with the exception that severe pancytopenia does not occur. Hyperglobulinaemia is common but other serum biochemistry tests are usually normal. Most cats are not concurrently infected with FeLV or FIV. Thoracic radiographs demonstrate a pattern of lung involvement similar to feline histoplasmosis; however, more discrete mass-like lesions and hilar lymphadenopathy also occur.

The diagnosis of feline blastomycosis is accomplished by finding the organism in cytological preparations or tissue biopsy specimens. The organism is usually found extracellularly and is a large (5–10 μm) budding yeast. Special fungal stains are useful to demonstrate *Blastomyces* in tissue sections. Serological tests for antibodies against *Blastomyces* are negative in most cats.

Feline blastomycosis is treated with amphotericin B and KTZ as previously described for histoplasmosis. These drugs do not penetrate the eye well and severely affected eyes should be enucleated. If the eye is considered savable, subconjunctival treatment with amphotericin B in a single dose of 125 µg has been recommended. The CNS is another protected site and successful treatment of CNS blastomycosis has not been reported. The prognosis for cats with blastomycosis is guarded to grave.

Coccidioidomycosis

Cats appear to be highly resistant to infection by *Coccidioides immitis* and only a few cases have been reported. Therefore, little is known about age, breed or sex predilections for this disease. Clinical findings have included respiratory signs, draining skin lesions, peripheral lymphadenopathy, and lameness due to osseous lesions. Haematological and clinical pathological findings have not been described. Thoracic radiographic findings should be similar to the other systemic mycoses.

Coccidioides organisms are large (10–80 µm), extracellular, double-walled spherules. Organisms are most likely to be recovered from lymph node aspirates and exudate from draining skin lesions. *Coccidioides* spherules are not abundant in affected tissues and it is often necessary to use fungal stains to find them in biopsy specimens. Serological testing (immunodiffusion, complement fixation) for antibodies against *Coccidioides* may be helpful in confirming a diagnosis although few cats have been evaluated.

The recommended treatment for feline coccidioidomycosis is KTZ alone at 10–15 mg/kg PO bid. ITZ may also be effective against this organism. Treatment should continue for 4–6 months or for at least 2 months following resolution of clinical signs and lesions. If complement fixing (CF) antibodies were present, the CF titre can be used in conjunction with evaluation of the clinical signs to monitor the response of the patient to treatment. The prognosis for cats with coccidioidomycosis is guarded.

Cryptococcosis

The age range of cats affected with cryptococcosis is 1 to 13 years with an average of 5.2 years. There is no apparent breed or sex predilection.

Clinical signs are most commonly associated with the respiratory tract, usually the nasal cavity and nasal sinuses. Infection induces the formation of granulomatous mass lesions in the nasal cavity and results in nasal discharge that ranges in character from mucopurulent to haemorrhagic. Local extension of the infection may cause facial ulcers or regional lymphadenopathy. Skin lesions and peripheral lymphadenopathy occur in approximately 35% of feline patients. The CNS may be invaded directly or by erosion of nasal infection through the cribriform plate. Clinical signs of CNS involvement can be quite variable and include depression, amaurotic blindness, ataxia, circling, paresis, paralysis, and seizures. Ocular lesions include optic neuritis, granulomatous chorioretinitis, retinal detachment, and anterior uveitis. *Cryptococcus* also occasionally affects the lung, bone and kidney. Cryptococcal infection is unusual in its failure to cause many signs of systemic illness. Malaise, anorexia and weight loss may be found in chronic cases. Fever is usually absent.

Haematological parameters are usually normal but leukocytosis and a degenerative left shift have been reported. Biochemistry profiles are usually normal; hyperproteinaemia is an occasional finding. Thoracic radiographs rarely reveal significant pathology. Examination of the cerebrospinal fluid of cats with CNS involvement has revealed increased cellularity, neutrophilia, and elevated protein concentrations. FeLV antigen and FIV antibody tests are usually negative.

Diagnosis is made by identifying the *Cryptococcus* organisms that are usually numerous in aspirates or impression smears made from affected tissues or body fluids. *Cryptococcus* appears as a 1–7 µm body surrounded by a non-staining 1–30 µm capsule. The capsule apparently shields the organism from the host immune system. Tissue biopsy specimens may be stained routinely or with special fungal stains. The latex cryptococcal antigen test is a sensitive and accurate method to detect capsular polysaccharide antigen in serum, urine and CSF. Cryptococcal antigen titres vary with the severity of the disease and can be used to monitor the response to therapy.

Treatment is recommended for all cats. KTZ at 10 mg/kg PO bid appears to be highly efficacious in the treatment of nasal and cutaneous disease. ITZ and another orally administered azole, fluconazole (2.5–5.0 mg/kg PO q12–24h), also have promise on the basis of clinical and experimental studies in man and laboratory animals. Fluconazole is commercially available and has the advantage of having fewer side effects in cats (e.g. anorexia, hepatotoxicity) than KTZ. It has the additional property of excellent penetration into the CNS and is preferred for CNS infections. The major drawback to fluconazole is its cost: it is approximately four times as expensive as KTZ.

Combination therapy with amphotericin B and flucytosine (feline dose: 100 mg PO qid) has been used in cats and is still used to treat some human patients with CNS cryptococcosis. Successful treatment of CNS cryptococcosis in cats has not been reported but this regimen or fluconazole is recommended for patients with retinal or CNS lesions.

The prognosis for nasal and cutaneous cryptococcosis is guarded to fair, depending on the stage of the disease and the degree of involvement. The prognosis for CNS cryptococcosis is grave.

Aspergillosis, mucormycosis, candidiasis and penicilliosis

The common feature of these fungal diseases in the cat is that they occur almost exclusively as opportunistic infections in immunosuppressed individuals. Immunosuppressive diseases predisposing to opportunistic fungal infection include feline parvovirus, feline leukaemia virus and feline immunodeficiency virus. The majority of affected cats (75%) are less than 3 years of age; there is no breed or sex predilection. Opportunistic fungal infections occur more commonly in Europe than in the United States and are more prevalent in colder climates and during the colder months of the year.

Clinical signs caused by opportunistic fungal infections are nonspecific and include depression, anorexia, weight loss and fever. Other signs may be present, depending on the primary cause of the immunosuppression. The fungal organisms usually gain entry to the body via the respiratory or gastrointestinal tract and cause signs depending on the specific sites of organ system involvement. The complete blood count usually demonstrates neutropenia or panleukopenia. Many cats affected with opportunistic fungi are concurrently FeLV- or FIV-infected. Other clinical pathological findings are variable.

Unfortunately, most of these opportunistic fungal diseases are not recognised prior to postmortem examination. Even if they are identified early, antifungal chemotherapy will not be effective in the face of immunosuppression.

Sporotrichosis

Sporothrix schenckii is a soil-borne, dimorphic fungus that causes skin infection and lymphadenitis following cutaneous inoculation. It has a worldwide distribution but disease is more common in Central and South America than North America, and is rare in Europe.

Sporothrix lesions are suppurative or granulomatous and are usually located on the distal limbs. Secondary cutaneous lesions can arise elsewhere on the body from direct transfer during self-grooming. Lymphatic dissemination occurs in some individuals but systemic involvement is rare. Laboratory findings from affected cats are usually unremarkable. Feline leukaemia virus and feline immunodeficiency virus do not appear to be major predisposing factors in the development of sporotrichosis; however, the presence of these retroviral diseases may increase the likelihood of dissemination and will make successful treatment more difficult.

The diagnosis of sporotrichosis is confirmed by identification of the ovoid *Sporothrix* organisms (3–8 μm) in macrophages during cytological examination of Wright's stained impression smears or aspirates from cutaneous lesions or lymph nodes. Fungal stains should be used to examine tissue biopsy specimens to avoid confusion with *Histoplasma*, which are similar in appearance.

Although *Sporothrix* lesions may regress spontaneously, treatment is recommended for all affected cats because of public health considerations and the danger of self-dissemination. Potassium or sodium iodide solution is the treatment of choice and is given at a dose of 20 mg/kg PO bid for 4 weeks. Cats are very sensitive to iodine compounds and signs of iodine toxicity include depression, anorexia, vomiting and cardiac failure. Ketoconazole has not been effective in the treatment of sporotrichosis; some of the newer azole compounds (itraconazole, fluconazole) may have promise but have not yet been evaluated for efficacy against this organism.

Humans can contract sporotrichosis from infected cats and immunosuppressed people are more likely to develop disseminated disease. Those who work with an affected cat should avoid contact with fomites bearing infectious exudates and wear protective clothing and gloves.

Dermatophytosis

The most common dermatophytes affecting domestic animals are those of the genera *Microsporum* and *Trichophyton*. Local conditions affect the frequency and distribution of the various fungi but, in general, *Microsporum canis* is responsible for most cases of feline dermatophytosis.

Dermatophyte spores are highly resistant to environmental degradation and may remain infectious for as long as 13 months. Infection is acquired from contact with spores in the environment or on infected individuals. Kittens are more susceptible to active infection than adult cats; adults are more likely to be asymptomatic carriers of infection. Mixed breed long-haired cats are less likely than mixed breed short-haired cats to have clinical disease but are more likely to be asymptomatic dermatophyte carriers. Purebreed cats, particularly Persian and Siamese, may have an increased risk of dermatophytosis. Stress, crowding, poor nutrition, concurrent disease and poor husbandry conditions increase the incidence and severity of dermatophyte infections and it is difficult to disassociate these factors from breed related factors when evaluating a purebred population.

The appearance of dermatophyte lesions is variable depending on the infecting strain of fungus, and the location, extent and duration of infection. Superficial *M. canis* lesions begin with a brief period of hyperaemia, followed by hair loss in the central part of the lesion. Hair death and breakage occur around the periphery of the lesion. The peripheral zone spreads laterally while the area of initial involvement clears and hair regrowth occurs. More deep seated disease can involve the vibrissae, eyelashes, nail beds and subcutaneous tissue.

Lesions caused by *M. canis* can often be identified by their characteristic 'apple green' fluorescence under Wood's lamp illumination. Infected hair and hair shafts are most likely to be found in the active, peripheral part of the lesion. Skin scrapings and hair plucked from lesions can be examined for fungal spores but these are often difficult to find. Fungal culture of infected hair on a dermatophyte test medium is somewhat more time consuming but is accurate, economical and practical for most practitioners.

Single superficial dermatophyte lesions can often be successfully treated with topical therapy alone. A number of effective commercial compounds are available for this purpose. Clipping the hair surrounding the lesion(s) will improve contact with topical medications and reduce environmental contamination with infectious spores. Cats with multifocal or deep seated lesions should receive systemic antifungal therapy in addition to topical treatments. Griseofulvin is given at a dose of 20–50 mg/kg PO sid for 6–8 weeks. Griseofulvin is embryotoxic and teratogenic, and should not be given to pregnant queens. Severe bone marrow suppression causing fatal pancytopenia has been reported as an idiosyncratic reaction and in a group of FIV-positive cats given griseofulvin. Griseofulvin-induced bone marrow suppression is potentially reversible if it is recognised early and drug treatment discontinued. Ketoconazole is very effective against dermatophytes but its use should be reserved for cases which are resistant to griseofulvin.

Control of dermatophytosis is a serious problem in catteries and other multiple cat environments. All affected cats (ideally, all cats in the environment) should be treated topically and simultaneously, clipping the whole body to improve the efficacy of treatment. Captan fungicide is an economical and effective topical treatment which is available as a 50% wettable powder under veterinary labelling or as a garden fungicide. Mix two tablespoons of captan powder with one gallon (4.5 litres) of water, shake well to suspend the powder, and saturate the hair and skin of affected cats thoroughly with this solution twice a week. Systemic antifungal treatment should be given to all cats with active lesions. Even this comprehensive approach to cattery treatment will not be effective unless fungal contamination of the environment can be eliminated and poor husbandry conditions are improved.

Other fungal infections

A number of miscellaneous soil-borne fungi occasionally cause cutaneous or subcutaneous infection following cutaneous inoculation. These include phaeohyphomycosis (*Stemphylium* spp, *Cladosporium* spp, *Drechslera spicifera*, *Exophiala jeanselmei*, *Alternaria alternata*, *Curvularia* spp, *Phialophora* spp), chromomycosis (*Phialophora verrucosa*, *Fonsecaea* spp, *Cladosporium carrioni*, *Rhinocladiella cerophilim*), paecilomycosis (*Paecilomyces fumosoroseus*) and trichosporonosis (*Trichosporon* spp). Diagnosis is based on identification of the organism during examination of exfoliative cytology or biopsy and in fungal culture. These fungi are variably susceptible to amphotericin B and azole antifungal drugs. Surgical excision of the lesion is the treatment of choice.

PROTOTHECOSIS

Prototheca wickerhamii is a colourless alga found as a saprophyte in moist environments. Cats develop subcutaneous infection following traumatic inoculation of the organism. The lesions are granulomatous but not exudative; numerous ovoid organisms (2–20 μm) can be found free and contained within giant macrophages in affected tissue. *Prototheca* is poorly responsive to medical therapy; amphotericin B and ketoconazole have been used in some patients with variable success. Complete surgical excision of the lesion is the treatment of choice.

RICKETTSIA

Q-Fever (coxiellosis)

Q-Fever is a disease of man caused by the rickettsial agent *Coxiella burnetii*. The cat is implicated in the spread of disease to man, by harbouring the agent whilst not showing signs of disease. An outbreak of Q-Fever pneumonia in a household was attributed to the pet cat who had just given birth: the organism is excreted in large numbers in placental fluids, and parturition can produce airborne transmission.

Haemobartonella felis

Haemobartonella felis is a rickettsial parasite of erythrocytes, and the causal agent of feline infectious anaemia or haemobartonellosis, a common disease of cats with a world-wide distribution. The organism attaches to the surface of erythrocytes and is pleomorphic when viewed in blood films, appearing as dots, rods, cocci, rings or chains.

The mode of transmission of *H. felis* is uncertain but blood-sucking arthropods (e.g. fleas), vertical transmission (intra-uterine, during parturition, or via the milk) and cat bites have all been proposed. Infected cats may exhibit cycles of parasitaemic episodes lasting for a few days, interspersed with periods of several days when few or no parasites are observed in the blood. The parasitaemic episodes are associated with progressive anaemia and occasionally death. A spontaneous recovery often occurs with resolution of the anaemia and parasitaemia, although chronic infection persists with occasional recurrent parasitaemic episodes.[14] The course of the disease will be influenced by many factors, including the route of transmission, the virulence of the organism, and the immune response of the host. It is likely that many naturally infected cats are exposed to relatively small numbers of the organism, and a chronic carrier state may be established without significant clinical signs. Such carrier cats may later develop disease, especially if there is a disturbance to the balance that exists between the host and the parasite.

Clinical signs may be acute or chronic and include lethargy, weakness, anorexia, splenomegaly and pale mucous membranes. Pyrexia and jaundice are inconsistent features. The disease can occur in any age group but is more common in male cats.[12] Although experimentally induced immunosuppression and artificially induced stress have failed to induce clinical disease in carrier cats, there is substantial evidence from clinical observations indicating that stress and immunosuppression are frequently important in the pathogenesis of the disease.[15] A positive association has been found between FeLV infection and haemobartonellosis, probably due to the immunosuppressive nature of the former infection.[4] In some cases, therefore, presenting clinical signs may relate to an underlying disease process in addition to the *H. felis* infection.

In uncomplicated *H. felis* infection the anaemia induced is regenerative, and typically macrocytic and hypochromic. Blood films may show polychromasia, anisocytosis and reticulocytosis. However, in many cases concurrent disease (e.g. FeLV or FIV co-infection) may complicate the haematological picture. Diagnosis is confirmed by the demonstration of organisms in a blood smear. Smears should be made from a fresh blood sample, and Giemsa or Wright stains are routinely used for diagnosis. Due to the intermittent nature of the parasitaemia, infection cannot be excluded if parasites are not observed, and examination of blood smears collected over several days improves diagnostic sensitivity. False positive results can also occur where artefacts on blood smears are mistaken for low numbers of *H. felis* organisms. The development of more sensitive and specific diagnostic tests is clearly highly desirable. When a diagnosis of haemobartonellosis is made, careful consideration should be given to the possibility of underlying disease, and investigations should include screening for FIV and FeLV infection.

Critical evaluation of specific chemotherapeutic agents in haemobartonellosis is lacking. Oxytetracycline (25 mg/kg PO tid) is suggested as the treatment of choice, but doxycycline (5 mg/kg PO sid) produces fewer gastrointestinal side effects and iatrogenic pyrexia. Assessment of response to such therapy is difficult due to the intermittent nature of the parasitaemia and the spontaneous clinical improvement that can be seen in affected cats. However, tetracyclines alone rarely appear effective. Due to the importance of immune-mediated mechanisms in the pathogenesis of the anaemia, it would seem appropriate to consider immunosuppressive glucocorticoid therapy in infected cats, although the possible adverse effects of such therapy should also be considered. Treatment of *H. felis* infected cats with a combination of prednisolone (2–4 mg/kg PO bid) and oxytetracycline has, subjectively, shown results far superior to oxytetracycline therapy alone. In severely anaemic cats, blood transfusions may be considered and may be life saving.

The prognosis for haemobartonellosis is usually related to any concurrent or predisposing disease. Generally the prognosis is good in uncomplicated cases, although most recovered cats probably remain chronic carriers and may develop recurrent episodes of disease. As infection can readily be transmitted by blood transfusion, any potential blood donor should be thoroughly screened for the presence of *H. felis* prior to being used.

PROTOZOAL INFECTIONS

Coccidian parasites

Toxoplasma gondii

Domestic cats and some other Felidae are the definitive hosts for *T. gondii*, which has a worldwide distribution. Almost all warm-blooded animals, including man, can act as intermediate host for the organism. Although *Toxoplasma* infections can result in significant disease and even mortality, most infections in cats and in intermediate hosts are subclinical.[7, 30]

Cats usually become infected indirectly by ingestion of cysts present in the tissues of an infected intermediate host; oocyst ingestion is an uncommon and less potent source of infection. Following ingestion, the parasite's replication in intestinal epithelial cells (an entero-epithelial cycle of infection) culminates in sexual reproduction and the shedding of oocysts in the faeces for a period of 1–3 weeks. Oocysts undergo sporulation in the environment after 1–5 days, prior to which they are not infectious. As well as the entero-epithelial cycle, there is an extra-intestinal cycle also in which the parasite is disseminated throughout the body in the form of rapidly dividing tachyzoites. An immune response arrests tachyzoite proliferation and the shedding of oocysts but, despite this, infection persists (in the form of encysted bradyzoites within body tissues) probably for the lifetime of the cat. Almost all previously unexposed cats will shed oocysts after ingestion of tissue cysts, but re-excretion after primary infection is very rare and epidemiologically unimportant. Oocysts are quite resistant; depending on environmental conditions, they may survive for well over a year. Intermediate hosts become infected by ingesting oocysts or tissue cysts, or by transplacental migration of tachyzoites. Only an extra-intestinal cycle of infection occurs in intermediate hosts, which results in the formation of tissue cysts.

The prevalence of *Toxoplasma* infection in cats depends on the availability of infected prey and the lifestyle of the cat. Stray and feral cats are more commonly infected than pet cats, and the prevalence rises with age.[5] Serological studies of domestic cats in the UK and the USA indicate a prevalence of infection of 30–40% or greater, but the incidence of oocyst shedding is generally less than 1%, which is explained by the short duration of oocyst production following infection. Most feline infections are asymptomatic but disease can develop if an inadequate immune response fails to arrest tachyzoite proliferation in body tissues, for example in young immunologically immature cats or in adults with impaired immune responses (e.g. those with FeLV or FIV co-infection). Chronic disease is seen more typically in older cats where it frequently arises as recrudescence of infection from encysted bradyzoites present from a primary infection earlier in life.

Most reports of clinical toxoplasmosis in cats arise from fatal cases which were diagnosed at post-mortem examination. Common clinical signs in these cases included lethargy, inappetence, pyrexia, weight loss and severe dyspnoea. Gastrointestinal, neurological and ocular signs, and lymphadenopathy were less common features. Non-fatal toxoplasmosis may present differently: in a recent study, which was not based on post-mortem diagnosis, ocular signs were present in 9/15 (60%) cases, including anterior uveitis in all nine cats.[22] Neonatal toxoplasmosis due to infection acquired *in utero* or shortly after birth usually results in acute generalised disease, and sudden death.

Diagnosis is based on a combination of clinical signs and serological tests, examination of faeces for oocysts, histopathological demonstration of tachyzoites in tissues, or biological assays (e.g. inoculation of body fluids or tissues into mice). The latter two may provide a definitive diagnosis but may be impractical in many situations. Faecal examination is an insensitive diagnostic aid as most cats do not develop clinical signs until after oocyst shedding has ceased, and *Toxoplasma* oocysts also

have to be differentiated from those of certain other feline coccidia.

Most serological assays measure primarily or exclusively the IgG class antibody response, but titres usually remain high for months or years following primary infection, regardless of whether cats develop disease, and thus the finding of a positive antibody titre provides little information. Also acute disease can sometimes develop prior to seroconversion. An IgM ELISA has recently been developed in the USA which is superior to IgG as titres are elevated only transiently following primary infection; thus a single high titre is very suggestive of recent infection, and titres may also increase again in recrudescent toxoplasmosis. Wider availability of IgM serology should be of significant benefit, although a diagnosis cannot be based on serology alone as both IgM and IgG responses are similar in ill and asymptomatic cats.

Clindamycin is probably the drug of choice for the treatment of feline toxoplasmosis, given either orally or parenterally at 25–50 mg/kg/day divided into two or three doses. Treatment should be continued for 2 weeks beyond resolution of clinical signs.

Toxoplasma is an important zoonosis. Although most infections in man are mild or asymptomatic, severe disease can occur in immunocompromised individuals, or from congenital infections acquired *in utero* when a previously unexposed woman contracts toxoplasmosis during pregnancy. In industrialised countries it is thought that most human infections are acquired by ingestion of tissue cysts in undercooked meat, or from poor meat hygiene. Studies have generally failed to show an association between owning (or having contact with) a cat and an increased risk of toxoplasmosis, and stray or feral cats are considered to be a more important source of oocysts than pet cats.[10] The following simple hygiene precautions can dramatically reduce the risk of human transmission:[1]

- Washing hands, implements and surfaces after handling raw meat.
- Cooking meat to at least 70°C throughout, and washing all vegetables.
- Careful daily disposal of cat litter by a non-pregnant person, and disinfection of the litter tray with boiling water.

- Wearing rubber gloves when gardening in potentially contaminated soil.
- Preventing cats from hunting or eating raw meat.
- Covering children's sand boxes.

Recently progress has been made in the development of prospective vaccines for use both in intermediate hosts and in cats (to prevent oocyst shedding). Such vaccines may play an important role in the future control of toxoplasmosis.[9]

Neospora caninum

Neospora caninum is a recently described protozoan parasite morphologically similar to *Toxoplasma gondii* but with an unknown life-cycle. It is now thought that many cases of toxoplasmosis previously described in dogs may have been due to neosporosis. *N. caninum* has been reported in many parts of the world including Europe, Australia and the USA, and infection has also been described in farm animals. Natural infections have not yet been described in cats[6] but they are susceptible to experimental infection, which may result in a spectrum of disease from subclinical infection to fatal encephalitis, myositis and hepatitis. Severe disease occurred in neonates or immunosuppressed adults.

Isospora spp

Isospora (Cystoisospora) felis and *I. (C.) rivolta* are the two most common coccidian parasites of the cat, the former being the more prevalent. Infection is most common in kittens and young cats. These parasites have a world-wide distribution, and it is suggested that nearly all cats become infected with *I. felis* at some point in their lives. Unsporulated oocysts are shed in the faeces of infected cats and a direct life-cycle follows ingestion of oocysts (after sporulation) by another cat. An indirect life-cycle can also take place through an intermediate host (e.g. rodent) which develops tissue cysts following ingestion of an oocyst. *Isospora* spp have a low pathogenic potential but heavy infestations may result in, or contribute to, gastrointestinal disease. Diagnosis is made by demonstration of oocysts in faecal samples. As spontaneous elimination of infection occurs, treatment is probably unnecessary. However, several drugs, including sulphonamides or sulphonamide/trimethoprim combinations, have been suggested as treatments.

Hammondia hammondi

This parasite has an obligatory two-host life cycle: domestic cats and the European wild cat are the definitive hosts; birds, rodents and other animals act as intermediate hosts. Oocysts shed in cat faeces are infective to intermediate hosts following sporulation in the environment. Structurally, *H. hammondi* is identical to *T. gondii*, and their oocysts are morphologically identical, but there is no extra-intestinal infection of cats with *H. hammondi*. The distribution of the latter parasite includes the USA and Europe but the prevalence of infection is uncertain as, for practical reasons, the oocysts of *H. hammondi* and *T. gondii* are rarely differentiated. Most surveys demonstrate a less than 1% prevalence of shedding of this type of oocyst in cat faeces, and it is likely that the majority of these are due to infection with *T. gondii*. *H. hammondi* is regarded as non-pathogenic for cats.

Besnoitia spp

Infection of cats with *B. darlingi* has been described in North America, *B. wallacei* in Hawaii and *B. besnoiti* in southern Europe and elsewhere. The life-cycle is similar to *H. hammondi*; intermediate hosts are rodents for *B. wallacei*, cattle for *B. besnoiti* and the Virginia opossum, lizards, rodents and bats for *B. darlingi*. The oocysts excreted by cats are difficult to distinguish from those of *T. gondii* but, as with *Hammondia*, *Besnoitia* spp are regarded as non-pathogenic for the cat.

Sarcocystis spp

Sarcocystis spp have a world-wide distribution, with cats serving as the definitive host for several species. The parasite is considered non-pathogenic to cats, which become infected by eating intermediate hosts including rodents, food-producing animals and many other mammals. Sporulated oocysts are passed in the faeces of infected cats. Extraintestinal dissemination of *Sarcocystis* has occasionally been reported in the cat and may be related to immunosuppression.

Cryptosporidium spp

Cryptosporidium is known to infect a broad host range, but it is uncertain whether these all represent infections with a single species. Epithelial cells of the small intestine are infected and oocysts are excreted in the faeces, but since sporulation occurs within the intestine some thin-walled oocysts cause autoinfection. The life-cycle is direct. Infection is world-wide, facilitated by the apparent lack of host specificity. Clinical disease is frequently reported in calves and lambs, and *Cryptosporidium* can be an important cause of human disease. Feline infections are uncommon and most are probably asymptomatic, although diarrhoea and weight loss have been reported. Signs may be more severe and prolonged in immunosuppressed individuals. Diagnosis is made by demonstration of the small oocysts in faeces. Most infected cats will eliminate infection spontaneously within a few weeks. No treatment is universally successful, although spiramycin has been efficacious in some human cases. Cryptosporidiosis can be a zoonosis or a reverse zoonosis (human to cat transmission).

Non-coccidian intestinal protozoa

Giardia spp

Giardia spp are important pathogens recognised throughout the world in man and a wide range of animals including cats. *Giardia* are binucleate flagellate extracellular parasites of the small intestine, where they are present as trophozoites.[20] The organism adheres to villi in the feline jejunum and ileum where it multiplies by binary fission. Trophozoites may become encysted and pass out in the faeces, and direct transmission occurs as a result of ingestion of these cysts. Feline giardiasis has been reported world-wide, and surveys generally show that up to 10% of cats may be shedding cysts, although some studies have found a higher prevalence than this. Young cats are probably more frequently infected, and the disease is more common in colony cats where transmission is more efficient. Specific immunity probably develops, leading to resolution of infection.

Infections with *Giardia* are frequently asymptomatic, but in other cases a malabsorption syndrome occurs, due in part to inflammatory cell infiltration of the intestine, stunting of villi and inhibition of digestive enzymes by the organism. In affected cats, acute or chronic, persistent or intermittent mucoid diarrhoea may develop. The faeces are usually pale and soft, and may be steatorrhoeic. There may also be weight loss or stunting of growth.

Diagnosis is made by demonstrating the cysts in faecal samples, employing the zinc sulphate centrifugal flotation method. (Trophozoites are rarely seen in faeces as they have a very short survival time.) As cyst excretion is sporadic, improved diagnostic sensitivity is achieved by examination of three faecal samples collected at 48-hour intervals. Diagnosis may also be made by demonstrating trophozoites in freshly examined small intestinal aspirates, although studies in other species suggest this may be a less sensitive diagnostic technique than faecal examinations. An ELISA has recently been developed at Cornell University (USA) to detect *Giardia* antigen in faeces which, if it performs as well as similar tests in humans, should enable improved diagnosis with excellent sensitivity and specificity.

Metronidazole is probably the treatment of choice for feline giardiasis at a dose of 10–15 mg/kg PO bid for 5 days. Attention should also be paid to improving hygiene where *Giardia* is identified in a colony of cats. The zoonotic potential of *Giardia* is uncertain at present but, unless proven otherwise, it is best to regard giardiasis as a zoonotic disease and to treat all cats where infection is detected, regardless of whether they are displaying clinical signs.

Entamoeba histolytica

Entamoeba histolytica is an amoebic parasite that can colonise the colon of both humans and animals. It is rare in developed countries. In cats, most cases are thought to be acquired from humans and infected animals may be asymptomatic or develop an ulcerative colitis. Treatment with metronidazole is recommended.

Non-intestinal protozoal infections

Cytauxzoon felis

Cytauxzoonosis is an uncommon disease of cats reported in the USA. The organism infects erythrocytes, monocytes and macrophages, causing a fatal disease characterised by anaemia and circulatory failure. The life-cycle and transmission of *C. felis* is uncertain, although ticks and other blood-sucking arthropods are thought to be the major source of infection to cats, with bobcats possibly acting as a natural reservoir of infection.

Intracellular pleomorphic piroplasms can be seen within erythrocytes in Wright- or Giemsa-stained blood films, and multiplication occurs in infected macrophages and monocytes. The course of the disease is usually less than a week, with signs including anaemia, lethargy, pyrexia, jaundice and splenomegaly progressing to dyspnoea, collapse and death. Diagnosis is confirmed by demonstration of the parasite in erythrocytes or macrophages. No treatment is successful.

Babesia felis

Babesiosis in the domestic cat is confined almost exclusively to South Africa, where it is an important disease. *Babesia felis* parasitises erythrocytes, causing a sometimes fatal anaemia. The parasitaemia is persistent in contrast to that seen in haemobartonellosis, and diagnosis is made by demonstration of the organism in blood films. Primaquine is reported to be the drug of choice for treatment.

INTESTINAL HELMINTHS

Cats may harbour a variety of intestinal helminths, the most common of which are *Toxocara cati*, *Toxascaris leonina*, *Dipylidium caninum* and *Taenia taeniaformis*. Studies in the UK have shown a prevalence of infection with *T. cati* and *D. caninum* of up to 60%, but with most helminths there are marked geographical variations in the distribution and prevalence of infections so that important parasites in some areas may be absent or rare in others. In many cases helminth infestation may be inapparent or cause minimal disease, although sometimes severe disease may result and additionally some of the parasites are of zoonotic importance.

Helminths of the stomach

Ollulanus tricuspis

Ollulanus tricuspis is a small trichostrongyle nematode (up to 1 mm long) which parasitises the stomach of domestic cats and certain other animals and has a world-wide distribution. The life-cycle is direct, with cats becoming infected by ingestion of vomitus containing adults or larvae (*O. tricuspis* is viviparous), so that infection is more common in colonies and ferals than in household cats. Infection is usually asymptomatic although anorexia, chronic vomiting and chronic fibrosing gastritis have been reported. Adults and larvae are rarely seen in faeces; therefore diagnosis is made by demonstrating their presence in vomitus or gastric lavage fluid. Experimental infections in kittens respond well to treatment with fenbendazole at 10 mg/kg PO for 2 days.

Physaloptera spp

Infrequent infections with these worms have been reported in the USA. Adults are found attached to the gastric mucosa, where they ingest blood and may cause gastritis. The life-cycle is indirect, with insects serving as intermediate hosts and rodents as paratenic hosts. Pyrantel pamoate (5 mg/kg PO) is reported to be effective.

Spirura rityopleurites

Infection with this worm has been reported in Europe, and the life-cycle is similar to *Physaloptera* spp. Infections are usually asymptomatic.

Gnathostoma spinigerum

This parasite has been reported in Asia and Australasia and infections are almost always fatal. A diverse range of animals can act as intermediate hosts, and widespread somatic migration occurs in cats before the adults encyst in the stomach wall, where they cause massive damage and intermittently shed eggs which are passed in the faeces.

Small intestinal ascarids

Toxocara cati

Toxocara cati is the most common intestinal helminth parasite of cats. It has a world-wide distribution, with young cats (those under a year of age) showing the highest prevalence of infection. Adult worms are present in the small intestine and shed eggs which are passed out in the faeces. Other cats may become infected either directly by ingestion of an embryonated egg or indirectly by ingestion of larvae in a paratenic host (rodents, birds, earthworms, beetles). Ingestion of embryonated eggs by cats results in somatic migration of larvae via the liver and lungs to the small intestine, where they mature into adults. Larvae may also migrate to and remain dormant in many tissues of the body, including mammary glands. Subsequently, following a pregnancy, larvae are excreted in the milk of an infected queen throughout lactation and serve as a potent source of infection to sucking kittens. Ingestion of larvae (via the milk or in the tissues of a paratenic host), in contrast to ingestion of embryonated eggs, does not result in somatic migration. Unlike *Toxocara canis* infection in dogs, transuterine infection does not occur with *T. cati*.

Toxascaris leonina

Infection with *T. leonina* is also prevalent in cats, although it is less common than *T. cati*. In Britain most surveys have shown less than 10% prevalence of infection with this species. Cats become infected either by ingestion of an embryonated egg or by ingestion of an intermediate host (rodents) with larvae encysted in their tissues. Infection of cats results in the larvae burrowing into the wall of the small intestine, where they mature and emerge as adults into the lumen. In contrast to *T. cati*, there is no somatic migration.

Clinical signs, diagnosis and treatment of ascarid infections

Clinical signs, which occur primarily in young kittens with heavy worm burdens, include failure to thrive, diarrhoea, vomiting, palpably thickened intestines, poor coat and a pot-bellied appearance. Diagnosis is based on the presence of eggs in the faeces, or observation of adults or larvae in faeces or vomitus. A variety of anthelmintics show good efficacy against ascarids; they include piperazine (110 mg/kg PO), fenbendazole (50 mg/kg daily PO for 5 days), and pyrantel pamoate (5 mg/kg PO). Treatment should always be repeated after 14 days due to the possibility of somatic migration with *T. cati*, and regular treatment of kittens is advisable until after weaning. *Toxocara cati* and *Toxascaris leonina* appear to be very rare causes of the zoonosis visceral larva migrans, which is usually associated with the larvae of *Toxocara canis*.

Cestodes

Cestodes are more prevalent in adult cats (over one year old) than in young cats, but the prevalence in any particular population will depend on many factors, including the availability of infected intermediate hosts and the life-style of the cats. Treatment of choice for all cestode infections is praziquantel at 5 mg/kg SC or PO.

Dipylidium caninum

Dipylidium caninum is the most common tapeworm infecting cats. Adults are present in the small intestine, often in large numbers, where they shed gravid proglottids containing numerous eggs. The proglottids may be passed in the faeces or, as they are motile, they may migrate out of the rectum on to the perineum. The eggs are ingested by an intermediate host which is usually a flea (the eggs being ingested by larval fleas) or may be biting lice (*Felicola subrostratus* or *Trichodectes canis*). Cats become infected by ingestion of an intermediate host during grooming. Infection is usually asymptomatic, but anal pruritus may sometimes be observed. Owners may become aware of infection when motile proglottids are seen in the perineal area or in the faeces. Fresh segments are approximately 1 cm in length and have a shape similar to a cucumber seed. Occasionally human *D. caninum* infection (usually in children) has been reported following inadvertent ingestion of an intermediate host.

Joyeuxiella spp and Diplopylidium spp

These cestodes are similar to *Dipylidium caninum* and have a geographical distribution including Australasia, Africa and the Middle East. Two intermediate hosts are involved in the life-cycle, insects being the first and reptiles or small mammals the second.

Taenia taeniaformis

Taenia taeniaformis is the most prevalent taenian tapeworm infection in cats. Adults in the small intestine may grow up to 60 cm in length, and shed flattened, bell-shaped, gravid proglottids. As with *Dipylidium caninum*, the proglottids may be passed in faeces or may migrate onto the perineal area. Intermediate hosts are rodents, primarily rats and mice, which become infected by ingesting eggs. Clinical signs due to taenian infections are rare, although gastrointestinal irritation and perforation have been reported. The diagnosis is based on the observation of the proglottids or eggs in faeces or on the perineal area.

Other taenian tapeworms

Cats may become infected infrequently with a number of other taenian tapeworms including *Taenia pisiformis* (intermediate hosts are primarily rabbits and hares), *T. hydatigena* (intermediate hosts include sheep, goats, cattle and pigs) and *Echinococcus multilocularis*, which is not present in the UK. Adult *E. multilocularis* worms are small (1.2–3.7 mm in length) with a wide range of definitive hosts, including cats and dogs; intermediate hosts are rodents. The main importance of this parasite is that occasional infections occur in humans: a hydatid cyst develops in the liver or elsewhere, causing eventual death.

Diphyllobothrium latum

Diphyllobothrium latum has a widespread geographical distribution in temperate areas but does not occur in the UK. It is considered to be primarily a human parasite, but cats occasionally act as the final host. Adults in the small intestine shed free eggs rather than proglottids, and two intermediate hosts are necessary for the life-cycle, the first being a copepod crustacean and the second a freshwater fish. Cats may therefore become infected by eating an infected fish. *Diphyllobothrium latum* absorbs vitamin B_{12}; this may result in anaemia in severely infected humans but the worm probably has a low pathogenic potential in domestic animals. Diagnosis is made by demonstration of eggs in faecal samples.

Spirometra spp

Spirometra spp are similar and related to *D. latum*. Infections have been reported in the USA, Australia and Asia. The life-cycle is similar to *D. latum* although the second intermediate hosts are frogs, snakes or mammals.

Hookworms

Ancylostoma tubaeforme and ancylostoma braziliense

These hookworms are prevalent in warm temperate, subtropical and tropical parts of the world including the USA, Australia and southern Europe. *Uncinaria stenocephala* may also rarely infect cats. The worms are 6–20 mm in length and have a direct or indirect life-cycle. Adults are frequently found partially buried in the mucosa of the small intestine. Eggs are passed in the faeces from which larvae emerge and develop in the environment. Infection of the definitive host occurs by ingestion of larvae (directly or via transport hosts such as rodents) or by cutaneous perforation by larvae. Larvae penetrating the skin migrate to local blood vessels, from where they are transported to the lungs and then migrate via the trachea and oesophagus to the intestine, where the adult develops.

Hookworm infection in cats is generally less severe than in dogs, but heavy infestations can result in a microcytic hypochromic anaemia due to loss of blood. Diagnosis is made by demonstrating eggs in fresh faecal samples. A variety of anthelmintics are effective, including fenbendazole (50 mg/kg PO daily for 5 days) and pyrantel pamoate (5 mg/kg PO). Treatment should be repeated after 14 days as migrating worms may not be killed, and environmental hygiene should also be considered. Hookworms can cause dermatitis in humans exposed to the larvae.

Threadworms

Strongyloides tumefaciens

This uncommon parasite of cats has been reported in some areas of the USA. Infection may cause small nodules in the large intestinal mucosa (containing adult female worms) and an associated inflammatory response may be seen, sometimes leading to chronic diarrhoea and weight loss. Diagnosis is made by demonstrating larvae in the faeces, and thiabendazole treatment has been reported to be effective.

Whipworms

Trichuris spp

Two species of *Trichuris* have been described affecting cats: *T. campanula* and *T. serrata*. Infection is apparently rare but has been reported in the USA, South America and Australia. The life-cycle is direct, with adult worms parasitising the caecum and large intestine. Infection with these worms is usually an incidental finding in cats.

Trematodes

A variety of flukes may occasionally parasitise the feline intestine as the adults lack host specificity. Infections are generally non-pathogenic unless very heavy burdens are carried. Intestinal fluke infections in cats have been reported in the USA, Australia and Europe. The flukes require two intermediate hosts for completion of the life-cycle, the first of which is a mollusc and the second usually a fish.

Hepatobiliary trematode infections are a more important though uncommon cause of disease in cats, with *Platynosomum concinnum* (reported in Australia, Africa, southern USA and elsewhere) and *Opisthorchis tenuicollis* (reported in central and eastern Europe, Asia, Canada and elsewhere) being the two most common. Final intermediate hosts are reptiles or amphibians for *P. concinnum*, and fish for *O. tenuicollis*. Infections may be asymptomatic or result in a hepatopathy with associated clinical signs such as anorexia, jaundice and ascites. Diagnosis is made by demonstrating eggs in faecal samples, and recommended treatments have included praziquantel at 20 mg/kg SC for 3 days or fenbendazole at 50 mg/kg PO bid for 5 days.

REFERENCES

1. August J.R., Chase T.M. (1987) Toxoplasmosis. *Vet. Clin. N. Am.* (*Small Anim. Pract.*) **17**(1): 55–71.
2. Barlough J.E., Stoddart C.A. (1988) Cats and coronaviruses. *J. Am. Vet. Med. Assoc.* **193**: 796–800.
3. Bennett M., Knowles J.O., McCracken C., Gaskell R.M., Gaskell C.J., Lutz H. (1989) Diagnosis of FIV infection. *Vet. Rec.* **124**: 520–521.
4. Bobade P.A., Nash A.S., Rogerson P. (1988) Feline haemobartonellosis: clinical, haematological and pathological studies in natural infections and the relationship to infection with feline leukaemia virus. *Vet. Rec.* **122**: 32–36.
5. Dubey J.P. (1986) Toxoplasmosis in cats. *Feline Practice* **16**(4): 13–45.
6. Dubey J.P. (1990) Neospora caninum: a look at a new Toxoplasma-like parasite of dogs and other animals. *Compend. Contin. Educ. Pract. Vet.* **12**: 653–663.
7. Dubey J.P., Beattie C.P. (1988) *Toxoplasmosis of Animals and Man.* CRC Press, Boca Raton, Florida.
8. Esh J.B., Cunningham J.G., Wiktor T.J. (1982) Vaccine-induced rabies in four cats. *J. Am. Vet. Med. Assoc.* **180**: 1336–1338.
9. Fishback J.L., Frenkel J.K. (1990) Prospective vaccines to prevent feline shedding of toxoplasma oocysts. *Compend. Contin. Educ. Pract. Vet.* **12**: 643–648.
10. Ganley J.P., Comstock G.W. (1980) Association of cats and toxoplasmosis. *Am. J. Epidem.* **111**: 238–246.
11. Gaskell R.M., Gaskell C.J., Evans R.J., Dennis P.E., Bennett A.M., Voyle C., Hill T.J. (1983) Natural and experimental pox virus infection in the domestic cat. *Vet. Rec.* **112**: 164–170.
12. Grindem C.B., Corbett W.T., Tomkins M.T. (1990) Risk factors for *Haemobartonella felis* infection in cats. *J. Am. Vet. Med. Assoc.* **196**: 96–99.

13. Harbour D.A., Ashley C.R., Williams P.D., Gruffydd-Jones T.J. (1987) Natural and experimental astrovirus infection of cats. *Vet. Rec.* **120**: 555–557.
14. Harvey J.W., Gaskin J.M. (1977) Experimental feline haemobartonellosis. *J. Am. Anim. Hosp. Assoc.* **13**: 28–38.
15. Harvey J.W., Gaskin J.M. (1978) Feline haemobartonellosis: attempts to induce relapses of clinical disease in chronically-infected cats. *J. Am. Anim. Hosp. Assoc.* **14**: 453–456.
16. Hopper C.D., Sparkes A.H., Gruffydd-Jones T.J., Crispin S.M., Muir P., Harbour D.A., Stokes C.R. (1989) Clinical and laboratory findings in cats with feline immunodeficiency virus. *Vet. Rec.* **125**: 341–346.
17. Hopper C.D. (1990) Comparison of antibody testing and virus isolation for the diagnosis of feline immunodeficiency virus. Proceedings of BSAVA Congress April 1990, p. 195.
18. Hosie M., Jarrett O. (1990) Serological responses of cats to feline immunodeficiency virus. *AIDS* **4**: 215–220.
19. Hosie M., Robertson C., Jarrett O. (1989) Prevalence of feline leukaemia virus and antibodies to feline immunodeficiency virus in cats in the United Kingdom. *Vet. Rec.* **125**: 293–297.
20. Kirkpatrick C.E. (1986) Feline giardiasis: a review. *J. Small Anim. Pract.* **27**: 69–80.
21. Kruger J.M., Osborne C.A. (1990) The role of viruses in feline lower urinary tract disease. *J. Vet. Intern. Med.* **4**: 71–78.
22. Lappin M.R., Greene C.E., Winston S., Toll S.L., Epstein M.E. (1989) Clinical feline toxoplasmosis, serologic diagnosis and therapeutic management of 15 cases. *J. Vet. Intern. Med.* **3**: 139–143.
23. Marshall J.A., Kennett M.L., Rodger S.M., Studdert M.J., Thompson W.L., Gust I.D. (1987) Virus and virus-like particles in the faeces of cats with and without diarrhoea. *Aust. Vet. J.* **64**: 100–105.
24. Martin W.B., Scott F.M.M., Lander I.M., Nash A. (1984) Pox virus infection of cats. *Vet. Rec.* **115**: 36.
25. Muir P., Harbour D.A., Gruffydd-Jones T.J., Howard P.E., Hopper C.D., Gruffydd-Jones E.A.D., Broadhead H.M., Clarke C.M., Jones M.E. (1990) A clinical and microbiological study of cats with protruding nictitating membranes and diarrhoea: isolation of a novel virus. *Vet. Rec.* **127**: 324–330.
26. Olsen C.W., Scott F.W. (1991) Feline infectious peritonitis vaccination – past and present. *Feline Health Topics for Veterinarians* (Cornell Feline Centre) **6**(3): 1–4.
27. Pedersen N.C., Boyle J.F., Floyd K., Fudge A., Barker J. (1981) An enteric coronavirus infection of cats and its relationship to feline infectious peritonitis. *Am. J. Vet. Res.* **44**: 229–234.
28. Pedersen N.C., Ho E.W., Brown M.L., Yamamoto J.K. (1987) Isolation of a T-lymphotropic virus from cats with an immunodeficiency-like syndrome. *Science* **235**: 790–793.
29. Reid-Sanden F.L., Dobbins J.G., Smith J.S., Fishbein D.B. (1990) Rabies surveillance in the United States during 1989. *J. Am. Vet. Med. Assoc.* **197**: 1571–1583.
30. Sparkes A.H. (1991) Toxoplasmosis in cats. In Grunsell C.S.G., Raw M.E. (eds) *The Veterinary Annual* **31** Blackwell Scientific Publications, Oxford. 186–191.
31. Sparkes, A.H., Gruffydd-Jones T.J., Harbour D.A. (1991) Feline infectious peritonitis: a review of clinicopathological changes in 65 cases and a critical assessment of their diagnostic value. *Vet. Rec.* **129**: 209–212.
32. Trimarchi C.V., Rudd R.J., Abelseth M.K. (1986) Experimentally-induced rabies in four cats inoculated with a rabies virus isolated from a bat. *Am. J. Vet. Res.* **47**: 777–779.
33. Wills J.M., Gruffydd-Jones T.J., Bourne F.J., Richmond S.J., Gaskell R.M. (1987) Effect of vaccination on feline *Chlamydia psittaci* infection. *Infect. Immun.* **55**: 2653–7.
34. Wills J.M., Howard P.E., Gruffydd-Jones T.J., Wathes C.E. (1988) Prevalence of *Chlamydia psittaci* in different cat populations in Britain. *J. Small Anim. Pract.* **29**: 327–339.
35. Yamamoto J.K., Sparger E., Ho E.W., Anderson P.R., O'Conner T.P., Mandell C.P., Lowenstine L., Munn R., Pedersen N.C. (1988) Pathogenesis of experimentally induced feline immunodeficiency virus infection in cats. *Am. J. Vet. Res.* **49**: 1246–1258.

FURTHER READING

Appel M.J. (1987) *Virus infections of vertebrates* Vol 1: *Virus infections of carnivores*. Elsevier Science Publishers, Amsterdam.

August J.R. (ed.) (1991) *Consultations in Feline Internal Medicine*. W.B. Saunders, Philadelphia. 535–596.

Chandler E.A., Gaskell C.J. and Hilbery A.D.R. (eds.) (1985) *Feline Medicine and Therapeutics* Part 2: *Infectious Diseases*, 251–317. Blackwell Scientific, Oxford.

Dunn A.M. (1978) *Veterinary Helminthology*, 2nd edn. William Heinemann, London.

Greene C.E. (1990) *Infectious Diseases of the Dog and Cat*. W.B. Saunders, Philadelphia. 453–632.

Grieve R.B. (1987) Parasitic Infections. *Vet. Clin. N. Am.* 17(6). W.B. Saunders, Philadelphia.

Holzworth J. (1987) *Diseases of the cat: medicine and surgery*, Vol 1. W.B. Saunders, Philadelphia.

Pedersen N.C. (1988) *Feline Infectious Diseases*. American Veterinary Publications Inc., Goleta, CA.

Povey R.C. (1985) *Infectious Diseases of Cats: A Clinical Handbook*. Centaur Press, Ontario.

Sherding R.G. (1989) *The Cat: Diseases and Clinical Management*, Vol 1. Churchill Livingstone, New York.

Soulsby E.J.L. (1982) *Helminths, Arthropods and Protozoa of Domesticated Animals*. 7th edn. Ballière Tindall, London.

Wills J.M. (1988) Feline Chlamydial Infection (Feline pneumonitis). In: E.A. Chandler (ed.) *Advances in Small Animal Practice* 1. Blackwell Scientific Publications. 182–190.

APPENDIX

List of abbreviations

ACh	acetylcholine
AChE	acetylcholine esterase
ACTH	adrenocorticotrophin
ADH	anitidiuretic hormone
AIHA	autoimmune haemolytic anaemia
ALP	alkaline phosphatase
ALT (SGPT)	alanine aminotransferase
ANA	antinuclear antibody
APTT	activated partial thromboplastin time
ARF	acute renal failure
AST (SGOT)	aspartate aminotransferase
AV	atrioventricular
AZT	3-azido-3-deoxythymidine
bid	twice daily
BSP	bromosulphthalein
BUN	blood urea nitrogen
CBC	complete blood count
CCHS	cholangitis-cholangiohepatitis syndrome
CCV	canine coronavirus
CF	complement-fixing
CITE	combined immunoassay technology
CMI	cell-mediated immunity
CNS	central nervous system
COLD	chronic obstructive lung disease
CP	conscious proprioceptive
CPK	creatinine phosphokinase
CRF	chronic renal failure
CSF	cerebrospinal fluid
CT	computed tomography
DAT	direct antiglobulin test (Coombs' Test)
DCM	dilated cardiomyopathy
DIC	disseminated intravascular coagulation
DM	dry matter
DMSO	dimethyl sulphoxide
DNA	deoxyribonucleic acid
DSH	domestic shorthair
DV	dorsoventral
ECG	electrocardiograph
eCG	equine chorionic gonadotrophin
EDTA	ethylenediamine tetra-acetic acid
EHBDO	extrahepatic bile duct obstruction
ELISA	enzyme-linked immunosorbent assay
FCRD	feline central retinal degeneration
FCV	feline calicivirus
FDPs	fibrin degradation products
FeCAHV	feline cell-associated herpesvirus
FECV	feline enteric coronavirus
FeLV	feline leukaemia virus
FeSFV	feline syncytium-forming virus
FeSV	feline sarcoma virus
FHV	feline herpesvirus
FIPV	feline infectious peritonitis virus
FIV	feline immunodeficiency virus
FSH	follicle stimulating hormone
FUS	feline urological syndrome
GFR	glomerular filtration rate
GGT	gamma glutamyltransferase
GH	growth hormone
GTT	glucose tolerance test
Hb	haemoglobin
HCM	hypertrophic cardiomyopathy
HCT	haematocrit
HIV	human immunodeficiency virus
IBD	inflammatory bowel disease
IFA	immunofluorescent antibody
IM	intramuscular
IP	idiopathic polyarthritis
ITZ	itraconazole
IV	intravenously
KOH	potassium hydroxide
KTZ	ketoconazole

LCAT	serum cryptococcal antigen titre		PPP	periosteal proliferative polyarthritis
LE	lupus erythematosus		PRA	progressive retinal atrophy
LH	luteinising hormone		PSVA	portosystemic vascular anomalies
LUTD	lower urinary tract disease		PT	prothrombin time
			PTH	parathyroid hormone
MCH	mean corpuscular haemoglobin		PTU	propylthiouracil
MCHC	mean corpuscular haemoglobin concentration			
MCV	mean cell volume		qid	every 6 hours
MDA	maternally derived antibody			
ME	metabolisable energy		RA	rheumatoid-like arthritis
MEA	mean electrical axis		RBC	red blood cell
MRI	magnetic resonance imaging		RNA	ribonucleic acid
NAD	nicotinamide adenine dinucleotide		SAP	serum alkaline phosphatase
NRC	National Research Council		SC	subcutaneously
NSAID	non-steroidal anti-inflammatory drugs		SCr	serum creatinine
			SG	specific gravity
			sid	once daily
oid	every other day		SLE	systemic lupus erythematosus
PCV	packed cell volume		TGEV	transmissible gastroenteritis virus
PE	pemphigus erythematosus		tid	every 8 hours
PF	pemphigus foliaceus		TPA	tissue plasminogen activator
PIE	pulmonary infiltrates with eosinophilia		TSH	thyroid stimulating hormone
PMEA	9-(2-phosphonomethoxyethyl) adenine		UPC	urine protein:creatinine ratio
PMN	polymorphonucleocyte (neutrophil)		URI	upper respiratory infection
PMSG	pregnant mare serum gonadotrophin		UTI	urinary tract infection
			UV	ultraviolet
PN	polyarteritis nodosa			
PO	*per os*, orally		VD	ventrodorsal
PPM	persistent pupillary membranes		VPC or PVC	ventricular premature complexes
			WBC	white blood cell

Index

Note: drugs are indexed under their main group headings; in addition, information is indexed under individual drug names.